The Little Black Book of
Primary Care

Series Editor: Daniel K. Onion

FIFTH EDITION

Daniel K. Onion, MD, MPH, FACP
Professor of Community and Family Medicine
Dartmouth Medical School
and
Director (Emeritus)
Maine–Dartmouth Family Practice
Residency Program
Augusta, Maine

JONES AND BARTLETT PUBLISHERS
Sudbury, Massachusetts
BOSTON   TORONTO   LONDON   SINGAPORE

World Headquarters

Jones and Bartlett
Publishers
40 Tall Pine Drive
Sudbury, MA 01776
978-443-5000
info@jbpub.com
www.jbpub.com

Jones and Bartlett
Publishers
Canada
6339 Ormindale Way
Mississauga, ON L5V 1J2
CANADA

Jones and Bartlett
Publishers
International
Barb House, Barb Mews
London W6 7PA
UK

Jones and Bartlett's books and products are available through most bookstores and online booksellers. To contact Jones and Bartlett Publishers directly, call 800-832-0034, fax 978-443-8000, or visit our website at www.jbpub.com.

Substantial discounts on bulk quantities of Jones and Bartlett's publications are available to corporations, professional associations, and other qualified organizations. For details and specific discount information, contact the special sales department at Jones and Bartlett via the above contact information, or send an email to specialsales@jbpub.com.

Library of Congress Cataloging-in-Publication Data
Onion, Daniel K.
    The little black book of primary care / Daniel K. Onion. — 5th ed.
        p. ; cm.
    Includes index.
    ISBN 0-7637-3459-4
    1. Primary care (Medicine)—Handbooks, manuals, etc.   I. Title.
    [DNLM: 1. Therapeutics—Handbooks.   2. Disease—Handbooks.
    3. Primary Health Care—methods—Handbooks.   WB 39 058L 2006]
    RC55.065 2006
    616—dc22

                                                                    2005019331
                                                                    6048

Production Credits
Executive Publisher: Christopher Davis
Production Director: Amy Rose
Associate Editor: Kathy Richardson
Production Assistant: Alison Meier
Associate Marketing Manager: Laura Kavigian
Manufacturing Buyer: Therese Connell

Composition: ATLIS Graphics
Cover Design: Anne Spencer
Cover Image: © Photos.com
Printing and Binding: Malloy, Inc.
Cover Printing: Malloy, Inc.

Printed in the United States of America
10   09   08   07   06   10   9   8   7   6   5   4   3   2   1

Contents

Notice

We have made every attempt to summarize accurately and concisely a multitude of references. However the reader is reminded that times and medical knowledge change, transcription or understanding error is always possible, and crucial details are omitted whenever such a comprehensive distillation as this is attempted in limited space. And the primary purpose of this compilation is to cite literature on various sides of controversial issues; knowing where "truth" lies is usually difficult. We cannot, therefore, guarantee that every bit of information is absolutely accurate or complete. The reader should affirm that cited recommendations are reasonable still, by reading the original articles and checking other sources, including local consultants as well as recent literature, before applying them.

Drugs and medical devices are discussed that may have limited availability controlled by the Food and Drug Administration (FDA) for use only in research study or clinical trial. The drug information presented has been derived from reference sources, recently published data, and pharmaceutical tests. Research, clinical practice, and government regulations often change the accepted standard in this field. When consideration is being given to use of any drug in the clinical setting, the clinician or reader is responsible for determining FDA status of the drug, reading the package insert, and prescribing information for the most up-to-date recommendations on dose, precautions, and contraindications, and determining the appropriate usage for the product. This is especially important in the case of drugs that are new or seldom used.

Co-Authors

Dermatology

Eleanor E. Sahn, MD
Clinical Associate Professor of Dermatology
Medical University of South Carolina
Charleston, South Carolina

Geriatrics

Karen Gershman, MD, CAQ in Geriatrics
Assistant Professor of Community and Family Medicine
Dartmouth Medical School
MaineGeneral Medical Center
Augusta, Maine

Infectious Diseases

Stephen D. Sears, MD, MPH
Adjunct Associate Professor of Community and Family Medicine
Dartmouth Medical School
MaineGeneral Medical Center
Augusta, Maine

Obstetrics and Gynecology

Russell N. DeJong Jr., MD
Assistant Professor of Community and Family Medicine
Dartmouth Medical School
MaineGeneral Medical Center
Waterville, Maine

Sports Medicine

James L. Glazer, MD, CAQ in Sports Medicine
Assistant Director, Division of Sports Medicine
Maine Medical Center, Portland, Maine
Assistant Professor, Community and Family Medicine
University of Vermont School of Medicine

Preface

Frontline doctors are the primary care physicians who still practice medicine the way it has been practiced through the millennia. They are the first and usually the only professional healer to see a person who decides he or she needs one. There is no filter, no screening. It is exhilarating and scary work. Exhilarating to fit the puzzle of a patient's problem and personality into the medical model and provide relief; scary because it is impossible to always fit it correctly, efficiently, and in a way that is satisfying to the patient. The knowledge and wisdom expected of a "real doc" seem impossibly infinite. Primary care is a humbling calling.

Nearly all physicians, as medical students or residents, start a "little black book" system of relevant medical facts and opinions sometime during their early training to try to encapsulate, master, and/or summarize that infinite and ever-changing sea of medical knowledge. Most abandon their attempts, either as they subspecialize or as volume overwhelms their systems for organizing and integrating new with older information.

This manual is intended as a "starter" notebook that students or residents in primary care may add to and modify as they encounter new information. It is NOT a comprehensive compilation of facts, for nobody's notebook could be; rather, it offers a framework for organizing clinical information from a variety of sources including lectures (place or person and date noted), journals (journal abbreviation, volume, and page or issue number noted), and texts (name and edition date noted). Thus it contains both "pearls" and literature-debated issues. Disease processes about which there is little current controversy or new information are treated briefly; the book assumes the user already knows the basics. Its 6000+ fact-specific references for virtually every aspect of clinical primary care are unique for a medical manual.

Clinicians may use this book both for references and for noting new data themselves. Most journal articles and many talks convey only a small bit of truly new information to the practitioner; hence a word or two plus the source reference is all the reader need note to update and personalize that section. Since not all articles, even in the best clinical journals, carry new information relevant to the practicing primary care physician, the size of my book has remained relatively constant over 35 years. My practice is to look for the kernel of relevant articles and talks and not to attempt to transcribe monographs.

The book is organized by medical specialty. I group diseases in related clusters to allow browsing among related diseases; where no obvious cluster exists, I have categorized them logically; for instance, the gi sections are organized mouth to anus. The danger of alphabetizing is that the reader and I may not use the same key word. I hope the index, which I have tried to make very complete, will put us on the same page. Most chapters have a miscellaneous section at the end for unclassifiable information in that area, brief comments about less important diseases, and for differential diagnoses not unique to one disease. When drugs are used for many diseases in a given section, relevant drug summaries appear at the beginning of chapters; otherwise, drugs specific to one or two diseases are discussed under those diseases. Liberal abbreviations ("doc talk") (see page xix) are used to save space and mimic clinical conversation; most should be familiar to American clinicians. Differential diagnoses of various signs, symptoms, and lab results are outlined in those (Sx, Si, Lab) sections, or under complications, as rule outs (r/o).

The book consists primarily of references and information about technical medicine and thereby de-emphasizes ideas and compilations focused on psychosocial issues, although such paradigms are obviously crucial to the application of technical knowledge. Some sections are less extensive than others, partly a reflection of my own training and experience, and partly because in some areas, like pediatrics, subjects that can be related to another specialty appear there rather than under pediatrics.

This edition incorporates many suggestions made by readers and reviewers as well as new references. In response to consistent requests to make the book truly small enought to fit in a white coat pocket, we are also producing it in electronic formats for personal digital assistants. Much clinical medicine is learned "on the hoof," so portability is essential.

I welcome readers'/users' suggestions and corrections.

Daniel K. Onion
email: Daniel.K.Onion@dartmouth.edu

Acknowledgments

Several physicians kindly reviewed and critiqued the various sections of this book; I have not always followed their advice as I made judgments about what a primary care physician might want to know, so the residual errors are mine. For their help, I am grateful.

Emergency Medicine
Steve E. Diaz, MD
MaineGeneral Medical Center
Waterville, Maine

Cardiology
John Sutherland, MD, FACC
Arizona Heart Institute
Phoenix, Arizona
            and
Michael LaCombe, MD, MACP
MaineGeneral Medical Center
Augusta, Maine

Dermatology
Eleanor E. Sahn, MD
    (coauthor)
Clinical Associate Professor of
    Dermatology
Medical University of South
    Carolina
Charleston, South Carolina

Gastroenterology
David W. Hay, MD
Adjunct Assistant Professor of
    Community and Family
    Medicine
Dartmouth Medical School
MaineGeneral Medical Center
Waterville, Maine

Geriatrics
Karen Gershman, MD, CMD,
CAQ in Geriatrics
    (coauthor)
Associate Professor of
    Community and Family
    Medicine
Dartmouth Medical School
MaineGeneral Medical Center
Augusta, Maine

Hematology/Oncology
Donald Magioncalda, MD
Adjunct Assistant Professor of
   Community and Family
   Medicine
Dartmouth Medical School
MaineGeneral Medical Center
Augusta, Maine

Infectious Disease
Stephen D. Sears, MD, MPH
   (coauthor)
Adjunct Associate Professor of
   Community and Family
   Medicine
Dartmouth Medical School
MaineGeneral Medical Center
Augusta, Maine
               and
Mark Rolfe, MD (HIV disease)
Medical Director, Central Maine
   Ryan White Project
MaineGeneral Medical Center
Augusta, Maine

Nephrology
Charles Jacobs, MD
Adjunct Assistant Professor of
   Community and Family
   Medicine
Dartmouth Medical School
MaineGeneral Medical Center
Waterville, Maine

Neurology
Alexander McPhedran, MD
Associate Professor of
   Community and Family
   Medicine (Emeritus)
Dartmouth Medical School
MaineGeneral Medical Center
Augusta, Maine

Obstetrics/Gynecology
Russell N. DeJong Jr., MD
   (coauthor)
Assistant Professor of
   Community and Family
   Medicine
Dartmouth Medical School
MaineGeneral Medical Center
Waterville, Maine

Ophthalmology
Maroulla Stavrinou Gleaton,
   MD
Adjunct Assistant Professor of
   Community and Family
Dartmouth Medical School
MaineGeneral Medical Center
Augusta, Maine

Pediatrics
Syd Sewall, MD
Associate Professor of Pediatrics
University of Vermont
Maine Medical Center
Portland, Maine

Psychiatry
David Moore, MD
Associate Clinical Professor
Department of Psychiatry
University of Louisville School
  of Medicine
Louisville, Kentucky

Pulmonary
Edward Ringel, MD
Adjunct Assistant Professor of
  Community and Family
  Medicine
Dartmouth Medical School
MaineGeneral Medical Center
Waterville, Maine

Rheumatology
Margaret A. Duston, MD
Adjunct Assistant Professor of
  Community and Family
  Medicine
Dartmouth Medical School
MaineGeneral Medical Center
Waterville, Maine

Sports Medicine
James L. Glazer, MD, CAQ
Assistant Director, Division of
  Sports Medicine
Maine Medical Center, Portland,
  Maine
Assistant Professor, Community
  and Family Medicine
University of Vermont School of
  Medicine

Urology
Pamela Ellsworth, MD
Associate Professor and Chief
  Division of Urology
University of Massachusetts
  Memorial Healthcare
Worcester, Massachusetts

I thank the many medical students, residents, and colleagues with whom I have had the pleasure of working over the last 30 years who have made multiple good suggestions including many for this fifth edition. I am particularly appreciative of the concise and helpful new sports medicine contributions by new co-author, James Glazer, a gifted medical writer.

I am deeply impressed with and grateful to the editors and staff of this book's new print publisher, Jones and Bartlett, including especially Chris Davis, Kathy Richardson, Alison Meier, and many others. Their cooperation with the technical staff, especially Jennifer Torres, Peter Tierney, and Bob Casinghino at the PDA electronic publisher, Skyscape, bodes well for this second attempt at dual media publication. And finally, I am grateful to Debbie Devoe, my secretary at the Maine-Dartmouth Family Practice Residency who has tirelessly helped me prepare this edition with its complex copyright permissions, for publication.

Daniel K. Onion

Text Abbreviations

A_2	Aortic (first) component of S_2	AI	Aortic insufficiency
AA	Alcoholics Anonymous	aka	Also known as
ab	Antibodies	Al	Aluminum
ABGs	Arterial blood gases	ALA	α-Levulinic acid
ac	Before meals	ALL	Acute lymphocytic leukemia
AC	Anticoagulate	ALS	Amyotrophic lateral sclerosis
ACE	Angiotensin-converting enzyme	ALT	SGPT; alanine transferase
ACEI	ACE inhibitor	AMI	Anterior myocardial infarction
Ach	Acetylcholine		
ACLS	Advanced cardiac life support	AML	Acute myelogenous leukemia
ACOG	American College of Obstetrics and Gynecology	ANA	Antinuclear antibody
		ANCA	Antineutrophil cytoplasmic autoantibodies
ACTH	Adrenocorticotropic hormone	AODM	Adult-onset diabetes mellitus
AD	Right ear		
ADH	Antidiuretic hormone	AP	Anterior-posterior
ADHD	Attention deficit hyperactivity disorder	AR	Aldose reductase
		ARA	Angiotensin receptor antagonist
ADLs	Activities of daily living		
AED	Automated external defibrillator	ARB	Angiotensin receptor blocker
AF	Atrial fibrillation	ARDS	Adult respiratory distress syndrome
AFB	Acid-fast bacillus		
Afib	Atrial fibrillation	AS	Aortic stenosis; left ear
Aflut	Atrial flutter	ASA	Aspirin
AFP	Alpha fetoprotein	asap	As soon as possible
ag	Antigen	ASCVD	Arteriosclerotic cardiovascular disease
AGN	Acute glomerular nephritis		

ASD	Atrial septal defect	BSOO	Bilateral salpingo-oophorectomy
ASHD	Arteriosclerotic heart disease	BUN	Blood urea nitrogen
ASLO	Antistreptolysin O titer	bx	Biopsy
ASO	Antistreptolysin O titer		
AST	SGOT; aspartate transferase	C′	Complement
asx	Asymptomatic	Ca	Calcium; cancer
atm	Atmospheres	CABG	Coronary artery bypass graft
ATN	Acute tubular necrosis	CAD	Coronary artery disease
AU	Both ears	cAMP	Cyclic AMP
AV	Arteriovenous; atrial-ventricular	cath	Catheterization
avg	Average	CBC	Complete blood count
AVM	Ateriovenous malformation	cc	Cubic centimeter
		CEA	Carcinoembryonic antigen
		cf	Compare
Ba	Barium	CF	Complement fixation antibodies; cystic fibrosis
bact	Bacteriology		
BAL	British anti-Lewisite	CHD	Congenital heart disease
bc	Birth control	chem	Chemistries
BCG	Bacille Calmette-Guérin	chemoRx	Chemotherapy
BCLS	Basic cardiac life support	CHF	Congestive heart failure
bcp's	Birth control pills	CI	Cardiac index
BE	Barium enema	CIN	Cervical intraepithelial neoplasia
bid	Twice a day		
BiPAP	Bi (2)-positive airway pressures	CIS	Carcinoma in situ
		Cl	Chloride
biw	Twice a week	CLL	Chronic lymphocytic leukemia
BJ	Bence-Jones		
bm	Bowel movement	CMF	Cytoxan, methotrexate, 5-FU
BM	Basement membrane		
BP	Blood pressure	CML	Chronic myelocytic leukemia
BPH	Benign prostatic hypertrophy		
		cmplc	Complications
BS	Blood sugar	CMV	Cytomegalovirus
BSE	Breast self-exam	CN	Cranial nerve; cyanide
		CNS	Central nervous system

c/o	Complaining of	DBCT	Double-blind controlled trial
CO	Cardiac output		
col	Colonies	D + C	Dilatation and curettage
COPD	Chronic obstructive lung disease	D + E	Dilatation and evacuation (suction)
cp	Cerebellar-pontine	DES	Diethyl stilbesterol
CP	Cerebral palsy	DHS	Delayed hypersensitivity
CPAP	Continuous positive airway pressure	DI	Diabetes insipidus
		dias	Diastolic
CPC	Clinical/pathologic conference	DIC	Disseminated intravascular coagulation
CPG	Coproporphyrinogen	dig	Digoxin
CPK	Creatine phophokinase	dip	Distal interphalangeal joint
CPR	Cardiopulmonary resuscitation	DJD	Degenerative joint disease
cps	Cycles per second		
CREST	Calcinosis, Raynaud's, esophageal reflux, sclerodactyly, telangiectasias	DKA	Diabetic ketoacidosis
		DMSA	Dimercaptosuccinic acid
		DNA	Deoxyribonucleic acid
CRH	Corticotropin-releasing hormone	d/o	Disorder
		DOE	Dyspnea on exertion
crit	Hematocrit	DPG	Diphosphoglycerate
CRP	C reactive protein	DPI	Dry powder inhaler
crs	Course	DPN	Diphosphopyridine nucleotide
c + s	Culture and sensitivity		
C/S	Cesarean section	DPNH	Reduced DPN
CSF	Cerebrospinal fluid	DPT	Diphtheria, pertussus, tetanus vaccine
CT	Computerized tomography		
Cu	Copper	DS	Double strength
CVA	Cerebrovascular accident	dT	Diphtheria tetanus adult vaccine
CVP	Central venous pressure		
		DTaP	Diphtheria, tetanus, acellular pertussis vaccine
d	Day(s)		
DAT	Dementia, Alzheimer's type	DTRs	Deep tendon reflexes
		DTs	Delirium tremens
dB	Decibel	DU	Duodenal ulcer

DVT	Deep venous thrombosis
dx	Diagnosis or diagnostic
EACA	ε-Aminocaproic acid
EBV	Epstein-Barr virus
ECM	Erythema chronicum marginatum
EF	Ejection fraction
eg	for example
EGD	Esophagogastro-duodenoscopy
EKG	Electrocardiogram
ELISA	Enzyme-linked im-munosorbent assay
E/M	Erythroid/myeloid
EM	Electron microscopy
EMG	Electromyogram
EMT	Emergency Medical Technician
Endo	Endoscopy
Epidem	Epidemiology
ER	Estrogen receptors; emergency room
ERCP	Endoscopic retrograde cholangio-pancreatography
ERT	Estrogen replacement therapy
ESR	Erythrocyte sedimentation rate
et	Endotracheal
et al	And others
etc	And so forth
ETOH	Ethanol
ETT	Exercise tolerance test
F	Female; Fahrenheit

FA	Fluorescent antibody; folic acid
FBS	Fasting blood sugar
Fe	Iron
FEV_1	Forced expiratory vital capacity in 1 second
FFA	Free fatty acids
FIGLU	Formiminoglutamic acid
fl	Femtoliter
FMF	Familial Mediterrranean fever
freq	Frequency
FSH	Follicle-stimulating hormone
FTA	Fluorescent treponemal antibody
FTT	Failure to thrive
f/u	Follow up
FUO	Fever of unknown origin
FVC	Forced vital capacity
fx	Fracture
g	Gauge
GABA	γ-Aminobutyric acid
gc	Gonorrhea
GE	Gastroesophageal
GFR	Glomerular filtration rate
GHRH	Growth hormone–releasing hormone
gi	Gastrointestinal
glu	Glucose
glut	Glutamine
gm	Gram
GN	Glomerulonephritis
GnRH	Gonadotropin-releasing hormone
GTT	Glucose tolerance test

gtts	Drops	HRIG	Human rabies immune globulin
gu	Genitourinary		
GVHD	Graft-vs-host disease	hs	At bedtime
		HSP	Henoch-Schonlein purpura
HBIG	Hepatitis B immune globulin		
		HSV	Herpes simplex virus
HCG	Human chorionic gonadotropin	HT	Hypertension
		5HT	5-Hydroxytryptophan
HCGrH	HCG-releasing hormone	HUS	Hemolytic uremic syndrome
HCl	Hydrochloric acid		
HCO_3	Bicarbonate	HVA	Homovanillic acid
hct	Hematocrit	hx	History
HDL	High-density lipoprotein		
H & E	Hematoxylin and eosin	I or I_2	Iodine
hem	Hematology	IADLs	Instrumental activities of daily living
hep	Hepatitis		
H. flu	*Hemophilus influenzae*	IBD	Inflammatory bowel disease
Hg	Mercury		
hgb	Hemoglobin	ibid	Same reference as last reference above
$HgbA_1C$	Hemoglobin A_1C level		
HGH	Human growth hormone	ICU	Intensive care unit
5-HIAA	5-Hydroxy indole acedic acid	I+D	Incision and drainage
		IDDM	Insulin-dependent diabetes melitus
Hib	*Hemophilus influenzae* B vaccine		
		ie	in other words
his	Histidine	IEP	Immunoelectrophoresis
HIV	Human immunodeficiency virus	IF	Intrinsic factor
		IFA	Immunofluorescent antibody
HLA	Human leukocyte antigens		
HMG-COA	Hydroxymethylglutaryl-coenzyme A	IgA	Immunoglobulin A
		IgE	Immunoglobulin E
h/o	History of	IgG	Immunoglobulin G
H+P	History and physical	IgM	Immunoglobulin M
hpf	High-power field	IHSS	Idiopathic hypertrophic subaortic stenosis
HPV	Human papillomavirus		
hr	Hour(s)	im	Intramuscular

incr	Increased	KUB	Abdominal X-ray ("kidneys, ureters, bladder")
INH	Isoniazid		
INR	International normalized ratio (protimes)		
IP	Interphalangeal	L	Liter; left
IPG	Impedance plethysmography	LA	Left atrium; long acting
		LAP	Leukocyte alkaline phosphatase
IPPB	Intermittent positive pressure breathing	LATS	Long-acting thyroid-stimulating protein
IPPD	Intermediate purified protein derivative		
		LBBB	Left bundle branch block
IQ	Intelligence quotient		
ITP	Idiopathic thrombocy-topenic purpura	LDH	Lactate dehydrogenase
		LDL	Low-density lipoprotein
IU	International units	LES	Lower esophageal sphincter
IUD	Intrauterine device		
IUGR	Intrauterine growth retardation	LFTs	Liver function tests
		LH	Luteinizing hormone
iv	Intravenous	LHRH	LH-releasing hormone
IVC	Inferior vena cava	LMW	Low molecular weight
IVP	Intravenous pyleogram	LP	Lumbar puncture
IWMI	Inferior wall myocardial infarction	LS	Lumbosacral
		LV	Left ventricle
		LVH	Left ventricular hypertrophy
J	Joule		
JODM	Juvenile-onset diabetes mellitus	lytes	Electrolytes
JRA	Juvenile rheumatoid arthritis	m	Meter(s)
		M	Male
JVD	Jugular venous distention	MAI	*Mycobacterium avium* intracellulare
JVP	Jugular venous pressure/pulse		
		MAO	Monamine oxidase
		MAST	Military antishock trousers
K	Potassium	mcp	Metacarpal-phalangeal joint
kg	Kilogram		
KOH	Potassium hydroxide	MD	Muscular dystrophy; physician
KS	Kaposi's sarcoma		

MDI	Metered-dose inhaler	Na	Sodium
meds	Medications	NAD	Nicotinamide adenine
MEN	Multiple endocrine		dinucleotide
	neoplasias	NADH	Reduced form of NAD
mEq	Millieqivalent	NCI	National Cancer Institute
mets	Metastases	ncnc	Normochromic
METs	Metabolic equivalents		normocytic
mg	Milligram	NCV	Nerve conduction
Mg	Magnesium		velocities
MI	Myocardial infarction;	neb	Nebulizer
	mitral insufficiency	neg	Negative
MIC	Minimum inhibitory	NG	Nasogastric
	concentration	NH	Nursing home
MID	Multi-infarct dementia	NH_3	Ammonia
min	Minute(s)	NICU	Newborn intensive care
MMR	Measles, mumps, rubella		unit
mOsm	Milliosmole(s)	NIDDM	Non-insulin-dependent
mp	Metocarpal phalangeal		diabetes mellitus
6MP	6-Mercaptopurine	nl	Normal
MR	Mitral regurgitation	nL	Nanoliter(s)
MRA	Magnetic resonance	nm	Nanometer(s)
	angiography	NMRI	Nuclear magnetic
MRFIT	Multiple risk factor		resonance imaging
	intervention trial	NMS	Neuroleptic malignant
MRI	Magnetic resonance		syndrome
	imaging	NNH	Number needed to harm
MRSA	Methicillin-resistant	NNT	Number needed to treat
	staphylococcus aureus	NNT-5	NNT over 5 years
MS	Multiple sclerosis; mitral	noninv	Noninvasive
	stenosis	NPH	Normal-pressure
MSH	Melanocyte-stimulating		hydrocephalus
	hormone	npo	Nothing by mouth
mtx	Methotrexate	NS	Normal saline
μ	Micron(s)	NSAID	Nonsteroidal anti-
μgm	Microgram(s)		inflammatory drug
Multip	Multiparous patient	NSR	Normal sinus rythmn
		NST	Nonstress test

Nullip	Nulliparous patient	PAT	Paroxysmal atrial tachycardia
NV+D	Nausea, vomiting, and diarrhea	patho-phys	Pathophysiology
O_2	Oxygen	Pb	Lead
OB	Obstetrics	PBG	Porphobilinogen
OCD	Obsessive-compulsive disorder	pc	After meals
		PCP	*Pneumocystis carinii* pneumonia
OD	Overdose; right eye	PCR	Polymerase chain reaction
OGTT	Oral glucose tolerance test		
OH	Hydroxy-	PCTA	Percutaneous transluminal angioplasty
OM	Otitis media		
op	Operative; outpatient	PCWP	Pulmonary capillary wedge pressure
O+P	Ova and parasites		
OPD	Outpatient department	PDA	Patent ductus arteriosus
OPV	Oral polio vaccine	PEG	Percutaneous endoscopic gastrostomy
OS	Left eye		
osm	Osmole(s)	PEP	Protein electrophoresis
OTC	Over the counter	PERRLA	Pupils equal round reactive to light and accommodation
OU	Both eyes		
oz	Ounce		
		PFTs	Pulmonary function tests
P	Pulse	PG	Prostaglandin
P_2	Pulmonary (second) component of S_2	PHLA	Post-heparin lipolytic activity
PA	Pernicious anemia; pulmonary artery	PI	Pulmonic insufficiency
		PID	Pelvic inflammatory disease
PABA	Paraminobenzoic acid		
PAC	Premature atrial contraction	PIH	Pregnancy-induced hypertension
PAF	Paroxysmal atrial fibrillation	pip	Proximal interphalangeal joint
PAN	Polyarteritis nodosa		
Pap	Papanicolaou	PMI	Point of maximal impulse of heart
PAP	Pulmonary artery pressure		
par	Parenteral	PMNLs	Polymorphonuclear leukocytes
PAS	p-Amino salicylic acid		

PMR	Polymyalgia rheumatica	q	Every
PND	Paroxysmal nocturnal dyspnea	qd	Daily
		qid	4 times a day
PNH	Paroxysmal hemoglobinuria	qod	Every other day
		qow	Every other week
po	By mouth	qt	Quart
PO4	Phosphate		
polys	Polymorphonuclear leukocytes	R	Right; respirations
		RA	Rheumatoid arthritis
pos	Positive	RAIU	Radioactive iodine uptake
post-op	Postoperative	RAST	Radioallergosorbent test
PP	Protoporphyrin	RBBB	Right bundle branch block
ppd	Pack per day	rbc	Red blood cell
PPD	Tuberculin skin test	RCT	Randomized controlled trial
PPG	Protoporphyrinogen		
pr	By rectum	RDBCT	Randomized double-blind trial
pRBBB	Partial right bundle branch block		
		RDS	Respiratory distress syndrome
pre-op	Pre-operative		
prep	Preparation	re	About
primip	Primiparous patient	rehab	Rehabilitation
prn	As needed	REM	Rapid eye movement
PROM	Premature rupture of membranes	RES	Reticuloendothelial system
PS	Pulmonic stenosis	retic	Reticulocyte(s)
PSA	Prostate-specific antigen	Rh	Rhesus factor
PSVT	Paroxysmal supraventricular tachycardia	RHD	Rheumatic heart disease
		RIA	Radioimmunoassay
pt(s)	Patient(s)	RIBA	Radio-immunoblot assay
PT	Protime	RMSF	Rocky Mountain spotted fever
PTH	Parathormone		
PTT	Partial thromboplastin time	ROM	Range of motion
		ROS	Review of systems
PUD	Peptic ulcer disease	RNA	Ribonucleic acid
PUVA	Psoralen + UVA light	RNP	Ribonucleoprotein
PVC	Premature ventricular tachycardia	r/o	Rule out
		RSV	Respiratory syncytial virus

RTA	Renal tubular acidosis	specif	Specificity
rv	Review	SPEP	Serum protein electrophoresis
RV	Right ventricle		
RVH	Right ventricular hypertrophy	SR	Slow release
		SRS	Slow-reacting substance
rx	Treatment	SS	Sickle cell disease
		SSI	Sliding-scale insulin
S_1	First heart sound	SSKI	Saturated solution of potassium iodide
S_2	Second heart sound		
S_3	Third heart sound, gallop	SSRI	Selective serotonin reuptake inhibitor
S_4	Fourth heart sound, gallop		
SAB	Spontaneous abortion	SSS	Sick sinus syndrome
SAH	Subarachnoid hemorrhage	staph	*Staphylococcus*
Sb	Antimony	STD	Sexually transmitted disease
SBE	Subacute bacterial endocarditis		
		strep	*Streptococcus*
sc	Subcutaneous	STS	Serologic test for syphilis
SD	Standard deviation	SVC	Superior vena cava
sens	Sensitivity	SVT	Supraventricular tachycardia
SER	Smooth endoplasmic reticulum		
		sx	Symptom(s)
serol	Serology		
SGA	Small for gestational age	$T°$	Fever/temperature
si	Sign(s)	T_3	Triiodothyronine
SI	Sacroiliac	T_4	Thyroxin
SIADH	Syndrome of inappropriate ADH	T+A	Tonsillectomy and adenoidectomy
		TA	Temporal arteritis
SIDS	Sudden infant death syndrome	tab	Tablet
		TAH	Total abdominal hysterectomy
SKSD	Streptokinase, streptodornase		
		tbc	Tuberculosis
sl	Sublingual	TBG	Thyroid-binding globulin
SLE	Systemic lupus erythematosus	TCAs	Tricyclic antidepressants
		tcn	Tetracycline
SNF	Skilled nursing facility	Td	Tetanus/diphtheria, adult type
soln	Solution		
s/p	Status post		

TEE	Transesophageal echocardiogram	U	Unit(s)
		UA	Urinalysis
TENS	Transcutaneous electrical nerve stimulation	UBO	Unidentified bright object
tfx	Transfusion	UGI	Upper gastrointestinal
THC	Tetrahydro-cannabinol	UGIS	Upper gastrointestinal series
TI	Tricuspid insufficiency		
TIA	Transient ischemic attack	URI	Upper respiratory illness
TIBC	Total iron-binding capacity	U.S.	United States
		US	Ultrasound
tid	3 times a day	USPTF	U.S. Preventive Task Force
TIPS	Transjugular intrahepatic portosystemic shunt		
		UTI	Urinary tract infection
tiw	Three times a week	UUB	Urine urobilinogen
Tm	Trimethoprim	UV	Ultraviolet
TM	Tympanic membrane	UVA	Ultraviolet A
Tm/S	Trimethoprim/sulfa	UVB	Ultraviolet B
TNF	Tumor necrosis factor		
TNG	Nitroglycerine	vag	Vaginally
TNM	Tumor, nodes, metastases	val	Valine
		VCUG	Vesico-urethrogram
TPA	Tissue plasminogen activator	VDRL	Serologic test for syphilis (Venereal Disease Research Lab)
TPN	Total parental nutrition		
TPNH	Triphosphopyridine reduced	VF or Vfib	Ventricular fibrillation
TRH	Thyroid-releasing hormone	VIP	Vasoactive intestinal peptide
TS	Tricuspid stenosis	VLDL	Very-low-density lipoprotein
TSH	Thyroid-stimulating hormone		
		VMA	Vanillymandelic acid
tsp	Teaspoon(s)	vol	Volume
TTP	Thrombotic thrombocy-topenic purpura	V/Q	Ventilation/perfusion
		vs	versus
TURP	Transurethral resection of prostate	VSD	Ventricular septal defect
		VT or Vtach	Ventricular tachycardia

V-ZIG	Varicella-zoster immune globulin	xmatch	Cross-match
		yr	Year(s)
w	With		
wbc	White blood cells; white blood count	ZE	Zollinger-Ellison syndrome
		Zn	Zinc
wk	Week(s)		
WNL	Within normal limits	>	More than
WPW	Wolff-Parkinson-White syndrome (short PR interval)	>>	Much more than
		<	less than
		<<	Much less than
W/s	Watt/second	→	Leads to (eg, in a chemical reaction)
w/u	Work up		

Journal and Other Reference Abbreviations

Acta Obgyn	Acta Obstetricia et Gynecologica Scandinavia
ACP J Club	American College of Physicians Journal Club supplement to Annals of Internal Medicine
Age Aging	Age and Aging
Am Fam Phys	American Family Physician
Am Hrt J	American Heart Journal
Am J Clin Path	American Journal of Clinical Pathology
Am J Dis Child	American Journal of Diseases of Childhood
Am J Med	American Journal of Medicine
Am J Obgyn	American Journal of Obstetrics and Gynecology
Am J Psych	American Journal of Psychiatry
Am J Pub Hlth	American Journal of Public Health
Ann EM	Annals of Emergency Medicine
Ann IM	Annals of Internal Medicine
Ann Neurol	Annals of Neurology
Ann Rv Public Health	Annual Review of Public Health
Arch Derm	Archives of Dermatology
Arch IM	Archives of Internal Medicine
Arch Phys Med Rehab	Archives of Physical Medicine and Rehabilitation
Arthritis Rheum	Arthritis and Rheumatism
BMJ	British Medical Journal
Brit J Rheum	British Journal of Rheumatology
Bull Rheum Dis	Bulletin of Rheumatic Diseases

Can Med Assoc J	Canadian Medical Association Journal
Circ	Circulation
Cleve Clin J Med	Cleveland Clinic Journal of Medicine
Clin Exp Rheum	Clinical and Experimental Rheumatology
Clin Ger Med	Clinics in Geriatric Medicine
Clin Orthop	Clinical Orthopedics
Clin Perinatol	Clinical Perinatology
Contraceptive Tech	Contraceptive Technology
Crit Care Med	Critical Care Medicine
Curr Concepts Cerebro Dis	Current Concepts of Cerebrovascular Disease
Diab Care	Diabetes Care
Diab Res Clin Pract	Diabetes Research and Clinical Practice
Eff Clin Prac	Effective Clinical Practice
Emerg Med Clin N Am	Emergency Medical Clinics of North America
Epidem Rev	Epidemiology Review
Fam Pract Recert	Family Practice Recertification
Fam Pract Survey	Family Practice Survey
FDA Bul	Federal Drug Administration Bulletin
Fertil Steril	Fertility and Sterility
GE	Gastroenterology
Ger Med Today	Geriatric Medicine Today
Gerontol	Gerontologist
Ger Rv Syllabus	Geriatric Review Syllabus
HT	Hypertension
Inf Contr Hosp Epidem	Infection Control and Hospital Epidemiology

Inf Dis Clin N Am	Infectious Disease Clinics of North America
Jama	Journal of the American Medical Association
J Am Acad Derm	Journal of the American Academy of Dermatology
J Am Coll Cardiol	Journal of the American College of Cardiology
J Am Ger Soc	Journal of the American Geriatric Association
J Cardiovasc Pharmacol	Journal of Cardiovascular Pharmacology
J Chronic Dis	Journal of Chronic Disease
J Clin Epidem	Journal of Clinical Epidemiology
J Clin Immunol	Journal of Clinical Immunology
J Fam Pract	Journal of Family Practice
J Gen Intern Med	Journal of General Internal Medicine
J Gerontol	Journal of Gerontology
J Ger Psych Neurol	Journal of Geriatric Psychiatry and Neurology
J Infect Dis	Journal of Infectious Disease
J Intern Med	Journal of Internal Medicine
J Investig Derm	Journal of Investigative Dermatology
J Lab Clin Med	Journal of Laboratory and Clinical Medicine
J Peds	Journal of Pediatrics
J Pharm Experim Ther	Journal of Pharmocology and Experimental Therapy
Mccvd	Modern Concepts of Cardiovascular Disease
Md State Med Assoc J	Maryland State Medical Association Journal
Med	Medicine
Med Aud Dig	Internal Medicine Audio Digest
Med Care	Medical Care

Millbank Q	Millbank Quarterly
MKSAP	American College of Physicians Medical Knowledge Self-Assessment Test
Mmwr	CDC Morbidity and Mortality Weekly Review
Mod Med	Modern Medicine
Nejm	New England Journal of Medicine
Neurol	Neurology
Obgyn	Obstetrics and Gynecology
Obgyn Cl N Am	Obstetrics and Gynecology Clinics of North America
Ophthalm	Ophthalmology
Ped Derm	Pediatric Dermatology
Ped Infect Dis J	Pediatric Infectious Disease Journal
Ped Rv	Pediatric Review
Peds	Pediatrics
Post Grad Med J	Postgraduate Medicine Journal
Psych Ann	Psychiatric Annals
Rev Inf Dis	Review of Infectious Disease
Rx Let	Prescribers Letter
Scand J Gastroenterol	Scandanavian Journal of Gastroenterology
Sci Am Text Med	Scientific American Textbook of Medicine
Semin Arth Rheum	Seminars in Arthritis and Rheumatology
West J Med	Western Journal of Medicine

Page Format

Below is outlined the uniform format of all disease pages:

Chapter (System/Specialty)

Disease Name (Other Names)

General references, reviews

Cause: Agent, if relevant; mechanism of dissemination, if relevant

Epidem: Epidemiologic information

Pathophys: Pathophysiology

Sx: Symptoms

Si: Signs

Crs: Course of disease

Cmplc: Complications, including differential diagnoses of diseases with similar presentations

Lab: Tests and interpretation of their results, eg, pathology, chemistries, hematologies, etc, with sensitivity and specificity data if available

Xray: Radiologic and other studies usually performed by radiology departments

Rx: Treatments:
Preventive if relevant
Therapeutic of existing disease, further divided into medical vs surgical if appropriate and of complications

Chapter 1

Emergencies

D. K. Onion

1.1   General Issues

Definition: Diagnosis and treatment too urgent to allow time to look things up; all diagnostic (hx and si) findings, workup (w/u), and treatment (rx) must be memorized

Medication Routes: Can give epinephrine, atropine, lidocaine, diazepam (Valium), and naloxone (Narcan) via endotracheal tube (ET) at 2-2.5 × the iv dose, chase w 10 cc sterile water

Pediatric Special Cases:
- Endotracheal tube sizes (internal diameter) = 3 mm for newborn, 3.5 mm for 6 mo, 4 mm for 18 mo, size thereafter = 4 + age/4 in mm (Nejm 1991;324:1477) or width of 5th fingernail (Ann EM 1993;22:530)
- Nasogastric and Foley tube sizes = 2 × ET tube size
- Fluid resuscitation: Intraosseous infusions, eg, of proximal tibia very effective and fast if < 5 yr old (technique: Nejm 1990;322:1579); 20-g needle w 300 mm Hg pressure can infuse 1500 cc/hr
- Weight estimates: Weight in kg = 2 × age + 8; blood volume = 80 cc/kg of weight (Nejm 1991;324:1477)

Table 1.1   Normal Vital Signs by Age

Age	Systolic BP*	Pulse	Respirations
Newborn	60-90	94-145	30-60
Infant	74-100	124-170	30-60
Toddler	80-112	98-160	24-40
Preschool	82-110	65-132	22-34
School age	84-120	70-110	18-30
Adolescent	94-140	55-105	12-16

*Or calculate lower limit (5th percentile) of normal = $70 + 2 \times$ (age in yrs) (Nejm 1991;324:1477).

1.2   Emergency Protocols

CARDIAC ARREST AND ARRHYTHMIAS

Cardiac Arrest

ACLS, Am Hrt Assoc 2004; Nejm 1992;327:1075

Si: No effective pulse or respiration (don't be fooled by agonal respirations); unconscious

Procedures: Chest thump, debatably (only if defibrillator not available)

CPR; chest compressions alone w/o ventilation is adequate and may be better than full CPR in 1st 5-10 min of arrest, esp if doing solo (Nejm 2000;342:1546). If circulation not restored within 20-25 min of adequate CPR and patient is normothermic (> 30°C), stop, since no survivors beyond that (Nejm 1996; 335:1473).

Defibrillation ASAP w AED or other device in 1st 10 min, the only intervention that prolongs life (Nejm 2004;351: 637,647); adding ACLS to it increases survival to hospital but not long term

Never quit CPR, whether EMD, Vfib, or asystole, *until normothermic* (see p 21); hypothermic rx @ 32°C × 24 hr improves morbidity and mortality (55% to 40%) (Nejm 2002;346: 549,612,557)

if **electromechanical dissociation** (pulseless electrical activity), then r/o or rx hypothermia, hypovolemia, tamponade, tension pneumothorax, hypoxemia, acidosis, hyperkalemia, drug OD (especially cardiac meds), and pulmonary embolus

Meds:

- Vasopressin (Pitressin) 40 U iv ×1, especially if asystole (Nejm 2004;350:105 vs ACP J Club 2004;141:2), then
- Epinephrine 1 mg of 1:10 000 iv or ET (in children, 10 μgm/kg, ie, 0.1 cc/kg of 1:10 000 iv or ET); higher doses show no benefit (Nejm 2004;350:1722)
  - $NaHCO_3$ no help, worsens by hyperosmolarity and paradoxical CNS acidosis (Ann EM 1990;19:1; Med Let 1992;34:30)
  - $CaCl_2$ not helpful unless has hyperkalemia (Med Let 1992;34:30)
  if **asystole:**
- Atropine 1 mg, repeat ×1 (in children, 0.03 mg/kg, 0.1 mg minimum dose)
- Vasopressin and epinephrine as above, then rx-specific conditions found (eg, Vtach, heart block, etc)

Heart Block

Hx: Loss of consciousness or weakness

Procedures: Pacemaker, external or temporary, although in-the-field use of external pacer doesn't increase survival (Nejm 1993; 328:1377)

Meds:

- Atropine 0.5 mg iv, repeat once if no response (in children, 0.01 mg/kg iv or ET but 0.1 mg is minimum dose no matter the weight)

- Dopamine 5-20 μgm/kg/min drip, or
- Epinephrine 2-10 μgm/min drip, or
- Isoproterenol 1 mg in 500 cc drip (in children, 0.02 μgm/kg/min drip, titrate up)

Supraventricular Tachycardias (PAT, AV Nodal Reentrant and AV Reentrant Tachycardias, atrial flutter, atrial fibrillation)

Hx: Dizzy, "fluttering"

Si: Narrow complexes on EKG; IF WIDE, RX AS VTACH

Procedures: Carotid sinus massage; cardioversion at 30-100 W/s synchronized; overdrive external pacing at 120 mA, at rate faster than SVT rate in 3-5 beat pulses (Ann EM 1993;22:1993)

Meds:
- Adenosine analog (Adenocard) 6 mg push ×1, then, if no conversion in 5 min, 12 mg (Ann IM 1991;114:513; Nejm 1991;325:1621) or in children 0.1 mg/kg, repeat w 0.2-0.3 mg/kg (Ann EM 1992;21:1499); 10 sec half-life; for PAT and AV reentrant types only, not Afib or Aflut (Med Let 1990;32:63), especially since it can cause enhanced a-v conduction, ie, Aflut at 2:1 or 3:1 can be converted to 1:1 conduction (Nejm 1994;330:288) though becoming controversial; most pts have angina-like chest pain w rx; ok in pregnancy (Am J Em Med 1992;10:54), avoid in asthma; or
- Verapamil 2.5-5 mg, repeat in 20 min at 5-10 mg iv (0.1 mg/kg in children), or
- Sotalol (Betapace) 1 mg/kg iv bolus (Nejm 1994;331:31), other β-blocker, or
- Digoxin 0.5 mg iv, then 0.25 mg iv q 4 hr to 1.5 mg total in 24 hr; becoming less popular

Ventricular Tachycardia

Hx: Loss of consciousness usually but not always

Si: Wide complexes

Procedures: Chest thump; cardioversion with 200 W/s synchronized; sedate if awake (in children, defibrillate at 2 J/kg, double if necessary)

Meds:

> 1st: Amiodarone (Cardarone) (Am J Cardiol 2002;90:853) 150-300 mg (5 mg/kg) iv over 10 min, then 1mg/min drip; or
>
> 2nd: Procainamide up to 1 gm over 20 min or until response, then drip at 2-4 mg/min; or
>
> 3rd: Magnesium sulfate 1-2 gm iv push (2-4 cc of 50% soln) in 50-100 cc D5W; or
>
> 4th: Lidocaine 75-150 mg (1-2 mg/kg) iv bolus, drip at 2-4 mg/min (in children, 1 mg/kg bolus iv or ET, then 0.03-0.04 mg/kg/min); or
>
> 5th: Sotalol 100 mg iv over 5 min, may be better than lidocaine (Lancet 1994;344:18)

Ventricular Fibrillation

Hx: Loss of consciousness

Procedures: Chest thump; defibrillation with 2-300 W/s

Meds:

- Epinephrine 1 mg of 1:10 000 iv or ET (in children, 10 μgm/kg, ie, 0.1 cc/kg of 1:10 000 iv or ET); or
- Vasopressin (Pitressin) 40 U iv ×1; then more defibrillations, and consider:
- Amiodarone (Nejm 1999;341:871) as above; clearly better than lidocaine (Nejm 2002;346:884)
- Procainamide as above, or
- Magnesium sulfate 1-2 gm iv, especially if looks like torsades de pointes
- Lidocaine as above

COMA/CONFUSION/SEIZURE

Seizure (p 726)

Hx: By observers of tonic-clonic activity, and postictal gradual recovery; possible h/o seizures

Si: Unconscious, lateral tongue bites, r/o cardiac arrest by checking pulses and respiration procedures: place prone, iv, oral airway; last resort, general anesthesia

Meds (Jama 1993;270:854) (see sz p 723): None at first. Wait; if doesn't resolve, may be status epilepticus; give iv thiamine and glucose, +

- Diazepam (Valium) 5-10 mg iv, may repeat (in children, 0.1 mg/kg, up to 0.5 iv, pr, or ET); or lorazepam (Ativan) 1-2 mg iv; or midazolam (Versed) 0.2 mg/kg (Crit Care Med 1992;20:483), used especially in children
- Phenytoin 15-20 mg/kg at 50 mg/min iv in rapid flow saline (no glucose) (in children, 10 mg/kg slowly ×1 or ×2 up to 30 mg/kg iv); or fosphenytoin (Cerebyx), new iv form, comes in phenytoin equivalents, can give much faster and safer iv, eg, 100-150 mg/min
- Phenobarbital 750-1500 mg iv slowly (in children, 5 mg/kg/dose up to 20 mg/kg total over 1 hr iv or im)
- Lidocaine iv as for Vtach above

of **Status epilepticus** (Nejm 1998;338:970): 65% successful for overt status, 25% for occult type (obtunded + positive EEG)

1st: iv thiamine 100 mg + glucose

1st: Lorazepam (Ativan) (best: Nejm 2001;345:631) 2 mg/min iv to 0.1 mg/kg; or diazepam (Valium) up to 20 mg iv, or as rectal gel 5 mg/cc in syringes for home use w repetitive sz's (Nejm 1998;338:1869); or midamozole (Versed) 0.2 mg/kg

2nd: Fosphenytoin 20 mg/kg iv over 10 min (can use phenytoin 1-1.5 gm over 30 min), repeat 10 mg/kg if still seizing

3rd: Phenobarbital 15 mg/kg at 100 mg/min iv (may need to intubate)

3rd: Lidocaine 100 mg bolus, 2 mg/min drip
4th: General anesthesia

Hypoglycemia

Hx: Insulin use or alcoholism

Si: Intoxication, coma

W/u: Draw blood sugar

Procedures: 25 gm (50 cc of 50% soln) glucose stat iv with 100 mg of thiamine (see below); may repeat ×1; in children, 2 cc of a 50% soln or 4 cc of a 25% soln (1 gm)/kg iv

Alcoholism

Si: Intoxication, coma

W/u: Blood alcohol, r/o other ODs w hx and levels

Meds:
- Thiamine 100 mg iv/im (Jama 1995;274;562) to avoid precipitating Wernicke's, continue × 3 d
- $MgSO_4$ 2 gm iv/im and continue 8-10 gm qd × 3 d if renal function ok

Intracranial Mass/Bleed

Hx: Trauma

Si: Eye si's including lateral gaze palsies, pupillary inequalities

W/u: CT or MRI; neurosurgical consult

Procedures: Burr hole, if deteriorating, on side of dilated pupil; elevate head of bed to 45°

Meds:
- Mannitol 1.5-2 gm/kg as 20-25% soln over 30-60 min
- Dexamethasone 5-10 mg iv push, efficacy?

Meningitis/Encephalitis

W/u: Lumbar puncture asap

Meds:

- Ceftriaxone or cefotaxime 2 gm iv (adult) or 50-75 mg/kg (child), plus vancomycin 1 gm iv (adult) or 10-15 mg/kg (child) to cover penicillin-resistant pneumococcus, plus ampicillin at age extremes to cover listeria
- Dexamethasone 0.15 mg/kg repeated ×3 q 6 hr in addition to antibiotics, in children

Dyspnea

Anaphylaxis (p 23)

Hx: Bee sting, penicillin et al. exposure less than 2 hr previously

Si: Shock, wheezes, w or w/o rash and hives

Procedures: Tourniquet if practical and sc or im source, iv, O_2

Meds:

- Epinephrine 0.5-1 mg im or sc (in children, 10 μgm/kg, ie, 0.01 cc/kg of 1:1000 sc), repeat q 30 min
- Diphenhydramine (Benadryl) 25-50 mg (in children, 1 mg/kg) iv/im; + cimetidine 300 mg iv
- Hydrocortisone 200-400 mg iv, or methylprednisolone 60-80 mg iv followed by prednisone 60 mg po qd × 2-3 d
- Aminophylline 9 mg/kg load, 0.7 mg/kg/hr perhaps if bronchospasm

Asthma/COPD (p 969, p 981)

Hx: Often presents w empty inhaler; usually long h/o similar problems

Si: Speaks in less than whole sentences, papilledema, wheezing but may be diminished as worsen, asterixis, accessory muscle use, P > 100, pulsus paradoxicus

W/u: Chest xray, ABGs or O_2 saturation, PFTs

Procedures: iv, D_5W if age > 50, otherwise D_5S to repair usually depleted state; O_2; intubation

Meds:

Primary meds:
- Albuterol 5 cc of 0.5% soln by nebulizer q 15-20 min × 3-4 or continuous (½ dose in children < 5 yr) w
- Ipratropium 500 μgm (250 in children < 5 yr); plus
- Hydrocortisone 200-400 mg iv bolus or methylprednisolone (Solumedrol) 60-100 mg, or equivalent (in children, methylprednisolone 0.5 mg/kg iv)

Other meds to consider:
- Terbutaline, in children 0.01 mg/kg sc up to 0.3 mg maximum; in adults, 1 mg sc or in neb
- Epinephrine (if age < 35) 0.5 mg sc or 1 mg in 500 D_5S (in children 10 μgm/kg, ie, 0.01 cc/kg of 1:1000 sc up to 0.3 cc)
- Aminophyllin load (if not on) and drip as above (in children, 6 mg/kg iv over 20 min then 1 mg/kg/hr)
- Heliox (helium oxygen gas mixture), which decreases turbulence
- Morphine 2-4 mg iv

Croup, Severe (p 886)

Meds:
- Racemic epinephrine 0.5 cc in 4 cc water via aerosol; admit if recurs within 30 min
- Dexamethasone (Decadron) 0.6 mg/kg iv/im

Epiglottitis (p 235)

Hx: Rapid onset

Si: Drooling, leaning forward, dysphagia; airway obstruction especially if stressed, eg, by looking in throat with tongue blade

W/u: Lateral neck xray

Procedures: Consider/prepare for intubation or tracheostomy

Meds:

- Ceftriaxone, or ampicillin 50 mg/kg (200 mg/kg/d) and chloramphenicol 25 mg/kg (100 mg/kg/d) iv
- Racemic epinephrine + dexamethasone (Decadron) as above

Foreign Body in Airway

Si: Dinner table aphonic dyspnea or young child eating small food (peanuts) or toys

Procedures: Heimlich maneuver, direct visualization, and extraction

Pulmonary Edema

Sx: PND, DOE

Si: Orthopnea, rales, edema, S_3, JVD, P > 100

W/u: EKG, chest xray

Procedures: D_5W iv; O_2; phlebotomy/tourniquets; Foley; noninvasive positive pressure respiration (Chest 1998;114:1185) w BiPAP (Nejm 1991;325:1825), CPAP, or endotracheal intubation

Meds:

- Morphine 2-5 mg iv
- TNG 0.4 mg sl or 10-20 μgm/min iv
- Furosemide 20-40 mg iv; or dobutamine 2.5-15 μgm/kg/min iv (250 mg amps) + nitroprusside 1-5 μgm/kg/min (50 mg amps)
- Captopril 12.5-25 mg po chewed and swallowed
- Digoxin, consider later

Pulmonary Embolus (p 13)

Tension Pneumothorax

Hx: Chest trauma or sudden onset with past history of pneumothorax

Si: Increased resonance, decreased breath sounds, cyanosis, tracheal deviation

W/u: Chest xray later

Procedures: Tap upper anterior chest in 2nd intercostal space, mid-clavicular line with over-the-needle catheter (Nejm 1991;324:1479); f/u chest tube

Fractures

Midfemoral Fracture

Hx: Fall, trauma

Si: External rotation, deformity, distal pulses may be compromised

W/u: Xray (later); type and cross

Procedures: Thomas (traction) splint; saline iv

Supracondylar Fracture of Humerus

Hx: Fall on elbow, most often in children

Si: Subtly short upper arm, pain, distal pulses may be compromised

W/u: Xray (later)

Procedures: Sling and downward traction with weight on it; immobilization splint

Cervical Fracture

Hx: Diving, fall from pickup tailgate, or any headfirst fall; consider in any head injury

Si: Pain, paresthesias, weakness

W/u: Xrays after immobilized; must include all of C_7, may require swimmer's view; or CT. Films unnecessary (NEXUS criteria: Nejm 2000;343:94,138) if (1) no midline cervical tenderness; (2) no focal neurol deficit; (3) normal alertness; (4) no intoxication; and (5) no distracting significant other injury. Canadian cervical spine rules more sens and specific (Nejm 2003;349:2510).

Procedures: Splint and in-line immobilization of neck before xrays

Meds: Methylprednisolone 30 mg/kg iv over 15 min w 5.4 mg/kg/hr iv × 24 hr for spinal cord injury (Nejm 1990;322:1405)

Flail Chest

Hx: Steering wheel injury

Si: Paradoxical motion

W/u: Xray later

Procedures: Bag breathe, then respirator; epidural block for pain control

Pelvic Fracture

Hx: Crush injury usually, male unable to void

Si: Rectal to look for high-riding prostate

W/u: Urethrogram; pelvic xray. Crit; type and cross

Procedures: MAST for transport; *do not catheterize* bladder until urethrogram; 2 large-bore iv's.

Shock with Chest Pain

Anaphylaxis (p 23)

Aortic Dissection

Hx: Back/neck pain; h/o hypertension

Si: Transiently absent pulses, bruits; BP differences between extremities

W/u: Chest xray, CT of chest; arteriogram

Meds:
- Nitroprusside iv (p 62) to BP < 100 systolic, and
- Metoprolol 5 mg iv, or
- Propranolol 1-2 mg iv or esmolol @ 50-200 μgm/min

Myocardial Infarction

p 86; Nejm 1999;341:625, 1991;325:1117; Jama 2001;285:190

Hx: Chest pain, substernal radiation in distribution of a tree, worse supine

Si: Gray, often middle-aged man, shock with relative bradycardia

W/u: EKG, chest xray

Procedures: iv, O_2; consider emergent referral for PCTA/CABG revascularization if available

Meds:

- Thrombolysis if sx < 6 hr old (perhaps up to 12 hr), pain, and ST elevations
- ASA 80-160 mg po
- Morphine, enough to decrease pain, up to 20 mg iv in divided doses
- Metoprolol (Lopressor) 5 mg iv × 3 within 24 hr unless heart block, hypotension, or severe bradycardia
- ACE inhibitor within 24 hr and for at least 6 wk
- Perhaps TNG 50 mg iv q 3-5 min or 10^+ μgm/min drip (3 mg in 20 cc = 0.15 mg/cc)
- Dopamine 2-10 μgm/kg/min (200 mg amp) and/or dobutamine (p 44) if shock
- Nitroprusside (p 62) if low cardiac output and BP allows

Pericardial Tamponade

Hx: Steering wheel trauma; possible acute inflammatory pericarditis

Si: Shock, although BP may be elevated in $^1/_3$ (Nejm 1992;327:463); paradoxical pulse > 20 mm Hg; JVP elevation

Procedures: Pericardiocentesis w 18-g spinal needle

Pulmonary Embolus

Hx: Bedridden, long trip, leg trauma, or positive family hx; cough, dyspnea

Si: No orthopnea or increased pain supine unlike MI

W/u: ABGs, chest xray, EKG, V/Q scan, IPG or Doppler ultrasound, PT, PTT, platelets, guaiac, crit

Procedures: iv, O_2

Meds:
- Heparin 5000 U bolus, 1000-hr drip, adjust q 12-24 hr; or weight-adjusted 80 U/kg bolus and 18 U/kg/hr
- Perhaps thrombolysis if severe sx

Sepsis/Septic Shock

Hx: Post-surgery, Foley, other predisposers

Si: BP decreased but relative bradycardia, fever sometimes, decreased urine output

W/u: Blood and other cultures; Gram stain buffy coat

Procedures: Saline or Ringer's based on CVP; in children, 20 cc/kg boluses until hemodynamically stable, may take 3-5 such boluses

Meds:
- Antibiotics: Ceftriaxone or ceftazidime 1 gm iv q 12 hr + gentamicin 5 mg/kg/24 hr iv in divided doses
- Pressors: Norepinephrine 0.05-0.25 μgm/kg/min titrated to BP is better than dopamine (Jama 1994;272:1354)

Volume Loss/Bleeding (including anaphylaxis, toxic shock, bleeding, spinal cord shock)

Hx: Postural sx sometimes (dizzy when stands)

Si: Systolic BP decreases ≥ 25 mm; P increases > 100 or ≥ 20/min when stand from supine position; in children especially: delayed capillary refill, altered consciousness, increased pulse and respirations before BP decreases

W/u: Type and crossmatch; clotting studies; lytes; guaiacs

Procedures: 2 large-bore iv's to transfuse blood and saline maximally, use fluid warmer if can; in children, 20 cc/kg saline, Ringer's, or fresh frozen plasma, may bolus up to 70 cc/kg in 1st hr (Jama 1991;266:1242); MAST trousers (warmed); 10 cc/kg packed rbc's, 20-g needle + 300 mm Hg pressure allows 70 cc/min of packed rbc infusion if diluted 1:1 w saline

Meds: Dopamine 10 μgm/kg/min drip, titrate up to BP or 25 μgm/kg/min

Transfusion Reactions

Histamine Transfusion Reactions (Anaphylaxis)

Hx: Pruritus, dyspnea

Si: Hives/rash, wheezing, fever

W/u: ABGs and/or central venous gases (Nejm 1989;320:1312)

Procedures: Stop transfusion; MAST trousers if shocky

Meds:
- Diphenhydramine (Benadryl) 25-50 mg iv or im
- Epinephrine 0.5-1 mg iv or sc
- Hydrocortisone 200-400 mg iv
- H_2 blockers (eg, cimetidine 300 mg iv)

Febrile Transfusion Reactions

Many or most due to interleukins in plasma that increase w age of the unit, not white cell antigens; more common (10-30%) w platelet transfusions than w rbc transfusions (Nejm 1994;331:625), r/o infected unit

Hx: Malaise, nausea

Si: Fever, chills, rigors

W/u: Culture bag and perhaps patient

Procedures: Stop transfusion or remove supernatant plasma

Meds: Diphenhydramine (Benadryl) as above or in bag

Hemolytic Transfusion Reactions (with renal shutdown)

Hx: Back pain

Cmplc: ATN with hemolysis

W/u: UA, repeat crossmatch, look at serum for free hemoglobin

Meds:
- Mannitol (1 amp) +
- NaHCO$_3$ (1 amp) in 1000 cc D$_5$W

HYPERTHERMIA

Malignant Hyperthermia

Jama 2005;293:2918; Nejm 1993;329:484; Nejm 1983;309:416

Cause: Genetic plus anesthesia or other stress; autosomal dominant

Epidem: Prevalence = 1/14,000 people can develop if stressed; a history of one safe anesthesia is no guarantee next will be ok

Pathophys: Abnormal calcium channel in muscles causes Ca^{++} release into muscles and intense contractions

Sx: None

Si: Intraoperatively tachycardia and tachypnea precede muscle rigidity and then high fever

Crs: High mortality

Cmplc: r/o neuroleptic malignant syndrome (p 17); cocaine OD (p 27); and simple **heat stroke** (Nejm 2002;346:1979) with T° > 40°C, impaired thermoregulation, cognitive impairment, and anhidrosis; 10% mortality; in the elderly or in healthy adults exercising in the heat (Nejm 1993;329:484)

Lab: *Chem:* Platelet ATP studies distinguish? (Letter: Nejm 1980;303:642)

Path: Muscle bx of relatives shows abnormality in vitro responses to drug stimulation if they are susceptible

Rx: Prevent by avoiding halogenated gases and muscle paralyzers; may try to prevent with dantrolene (Dantrium) 1 mg/kg po × 2 d prior to elective surgery; avoid calcium-channel blockers of acute attack: stop anesthesia; dantrolene (Dantrium) 1 mg/kg push, repeat up to response or 10 mg/kg

Neuroleptic Malignant Syndrome

Med Clin N Am 1993;77(1):185; Nejm 1993;329:485; Nejm 1985;313:163

Cause: Neuroleptic drugs (major tranquilizers) including phenothiazines, butyrophenones, thioxanthenes, loxapine, and rarely clozapine (Nejm 1991;324:746)

Epidem: 0.2-0.5% of patients given these drugs will develop; unrelated to dose; 96% of cases occur within 30 d of starting the drug; 30% of those who have had before will get again if reexposed. Incidence is increased with exhaustion, dehydration, organic brain syndrome, and depot phenothiazines.

Pathophys: Diminished CNS dopamine

Sx: 1-3 d onset, up to 5-10 d after drug stopped, or 10-30 d after im depot types

Si: Fever (> 38°C/100.4°F in 87%), rigidity and hypertonia ("lead pipe") (97%), changes in mental status (97%), autonomic instability (pallor, diaphoresis, BP changes, tachycardia, arrhythmias), akinesia, involuntary movements, tremor

Precipitated by dopamine agonists like metaclopramide (Reglan), or amoxapine (Asendin) sometimes

Crs: 10% mortality in 3-30 d; before 1984 and aggressive rx, mortality was ~25%

Cmplc: Respiratory failure, myoglobinuric renal failure, cardiovascular collapse, arrhythmias, pulmonary embolus

r/o **heat stroke** (Med Let 2003;47:58; Ann IM 1998;129:173): fever > 40.6°C (105°F), altered mental status (100%), anhidrosis; associated w exertion or infection in elderly, drug use (phenothiazines, anticholinergics, diuretics, β-blockers, alcohol) in presence of hot humid weather; cmplc include DIC (50%) and renal insufficiency, 20% in-hospital mortality; prevent w fluids and air conditioning, rx w cooling

Also malignant hyperthermia (above), idiopathic **acute lethal catatonia,** drug interactions with MAO inhibitors, central anticholinergic crisis that responds to iv physostigmine, tetanus, stiff man syndrome (p 577), myotonia, meningitis or encephalitis, thyroid storm, cocaine OD (p 27)

Lab: *Chem:* CPK elevated, may be > 16,000 IU; aldolase elevated; elevated LFTs (due to pyrexia-induced fatty changes?)
Hem: Wbc 15,000-30,000 with L shift
Urine: Myoglobinuria (67%)

Rx: Stop neuroleptics then give
- Dantrolene (Dantrium) 1-2 mg/kg iv initial dose, then up to 10 mg/kg/d iv or po divided in q 6 hr doses; beware of concomitant calcium-channel blocker use +
- Bromocriptine 2.5-10 mg po tid, or amantadine 100 mg po bid, or perhaps L-dopa

  Nitroprusside iv/minoxidil po worked in 1 patient when dantrolene failed, controlled fever and BP (Ann IM 1986;104:56)

  Prevent myoglobinuric ATN by iv fluids, mannitol infusion, and $NaHCO_3$ iv to alkalinize the urine

Serotonin Syndrome

Nejm 2005;352:1112

Cause: Excessive serotonin, usually caused by prescription or illicit drugs including:
- Antidepressants like MAOIs, tricyclics, SSRIs, trazodone, nefazodone (Serozone), buspirone (Buspar), clomipramine (Anafranil), venlafaxine (Effexor)
- Opiates, especially meperidine, fentanyl (Duragesic), tramadol, dextromethorphan (OTC), pentazocine
- Dietary supplements: tryptophan, St. John's wort, ginseng
- Abused drugs: LSD, ecstasy, foxymethoxy

- Antiemetics: odansetron, granisetron, metoclopramide
- Others: valproate, sumatriptan, linezolide (Zyvox), lithium

Epidem: Present in 15% of SSRI overdoses; 1000's of cases/yr in U.S., often undiagnosed

Pathophys: Excessive serotonin peripherally and in CNS causes sx. Onset can occur when the 2nd precipitating drug is added even weeks after stopping 1st drug, eg, w fluoxetine.

Sx: After precipitating drug taken, rapid onset of anxiety, diaphoresis, shivering

Si: (* = most important si and, if present, dx is likely)
Mild: tachycardia, diaphoresis, shivering, mydriasis (dilated pupils), tremor, myoclonus, hyperreflexia*
Moderate: above plus hypertension, hyperthermia to 40+°C, hyperactive bowel sounds, clonus* especially in lower extremities or ocular, agitation/hypervigilance, pressured speech, repetitive head turning w neck in extension
Severe: big hypertension and tachycardia leading to shock, agitated delirium, muscle rigidity* and hypertonia especially in lower extremities, fever > 41°C, metabolic acidosis, rhabdomyolysis, seizures

Cmplc: DIC, shock, renal failure; all due to uncontrolled hypertension?
r/o Diagnoses listed above under NMS and malignancy hyperthermia

Lab: *Chem:* CPK, AST (SGOT), creatinine elevations

Rx: Supportive iv fluids
Diazepam or other iv benzodiazepines
Cyproheptadine po or via ng tube, 12 mg ×1, then 2 mg q 2 hr until better up to 32 mg/day, 8 mg po q 8 hr maintenance until causes cleared
Chlorpromazine 50-100 mg im
Olanzapine 10 mg sl?

of fever: no antipyretics; general anesthesia and intubation (avoid succinylcholine) if can't control fever and if necessary to eliminate muscle rigidity

DROWNING/HYPOTHERMIA

Drowning

Nejm 1992;328:53

Cause: Water inhalation/immersion

Epidem: 7000 drowning deaths/yr in U.S.; majority are freshwater; $^1/_4$ are teenagers

Pathophys: Pulmonary edema, metabolic acidosis, and hypoxia with very rapid changes in V/Q ratios and lung elasticity occur. Fresh water may enter the circulation and cause hypervolemia and hemodilution with red cell lysis, which in turn causes hyperkalemia leading to Vfib and death, or hemoglobinemia/uria leading to renal damage; lung cells also lysed. Salt water pulls plasma into the alveoli and thus causes hypovolemia and hemoconcentration leading to pulmonary edema, anoxia, and death. Surfactant changes cause decreases in lung compliance.

Sx:

Si: ARDS with decreased lung compliance and consequent blood gas changes

Crs: If comatose, 40-50% recover, 10-20% die, and 30-50% survive w brain damage

Cmplc: Hypothermia (p 21); ATN from hypotension and myoglobinuria; anoxic neurologic damage; diminished platelet numbers and/or function; DIC within hours in freshwater drowning (Ann IM 1977;87:60); ARDS; Vfib; hypoglycemia; hyperkalemia; impaired drug clearance

Lab:
Chem: if $K^+ > 2\times$ normal, universally fatal
Hem: Crit decreases over the first 1-2 hr

Path: At postmortem, in freshwater drowning, lungs show intra-alveolar and interstitial edema as well as altered surface tension. In saltwater drowning, major finding is pulmonary edema and only slight changes in surface tension.

Rx: CPR, CPAP/PEEP, rx pH < 7.1 w bicarb; avoid too high O_2 concentrations, which can further decrease surfactant; treat hypothermia (p 21); antibiotics only if gastric aspiration or dirty water aspiration occurred. Initial abdominal thrust no use unless airway obstruction suspected.

Hypothermia

Nejm 1994;331:1756; Postgrad Med 1990;88:55

Cause: Drowning, outdoor exposure, often associated with alcohol/drugs/overdoses, bacteremia in the aged, CVA, DKA, pancreatitis, hypothyroidism, hypoadrenalism

Epidem:

Pathophys: "Cold diuresis" occurs because of peripheral vasoconstriction and/or renal inability to resorb water. Hypoxic damage as hemoglobin dissociation curve shifted to left, releasing less O_2 to tissues.

Sx: Decreased cold perception

Si: Must use special thermometer that can register $< 95°F$ (35°C)

Mild = 35-32.2°C (95-90°F); moderate = 32.2-28°C (90-82.4°F); severe = $< 28°C$ (82.4°F)

$< 95°F$ (35°C) causes ataxia, slowed reflexes, sinus bradycardia (don't do CPR as long as you can feel a pulse, even if it is very slow), hypotension; $< 82.4°F$ (28°C) unconciousness occurs, fixed and dilated pupils

Crs:

Cmplc: DIC within hours; Vfib; hypoglycemia; hyperkalemia; impaired drug clearance. Late cardiomyopathy due to multiple micro infarcts.

Lab:

Chem: Screens for above causes; if $K^+ > 2\times$ normal, universally fatal

Noninv: EKG shows Osborn J waves (wide, upright slur in terminal QRS) (see Figure 1.1) (Nejm 1994;330:680; Am J Physiol 1953; 175:389), which are pathognomonic for hypothermia, occur at $< 80°F$ ($27°C$); general QRS widening follows and predicts ventricular fibrillation

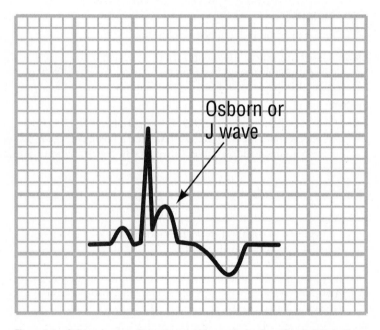

Figure 1.1 Osborn J waves. Reproduced with permission from Garcia T, Holtz N. The 12 Lead EKG, The Art of Interpretation. Sudbury, MA: Jones & Bartlett, 2001, p214.

Rx   (Med Let 1994;36:116): Rewarm core first
    if 85-90°F (34-36°C) and cardiovascularly stable, use
warmed blankets, warmed D$_5$ saline, and O$_2$/air (104°F, 41.6°C)
    if < 85°F (< 34°C) (Vfib risk) and/or unstable, then use
warm lavages via Foley catheter, NG tubes, rectal tubes; intraperitoneal lavage (can raise by 2°C/hr); pleural continuous
warm lavage (Ann EM 1990;19:204) can raise by 20°C/hr; or
extracorporeal cardiopulmonary bypass, which is very effective
(Nejm 1997;337:1500), consider transferring to get it
    if in Vfib or standstill, rewarm to 90°F before cardioverting
or quitting; beware of impaired lidocaine metabolism
    Antibiotics pending culture workup
    Avoid heating blankets, which can rewarm periphery before
core and cause shock and hyperkalemia, although active rewarm-
ing of trunk alone may be ok
    Avoid insulin for hyperglycemia since insulin resistance is
present at hypothermic temperatures but will act later, causing
hypoglycemia

OVERDOSES, STINGS, AND POISONINGS

Anaphylaxis

Cause: Aspiration, ingestion (Nejm 1992;327:380), or parenteral use
    of drugs and other haptens, eg, penicillin, anesthetics, radiocon-
    trast agents, ACE inhibitors, NSAIDs (Nejm 1994;331:1282);
    foreign antigens, eg, insect stings (Nejm 1994;331:523) including
    fire ants (Ann IM 1999;131:424), desensitization shots, semen
    (Ann IM 1981;94:459), peanuts (Nejm 2003;348:986); polysac-
    charides, eg, dextran. Sulfa antibiotic allergy does not increase
    likelihood of sulfa non-antibiotic reaction (Nejm 2003;
    349:1628).

Epidem: Increased incidence in atopic persons

Pathophys: Respiratory distress due to both upper tract edema and
    lower tract bronchospasm perhaps due to leukotrienes (Ann IM

1997;127:472), previously called slow-reacting substance (SRS). Hypotension due to histamine, kinins, and perhaps leukotriene release. Diarrhea and gi sx may be due to serotonin. Several drug-induced types of reactions are not IgE mediated, eg, those by radiocontrast agents, ACE inhibitors, and NSAIDs (Nejm 1994;331:1282).

Sx: Respiratory distress; vascular collapse; cutaneous rash/itch; gi nausea, vomiting, diarrhea, and pain especially if antigen taken po

Si: Upper or lower airway obstruction; vascular collapse; rash

Crs: Onset in ½-3 min, die in 15-120 min if going to; recurs in 28% if rechallenged (Ann IM 1993;118:161)

Cmplc: Respiratory or vascular collapse, death

Lab:

Chem: Serum tryptase increased? (Nejm 1987;316:1622)

Serol: RAST testing, 20% false neg compared to skin testing

Skin tests: Pos test is very specific at 0.1-1 μgm/cc if anaphylaxis truly present (Nejm 1994;331:523); whole-insect preparations no use, pure venom very specific. Passive transfer: patient's serum sc to animal or volunteer, challenge at 24 hr.

Histamine release from basophils in vitro very specific, 20% false neg, expose to 0.1 μgm/cc venom

Rx: Emergent:
- Tourniquet if practical and sc or im source; ice packs
- Support vital signs w iv fluids, O_2, neb
- Epinephrine 0.5-1 mg iv, im, or sc (in children, 10 μgm/kg, ie, 0.01 cc/kg of 1:1000 sc) or smaller iv doses, repeat q 30 min
- Diphenhydramine (Benadryl) 25-50 mg (in children, 1 mg/kg) iv/im + cimetidine 300 mg iv
- Hydrocortisone 200-400 mg iv, or methylprednisolone 60-80 mg iv followed by prednisone 60 mg po qd × 2-3 d
- Aminophylline 9 mg/kg load, 0.7 mg/kg/hr perhaps if bronchospasm

Preventive options:
- Epipen home sc epinephrine kit
- Desensitize with venom (Nejm 2004;351:668) for pts w systemic reaction (uriticaria, angioedema, or mre); 95% effective, × 3-5 yr then stop; better than whole-body extracts (Nejm 1990;323:1627). Most helpful in children, probably worth doing in adults in whom half will have a systemic (not just large local) reaction after a first event if stung again.
- Steroids: for IVP dye reaction (not true anaphylaxis since doesn't always recur after previous episode), 150 mg prednisone divided q 24 hr beginning 18 hr before and continuing 12 hr after procedure helps (Ann IM 1975;83:159); or methylprednisolone 32 mg po 12 hr and 2 hr before dye exposure helps some but not all (Nejm 1987;317:845); or diphenhydramine 50 mg im × 1 (Ann IM 1975;83:277). New hyperosmolar agents 20× as expensive but less vagal and cardiac depression and perhaps less anaphylactoid (rv:Nejm 1992;326:425, 431).
- Experimental anti-IgE monoclonal antibody (Nejm 2003; 348:986) sc q 1 mo is effective against peanut anaphylaxis
  For idiopathic anaphylaxis, prednisone 60 mg qd × 1 wk, then qod and decrease to 5-10 mg qod; plus hydroxyzine 25 mg tid helps decrease frequency and severity (Ann IM 1991;114:133)

1.3 Overdoses/Poisonings

General rx (Jama 1999;282:1113; in children: Nejm 2000;342:186)
Call poison control center
Activated charcoal 1-2 gm/kg up to 75-100 gm po or via NG tube q 2 hr × 3 doses w cathartic like sorbitol; contraindicated if no bowel sounds, or if patient stuporous and not intubated; ineffective for boric acid, alcohols, alkalis, cyanide, heavy metals, and mineral acids. Adv effect: aspiration pneumonia.

if altered mental state or unconscious, give naloxone 2 mg iv +
    amp (50 cc) of 50% glucose iv + thiamine 100 mg iv/im
if pinpoint pupils, give naloxone 2 mg iv (0.05-0.4 if an addict)
    and r/o hypothermia. Empty stomach, unless ingestions of
    corrosives, high viscosity or < 2 cc/kg of low-viscosity petro-
    leum distillates, with:
Gastric lavage with large-bore Ewald tube in L lateral
    Trendelenberg position
Ipecac po, 30 cc for adults, 15 cc for children age 1-12, or 10 cc
    age 6 mo-1 yr; rarely used even as prehospital rx in U.S.
    since emesis may result in inability to give charcoal soon;
    but completely empties stomach 70% of the time, unlike
    lavage, which does so 12% of the time (J Roy Soc Med
    1991;84:35)

Aspirin OD (p 36)

Acetaminophen (Tylenol) OD (p 33)

Arsenic Poisoning (p 34)

β-Blocker OD

Rx: Glucagon 5-10 mg iv w saline, titrate to normal vital si's; 2-10
    mg/hr maintenance

Barbiturate OD

Sx: Bullae on hands (Nejm 1970;283:409)

Rx: iv fluids; HCO_3 to alkalinize urine especially with phenobarb (a
    weak acid); activated charcoal decreases half-life from 110 hr to
    45 hr (Nejm 1982;307:676, 692), po 50-100 gm × 1 then 20-60
    gm q 4-12 hr

Bee Sting (p 23)

Benzodiazepine OD

Rx: Supportive care
Flumazenil (Romazicon) 1 mg iv over 3 min (an antagonist)
q 1 hr (BMJ 1990;301:1308), may not reverse the respiratory
depression and may precipitate seizures (Med Let 1992;34:66)
especially in mixed ODs w cocaine or cyclic antidepressants

Butanediol

Purported dietary supplement for weight loss, muscle building,
and sexual enhancement; mutiplelethal and near lethal responses
reported (Nejm; 2001;344:87)

Chloroquine Toxicity/OD

Sx: > 5 gm fatal without rx

Rx: Ventilation, diazepam (Valium), and epinephrine produce >
90% survival (Nejm 1988;318:1)
Cardiac monitor × 6+ hr
No ipecac

Cocaine Use

Med Let 1996;38:43, Nejm 1996;334:965, 1995;333:1267

Sx: Used nasally or iv, or smoked as "free base" or "crack"

Pathophys: Overt and silent CNS (Jama 1998;279:376) and cardiac
(Nejm 2001;345:351) vasoconstriction; impaired perceptions of
overheating (Ann IM 2002;136:785)

Cmplc: Neurologic: Delirium, seizures, ischemic and hemorrhagic
CVAs (Nejm 1990;323:699)
Hyperthermia
Cardiac: MIs and arrhythmias (Nejm 1986:315:1438,1495),
premature atherosclerosis, silent ST elevations on Holter even

3 wk after discontinuation (Ann IM 1989;111:876), false pos CPK-MB elevations, EKG changes of MI only in 36% when actually present

r/o similar but longer-acting (12+ hr) methamphetamine abuse ("speed, crystal, ice") (Med Let 2004;46:62) and w which must avoid haloperidol which may impede metabolism

Rx:

of Agitation: iv benzodiazepines

of Chest pain: Nitrates plus O_2 and ASA; if not enough, use phentolamine, verapamil, or thrombolytics; avoid lidocaine (Med Let 1990;32:93) and labetolol as well as other β-blockers, which can result in unopposed α-stimulation

Cyanide Poisoning (p 39)

Digitalis Toxicity/OD

Rx: Fab fragments (Digibind) 40 mg/0.6 mg taken of digoxin or digitoxin, iv (Nejm 1992;326:1739); $MgSO_4$ 2 gm iv while waiting

Ethylene Glycol Antifreeze Ingestion

Nejm 1981;304:21

Pathophys: Alcohol dehydrogenase (ADH) converts to glycolic acid, which causes acidosis and is metabolized into oxalate; this produces high osmolar gap

Lab: High osmolar gap = measured osmoles − calculated osmoles (calculated = 2 × Na + glucose/18 + BUN/2.8); r/o methanol and/or ethanol ingestion

Rx: Ethanol po or iv continuous to levels of 100-125 mg %; to inhibit alcohol dehydrogenase

Fomepizole (Antizol) (Nejm 1999;340:832) 15 mg/kg iv load, then 10 mg/kg q 12 hr × 48 hr, then 15 mg/kg q 12 hr until ethylene glycol level < 20 mg %; cost: $4000/rx

Hemodialysis especially if large ingestion, acidotic, level $>$ 50 mg %, or renal failure

Thiamine 100 mg iv + pyridoxine 2-5 gm

Iron OD (p 41)

Isoniazid (INH) OD

Rx: Pyridoxine gm for gm; if unknown amount, start with 5 gm iv

Kerosene/Gasoline/Camphor Ingestion

Rx: Remove clothing soaked w substance and wash skin to decr dermal absorption

Avoid emesis/lavage if can because of aspiration risk

Gastric aspiration or lavage if $>$ 2 cc/kg since that amount can cause CNS, liver, and renal damage; charcoal

Lithium OD (p 948)

Rx: Na polystyrene SO_4 (Kayexalate) absorbs Li and other cations like K^+

Lye Ingestion

Rx: Do not induce emesis or place NG tube; steroids do not prevent strictures (Nejm 1990;323:637); charcoal not useful; dilution controversial

Marine Sting Injuries

Ann IM 1994;120:665; Nejm 1992;326:486

Cause: Man-of-war, jellyfish, anemones, and corals (all coelenterates); sting ray; stone, lion, and scorpion fish

Pathophys: Nematocysts inject polypeptide toxin-coated threads

Sx & Si: Local inflammation, vesicles

Cmplc: Anaphylaxis, acute renal and/or hepatic failure, persistent reactions, mononeuritis multiplex

Rx: Warm water (T° ≤ 113°F) irrigation × 30-90 min to denature the venom

Mercury Poisoning (p 45)

Methanol Ingestion

Pathophys: Converted by alcohol dehydrogenase to formic acid, which causes brain and optic nerve toxicity and acidosis

Lab: Methanol level > 20 mg %; high osmolar gap (see ethylene glycol above), r/o ethylene glycol and/or alcohol ingestion

Rx: • Alcohol dehydrogenase inhibition w ethanol iv, or fomepizole (Antizol) (Nejm 2001;344:424) 15 mg/kg iv over 30 min then 10 mg/kg q 12 hr × 4 doses then 15 mg/kg q 12 hr
  • Bicarb and supportive rx
  • Folate 1 mg/kg iv q 4 hr × 6
  • Hemodialysis for large ingestions, levels > 50 mg %, acidosis (pH < 7.1), sx

Mushroom Poisoning (p 46)

Neurotoxic Shellfish Poisoning

Am J Pub Hlth 1991;81:471

Cause: Ingestion of shellfish contaminated with dinoflagellate (red tide) neurotoxin; when occurs with fish is called ciguatera poisoning (see scombroid below)

Epidem: Occurs in epidemics

Sx: Cooking does not prevent; onset in $1/2$-10 hr. Paresthesias (81%); reversal of hot/cold sensations (17%); vertigo (60%); myalgias; abdominal pain (48%); nausea (44%); rectal burning; headache (15%).

Si: Ataxia (27%); bradycardia; dilated pupils

Crs: 8-48 hr

Rx: Charcoal, respiratory support; mannitol 1-2 gm/kg; possibly calcium-channel blockers, lidocaine

Organophosphate Poisoning

eg, malthion, diazinon, parathion, and "nerve gas" (Med Let 1995;37:43)

Pathophys: Acetylcholinesterase inhibitors

Sx: H/o pesticide acute exposure

Si: Increased bronchial nasopharyngeal and gi secretions, muscle twitching and weakness, seizures, garlic breath (r/o arsenic)

Rx: Atropine 2-6 mg iv/im, then more q 5 min until secretions decrease, may take 15-20+ mg

Pralidoxime HCl 1 gm iv over 15-30 min, may repeat × 1 in 1 h, or iv infusion of 500 mg/hr

Diazepam 5-10 mg iv if seizures likely

Pennyroyal Herb Poisoning

Ann IM 1996;124:726

Sx: Used as an abortion inducer; nausea and vomiting within 1 hr of ingestion

Si: Shock, metabolic acidosis

Cmplc: Hepatic necrosis, DIC, hypoglycemia

Rx: Lavage

Psychedelic Drug Use/OD

Med Let 2002;44:21; Ann IM 1979;90:361

Amphetamines including Ecstasy; cause seizures, hyperthermia (rx w dantrolene), HT, rhabdo, DIC, arrythmias, CVAs, chronic psych changes; rx sx with diazepam (Valium) (Med Let 1990;32:93), hydration; avoid phenothiazines, which decrease seizure threshold

Cocaine use (p 27)

LSD and other hallucinogens; rx by decreasing sensory stimulation (dark, quiet room), companion, benzodiazepines prn

Marijuana (Nejm 1972;287:310); long-term recreational use impairs cognitive function (Jama 2002;287:1123)

Glue sniffing; ATN and hepatitis with hydrocarbon inhalation (Ann IM 1970;73:713), arrythmias

Sedative hypnotics: gamma hydroxybutyrate, "roofies" (flunitrazepam [Rohypnol]), and other date-rape drugs

Salt (NaCl) OD

Rx: Dialysis preferable; if can't, use D_5W with 100 mg furosemide (Lasix) q 1 hr and watch Ca^{2+} and pH

Scombroid Fish Poisoning

Nejm 1991;324:716

Cause: Ingestion usually of spoiled tuna, mackerel, bonito, bluefish, mahi mahi, et al.

Epidem: Most common type of fish poisoning in U.S.

Sx & Si: Peppery metallic taste to fish when eaten; headache, flushing, diarrhea within 10-30 min of ingestion; cooking does not prevent

Crs: 3 hr without rx; faster with rx

Cmplc: r/o **ciguatera (fish) poisoning** (Ann IM 1995;122:113) from dinoflagellate ingestion by fish; cooking does not prevent; sx of diarrhea, neuralgias, "loose teeth," dysphagia, loss of temperature sensation, et al., may last mos-yrs; rx like red tide poisoning (p 30)

Rx: Diphenhydramine (Benadryl) 50 mg iv/im/po

Theophylline Toxicity/OD

Ann IM 1984;101:457

Si & Sx: Seizures (15%), Vtach (20%) in all > 60 μgm/cc, low K^+ (100%), elevated glucose (98%), low PO_4 (80%), low Mg^{2+} (75%)

Lab: Toxicity with levels > 35 μgm/cc

Rx: Charcoal; hemoperfusion over charcoal if level > 100 μgm/cc in acute, > 40-60 μgm/cc in chronic toxicity, one of few indications for hemoperfusion (Med Let 1986;28:80); dialysis if hemoperfusion not available

of tachycardia, hypotension, and ventricular arrhythmias: esmolol; or low-dose propranolol, eg, 0.5 mg iv in adults (0.01 mg/kg to max of 1 mg/dose in children), repeat in 5-10 min if BP and P not decreased; complete β blockade occurs at 0.2 mg/kg

Tricyclic and Tetracyclic Antidepressant OD

Pathophys: Anticholinergic effects and fast-channel blockade

Lab: Monitoring EKG × 24 hr adequate (Jama 1985;254:1772); drug levels not predictive of cmplc (Nejm 1985;313:474); seizures predicted (in 34%) by QRS > 0.10 sec, Vtach/Vfib predicted (in 50%) by QRS > 0.16 sec (Nejm 1985;313:474), or R_{aVR} > 3 mm has best predictive (43%) value for seizure or ventricular arrhythmias (Ann EM 1995;26:195)

Rx: Supportive usually is all that is needed; rx arrhythmias or wide QRS w bicarb 1-2 mM/kg iv if heart block or ventricular arrhythmia (B. Higgins, ME Med Ctr 10/92)

Acetaminophen (Tylenol) OD

Nejm 1988;319:1557

Cause: Acetaminophen po

Epidem: Common overdose and common co-ingested drug

Pathophys: Toxic metabolite causes liver failure; can occur at "nontoxic" levels in alcoholics (Ann IM 1986;104:398) and be inadvertent (Nejm 1997;337:1112)

Sx: h/o OD > 10 gm (> 140 mg/kg), usually ≥ 15 gm (4 gm/d is maximal therapeutic dose) within 24 hr but can occur at just 4 gm/d in alcoholics (Med Let 1996;38:55). May have no sx for 72 hr.

Si: None

Crs: Most hepatitis is transient, but it can be fatal

Cmplc: Hepatitis more commonly if fasting and/or concomitant ethanol ingestion (Jama 1994;272:1845), and/or hepatic enzyme-inducing drugs like seizure medications

Lab:

> *Chem:* Acetaminophen level initially on all drug ODs and, if positive, at 4, 8, and 12 hr after OD and plot on nomogram (see Figure 1.2) (Nejm 1988;319:1558); if 4-hr level > 200 μgm/cc or 12-hr level > 50, hepatic toxicity likely; if half-life > 4 hr then hepatitis likely, if > 12 hr then encephalopathy likely

Rx: Acetylcysteine 140 mg/kg load, 70 mg/kg × 17 doses q 4 hr po or via NG tube; or 300 mg iv over 20 hr, probably not as good as po. Treat levels of > 150 μgm/cc at 4 hr, > 50 at 8 hr (see nomogram). Works regardless of level, probably by increasing tissue O_2 delivery (Nejm 1991;324:1852). Best result if start within 4-8 hr but still worth doing up to 24 hr postingestion. Activated charcoal binds acetylcysteine but 1 dose ok since have 12 hr to start acetylcysteine and 1 dose may help adsorb some of the acetaminophen and other drugs taken concomitantly; if did get charcoal, consider increasing initial acetylcysteine dose by 20-40%. Odansetron 4 mg iv can help nauseated pts tolerate.

Arsenic Poisoning (Acute and Chronic Types)

Cause: Insecticides and herbicides, especially crabgrass killers

Epidem:

Pathophys: Blocks Krebs cycle

Sx: Acute: Nausea, vomiting, and diarrhea with esophageal and epigastric pain; immediate "rice water," then bloody stool; CHF

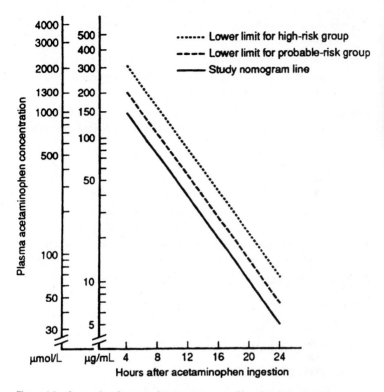

Figure 1.2 Acetaminophen overdose nomogram. Risk of serious hepatitis based on plasma Tylenol levels. (Reproduced with permission from Smilkstein MJ, et al. Efficacy of oral N-acetylcysteine in the treatment of acetaminophen overdose. New Eng J Med 1988;319:1558. Copyright 1988, Mass. Medical Society, all rights reserved.)

(myocardiopathy) immediate with increased QT and torsades de pointes, Vtach, rx with pacer or $MgSO_4$ (p 109)

Chronic: Vague malaise

Si: Chronic: Mees' lines in nails after 4-6 wk of chronic exposure (r/o INH, thallium); hematuria especially in children; increased skin pigmentation with spared spots = "raindrops on a dusty table"; keratosis

Crs: After several days mucous membrane inflammation, rashes, hematologic, ATN, encephalopathy, painful peripheral, sensory, and motor neuropathy after 7-14 d

Cmplc: Lung cancer incidence increased (Jama 2004;292:2984)
r/o similar toxicity from arsine gas from industrial exposure in semiconductor industry

Lab:

Chem: in acute, spot urine level
in chronic, arsenic (As) tissue levels in bone, nails, hair (pubic best since fast growing and sweat adds) normal levels = 3-13 μgm/100 gm; 24-hr urine arsenic level, fewer false positives than blood levels but will be back to normal when presents with neuropathy but can bring it out with dimercaprol

Xray: KUB shows radiodense cast of stomach or gi tract acutely

Rx: Dimercaprol (BAL, British anti-Lewisite) 3-5 mg/kg im q 4 hr × several days; within first 24-36 hr to chelate As and reverse sx's. Few cmplc's at these doses in adults or children
Succimer (DMSA) may be an alternative po rx

Aspirin (Salicylate) OD

Ann IM 1976;85:745

Cause: ASA ingestion of > 10 gm (120 mg/kg), > 500 mg/kg usually fatal, acutely or chronically build level up

Epidem: Common in children, adult suicides, and the elderly treating various medical illnesses with ASA (insidious, high morbidity and mortality)

Pathophys: Respiratory stimulation via respiration centers and chemoreceptors; oxidative metabolism uncoupling. Direct CNS stimulation; gastric irritant.

Sx: Dizziness; can be precipitated by steroid withdrawal; nausea, tinnitus, emesis

Si: Fever and hypermetabolism; respiratory alkalosis then metabolic acidosis; confusion evolving into convulsions

Crs:

Cmplc: CNS damage with seizures, from anoxia; coma; shock
Pulmonary edema even as ASA level decreasing due to increased capillary permeability, especially in smokers (Ann IM 1981;95:405)

Lab:
Chem: Salicylate level initially and 6 hr postingestion; > 70 mg % (indicates 10-30 gm ingested); therapeutic levels in RA ≤ 30 mg %; lytes show respiratory alkalosis evolving into metabolic acidosis or a combination of both
Hem: Protime increased
Urine: 10% FeCl$_3$ to 1 cc of urine shows a purple color

Xray: KUB may show size of pill bolus in gi tract

Rx: Respiratory alkalosis alone usually requires no rx
Glucose iv to avoid ASA-induced hypoglycemia (Nejm 1973;288:1110)
of metabolic acidosis: supportive care and respirator; correct lyte imbalances, eg, acidosis; dialyze soon; NaHCO$_3$ 1 mM/kg w 20 mEq Kcl diluted in 500 D$_5$$\frac{1}{2}$S at 2-3 cc/kg/hr iv to alkalinize urine or as iv push without increasing fluids probably best (BMJ 1982;285:1383)
Vitamin K for protime prolongation
Hemodialysis if initial salicylate level > 120 mg % or 6-hr level > 100 mg %, or renal failure, or hypoxia, CHF, pulmonary edema, or persistent CNS changes (seizures, coma, confusion)

Carbon Monoxide Poisoning

Nejm 1998;339:1603

Cause: Carbon monoxide: $O{=}C \leftrightarrow O^-{=}C^+$

Epidem: Oxidation of fuels in presence of insufficient O_2 forms carboxyhemoglobin, eg, car exhaust, fire smoke, gas appliances in campers and enclosed-cabin pleasure boats (Jama 1995;274:1615), especially at high altitudes (Sci Am Text Med 1982). Rarely from methylene chloride, absorbed cutaneiously from paint thinner and metabolized to CO in liver. 600 accidental and 3000-6000 intentional suicidal deaths/yr in US.

Pathophys: $C{=}O$ binds with 2 electrons to Fe^{++}, just as O_2 does, to bring its total electron complement to a stable 36. Carboxyhemoglobin has a high association rate but a slow dissociation rate ($200\times$ oxygen's affinity to bind to hemoglobin), ie, it shifts the hemoglobin dissociation curve to the left (increased affinity) and thus decreases hemoglobin's carrying capacity despite normal pO_2. Since CO also greatly increases the other 3 hemes' affinity for O_2, even 1 CO per hemoglobin molecule really slows O_2 dissociation. Also poisons mitochondrial cytochrome cellular respiration system.

Children physiologically more susceptible to injury.

Sx: If > 10% of hemoglobin is carboxyhemoglobin, sx include headache and dizziness; get level in patients with these sx if others in house have similar sx and home heating system would be compatible with carbon monoxide poisoning (Ann IM 1987;107:174)

If 30-40% carboxyhemoglobin: severe headache, easy fatigability

If 40-60% carboxyhemoglobin: unconscious

Si: Retinal hemorrhages, flame-shaped (Sci Am Text Med 1982); pink skin and mucous membranes

Crs: Recovery may take months

Cmplc: CNS damage including permanent memory loss and seizures, and peripheral neuritis from the anoxia, hyperthermia from sweat gland necrosis; precipitation of ischemic heart disease (Nejm 1995;332:48). Delayed (3-240 days) neuropsych sx and si, including personality changes, dementia, incontinence, psychosis, all w 50-75% 1 yr recovery

r/o cyanide poisoning from combustible plastics in burn patients w oxygen refractory acidosis

Lab:

ABGs: Normal pO_2; depressed O_2 saturation, but not pulse oximetry, which is falsely high (Ann EM 1994;24:252); metabolic acidosis if severe

Chem: Carboxyhemoglobin level > 10-15%; can be up to 15% in smokers

Rx: Prevent w home CO detectors (Jama 1998;279:685)

Support oxygenation with 100% O_2 as soon as suspected, at 1 atm pressure allows 2 vol% O_2 to be carried in plasma alone

Hyperbaric chamber (Nejm 2002;347:1057 [NNT = 6], 1105, vs no help: Med J Austr 1999;170:203) if available and practical, tid 100% O_2 at 3 atm results in plasma carrying 6 vol%; consider especially if levels > 25%, pregnant, unconscious, angina, other mental status changes

Exchange transfusion?

Cyanide Poisoning

Cause: Cyanide

Epidem: Ingestion, accidental or suicidal; may be absorbed through the skin. Inhalation in house fires is very common, from burning wood, wool, plastics, polyurethane, etc (Nejm 1991;325:1761); acetonitrile in nail glue remover; also in cyanogenic plants, eg, laetrile; nitroprusside metabolized to cyanide and builds up w high-dose infusions, renal failure or prolonged use

Pathophys: Cytochrome oxidase poisoning kills by cellular hypoxia, usually (diaphragmatic paralysis causes respiratory failure)

Sx: Nonspecific flushing, dizziness, headache intially, then agonal/stridorous breathing, coma, seizures

Si: Bitter almond smell to breath; retinal arteries and veins appear same color (elevated venous oxygen levels); tachycardia, later bradycardia; late cyanosis, poor respiratory effort, confusion/stupor, coma

Crs:

Cmplc: Chronic exposure from smoking can cause vitamin B_{12} deficiency, amblyopia, psychosis, thyromegaly, ataxia

Lab:

   Chem: Low HCO_3 and pH from lactic acidosis; also seen in carbon monoxide poisoning; lactate levels > 10 mM/L. Blood cyanide levels > 40 mM/L. Venous blood gas has abnormally high O_2 saturation and pO_2. Lee-Jones spot test on gastric aspirate.

Rx: Supportive care including oxygen, iv fluids, and pressors
Cyanide antidote kit contains:
- Amyl nitrite inhalation to enhance methemoglobinemia because CN^- binds strongly to Fe^{+++} of methemoglobin too; but may be dangerous if carbon monoxide poisoning concomitantly (J Pharm Experim Ther 1987;242:70) or hemoglobinopathy. Methylene blue is also in kit to reverse methemoglobinemia; shouldn't be used.
- Sodium nitrite ($NaNO_2$) 0.2 cc/kg of 3% soln iv to max of 10 cc
- Sodium thiosulfate ($Na_2S_2O_3$) to form SCN^- that can be excreted; 12.5 gm/amp
   Alternative: hydroxocobalamin, which combines with CN^- (Nejm 1991;325:1761); suitably concentrated form not available in U.S. yet

Iron Overdose, Acute

Cause: Ferric or ferrous iron; sx if > 20 mg/kg, serious if > 40 mg/kg, potentially lethal if > 60 mg/kg

Epidem: Accidental or suicidal poisoning; most common kind of accidental poisoning in children

Pathophys: Direct corrosive effect on gi mucosa causes markedly increased absorption of iron salts, which are hepatotoxic; subsequently iron and ferritin are released from periportal cells, leading to vasodepressor effect and shock

Sx: Nausea, vomiting, abdominal pain, diarrhea. Seizures, then 2-3 hr respite, then fatal seizures.

Si: gi bleeding

Crs:
Stage 1 ($\frac{1}{2}$-6 hr postingestion) = nausea, vomiting
Stage 2 (6-24 hr) = latent, though may be absent in severe OD
Stage 3 (4-40 hr) = systemic toxicity, including shock, seizures, and death
Stage 4 (2-5 wk) = late cmplc like gi strictures/obstruction

Cmplc: Gastric perforation, later strictures, intestinal obstruction; shock, coma, coagulopathy, heptatic failure, acidosis

Lab:
Chem: Serum iron level 4-6 hr after ingestion but not later because redistribution will falsely depress levels then at 10 hr in case delayed absorption; within 1-2 hr if chewable/liquid forms ingested; > 300 μgm % causes mild toxicity; > 500 μgm % causes serious toxicity; >1000 μgm % often fatal Glucose often > 150 mg %
Hem: WBC often > 15,000; TIBC no help
Urine: Deferoxamine challenge test occasionally used, urine may be rose-colored if serum-free iron is present

Xray: KUB, iron tablets often apparent unless ingested liquid, chewable or multivitamin preparations

Rx: Perhaps ipecac prehospital; lavage stomach w saline, although there is danger of perforating an already eroded stomach, or lavage whole bowel w PEG; fluids for shock. No charcoal.

Deferoxamine 1 gm stat, 0.5 gm q 4-12 hr up to 6 gm qd im, or iv if in shock, at 10-15 mg/kg/hr (higher doses precipitate shock) up to 6 gm qd total; cannot use via gastric lavage; may have cytoprotective effects independent of chelation.

Maybe someday L_1, an oral iron chelator, 1st choice (Clin Pharmacol Ther 1991;50:294)

Lead Poisoning, Chronic

Cause: An acquired porphyria due to elemental Pb ingestion; paint ingestion esp in children (Nejm 1974;290:245), battery fumes, moonshine (Nejm 1969;280:1199), pottery glazes commercial and homemade (Nejm1970;283:669), air contamination from smelter (Nejm 1975;292:123), indoor firing range users (Am J Pub Hlth 1989;79:1029), and radiator repair mechanics (Nejm 1987;317:214). Tetraethyl Pb from gas results in encephalopathy, without porphyria or blood changes.

Epidem: Common in young children; adult exposures usually occupational, eg, rehab'ing old buildings. Inversely correlated w vitamin C intake (Jama 1999;281:2289).

Pathophys: Pb inhibits by chelating sulfhydryl (SH) groups of ALA dehydrogenase (ALA → PBG), ferrochelatase (PP → heme), and possibly ALA synthetase. In adults, gout and gouty nephropathy; latter always associated with overt or silent lead intoxication (Nejm 1981;304:520).

Sx: In severe poisoning, abdominal colic, relieved by palpation; h/o family pet illness, eg, dog (Am J Pub Hlth 1990;80:1183)

Si: In severe poisoning, anemia, gingival margin lead line, motor peripheral neuropathy, eg, wrist drop, neuroses, and psychoses

Crs: Progressive, si and sx roughly correlate w blood lead levels; cognition deficits only partially reverse w long-term rx (Jama 1998;280:1915)

Cmplc

- Antisocial/delinquent behaviors long term (Jama 1996;275:363)
- Renal impairment (Ann IM 1999;130:7; Jama 1996;275:1177)
- Gout and gouty nephropathy
- Encephalopathy, mortality without rx is 50%, with rx is 3%
- Mental deficiencies and neurologic abnormalities even at blood levels < 50 μgm % (Nejm 1988;319:468) and long term in children with elevated lead in teeth representing old exposure (Nejm 1990;322:83) or with umbilical cord lead levels $\geq$ 10 μgm/cc (Nejm 1987;316:1037). Measurable behavioral problems at levels $\geq$ 15-50 μgm % (Am J Pub Hlth 1992;82:1356); before age 3, eventual IQ impaired even at average blood levels < 10 μgm % (Nejm 1992;327:1279).
- Hypertension, "essential hypertensives" with creatinine > 1.5 mg % often are really lead toxic (Jama 2003;289:1523, 1996;275:1171; Am J Pub Hlth 1999;89:330)
- Dental caries (Jama 1999;281:2294)

Lab:

Chem: Whole blood lead levels, even levels of 5-6 μgm % may indicate chronic lead load and may benefit from rx if creatinine > 1.5 mg % (Nejm 2003;348:277); tooth levels (deciduum) can be used for epidemiologic studies (Nejm 1974;290:245)

Hem: Rbc stippling (RNA and mitochondria), siderocytes. Free erythrocyte protoporphyrin no longer used as screening test because only sensitive down to 30-40 μgm % and levels lag by weeks

Urine: Increased coproporphyrins and protoporphyrins, no PBG elevations; Pb levels elevated; EDTA mobilization tests

Xray: KUB may show Pb opacities in gut; bones show lead lines at metaphyseal calcification line in children due to increased calcium laid down at zone of provisional calcification in rapidly growing bones, not in adults

Rx: Primary prevention by decreasing exposures is best health policy since now even levels < 10 µgm % are shown to significantly affect IQ of children (Nejm 2003;348:1515,1517,1527)

Screen all children with serum lead levels at 6-12 mo and q 6-12 mo to age 24 mo, screen older children only if high risk (Med Let 1991;33:78)

Table 1.2   Lead Poisoning Protocol

Level	Plan
<10 µgm %	Repeat per above schedule
10-25 µgm %	Repeat, improve environment, give po Fe, which decreases Pb absorption
25-45 µgm %	Aggressive rx of environment, po Fe; chelation not effective (Nejm 2001;344:1421,1470)
45+ µgm %	Refer for chelation w succimer

Chelation w (none have been shown to improve neurologic function aside from seizures):
- Succimer (DMSA, dimercaptosuccinate) po (Jama 1991;265:1802) if no gi toxicity or encephalopathy, or
- BAL (dimercaprol) im if level > 100 µgm/cc and/or sx; contraindicated in peanut allergy; followed not sooner than 4 hr (to avoid encephalopathy) by
- EDTA iv 1 gm weekly, does abort nephropathy (Nejm 2003;348:277)
- Vitamin C perhaps (Jama 1999;281:2289,2340)

Mercury Poisoning

Nejm 2003;349:1731

Cause: Inhalation of inorganic Hg or vaporized Hg; ingestion of Hg, inorganic mercuric/ous ions or salts, or organic mercurials (eg, methyl, alkyl)

Epidem: Inorganic: In miners, hatters, mirror makers, mercury factory or lab workers

Organic: Fish are major converters to methyl Hg when exposed to inorganic Hg, eg, in Minamata Bay; mercurial fungicides; low levels found in all fish may not impair childhood development (Jama 1998;280:701 vs 737). Organic Hg preservatives in interior latex paint, now removed (Nejm 1990; 323:1096).

Pathophys:

Sx: Hg vapor inhalation: Acutely chemical pneumonitis, gingivostomatitis, noncardiac pulmonary edema; chronically neuropsych sx, tremor, acrodynia

Inorganic salt ingestion: Gradual onset (mos-yrs) abdominal pain, gi bleeding, nausea, vomiting, diarrhea, shock, renal failure, CNS toxicity including erethism (shyness, decreased attention, decreased memory, decreased intellect)

Organic (see case report of fatal minor spill exposure of Dartmouth chemistry prof: Nejm 1998;338:1672): Rapid onset (day-mo), dysarthria, ataxia, leg cramps, restricted visual fields, muscle weakness, personality changes, desquamative rash, occasional gastroenteritis

Si: Inorganic: Fine tremor of face and tongue, may progress to coarse

Crs:

Cmplc: Inorganic: Nephrotic syndrome; perhaps ALS syndrome
Organic: Nephrotic syndrome (Ann IM 1977;86:731)

Lab:
    Chem: For elemental and inorganic exposures: whole blood urine levels followed by 24 hr urine collection for Hg (> 100-200 μg/L significant) and creatinine
        Organic: Blood Hg; urine as above; and hair analysis, but commercial lab heavy metal results unreliable (Jama 2001;285:67)

Xray: Head CT may show brain atrophy in chronic exposure

Rx: of elemental: Succimer may help
        of inorganic: BAL until enteritis resolves, succimer
        of organic: Succimer, possibly vitamin E as an antioxidant

Mushroom Poisoning

Ann IM 1979;90:332; Med Let 1984;26:67

Cause:
    Potentially fatal (PF) types: *Amanita sp*, *Galerina sp*
    Usually nonfatal (NF) types: *Amanita sp*, etc

Epidem: Ingestion

Pathophys:
    PF: Cyclopeptides
    NF: Gi irritants, muscarinics, et al.

Sx:
    PF: Onset in 6-20 hr; gi sx initially, transient improvement then potentially fatal liver and renal failure
    NF: Onset in min, < 8 hr maximum; hallucinations, Antabuse-like sx; sympathetic/parasympathetic sx; gi sx

Si:

Crs:
    PF: Severe, 40-80% fatal
    NF: Usually benign

Cmplc:
> PF: Renal and hepatic failure
> NF: Volume depletion, aspiration of vomitus

Lab:

Xray:

Rx:
> PF: Consult poison control. Acetylcysteine, penicillin, silibinin, cimetidine?
> Ipecac; and activated charcoal even late may help if in enterohepatic circulation

Narcotic Addiction, Withdrawal, OD, Heroin OD

OD: Ann IM 1999;130:584

Cause: Opium derivatives and synthetic opioids including propoxyphene (Darvon)

Epidem: Increased prevalence in urban areas, physicians (Nejm 1970;282:365)

Pathophys: Psychic dependence much greater problem than very real, though less common, physical dependence (Nejm 1983;308:1096)

Sx: of withdrawal: in first 48 hr restless, yawning, chills, increased pilomotor activity ("cold turkey"), progresses over 24 hr to cramps, diarrhea, sweating, vomiting, tachycardia, hyperventilation, hypertension, seizures (neonates)

Si: of OD: Small pupils, somnolence, and hypoventilation (if all 3 present, 92% sens, 76% specificity); needle tracks
> of withdrawal: Jerky respirations leading to muscle twitching

Crs:

Cmplc: Hepatitis B; pulmonary edema (Ann IM 1972;77:29); endocarditis especially right-sided (Ann IM 1973;78:25); nephrotic syndrome and renal failure (Nejm 1974;290:19)
> of OD: Hypostatic pneumonia, pulmonary edema

Lab: *Urine:* Opiate screen, r/o false pos results from quinolone antibiotics (Jama 2002;286:3115); will miss methadone, oxycodone, and propoxyphene, which require "confirmation" gas chromatography

Rx (Ann IM 1999;130:584)

of OD: Observe, rx depressed respirations w naloxone (Narcan) 0.4 mg or less challenge test if addiction suspected, if no w/drawal then 2 mg iv (or sc/im), then 2 mg iv q 2-3 min up to 10 (in children, 0.01 mg/kg iv or ET; repeat q 3 min until respond, then q 20 min); or more expensive nalmefene (Revex) (Med Let 1995;37:95) 0.5 mg iv then 1 mg 2-5 min later, use 0.1 mg challenge dose first if suspect addiction

of withdrawal: Clonidine 0.1 mg b-qid helps gi NV + D and cramps (Ann IM 1984;101:331), but methadone 1st choice at 40-100 mg po qd (Jama 1999;281:1000)

of addiction (Nejm 2000;343:1290) (available through addiction treatment clinics):

- Methadone 80-120 mg qd po results in less severe withdrawal sx; helps up to 50% come off, better than rehab (Jama 2000;283:1303,1337,1343); 50 mg po qd may be enough for maintenance (Ann IM 1993;119:23)
- Naltrexone 100-150 mg tiw, $2/50 mg, Antabuse approach, blocks narcotic effect (Med Let 1985;27:11); or iv × 8 hr w general anesthesia then discharge w sc naltrexone pellet being done in for-profit detox clinics (Jama 1998;279:229, 1997;277:363) vs 2005;294:903)
- Buprenorphine (Subutex) 8-32 mg sl qd-tiw; or as combined buprenorphine-naloxone (16 mg/4 mg) (Suboxone) sl (Nejm 2003;349:928,949, 2003;348:82; Med Let 2003;45:13; Am J Drug Alcohol Abuse 2002;28:231); naloxone prevents iv abuse, 50% 1 yr "cures"; FDA approved w 8 hr CME (http://buprenorphine.samhsa.gov, 866-287-2728); $5-10/d or 3 mg sl qd ×3, then clonidine 0.1-0.2 mg po q 4 hr prn sx, plus naltrexone 25 mg po qd ×2, 80% successful OP detox at 1 wk (Ann IM 1998;127:526); $300/mo

Chapter 2
Cardiology

D. K. Onion

2.1 Medications

Anticoagulants

Antiplatelet Drugs:

- Acetylsalicylic acid (aspirin, ASA) (Nejm 1994;330:1287) 80-325 mg po qd (Med Let 1998;40:59, 1995;37:14); inhibits platelet stickiness; can be used safely w warfarin (Nejm 1993;329:530); adverse effects: gastric intolerance only at doses ≥ 30 mg qd (Ann IM 1994;120:184), asthma, increased bleeding time for 2 d, platelet dysfunction for 7-10 d; cheap

- Clopidogrel (Plavix) (Med Let 1998;40:59) 75 mg po qd for anticoagulation alone or w ASA for high-risk CAD pts for up to 1 yr (Ann IM 2005;142:251) or TIAs, 300 mg po load then 75 mg qd × 3-12 mo, w ASA + heparin marginally better for unstable angina (Nejm 2001;345:494, 1998;338:1488, 1498,1539; Ann IM 1998;129:394); as good as ASA or ticlopidine without neutropenia of latter; takes days to take full effect, hepatic metabolism; gi bleeding 10× as frequent as w ASA and PPI (Nejm 2005;352:238), rare TTP (Nejm 2000; 342:1773), so use only if truly ASA intolerant (Nejm 2002; 346:1800); $87/mo

- Ticlopidine (Ticlid) (Med Let 1998;40:59) 250 mg po bid; antiplatelet effect different from that of aspirin's; can be used if aspirin intolerant or w aspirin if need extra antiplatelet effect as w coronary stents × 1 mo (Nejm 1996;334:1084), decreases restenosis rates after peripheral revascularizations (Nejm 1997;337:1726) or for TIAs (Med Let 1992;34:65); adverse effects: agranulocytosis (1%), reversible, occurs in first 3 mo; marrow aplasia; cholestasis, TTP (Ann IM 1998;128:541) in 0.02% (Jama 1999;281:806); $114/mo

Platelet Glycoprotein IIb/IIIa Receptor Antagonists (Med Let 1998;40:89):

All useful peri-stenting (ACP J Club 2002;136:41-44; Nejm 2001;344:1879,1888,1895,1937) and probably in unstable coronary syndromes on way to cath lab; all increase risk of bleeding and cost ~$2000/crs

- Tirofiban (Aggrastat) (Nejm 1998;338:1488,1498,1539) as part of triple rx of unstable angina; effects last < 4 hr
- Eptifibatide (Integrilin) (Nejm 1998;339:436); effects last < 4 hr
- Abciximab (ReoPro); effects last < 48 hr; used w coronary artery angioplasty stenting (Nejm 1999;341:319), not helpful post thrombolysis (Jama 2005:293:175a)

Heparins:

- Low-molecular-weight heparins (Am J Med 1999;106:660; Nejm 1997;337:688; Med Let 1997; 39:94, 1993;35:75); despite costs, are clearly better with less bleeding (5%: Ann IM 1994;121:81) for rx of acute pulmonary emboli and acute DVT (Arch IM 2000;160:229; Nejm 1997;337:657,663, 1996;334:672,682,724), overlap w Coumadin × 5 d or 2 d of PT INR > 2 to prevent paradoxical thrombosis; and better DVT/PE prevention at 40+ mg sc qd over 6 d (Nejm 1999;341:793, 1996;335:701, 1992;326:975; Ann IM 1992;117:353); also work for unstable angina and are better than unfractionated @ 1 mg/kg q 12 hr (Jama 2000;284:835); much less thrombocytopenia (Med Let 2001;43:11), and less osteoporosis than unfractionated heparin; $23/d for qd dosing

- Enoxaparin (Lovenox) (Nejm 1996;334:677) 30 mg or 1 mg/kg or 3000 anti-Xa U sc bid; or
- Tinzaparin (Innohep) (Med Let 2001;43:14; Nejm 1997;337: 657,663) 175 U sc qd
- Dalteparin (Fragmin) 2500 anti-Xa U sc qd
  Other new types approved for DVT prophylaxis only; can be used to anticoagulate pts w heparin-induced thrombocytopenia (Med Let 2001;43:12)
- Reviparin sc qd-bid (Nejm 2002;347:726)
- Ardeparin (Normiflo) 50 anti-Xa U/kg q 12 hr
- Danaparoid (Orgaran) 750 anti-Xa U bid
- Fondaparinux (Arixtra) (Med Let 2002;44:43; Nejm 2001;345:1298,1305,1340) 2.5 mg sc qd for prophylaxis, 5-10 mg (based on kg) sc qd for rx of PE; polysaccharide factor Xa inhibitors; no increase in PT or PTT; better than enoxaparin for DVT prophylaxis post ortho surgery; no platelet suppression; cost $44/d
- Heparin, unfractionated (Nejm 1991;324:1565) prophylactic regimen = 5000 U iv q 12 hr (Am Hrt J 1980;99:574) or sc (Mod Concepts Cardiovasc Dis 1976;45:105), therapeutic regimen = 5000 U load then 1200 U/hr iv (Nejm 1986;315:1109) continuous infusion (or 80 U/kg bolus and 18 U/kg/hr: Ann IM 1993;119:874) getting q 6 hr PTT until stable at 1.5-2 × control. Circadian increases in PTT of 50% in the evening complicate adjusting dose more often than daily (Arch IM 1992;152:1589; BMJ 1985;290:341); PTTs also vary by lot and manufacturer by 50% (Ann IM 1993;119:104). Reversible with protamine at 1 mg/100 U of heparin given in the past 4 hr (Ann IM 1989;111:1015). Strong organic acid that binds activated factor II (prothrombin) and so blocks fibrin formation and factor XI activation of factor IX; also inhibits activated prothrombin-platelet interaction; renal excretion, half-life = 105 min; works for venous and arterial thrombosis; can use in pregnancy because does not cross placenta; adverse effects: bleeding

CARDIOLOGY

especially when given with probenecid or in renal failure, excessive prothrombin prolongation, immune platelet clumping from ELISA platelet factor 4 antibodies (Ann IM 2002; 136:210) leading to thrombosis and thrombocytopenia with iv or sc prophylactic rx in 1% after 5 d, reversible (Nejm 2001; 344:1286, 1995;332:1330, 1987;316:581; Ann IM 1984;100: 535) but 60% have ischemic damage and 25% mortality despite early cessation (Am J Med 1999;106:629) and f/u warfarin rx may precipitate limb gangrene (Ann IM 1997;127: 804), frequently not looked for or recognized, often re-present 1+ wk out w thromboembolic disease, which is then disastrously rx'd w more heparin (Ann IM 2002;136:210)—should rx w a hirudin instead.

Hirudins:

- Argatroban (Med Let 2001;43:11) 2 μgm/kg/min, increase or decrease on PTTs; hepatically metabolized, used if heparin-induced thrombocytopenia, a little cheaper than lepirudin
- Bivalirudin (Angiomax) (Med Let 2001;43:37) used in unstable angina instead of heparin when angioplasty planned
- Lepirudin (Refludan) (Med Let 1998;40:94) 0.4 mg/kg bolus then 0.15 mg/kg/hr iv; use when can't use heparin because of thrombocytopenia; $3900/wk

Thrombin Inhibitors:

- Warfarin (Coumadin) (Nejm 1991;324:1865) prophylaxis w 1 mg po qd prevents venous thrombosis without increasing the PT, eg, with indwelling catheters (Ann IM 1990;112:423); 10 mg po qd first 2 d, then adjust on day 3 and 5 (Ann IM 2003;138:714) to a PT INR = 2-3 for routine anticoagulation, 3-4 for artificial valves (J Am Coll Cardiol 1998;32:1486; ACP J Club 1994;120[suppl 2]:52). Prolonged PT 2-5 d with heparin as switchover (Nejm 1996;335:1822) because warfarin inhibits liver synthesis of factors X (3-d half-life), IX (1.25 d), VII (7 hr), and II (4 d); PT measures factor VII because it has the shortest half-life, thus takes at least 2 d after PT is in range for factor II to come down and the hypercoaguable state w low protein C induced by warfarin to reverse (Nejm 1996;335:1822).

Adverse effects: rare cholesterol emboli with blue toes (Circ 1967;35:946); or perhaps related skin necrosis especially in pts w protein C heterozygous state, requires emergent vitamin K, heparin + protein C rx (Nejm 1994;331:1282); bleeding especially due to drug interactions, risk of serious bleeding rx (Ann IM 1996;124:970) = 2%/yr in therapeutic range (4.5%/yr over age 80), correlates w higher PTs and 1st 3 mo of rx, not age or gender (Ann IM 1993;118:511); risk of intracranial bleed = 2%/yr w PT 2 × control, much higher if PT higher (Ann IM 1994;120:897)

Potentiated by foods and drugs (Ann IM 1994;121:676) that either displace from carrier protein or compete for degradation enzyme including acetaminophen (Tylenol) (Jama 1998;279:657), allopurinol (Nejm 1970;283:1484), amiodarone, disulfiram (Antabuse), ASA, cimetidine (Ann IM 1979;90:993), clofibrate, COX-2 NSAIDs, erythromycin, ethacrynic acid, flu shots peaking at 1 wk (Nejm 1981;305:1262), fluconazole, glucagon (Ann IM 1970;73:331), indomethacin, INH, metronidazole (Nejm 1976;295:355), miconazole, nalidixic acid, nortriptyline (Nejm 1970;283:1484), omeprazole, phenylbutazone, phenytoin, piroxicam (Feldene), propranolol, quinidine (Ann IM 1968;68:511), sulfa drugs (Med Let 1977;19:7), vitamin E, desiccated thyroid, tolbutamide, trimethaprim/sulfa (Ann IM 1979;91:321)

Counteracted by avocados, barbiturates, carbamazepine, chlordiazepoxide (Librium), cholestyramine, ethanol, ginseng (Ann IM 2004;141:23), glutethimide, griseofulvin, sucralfate, vitamin K 1 mg po (not sc) reverses > 50% in 16 hr (DBCT Ann IM 2002;137:251; Lancet 2000;356:1551), and locally with dental surgery by tranexamic acid mouthwash (Nejm 1989;320:840)

Perioperatively hold × 4 doses until INR < 1.5, resume day after surgery; rarely need heparin coverage (Nejm 1997;336:1506); no need to hold prior to dental surgery if in therapeutic range

- Ximelagratran (Exantra) (Jama 2005;293:681,690,699,736; Nejm 2003;349:1704,1713,1762) 36 mg po bid; better than warfarin for DVT rx and prophylaxis, AF prophylaxis; no INR's needed; adverse effects: LFT elevations (10%) w rare hepatic failure, 1% increase MI rate?

Antiarrhythmics

Ann IM 1995;122:705; Med Let 1991;33:55

Transient Vasoconstrictors:

- Adenosine (Adenocard) 6 then 12 mg iv for SVT (not Aflut or Afib), converts 91% (Ann IM 1990;113:104) to 99% (Ann IM 1997;127:417), effect gone in 10 sec; theophylline inhibits effect; adverse effects: Afib in 12%, which could be dangerous if WPW present, resulting in ventricular response > 240/min
- Ibutilide (Corvert) (Med Let 1996;38:38) 1 mg iv over 10 min, repeat × 1 if need to; converts 20-40% of Afib and 40-70% of Aflut to NSR; adverse effects: long QT torsade de pointes syndrome

Class IA: All cause torsades de pointes Vtach

- Disopyramide (Norpace CR) (Ann IM 1982;96:337) 150-300 mg bid; renal excretion; adverse effects: strongly negative inotrope causes CHF (Nejm 1980;302:614), is an anticholinergic and so causes urinary retention
- Procainamide (Pronestyl) 0.5-2 gm SR po t-qid, or 100 mg iv push q 5 min up to 1 gm, then 2-4 mg/min drip; used for ventricular arrhythmias; renal excretion; adverse effects: ANA-positive in 50-80% at 6 mo, clinical SLE in 10-20%; 21% Coombs-positive, 3% with clinical hemolytic anemia (Nejm 1984;311:809), thrombocytopenia

- Quinidine (Nejm 1998;338:35) 400-1600 mg po, or 100 mg iv q 3-6 hr; rarely need now, for supraventricular tachycardias primarily, but ventricular antiarrhythmic effect as well; decreases conduction velocity, which increases the depolarization time, which in turn increases the QT and QRS intervals (if > 150% of baseline, should stop); renal excretion, need stomach acid to absorb; adverse effects: increases digoxin levels (Nejm 1979;300:1238), diarrhea, long QT syndrome w sudden death

Class IB:

- Moricizine (Ethmozine) (Nejm 1992;327:227; Ann IM 1992; 116:375,382; Med Let 1990;32:99) suppresses PVCs but increases sudden death
- Phenytoin (Dilantin) 100 mg iv q 5 min up to 1 gm load, then 400 mg/d iv or po; good vs ventricular and supraventricular arrhythmias, especially in digoxin toxic state since it causes no further prolongation of AV conduction; hepatic metabolism; adverse effects: folate deficiency, potentiates warfarin (and vice versa) via competition for hepatic metabolism, inhibits insulin release (Nejm 1972;286:339), vitamin D antagonism (Nejm 1972;286:1316), hypotension when given iv because it comes in a strongly basic diluent
- Lidocaine 100-150 mg iv then 1-4 mg/min drip (Nejm 1967;277:1215); depresses pNa in all heart tissue decreasing automaticity, excitability, and conduction velocity (no help), and increasing refractory period unrelated to membrane potentials; for ventricular arrhythmias mainly; metabolized exclusively in liver; no cross-allergy with procaine; half-life = 1.5 hr, increased to 3.5 hr after 24 hr; levels increased by cimetidine (Ann IM 1983;98:174); adverse effects: mildly negative inotrope, hypotension, seizures and confusion, occasional increase in AV block
- Mexiletine (Mexitil) (Med Let 1986;28:65; Nejm 1987;316:29) 100-400 mg po q 8 hr; like lidocaine, used for

PVCs, but can worsen them; hepatic metabolism; adverse effects: like lidocaine; ~$40/mo

Class IC All prolong QT at standard doses

- Flecainide (Tambocor) and encainide (withdrawn in 1994); shown to increase sudden death by increasing Vtach, Vfib, and post-MI shock (Nejm 1991;324:781), especially in the face of depressed LV function (Ann IM 1990;113:671); may be useful for paroxysmal SVT and PAF if other drugs fail (Med Let 1992;34:71)
- Propafenone (Rythmol) (Nejm 1990;322:518; Med Let 1990;32:37) 2 mg/kg iv push, 150-300 mg po tid; for PAT, Afib (Ann IM 1997;126:621) and other SVTs including reentrant types like WPW (Ann IM 1986;105:655) and ventricular arrhythmias (Ann IM 1991;114:539)

Class II-β Blockers: Generic price $1.50/mo, rest all about the same, $15-30/mo (Med Let 2001;43:9). Lipid solubility (*) causes fatigue, nightmares, worsens triglycerides but may help LDL/HDL ratios (Ann IM 1995;122:133), and increases drug interactions

Non-b-1 (Cardiac) Selective:

- Carteolol* (Cartrol) similar to pindolol but half the price
- Naldolol (Corgard) (Nejm 1981;305:678) 40-160 mg po qd single dose; 70% renal excretion, thus should decrease the dose in renal failure
- Penbutolol* (Levatol) similar to pindolol but half the price
- Pindolol* (Visken) (Med Let 1989;31:69; Nejm 1983;308:940) 20 mg po bid; some sympathomimetic effect, hence less bradycardia; adverse effects: can increase angina (BMJ 1984;289:951) and perhaps cardiac mortality (ACP J Club 1992;116[suppl 2]:1) so not protective post-MI; $42/mo
- Propranolol* (Inderal) 20-600+ mg po divided b-qid or 1-5 mg iv; adverse effects: half-life prolonged by cimetidine (Nejm 1981;304:692); CHF, asthma, hyperkalemia (Nejm 1980; 302:431), rebound PVCs and other malignant arrhythmias

with abrupt cessation, prolongs lidocaine half-life, suicide (Am J Psych 1982;139:92)

- Sotalol (Betapace) (Med Let 1993;35:27) 80-160 mg po bid or 1 mg/kg bolus; class IIB and III effects; useful in SVTs as well as Vtach where may be better than lidocaine (Lancet 1994;344:18), and can be used to prevent Vtach and decrease automatic defib discharge frequency (Nejm 1999;340:1853); no negative inotropism; adverse effects: prolonged QT, hence torsades de pointes (Nejm 1994;331:31), increases mortality if LV dysfunction present (Lancet 1996;348:7)
- Timolol* (Blocadren) 10-20 mg po bid

β-1 Selective: Use, if must, in smokers, Raynaud's, diabetes; avoid in migraine
- Atenolol (Tenormin) 50-100+ mg po qd single dose; renal excretion
- Betaxolol (Kerlone) (Med Let 1990;32:61) 5-10 mg po qd
- Bisoprolol (Zebeta) (Med Let 1994;36:23) 1.25-10 mg po qd-bid; $24/mo
- Esmolol (Brevibloc) (Med Let 1987;29:57) 0.5 mg/kg iv; like propranolol but shorter, 10-20 min half-life; used especially for rapid rx of Afib
- Metoprolol* (Lopressor) (Med Let 1978;20:97; Nejm 1979;301:698) 10-400 mg po qd divided b-tid, or as CR/XL qd (Jama 2000;283:1295); β-1 selective at doses <100 mg qd

Non-β-1 (Cardiac) Selective w α Blocking (Cir 2000;101:558): Most Useful in CHF
- Carvedilol (Coreg) (Nejm 1998;339:1759, 1996;334:1349; Med Let 1997;39:89) 3.125-25 mg po bid; has β-blocker and α-blocker vasodilatory effect, used in CHF; adverse effects: dizziness, bradycardia, edema, diarrhea, blurred vision; many drug interactions, eg, w digoxin, cimetidine, SSRIs
- Labetalol (Normodyne) (Med Let 1984;26:83) 100-600+ mg po; creates an α blockade too that helps cardiac output;

adverse effects: postural hypotension, rare hepatotoxicity (Ann IM 1990;113:210), and the worst sexual dysfunction of all the β blockers

Class III: Prolong repolarization; all can cause long QT and torsades de pointes, especially in pts w low EF

- Amiodarone (Cordarone) (Ann IM 1995;122:689; Nejm 1981;305:539; Ann IM 1984;101:462; Med Let 1995;37:114 [iv], 1986;28:49 [po]) 150 mg iv bolus in 10 min then 1 mg/min × 6 hr then $^1/_2$ mg/min until can give po, repeat bolus if VF/VT recurs; or < 800 po qd × 1-3 wk, then decrease to 200-400 mg po qd; 35 d half-life; for life-threatening VF and VT resistant to other rx or post-MI for 1 yr (Ann IM 1994; 121:529; Circ 1993;87:309), 75% effective by survivals and does not worsen arrhythmias, also used for Afib and PAT (Ann IM 1992;116:1017) in lower doses like 100-200 mg qd (J. Love 10/94), may help CHF and arrythmias prophylactically post-MI (Lancet 1997;1417; Circ 1997;96:2823); weeks-long half-life, and drug interactions (Nejm 1987;316:455); adverse effects: sun-induced blue skin (picture: Nejm 2001;345:1464), severe hepatotoxicity (Nejm 1984;311:167), hypo- (22%) or hyperthyroidism (10%) (Ann IM 1997;126:63: monitor w TSH and T_4 q 3 mo); elevated cholesterol independent of the TSH effect (Ann IM 1991;114:128); constipation and anorexia; insomnia; ataxia; pulmonary fibrosis in 10% (Chest 2003;123:646); increased digoxin levels; irreversible shock with anesthesia sometimes (Mod Concepts Cardiovasc Dis 1983;52:31); reversible and irreversible visual loss; iv doses can cause hypotension, bradyarrhythmias, and occasionally long QT syndrome

- Bretylium (Ann IM 1979;91:229; Nejm 1979;300:473; Med Let 1978;20:105) 5-10 mg/kg iv, then 1-2 mg/min drip; sympathetic blocker, for resistant Vtach and Vfib, contraindicated in digoxin toxicity and aortic stenosis

- Dofetilide (Tikosyn) (Med Let 2000;42:41; Nejm 1999;341: 858) 250-500 μgm po bid; for Afib conversion or maintenance, especially in CHF; renal clearance; interacts w long QT drugs, cimetidine, ketaconazole, trimethoprim, Compazine, megestrol, etc, but not digoxin or warfarin; adverse effects: long QT and torsades de pointes in 3% so start in hospital
- Ibutilide (Corvert) (Nejm 1999;340:1849); 1 mg iv; sometimes converts but always facilitates electrical cardioversion of Vfib and Afib at lower joules; adverse effects: long QT and Vtach
- Sotalol (Betapace) (p 57)

Class IV: Calcium Channel Blockers (Nejm 1999;341:1447; Med Let 1999;41:23, 1997;39:13,103): Adverse effects: diltiazem and verapamil slow AV conduction and decrease myocardial contractility; metabolism of many of these drugs inhibited by grapefruit (Med Let 1995;37:73); increased MIs, sudden death, and atherosclerosis, at least w short-acting types (Jama 1996;275;785,829) and/or in diabetics; all about $1/d at similar doses (Med Let 1991; 34:99) except generic verapamil, which is $4/mo, or $12/mo as slow release

- Diltiazem (Cardizem) (Med Let 1983;25:17) 0.25 mg/kg iv bolus then 5-10 mg/hr; or 120-480 mg po qd as long-acting form; use for rapid AF, Prinzmetal's angina although all calcium-channel blockers work; 4-8 hr half-life; less AV block than verapamil; less peripheral vasodilatation than nifedipine; most expensive po; precipitates CHF more often the lower the ejection fraction is (Circ 1991;83:52)
- Verapamil (Calan) (Med Let 1987;29:37) 5-10 mg iv over 1-2 min, repeat in 30 min, 4-6 hr half-life; long-acting 120-480 mg qd to bid; for supraventricular tachycardias, angina, IHSS, hypertensive crisis; adverse effects: increased digoxin levels, heart blocks, avoid in WPW (Med Let 1982;24:56; Ann IM 1982; 96:409), decreased insulin secretion and glucose tolerance, negative cardiac inotrope (decreases cardiac output), hypotension

CARDIOLOGY

when given after quinidine (Nejm 1985;312:167), constipation, increased effect and decreased clearance in elderly (Ann IM 1986;105:329)

Dihydropyridines: Potent vasodialators; cause reflex tachycardia, peripheral edema

- Amlodipine (Norvasc) 5-10 mg po qd; may be ok for pts w CHF (Nejm 1996;335:1107)
- Felodipine (Plendil) (Med Let 1991;33:115) 5-20 mg po qd; good for hypertension, first-pass metabolism so levels increased by liver disease, cimetidine, and grapefruit juice; adverse effects: like other dihydropyridines, including gingival hyperplasia; cheapest
- Isradipine (DynaCore) 2.5-5 mg po bid (Med Let 1991;33:51)
- Nicardipine (Cardene) (Med Let 1989;31:41) 20+ mg timed release bid; good for angina and hypertension, very like nifedipine, but little negative inotropic effect; adverse effects: gum hypertrophy and gingival hyperplasia; cheaper than diltiazem
- Nifedipine (Procardia) 10-40 mg po t-qid, or 30-120 mg XL qd; least variable (Med Let 1982;24:39) pharmacokinetics compared to diltiazem and verapamil over time, minimal negative inotropic effect, no AV block effect, use for angina, hypertension (not crisis); adverse effects: peripheral edema, hypotension, flushing, and dizziness from peripheral venodilatation; possibly increased rate of MIs, esp w higher doses and short-acting formulations (Jama 1996;275:423) as w other dihydropyridines (Jama 1995;244:360,654)
- Nisoldipine (Sular) (Med Let 1996;38:13) 20-60 mg po qd; for HT; adverse effects: headache, edema, dizziness; toxicity increased by cimetidine, fatty meals, and grapefruit juice (Med Let 1995;37:73)

Diuretics

Nejm 1998;339:387; Med Let 1999;41:23, 1995;37:45

Thiazides: NSAIDs decrease effectiveness (Med Let 1987;29:1), worsen LDL/HDL ratios (Ann IM 1995;122:133); many different kinds, most commonly used:

- Chlorthiazide; chlorthalidone; trichlormethiazide
- Hydrochlorothiazide 12.5-25 mg po qd; adverse effects: hypokalemia especially with steroids but use w K-sparing diuretics prevents MRFIT study-type hypo-K and hypo-Mg mortality (Nejm 1994;330:1852), pancreatitis, rashes, elevated levels of lithium, LDL cholesterol, uric acid, calcium, and blood sugar
- Indapamide (Lozol) 1.25-2.5 mg po qd; perhaps less adverse lipid effect than hydrochlorothiazide, works even in renal failure; $0.50/pill, not worth it (Med Let 1990;31:103)

Potassium-Sparing Distal Diuretics: Beware of hyperkalemia with po KCl, IDDM, renal failure, salt substitutes, and ACE inhibitors

- Amiloride (Midamor) (BMJ 1983;286:2015; Med Let 1981;23:109) 5-20 mg po qd; K^+ sparer, but not aldosterone antagonist; does have an antihypertensive effect, causes low uric acid; adverse effects: potentiates warfarin; causes elevated BUN when used with triamterine
- Eplerenone (Inspra) (Med Let 2003;45:39; Nejm 2003;348:1309,1380) 25-200 mg po qd; an aldosterone antagonist helpful in HT and CHF survival like spironolactone w/o its estrogen-like effects
- Spironolactone (Aldactone) 50-100 mg po qd; an aldosterone antagonist; adverse effects: hyperkalemia, gynecomastia, and impotence due to increased testosterone metabolism into estrogens (Ann IM 1977;87:398)
- Triamterene (Dyrenium) 25-50 mg bid po; K^+ sparer but not aldosterone antagonist and no antihypertensive effect

CARDIOLOGY

Loop Diuretics:

- Bumetanide (Bumex) (Med Let 1983;25:61) 1-5 mg po iv or im, 1 mg comparable to 40 mg of furosemide; adverse effects: like furosemide
- Ethacrynic acid (Edecrin) 25-100 mg po iv, rarely used now
- Furosemide (Lasix) 20-320 mg po iv or im as single dose or divided; works even in renal failure when resistant to thiazides, rapid onset, short half-life; adverse effects: hypokalemia, severe volume depletions possible, direct and indirect decreases in preload, elevates uric acid, blood sugar, and pH; for 40 mg qd, $2/mo generic, $6.50/mo as Lasix
- Metolazone (Zaroxolyn) 2.5-10 mg po qd or qod; works even in renal failure, long-acting, some proximal tubule effect; adverse effects: severe electrolyte imbalances
- Torsemide (Demadex) (Med Let 1994;36:73) 2.5-20 mg po/iv; lower doses as good as thiazides for HT; half-life twice that of furosemide; no drug interactions; adverse effects: same as furosemide; $14/mo for 10 mg qd

Vasodilators

Nitrates (Nejm 1998;338:520; Med Let 1994;36:111):

- Nitroglycerine 0.3-0.4 mg sl or spray (Med Let 1986;28:59) prn pain, or isosorbide dinitrate (Isordil) 5-20 mg po tid, or isosorbide 5-mononitrate (Ismo or Monoket) 20 mg po bid at 8 am and 3 pm (Ann IM 1994;120:353) ($40/mo), or as long-acting (Imdur) 30-120 mg po qd ($20+/mo), or as patch or 2% paste; decreases preload and causes coronary artery dilatation, tolerance, and tachyphylaxis if used continuously 24 hr/day, so nights off necessary for continued effect (Med Let 1994;36:13; Ann IM 1991;114:667; Nejm 1987;316:1635,1440)
- Nitroprusside (Nipride) 0.5-8 µgm/kg/min iv; mixed pre- and afterload reduction; use for hypertensive crises, acute mitral regurgitation and VSDs, pulmonary edema with hypertension,

normotension, or even mild shock; adverse effects: thiocyanate toxicity after 48 hr, especially if renal failure

Natriuretic Peptides: Nesiritide (Natrecor) (Med Let 2001;43:100) iv bolus followed by drip; used for NY Hrt Assoc Class IV pts; adverse reactions: shock; cost = $500/d

Angiotensin-Converting Enzyme Inhibitors (ACEIs) (Med Let 1996;38:104): All may show slowly progressive renal disease (Ann IM 1989;111:503) even in face of early renal failure (BMJ 1994;309:833); less effective in blacks (Nejm 2001;344:1351), but still much better than Ca^{++}-channel blockers (Jama 2001;285:2719); avoid in pregnancy because of potentially fatal effects in 2nd and 3rd trimesters (Jama 1997;277:1193, Med Let 1997;39:44); adverse effects: rare severe angioedema (Jama 1997;278:232); mania, anxiety, hallucinations (Med Let 2002;44:59)

- Benazepril (Lotensin) 10-40 mg po in 1-2 doses qd
- Captopril (Capoten) (Nejm 1988;319:1517; Med Let 1982;24:89) 12.5-100 mg po bid, ineffective if creatinine > 2.8 mg % (Ann IM 1986;104:147); mixed pre- and afterload reduction, positive effects on quality of life in contrast to enalapril, α-methyldopa, and propranolol (Nejm 1993;328:907); adverse effects: hypotension, especially if on diuretics (decrease dose of latter before starting); renal failure (20%) if systolic BP < 90 especially in summer and/or w renal artery stenosis, usually reversible (Ann IM 1991;115:513, 1987;106:346); hyperkalemia, especially in diabetics; cough (5-20%), often prominent and disabling (Ann IM 1992;117:234), treatable with indomethacin 50 mg po bid or nifedipine XL 30 mg po bid (J Cardiovasc Pharmacol 1992;19:670); nephrotic syndrome (1%); agranulocytosis; loss of taste; rash (Med Let 1980;22:39); cholestatic jaundice (Ann IM 1985;102:56); $106/mo for 50 mg tid
- Enalapril (Vasotec) (Med Let 1986;28:53) 2.5-40 mg po qd or bid, same doses in CHF (Nejm 1987;316:1429); activated in

liver, excreted in kidney, 24-hr effect; adverse effects: hyper-kalemia and elevated creatinine (Nejm 1986;315:847); $40/mo for 20 mg qd

- Fosinopril (Monopril) 10-40 mg po qd in 1-2 doses qd
- Lisinopril (Zestril or Prinivil) (Med Let 1988;30:41) 10-40 mg po qd; similar in most respects to captopril; $23/mo for 5 mg bid
- Moexipril (Univasc) 7.5-30 mg po qd; $15/mo for 7.5 mg qd
- Peridopril (Aceon) (Med Let 1999;41:105) 4-8 mg po qd or split bid
- Quinapril (Accupril) 5-80 mg po qd or divided bid; $27/mo for 20 mg qd
- Ramipril (Altace) 2.5-10 mg po bid; $21/mo for 2.5 mg po qd
- Trandolapril (Mavik) 1-4 mg po qd; $18/mo

Angiotensin Receptor Blockers (ARBs) (Med Let 2002;44:69):
Cardiac and renal protective effects like ACEIs (Ann IM 2004;141:693; Nejm 2001;245:851,861,870,910); try when intolerant of ACEIs, eg, cough or angioedema, though some cross-reactivity; less effective in blacks; avoid in pregnancy because of 2nd- and 3rd-trimester fetal damage (ACP J Club 1996;124:10, HT 1995;25:1345); all $40/mo for minimal dose (Med Let 1999;41:105), $5-10/mo more than ACEIs

- Candesartan (Atacand) (Med Let 1998;40:109) 16-32 mg po qd, less if volume depleted and/or on other antihypertensives
- Eprosartan (Teveten) 600-800 mg po qd
- Irbesartan (Avapro) 150-300 mg po qd
- Losartan (Cozaar) (Med Let 1995;37:57) 25-50 mg po qd-bid or w 12.5 mg of hydrochlorothiazide (Hyzaar) 1 tab po qd-bid
- Olmesartan (Benicar) 20-40 mg po qd
- Telmisartan (Micardis) 40-80 mg po qd
- Valsartan (Diovan) (Med Let 1997;39:44) 80-320 mg po qd; $34/30 d

Direct Vasodilators (Med Let 1995;37:45):

- Diazoxide (Hyperstat) (Curr Concepts Cerebro Dis 1982;17:5; Nejm 1976;294:1271) 300 mg iv push over 10-20 sec for hypertensive crisis but no longer 1st choice (nitroprusside w propranolol instead); effects last 3 hr; give with furosemide; protein-bound; get other drugs in soon; adverse effects: rarely can cause hypotension, CNS infarcts
- Hydralazine (Apresoline) 25-50 mg qid po or iv; afterload reduction, used often w isosorbide chronically to get combined pre- and afterload reduction; adverse effects: SLE, especially in women at > 200 mg qd, occurs in 5% of males and 20% of women after 3 yr at 200 mg qd (BMJ 1984;289:410); reflex tachycardia
- Minoxidil (Loniten) (Med Let 1980;22:21; Nejm 1980;303:922) 5-20 mg po bid; afterload reduction, "an oral nitroprusside"; adverse effects: hirsutism
- Morphine 2-5 mg iv; pre- and afterload reductions
- Dihydropyridine calcium-channel blockers (p 60)

α-Adrenergic Receptor Blockers (Med Let 1999;41:23, 1995;37:45):

- Prazosin (Minipress) (Ann IM 1982;97:67; Nejm 1979;300:232) 1-30 mg po qd divided b-tid; mixed pre- and afterload reduction, like nitroprusside, no reflex tachycardia; used for hypertension, CHF, and Raynaud's; 1st dose may cause hypotension often; tachyphylaxis not a problem in hypertension but is with CHF (Nejm 1986;314:1547); $2/mo generic
- Doxazosin (Cardura) 1-16 mg po qd hs (Med Let 1991;33:15); not as good as thiazides (Jama 2000;283:1967); $30/mo
- Terazosin (Hytrin) (Med Let 1987;29:112) 1-20 mg po qd; similar to prazosin; $52/mo

Other Antihypertensives

Med Let 1995;37:45, 1991;33:33

- α-Methyldopa (Aldomet) 0.5-3 gm po qd divided; central sympathetic action; adverse effects: sedation, hemolytic anemia, impotence, hepatitis, increased haloperidol (Haldol) and lithium toxicities

- Clonidine (Catapres) (Med Let 1985;27:95; Nejm 1975;293:1179) 0.1+ mg po bid ($13/mo) or patch q 1 wk ($25/mo); central sympathetic block; adverse effects: severe rebound hypertension when stop; sedation, dry mouth, retinopathy, blocked by tricyclics, patch causes skin reactions
- Fenoldopam (Corlopam) (Med Let 1998;40:57) 0.1-1.6 μgm/kg/min; dopamine-1 receptor antagonist; useful for rx of HT crisis, as good as nitroprusside, can increase intraocular pressures
- Guanfacine (Tenex) (Med Let 1987;29:49) 1-3 mg po qd; like clonidine
- Reserpine 0.1-0.25 mg po qd; acts via peripheral sympathetic blockade; adverse effects: depression, acid peptic disease

Inotropes

- Amrinone (Inocor) (Nejm 1986;314:350) 0.75 mg/kg bolus and drip at 5-10 μgm/kg/min; vasodilator and inotrope, no better than dobutamine and digoxin, may be worse (Ann IM 1985;102:399); adverse effects: depressed platelets, fever, hypotension
- Digoxin (Mod Concepts Cardiovasc Dis 1990;59:67; Nejm 1988;318:358); daily maintenance dose 0.25-0.5 mg po, or 0.125-0.25 mg iv; digitalizing dose is 2-3 mg po, or 1-2 mg iv over 24 hr; major effects are AV block and positive inotropy without increasing O_2 demand; ~80% gi absorption; 60% renal excretion so decrease the dose in renal failure; therapeutic blood level = 0.5-2 μgm %, which is increased by quinidine (Nejm 1981;305:209), verapamil, amiodarone, nifedipine, all NSAIDs including ASA (Mod Concepts Cardiovasc Dis 1986;55:26), antibiotics via increased absorption (Nejm 1981;305:327); decreased effect or levels with hypocalcemia (Nejm 1977;296:917), decreased absorption because of

antacids especially Mg trisilicates, Kaopectate, Dilantin (Nejm 1976;295:1034); misleadingly low levels in achlorhydrics and pts on omeprazole because higher % of active drug is absorbed (Ann IM 1991;115:540); digoxin overdose toxicity treatable with Fab fragments (Nejm 1982;307:1357), not dialyzable; adverse effects: neurologic including nausea and vomiting, visual distortions even at therapeutic levels (Ann IM 1995;123:676), confusion, gynecomastia, cardiac including PVC, AV, and other exit blocks, PAT with block, junctional tachycardia, bidirectional AV tachycardias

- Dobutamine (Dobutrex) (Ann IM 1983;99:490) 2-15 μgm/kg/min; predominantly inotrope; especially used in cardiovascular shock when the pulse rate is already maxima
- Dopamine 2-25 μgm/kg/min; ino- and chronotropic, renal blood flow sparing at these doses? (not so: Chest 2003;123:1266; ACP J Club 2002;136:3); used for shock
- Milrinone (Primacor)

Thrombolytics

- Anistreplase (Eminase) (Med Let 1989;31:15), similar to streptokinase
- Streptokinase 1.5 million U iv over 30 min + ASA 100-160 mg po qd + iv β-blocker (Ann IM 1991;115:34); like urokinase, causes plasmin activation; used for MI and in higher longer doses for pulmonary emboli and DVT; adverse effects: more allergic reactions than urokinase with repeat administrations so can't reuse at least within 6 mo; < 10% bleed, stroke rate < 1% but much higher if diastolic BP > 110 at time of administration (Nejm 1992;327:1); $200/treatment
- Tissue plasminogen activator (TPA) (Nejm 1997;337:118, 1993;329:673,1615; Ann IM 1991;114:417); all followed by or coincident w continuous iv heparin 60 U/kg then 12 U/hr (not more than 4000 U bolus and 1000 U/hr), for at least 1 d + ASA 100-160 mg po qd + iv β-blocker (Ann IM

1991;115:34); adverse effects: bleeding < 10%, stroke rate < 2%, but 4/1000 more than for streptokinase (Nejm 1992;327:1); $2750/treatment, especially in anterior MI and the elderly (Nejm 1995;332:1418)

- Alteplase (TPA, Activase), 100 mg iv over 1.5 hr, $^2/_3$ in 1st 30 min (Jama 2005;293:1746)
- Reteplase (Retavase) 10 U bolus q 30 min × 2; recombinant mutant TPA, cleared more slowly than natural TPA (alteplase), hence can give as bolus
- Tenecteplase (TNKase) (Med Let 2000;42:106) 30-50 mg (based on wt, 30 mg if < 60 kg, 50 mg if > 90 kg) iv bolus over 5 sec, half-life = 25 min
- Urokinase 4400 U/kg load in 10 min, then same/hr × 24 hr; $50/100,000 U

2.2 ASHD

Atherosclerosis

Nejm 1993;329:247 (women)

Cause: Multiple, including elevated cholesterol (Nejm 1981;304:65); smoking, passive (Nejm 1999;340:920) and active, correlates most w pack-years not w quitting (Jama 1998;279:119); hypertension; genetic, especially in women; HgbA$_1$C level > 5 (Ann IM 2004;141:413,421,475). Possibly induced by *Chlamydia pneumoniae* endovascular infection (Jama 1999;281;427,461; Lancet 1997;350:404; Ann IM 1996;125:979, 1992;116:273) or other causes of inflammation indicated by elevated C-reactive protein levels (Nejm 2002;347:1557,1615; Jama 1999;282:2131,2169) and interleukin-6 (Jama 2002;288:980); but no correlation between chlamydial IgG titers and ASHD found in women (Ann IM 1999;131:573)

Epidem: Increased incidence in Western countries although it has decreased in last 25 yr, half due to decrease in risk factors and half due to medical rx (Nejm 1996;334:884) w improving post-MI survival (Nejm 1998;339:861)

Increased in diabetes, hypertension, obesity (Nejm 1990;322:882), inflammation as measured by sCRP and h/o acute infections (Nejm 2004;351:2599,2611), smokers perhaps via inflammation (CRP) and homocysteine levels (Ann IM 2003;138:891), pseudoxanthoma elasticum, myotonic dystrophy, alkaptonuria, and ochronosis; homocystinuria/emia (p 317) and other causes of mild homocystinuria/emia like B_{12}, folate, and pyridoxine deficiencies, prevent w vitamin supplements (Nejm 1995;332:286) although unclear if mildly elevated homocysteine levels are cause or effect of ASCVD (Jama 1995;274:1526); hyperlipidemias (p 276), especially LDL elevations, often associated w apolipoprotein (epsilon) E4 allele (Jama 1994;272:1666), and w elevated lipoprotein (α) (Jama 1996; 276:544); sleep disorders (Am J Med 2000;108:396)

Weak (ACP J Club 1998;129:50) or no association w triglyceride elevations alone, although they are markers for other risk factors (Nejm 1993;328:1220)

Decreased in moderate (7-20 drink/wk) alcohol drinkers (Jama 1999;282:239; Nejm 1997;337:1705; Ann IM 1997;126:372; Nejm 1995;332:1245, 1993;329:1829), via increased TPA as well as HDL (Jama 1994;272:929) and flavins in red wine, which appear to decrease cancer mortality in addition (Ann IM 2000;133:411); in runners (Nejm 1980;303:1159) and otherwise regularly exercising men (Nejm 1998;338:94, 1993; 328:533,538,574, 1993;329:1829) and women (Jama 2001;285: 1447) via protective elevations of HDL cholesterol component; with high-fiber diets (20+ gm qd) (Jama 1999;281:1995) like those high in fruits and vegetables (Ann IM 2001;134:1106); with increased fish intake of omega-3 or N-3 fatty acids (see below); Mediterranean diet (Nejm 2003;348:2599)

Pathophys (Nejm 1999;340:115): Wall stress causes fibrous plaques, which later infiltrate with cholesterol; impaired fibrinolysis may

CARDIOLOGY

also play a role in genesis. Onset by age 18 yr (Nejm 1986;314:138). Hemorrhage into plaque causes sudden occlusions,

Sx: Claudication, angina, MI, sudden death, TIA/CVA, abdominal angina

Si: Renal hypertension; bruits, absent peripheral pulses; CVAs; arcus senilis in Caucasians age < 50 yr (Nejm 1974;291:1323) is a risk factor independent even of cholesterol levels (Am J Pub Hlth 1990;80:1200); retinal fundal vessel plaques, arterial narrowing correlates w MI risk in women but not men (Jama 2002;287:1153)

Crs:

Cmplc: All of above

Lab:

> *Chem:* Cholesterol (p 277). Apolipoprotein A_2 (Nejm 2000;343:1149) or A_1 (Nejm 1983;309:385) (components of HDL) may be better predictors.
>
> *Path:* Lipid in foam macrophages and smooth muscle; free cholesterol crystals between intima and media

Xray: Electron-beam CT screening of unproven value (Nejm 1998;339:1964,1972,2014,2018)

Rx: Prevent (Ann IM 2005;142:393)
- Stopping smoking
- Cholesterol LDL elevation rx (p 276) to get < 100 mg % (Nejm 1997;336:153; Circ 1994;89:1329) at least in pts w ASHD; helps both by decreasing plaques and by preventing coronary artery spasm (Nejm 1995;332:481,488); low-saturated-fat rather than low-total-fat diet (Jama 2002;288:2519), increased fruits, vegetables, and whole grains; Indo-Mediterranean diet (Lancet 2003;360:1455; Nejm 2003;348:2599)
- Cholesterol HDL depression; try to get over 60, at least over 40

- Alcohol @ 2-3 drinks qd decreases mortality by 25% (Am J Pub Hlth 1993;83:805)
- Omega-3 or N_3 fatty acids, as qd capsule (Lancet 1999;354:447) or 1 fatty fish meal/day-mo decreases incidence of cardiac arrest by up to 50% (Jama 2002;287:1815; ACP J Club 2000;132:6; Nejm 1997;336:1046), which also decreases stroke risk by 50% (Jama 2001;285:304) and sudden death risk (Nejm 2002;346:1113); counteracted by mercury content of fish (Nejm 2002;347:1747)
- Exercise (Jama 2001;285:1447, 1998;279:440) moderate (2-3 mi/hr) walking 1-2 hr/wk; total more important than intensity; increases fibrinolysis (Nejm 1980;302:987)
- Rx of diabetes and hypertension
- ASA 80-320 mg (Nejm 2005;352:1293 [women]; USPSTF in Ann IM 2002;136:157; ACP J Club 2001;135:88) po qd decreases MIs (men) and CVAs (women) especially if CRP chronically elevated (Nejm 1996;336:973,1014); effect is counteracted by ibuprofen but not acetaminophen or diclofenac (Voltaren) (Med Let 2004;46:61)
- Folic acid (Nejm 2001;345:1593; Jama 2001;286:936) 0.5-1 mg po qd; now "in the flour" (Nejm 1999;340:1449) or other anti-homocysteinemia (p 317) meds to keep levels < 10 μM/L like pyridoxine and/or B_{12}, esp for pts w established ASHD (DBCT: Jama 2002;288:973) though may worsen restenosis of stents (Nejm 2004;350:2673)
- ACE inhibitors in pts w diabetes or vascular disease and other risk factors decrease MI, sudden death, and CVA, even if normal EF, NNT-4 = 14 (Nejm 2000;342:454)
- No help from:
  - Vitamin E, antioxidant, prevents LDL oxidation but DBCTs show no or deleterious CHF effect (Jama 2005;293:1338; Nejm 2001;345:1583, 2000;342:154; Jama 2002;288:2432). No stroke reduction either (Ann IM 1999;13:963).
  - EDTA chelation of various heavy metals (Med Let 1994;36:48)

- β-Carotene (Nejm 1996;334:1145,1150,1189; Jama 1996;275:693,699: ERT (p 838)

  Rx of disease; various tertiary maneuvers to fix damage especially surgery, eg, angioplasty/CABG, femoral-popliteal bypass; plus dietary measures, eg, "Mediterranean diet" reduces subsequent mortality from 5% to 1% (Arch IM 1998;158:1181; Lancet 1994;343:1454) and can reverse ASHD vessel diameter narrowing (Jama 1998;280:2001; Ann IM 1994;121:348)

Angina

Cause: Atherosclerotic heart disease; "microvascular angina" caused by impaired vasodilatation capabilities in all arterioles seen in hypertension patients, causes 10-20% of angina (Nejm 1988;319: 1302, 1987;317:1366); rarely amyloidosis (Ann IM 1999;131: 838), which looks like microvascular angina because angiography normal, progresses to CHF. Chronic, asymptomatic CMV infection may increase rate of progression (Nejm 1996;335:624).

Epidem: 80% of ischemic events are asx, hence angina is the tip of the ischemic iceberg (Mod Concepts Cardiovasc Dis 1987;56:2; rv of silent isch w/u and rx: Nejm 1988;318:1038); mental stress is as good an inducer of angina as exercise (Nejm 1988;318:1005)

Pathophys: Spasm may occur even when there is no fixed lesion if vessel wall mast cell nests are present (Nejm 1985;313:1138). Unstable angina usually due to platelet thrombus (unlike red thrombus of MI: Nejm 1992;326:287) or fracture of plaque at the site (Nejm 1986;315:913). Paradoxical vasoconstriction with stress may occur because plaque prevents normal endothelial cell induction of coronary dilatation (Nejm 1991;325:1551).

Sx: Onset with first exercise after rest, more frequently in unfamiliar settings, worse supine, worse outdoors (B. Lown, 1985). Relieved by Valsalva maneuver, carotid sinus pressure, and TNG promptly (r/o esophogeal spasm pain; and doubts about its dx helpfulness: Ann IM 2003;139:979,1036).

Si: S_4; mitral regurgitant murmur during pain

Crs: ST depressions > 1 mm, especially those lasting > 60 min, at rest or asx are associated with MI within 6 mo in 15% of cases (Nejm 1986;314:1214) even when medically rx'd

Cmplc: MI

r/o esophageal reflux, which can clinically mimic exactly (Ann IM 1992;117:824), but value of dx studies questionable once ischemia is r/o (Ann IM 1996;124:959); carbon-monoxide induction if onset at home in winter (Nejm 1995;322:48); **syndrome X:** anginal/ischemic sounding chest pain and ST depressions w normal coronaries usually in women (Nejm 2000;342:829,885) associated w demonstrable subendocardial hypoperfusion (Nejm 2002;346:1948), responsive (50%) to imipramine 50 mg po hs (Jama 1995;273:883; Nejm 1994;330:1411, 1993;328:1659,1706), prognosis is good? (Jama 2005;293:117 vs Nejm 1977;297:916)

Lab:

Chem: CPK-MB may elevate mildly, but subsequent mortality is increased by any elevation above upper limit of normal (Jama 2000;283:247); troponin T levels elevated > 0.06 μgm/L (Nejm 2000;343:1139, 1992;327:146)

Hem: sCRP levels > 1.55 mg/L, of doubtful utility (Nejm 2004;350:1450)

Noninv: EKG normal in 50% when asx, 30% when sx (B. Lown, 1985); **Wellens' syndrome** (Am Hrt J 1982;103:730): evolving anterior T inversions w/o enzyme or Q-wave changes, associated w severe LAD lesions

Exercise testing (see Table 2.1) (Nejm 2001;344:1840, 1999;340:340; ACC/AHA guidelines J Am Coll Cardiol 1997;30:260; Mayo Clin Proc 1996;71:43). Contraindicated in CHF, aortic stenosis, IHSS, unstable angina; can't interpret ST changes in face of LBBB, WPW, digoxin, pacing, resting ST depressions > 1 mm, LVH, or lack of changes w submaximal test (< 85% maximal pulse achieved). Use 1+ mm ST depressions if downsloping or horizontal at 0.06 sec after J point, or 1.5 mm ST depressions if upsloping at 0.08 sec after J point; or if ST depression at rest, positive if STs depress ≥ 2 mm more; severity worse if depressions go from 0.5 mm to > 2 mm and start in first 3 min, or last 8+ min (Nejm 1979;301:230), and/or hypotension during ETT. Sensitivity 66% but sens/specif depend on pretest probability (Nejm 1979;300:1350); scoring system predicts 5-yr survival and annual mortality (Nejm 1991;325:849). ST depression not predictive of anatomic site, rarer ST elevations are (Ann IM 1987;106:53). If induce paired PVCs or PVCs are > 10% of all beats, 10-yr mortality incr 10% over baseline (Nejm 2000;343:826).

Nuclear (sestamibi and/or thallium) scan at peak exercise compared to resting, about 75% sens/specif (Nejm 2001;344:1840); a better predictor of long-term outcome than ETT or Holter monitoring (Jama 1996;277:318; Ann IM 1990;113:575); increased lung uptake predicts poor 5-yr outcome (Nejm 1987;317:1485). Nonexertional testing w dipyridamole (Persantine), dobutamine, arbutamine (Med Let 1998;40:19), or adenosine (Jama 1991;265:633) iv thallium test as good as ETT; theophylline blocks and reverses effect of dipyridamole (Med Let 1991;33:87); used when pt cannot walk on treadmill.

Echocardiogram w dobutamine stress (Am J Cardiol 1993;72:605); about same sens/specif as Persantine thallium; done w progressive 5-40 μgm/kg/min dobutamine infusion; can also distinguish whether a reversible perfusion defect is also associated w a reversible contraction abnormality, often an issue w reversible thallium defects next to an old infarct; < ¹/₂ the cost of nuclear stress but dependent on operator experience

Table 2.1 Attributes and Limitations of the Various Stress Modalities

Factor	Standard TET	Myocardial Perfusion Imaging	Radionuclide Angiography	Stress Echocardiography
Sensitivity for detecting CAD[1]	65–70%	80–85%	80–85%	80–85%
Accuracy if resting ECG findings are abnormal	Poor	Good	Good	Good
Ability to localize ischemia	Poor	Good	Good	Good
Additional information compared with standard TET	—	Resting LVEF,[2] lung uptake,[3] quantification of infarct size, qualitative assessment of LV size	Rest and exercise LVEF, rest and exercise regional wall motion, rest and exercise LV volumes, RV function	Rest and exercise LVEF, rest and exercise regional wall motion, rest and exercise LV volumes, RV function, wall thickness, valve status

Table 2.1 continued

Factor	Standard TET	Myocardial Perfusion Imaging	Radionuclide Angiography	Stress Echocardiography
Validation and value for for detecting left main or 3-vessel CAD	Well validated; modest value	Well validated; good value	Well validated; good value	Limited data
Validation and value for prognosis	Well validated; good value	Well validated; good value	Well validated; good value	Limited data
Accuracy for ischemia in the presence of resting regional wall motion abnormalities	—	Good	Modest	Modest
Clinical situations in which technical limitations occur	—	Some obese patients, some women with large breasts	Irregular heart rhythm	Some patients with COPD or obesity
Cost[4]	1+	4+	3+	2+

1. Specificity is difficult to determine accurately because most patients with normal results do not undergo coronary angiography.
2. Tc sestamibi.
3. Thallium-201.
4. Based on scale ranging from 1+ (least expensive) to 4+ (most expensive).
(Reproduced with permission from Mayo Clin Proc 1996;71:50)

Rx: Stopping smoking decreases mortality ×2.8 (Nejm 1984;310:951; BMJ 1983;287:324)

Maximize 1 drug before adding a 2nd drug (Nejm 1989;320:709)

ASA 75-325 mg po qd prevents MI but causes mild increase in stroke risk (Lancet 1992;340:1421; Ann IM 1991;114:835); effect is counteracted by ibuprofen but not acetaminophen or diclofenac (Voltaren) (Med Let 2004;46:61)

Aggressive lipid lowering in chronic stable angina w normal EFs w atoravastatin 80 mg qd as effective than angioplasty (Jama 2004;291:1071,1132; Nejm 1999;341:70)

Primary care management (Rv/guidelines: Ann IM 2004;141:562); no need for repeat w/u within 3 yr after neg w/u unless changing sx or EKG

Antianginal Meds (Med Let 1994;36:111):

- Nitrates to dilate spasms, increase collaterals, and decrease platelet adhesion; po, sl, buccal, or paste tid; tolerance develops so avoid hs or 24 hr rx (Nejm 1987;316:1635), also helpfully decreases gi bleeding if on NSAIDs (Nejm 2000;343:834); adverse effects: hypotension, especially if recent sidenafil (viagra) rx. Costs (Med Let 1987;29:39).

- β-Blockers decrease pulse, BP, platelet adhesion; avoid in Prinzmetal type because can increase spasm

- Calcium-channel blockers dilate spasm and decrease afterload but are 2nd choices after above of unstable angina (Nejm 2000;342:101; Am J Med 2000;108:41): ASA 75-325 mg po qd (Nejm 1992;327:175) w TNG (Nejm 1988;319:1105) and LMW heparin, eg, enoxaparin 1 mg/kg sc bid (J Am Coll Cardiol 1995;26:313) better than plain heparin if definitive invasive rx > 24 hr away (Jama 2004;292:45,89,55,101; Nejm 1997;337:447); w glycoprotein IIb/IIIa inhibitors (Jama 2000;284:1549) like tirofiban (Aggrastat) iv (Nejm 1998;338:1488,1539) or eptifibatide (Integrilin) iv (NNT =

75) (Nejm 1998;339;436), or abciximab (reoPro) (Med Let 1998;40:89) iv; then rapid invasive study. Thrombolysis no help (Circ 1994;89:1545); avoid transfusions (Jama 2004;292:1555).

Surgical:

- Angioplasty (Nejm 1994;331:1037,1044, 1994;330:981) w or w/o stenting (Nejm 1997;336:817); works for stable and unstable angina as well (Nejm 1985;313:342), in elderly even age > 80 yr (Ann IM 1990;113:423); also useful for single-vessel disease but more complications than medical rx (Nejm 1992;326:10); outcome similar to CABG except more reoperations (Lancet 1995;346:1179,1184); but when combined w stent placement (Nejm 1999;341:1949,1957,2005, 1998;339:1672) and clopidrogen or ticlopidine/ASA × 1 mo (Nejm 1998;339:1665), restenosis rate much less but costly (Nejm 1998;339:1702; Lancet 1998;352:87); avoid in diabetics and pts w multivessel disease who should get CABG. Invasive rx results in better outcomes (Am Col Cardiol 2002;40:1902; ACP J Club 2003;138:32, 2003;139:30), even in elderly (> 75 yr) (Heart 2001;86:317; Lancet 2001;358:951).
- CABG increases survival significantly in left main disease, patients with abnormal ETT, and 3-vessel disease in pts with ejection fx > 30% (Nejm 1988;319:332, 1987;316:981), and perhaps older pts; minimal increased survival in other pts with stable angina or asx post-MI with bypassable lesions (Lancet 1994;344:563; ACP J Club 1995;122:29). $^{2}/_{3}$ develop significant disease in grafts in 10 yr (Nejm 1984;311:1329). Significant cognitive decline in 50% @ hosp d/c, 24% @ 6 mo, but 42% @ 5 yr (Nejm 2001;344;395,451).
- Atherectomy (Nejm 1993;339:221,228,273) for eccentric lesions of unstable angina
- Experimental transmyocadial laser revascularization? (Nejm 1999;341:1021; Lancet 1999;354:885)/enhanced external counterpulsation (Am Hrt J 2003;146:453)

Myocardial Infarction

Cause: Atherosclerotic (85%), including spasm (Nejm 1983;309:220) with superimposed thrombus in 90% of those; emboli (15%: Ann IM 1978;88:155); occasionally cocaine-induced spasm when used as anesthesia or as recreational drug (Nejm 1989;321:1557)

Epidem: Increased incidence with h/o:

- Concurrent BCP use increases risk ×2 (Nejm 2001;345:1787)
- Carbon monoxide acute exposures, eg, firefighters; and chronic CS_2 exposures, eg, disulfiram (Antabuse) use, rayon manufacturing
- Cholesterol elevations of total and/or LDL, often with presence of arcus senilis (Nejm 1974;291:1382)
- Cocaine use or withdrawal (Ann IM 1989;111:876; Nejm 1986;315:1438,1495)
- Coffee, high decaffeinated but not regular coffee intake (Nejm 1990;323:1026); later study found no increased incidence w either (Jama 1996;275:458)
- Exercise test showing ischemia (Nejm 1983;309:1085)
- Family h/o MIs prematurely (age < 55 or 65 yr) (Nejm 1994;330:1041)
- Homocysteine levels > 15 μM/L correlate w worse prognosis (Nejm 1997;337:230)
- Hypertension
- Menopause if surgical and patients not placed on estrogen; but no sharp increase in natural menopause
- Sedentary work; in longshoremen, MIs but not CVAs increased, thus not a general ASCVD effect (Nejm 1975;292:545)
- Sexual activity increases risk slightly but not at all if regular (eg, 3×/wk) exercise (Jama 1996;275:1405)
- Smoking increases risk ×3, but risk decreases to normal over 2 yr after stop (Nejm 1985;313:1511), increases risk ×5 if > 1 ppd, ×2 if 1-4 cigarettes qd in women (Nejm 1987;317:1303)

- Stress, day to day (Jama 1997;277:1521) but not type A personality? (Nejm 1988;318:65,110)
- Viral URI in past 2 wk (Ann IM 1985;102:699) or chronic *Chlamydia pneumoniae* infections? (Ann IM 1996;125:979, 1992;116:273)

   Decreased incidence with: exercise, > 6 METs > 2 hr/wk divided t-qiw (Nejm 1994;330:1549); fish intake 1-4×/mo (Jama 1995;274:1363; Nejm 1995;332:977, 1985;312:1205,1254); 1-3 alcoholic drinks qd (Nejm 2003;348:109; Ann IM 1991;114:967) in men, vs 2-3/wk in women (Nejm 1995;332:1246); better control of hypertension, cholesterol, etc, in U.S. (Nejm 1985;312:1005,1053)

Pathophys: Platelet aggregations and thrombi (Nejm 1990;322:1549) on plaque fissures cause thrombosis w or w/o spasm (Nejm 1991;324:688; 1984;310:1137); or paradoxical vasoconstriction w stress because plaque prevents normal endothelial cell induction of coronary dilatation (Nejm 1991;325:1551)

Sx: Chest pain, substernal, in "distribution of a tree," worse supine; diaphoresis, dyspnea; associated with heavy exertion 5-40× more frequently depending on conditioning state (Nejm 1984;311:874); CNS sx are the presenting sx in 50% of pts age > 60 yr. No recognizable sx ("silent") in ±25% (Ann IM 2001;135:801, 2001;134:1043 vs 33%: Ann IM 1995;122:96) or half of these are asx, yet prognosis just as bad (Framingham-Nejm 1984;311:1144)

Si: Pericardial rub on day 2+, usually without ST changes (Nejm 1984;311:1211); S_4 gallop; fever < 103°F; transient S_2 paradoxical split

   Right ventricular infarct syndrome (Nejm 1998;338:978, 1994;330:1211): acute inferior MI, Kussmaul's si (paradoxical increases in JVP with inspiration) (Ann IM 1983;99:608), high CVP with low PAPs and PCWPs so all nearly equal, like pericardial tamponade (Nejm 1983;309:39,551), low cardiac output;

occurs in 50% of IWMI pts (Nejm 1993;328:982) but clinically significant in 30% (Nejm 1988;338:978) and nearly 100% of those w CPK levels > 2000 IU (J. Sutherland 1/96); reversible w reperfusion rx (Nejm 1998;338:933)

Rectal exam important for guaiac and detection of BPH (Nejm 1969;281:238; 1970;282:167)

Crs: 15% in-hospital mortality before thrombolytics, now 7-10%; 10% of survivors get severe pump failure, another 10% get persistent angina, 10% "flunk" discharge mini-ETT, another 10% "flunk" maximal ETT at 6 wk; remaining 50% do fine (Nejm 1986;314:161)

Prognosis is similar for Q-wave and non–Q-wave infarcts (Am J Med 2000;108:381) although non–Q-wave MIs are followed by more infarcts and angina but are associated w less CHF (Jama 1992;268:1545); is not affected by 1st-degree heart block, PVCs, or Vtach (Ann IM 1992;117:31), RBBB (Ann IM 1972;77:677), or type A personality (Nejm 1985;312:737); better prognosis if preinfarction angina preceded (Nejm 1996;334:7)

Age-adjusted 6 mo survival for women age < 75 yr is 15% worse than for men (Nejm 1999;341:217, 1998;338:8; Jama 1998;280:1405) primarily because they have worse MIs

Concomitant RV infarct increases IWMI mortality from 6% to 30% (Nejm 1993;328:982); mitral regurgitation, when severe, is associated w 50% 1-yr mortality despite all interventions (Ann IM 1992;117:18)

In elderly, aggressive invasive study and rx do not improve mortality (U.S. vs Canadian 65+-yr-olds: Nejm 1997;336:1500)

Cmplc:
- Aneurysm of left ventricular, develops in first 48 hr, leads to emboli, CHF, and PVC, 60% 1-yr mortality (Nejm 1984;311:100), though rate may be lower now w thrombolysis
- Arrhythmias, esp PVCs and Vtach
- CHF

- Dressler's syndrome (Arch IM 1959;103:38); transient post-MI/CABG pericarditis
- Heart block (p 102) (Mod Concepts Cardiovasc Dis 1976;45:129) occurs in 5% of inferior MIs, 3% of anterior MIs, and in 100% with anterior MI + RBBB causing a 75% mortality
- Mural thrombi without aneurysm in 11% of acute MIs, 2% of others (J Am Coll Cardiol 1993;22:1004)
- Papillary muscle rupture causes CHF with a normal-sized left atrium by TTE or TEE, occurs most often with inferior MIs (Nejm 1969;281:1458), rx with nitrites (Ann IM 1975;83:313,422) and other afterload reduction, and surgery (Ann IM 1979;90:149)
- Pericardial tamponade from inflammation (r/o RV infarct: Nejm 1983;309:39,551) since both functionally acutely constrict pericardial space by fluid or dilated RV (J. Love 3/95)
- Rupture of septal wall, usually day 3-5, to create a VSD (Circ 2000;101:27; Nejm 2002;347:1426), which must be repaired asap, or rupture into pericardial sac, causing tamponade (Nejm 1996;334:319)
- Shock (7.5%: Nejm 1991;325:1117); immediate revascularization improves survival (Jama 2001;285:190)
- Stroke, esp if EF < 28% post-MI (Nejm 1997;336:251), prevent w warfarin anticoagulation
- r/o transient LV apical ballooning syndrome in postmenopausal women w mild sc and transient ST elevations; benign (Ann IM 2004;141:858)

Lab:

Chem: Enzymes (Ann IM 1986;105:221):
- CPK and fractions up in 12 hr, peak at 2 d, last 4 d; CPK-MB subfractions MB2 and MB1 in 1st 6 hr after onset of pain have 95% sens/specif and may be used to send home from ER (Nejm 1994;331:561,607); total CPK correlates with MI size; may double in MI but still be less than upper limit of normal (Am J

Cardiol 1983;51:24); MB band is increased also by increased death and regeneration of skeletal muscle (Ann IM 1981;94: 341) and by decreased clearance in myxedema; MM is increased by hypothyroidism, myopathy; BB band is increased by CNS and/or smooth muscle damage (Bull Rheum Dis 1983;33:1)

- Troponin I and T levels elevate over first 8 hr (84-96% sens, 80-95% specif) (J Fam Pract 2000;49:550) and stay up for 7-10 d; "false pos" levels really represent ischemia (Nejm 1997;337:1648,1687); levels correlate w worse outcomes (Nejm 1996;335:1333,1342,1388); also useful perioperatively when surgery may increase CPK (Nejm 1994;330:670). But r/o nonthrombotic causes of elevations (Ann IM 2005;142:786)
- LDH and fractions: Isoenzymes 4 and 5 (rapidly migrating) increased, r/o renal and red cell source
- AST (SGOT) up in 24 hr, peaks at 2-4 d, lasts up to 7 d
- Malondialdehyde (MDA)-modified LDL > 0.85 mg % (Jama 1999;281:1718), 95% sens and specif for unstable angina or MI; combined w troponin I, is 99% sens and specif
- Myeloperoxidase level on admission perhaps (Nejm 2003;349:1595) but has a fairly continuous rise w ischemia likelihood, not the step up of CPK or troponin levels

Noninv Lab (Ann IM 1989;110:470):

- Echo for mitral regurgitation, aneurysm, EF estimation, and mural thrombi with 77% sens and 93% specif (Nejm 1982;306:1509)
- EKG (p 161) may show ST elevations (50% sens), duration of elevation correlates with extent of injury (Nejm 1969;280:123), T inversions much less specific (r/o acute cholecystitis: Ann IM 1992;116:218). In RV infarct, ST elevations present in V_1, or $V_{3-6}R$, especially V_4R w 80+% sens/specif (Nejm 1993;328:981).
- New RBBB or LBBB indicates occlusion of anterior descending proximal to 1st septal branch (Nejm 1993;328:1036); both worsen prognosis (Ann IM 1998;129:690)

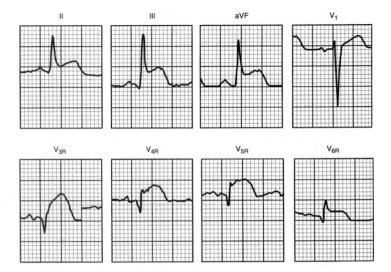

Figure 2.1 EKG from a patient with an inferior MI and right ventricular infarction. Reproduced with permission from Kinch JW, Ryan TJ. Current concepts: right ventricular infarction. New Eng J Med 1994;330:1214. Copyright 1994 Mass. Medical Society, all rights reserved.

- ETT (Circ 1996;94:2341): estimates prognosis (Nejm 1979;301:341), or more often with thallium (85% sens/specif-Ann IM 1990;113:684,703); predicts 5-yr survival (Ann IM 1987;106:793)

Xray:

Rx: Primary preventive interventions:
- ASA tab qod (Nejm 1992;327:175, 1989;321:129) or qd 75-325 mg (Ann IM 1996;124:292; Med Let 1995;37:14) after angina or MI, or as part of rx of HT (Lancet 1998;351:1755); effect is counteracted by ibuprofen but not acetaminophen, or COX-2s (Nejm 2001;345:1809)

- Dietary interventions like lowering cholesterol as does American Heart Association diet (BMJ 1992;304:1015) and "Mediterranean diet" (p 72). As primary prevention, NNT-5 = 53; as secondary prevention, NNT-5 = 16 (J Fam Pract 1996;42:577).
- Perioperative β-blockers like atenolol 5-10 mg iv pre- and post-op + 50 mg po bid during hospitalization decrease risk of cardiac morbidity/mortality by 11% (Nejm 1996;335: 1713,1761)
- Smoking cessation decreases risk to baseline in 3 yr (Nejm 1990;322:213); probably ok to use nicotine patch post-MI (Nejm 1996;335:1792)
- Statin rx if 3+ risk factors helps (NNT-3 = 53) even if no hyperlipidemia (Lancet 2003;361:1149)

Secondary preventive interventions (post-MI): above, plus

- β-Blocker within 24 hr of MI and continued indefinitely (BMJ 1999;318:1730; Jama 1998;280:623), improves survival even if elderly, low EF, non–Q-wave MI, or have COPD (NNT-2 = 10) (Nejm 1998;339:489: but not RCT); eg, metoprolol 5 mg iv q 5 min × 3 then 50 mg po bid × 1 d then 100 mg bid, or atenolol 50-100 mg po qd, helps prevent recurrent MI (Circ 1994;90:762; TIMI study: Nejm 1989;320:618) and fatal ventricular arrhythmias; use in elderly as well (Jama 1997;277:115); in post–Q-wave MI, increases survival for 6+ yr (timolol: Nejm 1985;313:1055), all work (Med Let 1982;24:44)
- ACE inhibitors within 24 hr of MI (Circ 1998;97:2202) especially if anterior MI, CHF, elevated pulse; and for 6 wk (Lancet 1994;343:1115); continue indefinitely if EF < 40% (J Am Coll Cardiol 1996;27:337; Ann IM 1994;121:750; Nejm 1992;327:669, 1992;327:629,685); eg, captopril 50 mg tid, increases ETT performance and decreases LV size (Nejm 1988;319:80), or ramipril 2.5-5 mg po bid (Lancet 1997;349:1493); prolongs life after MI even if no sx (Med Let

1994;36:69) but only if EF < 40% (Nejm 2004;351:2058). Unclear if ARBs equally safe/effective (Lancet 2003;360:752 vs ACP J Club 2003;138:65).

- Statin (HMG-CoA) lipid rx post-MI reduces further MIs and mortality (NNT-5 = 30-33: Nejm 1996;335:1001; Lancet 1994;344:1383; or better, NNT-1 = 25: Jama 2001;285:430); rx LDL to < 100 mg % (Jama 1997;277:1281; Nejm 1997;336:153) or even lower helps more (Nejm 2004;350:1495); helps in elderly age 65-75 (Ann IM 1998;129:681)
- Fibrate rx of HDL < 40 mg %, eg, w gemfibrosil (Nejm 1999; 341:410); for MI, NNT-5 = 23 (ACP J Club 2000;132:44)
- In all diabetics, continuous iv insulin × 24 hr then qid sc × yrs, improves survival, NNT-1 = 13 (J Am Coll Cardiol 1995;26:57)

of acute MI:

- ASA 325 mg po stat helps survival dramatically (Nejm 1997;336:847)
- Clopidogrel (Plavix) 300 mg × 1 then 75 mg po qd; improves outcomes (NNT = 14-33) (Nejm 2005;352:1179)
- LMW heparin alone or in combination w other interventions improves outcome (NNT = 75±) even in developing countries (Jama 2005;293:427)
- Angioplasty (PCTA) of evolving acute MI as acute primary rx w stenting, rather than thrombolysis, preferable if available (Nejm 2000;343:385; even in elderly: Jama 1999;282:341), in high-volume centers (Nejm 2002;346:957) and community hospitals by stat transfers w abciximab alone or w half-dose thrombolysis (Nejm 2004;291:947,1000) to cath labs w or w/o surgical backup (Jama 2002;287:1943) if can do within 2 hr of onset (Lancet 2003;361:13; Nejm 2003;349:733); "ischemia-guided rx" no longer the standard (Lancet 2004;364:1045) even in elderly (> 75 yr) (Circ 2004;110:1213); better success in high-volume centers (Nejm 2000;342:1573)

- Thrombolysis w streptokinase, TPA, etc (p 67) helps all pts including those > age 75 yr (Nejm 1992;327:7) although intracranial bleeding risk increases from < 0.5% under 65, to 2.5% over 75 (Ann IM 1998;129:597), hence still unclear if should use over age 75 (Circ 2000;101:2239); if systolic BP ≥ 175 or diastolic ≥ 100, bleeding risk is doubled (Ann IM 1996;125:891); use if pain is < 6 hr duration, or if 6-12 hr and STs still elevated (Lancet 1996;348:771, 1993;342:759,767) or LBBB and good story (Jama 1999;281:714; Ann IM 1998;129:690); does not help ST depressions, which should be rx'd as unstable angina (p 77). Give concomitantly or follow either with heparin iv × 1+ d (Nejm 1990;323:1433) + ASA 160 mg po qd + β-blocker (Ann IM 1991;115:34). CPK-MB and troponin T levels should rise 5× at 60 min and 5-10× at 90 min to indicate reperfusion (90% sens, ~65% specif) (J Am Coll Cardiol 1998;31:1499)
- β-Blocker and ACEI rx as above
- Nitroglycerine, as patch or iv if volume ok especially if continued pain, perhaps even if no pain; especially helpful if any element of CHF or if large anterior MI; avoid if recent sildenafil (Viagra) use
- Insulin iv w glucose and KCl no benefit (Jama 2005;293:437,489)
- Rehab programs probably help (ACP J Club 1999;131:41) over 3 mo if 3 wk post-MI ETT achieves < 8 METs (Ann IM 1988;109:650,671). Get 3-wk post-MI ETT and return to work at 4 wk unless severe ischemia (Ann IM 1992;117:383; Nejm 1992;327:227).
- CABG after angiography if low EF (21-49%) and multivessel disease, or left main disease; can do it 1 mo post-MI (Nejm 1982;307:1065)

of complications:

- Bradyarrhythmias: rx in IWMI only if pain, PVCs, CHF, or pulse < 45/min and unstable, then pace (Nejm 1975;292:572);

in anterior MI, pace to prevent 20-40% evolving to complete heart block if anterior MI + RBBB, RBBB + left anterior hemiblock, RBBB + left posterior hemiblock, or LBBB; bifascicular block evolving into trifascicular block during MI needs permanent pacer even if returns to normal later (Mod Concepts Cardiovasc Dis 1976;45:129)

- CHF/shock: Dobutamine (Nejm 1980;303:846) + nitroprusside acutely; or early revascularization to improve on 60% mortality (Nejm 1999;341:625); ACE inhibitors as above
- Mural thrombi in anterior MI: Prevent with heparin to PTTs ~48 sec for 10 d, sc not enough (Nejm 1989;320:352)
- Papillary muscle rupture acutely: Surgery sooner not later (Nejm 1996;335:1417)
- Pericarditis: Should not be rx'd with indomethacin, which can cause spasm (Nejm 1981;305:1171); other NSAIDs better
- RV infarct: Increase preload w iv saline, avoid nitrates and diuretics (lower preload), dobutamine drip, nitroprusside drip, sequential pacing, isoproterenol to unload RV (Nejm 1993;328:982)
- Ventricular arrhythmias: Amiodarone or implantable defibrillator for sudden death survivors (Circ 1995;91:2195) or perhaps all w EF < 30%? (Nejm 2002;346:877,931)
- Wall rupture or VSD development: Surgery if slow (Nejm 1983;309:539)

Congestive Heart Failure

Nejm 2003;348:2007

Cause: ASHD, dilated (systolic dysfunction), or hypertensive (diastolic dysfunction) cardiomyopathy; occasionally valve disease; and more rarely, high-output types, eg, AV malformations, Paget's disease, hyperthyroidism, beriberi, severe anemia as w pernicious anemia; tocolytic rx of premature labor (Ann IM 1989;110:714), NSAIDs in elderly

Epidem: In U.S., incidence is 400,000/yr

Increases w HT, in 40% of men and 60% of women (Jama 1996;275:1557), systolic BP > 160 just as significant as a diastolic > 95; obesity (Nejm 2002;347:305); homocysteine levels (Jama 2003;289:1251)

Decreased incidence by $\frac{1}{2}$ in regular alcohol users, even heavy users (Framingham-Ann IM 2002;136:181)

Pathophys (Ann IM 1994;121:363; Nejm 2004;351:1097 [diastolic type]):

Most CHF is due to systolic dysfunction, but > 30% is due to diastolic dysfunction (Nejm 2440;350:1953) and > 50% in elderly (p 435), eg, chronic systemic HT, mitral stenosis, constrictive pericarditis, IHSS, etc, conditions that prevent normal diastolic filling. Hypertrophy in response to load creates dysfunctional myocardial cells (Ann IM 1994;121:363). ACEIs, β-blockers, and calcium-channel blockers may help relax hypertrophic myocardium as well as decrease afterload (Ann IM 1992; 117:502; Nejm 1991;325:1557). Compensatory production of natriuretic peptide, atrial and ventricular B type, promotes diuresis (Nejm 2004;350:718, 1998;339:321).

Cardiac "asthma" is due to bronchial edema and hyperresponsiveness (Nejm 1989;320:1317)

Sx: Dyspnea on exertion, orthopnea, paroxysmal nocturnal dyspnea, ankle edema, bowel bloating and sense of fullness pc, nocturia

NY Heart Association Classification

I: No dyspnea on moderate exertion
II: Dyspnea w moderate exertion; 25% 4-yr mortality
III: Dyspnea w mild exertion; 50% 4-yr mortality
IV: Dsypnea at rest; 50%/yr mortality

Si: JVD, S_3 gallop (techniques: Nejm 2001;345:612) in systolic dysfunction; both correlate w worse prognosis (Nejm 2001;345:574); S_4 in diastolic dysfunction

Pulse > 100 (pulse > diastolic BP = 53% sens, 80% specif: BMJ 2000;320:220); displaced point of maximal impulse, dullness in L 5th intercostal space ≥ 10.5 cm from sternum (Am J Med 1991;91:328); pleural effusions R > L (Nejm 1983;308:696)

Central apnea in 45%, especially Cheyne-Stokes respirations from increased sens to pCO_2 (Nejm 1999;341:949,985), rx w theophylline 250 mg po bid (Nejm 1996;335:562)

Crs: > 70% 5-yr mortality if due to hypertension (Framingham-Jama 1996;275:1557), 50% 1-yr mortality after start medications; over age 70, 70% 2-yr mortality after pulmonary edema (Ann IM 1971;75:332)

Cmplc: Sleep apnea (Ann IM 1995;122:487)

Lab:

Chem: Hyponatremia due to inappropriate ADH (Nejm 1981;305:263)

Ventricular type B natiuretic peptide > 100 pgm/cc has 90% sens and 75% specif by rapid fluorescent immunoassay, so run stat to r/o CHF in acute SOB or if > 500 pgm/cc can rule in to allow rapid aggressive rx (Nejm 2004;350:647, 2002;347:161; ACP J Club 2002;136:68)

Hem: ESR low when acute and severe, correlates with fibrinogen levels (Nejm 1991;324:353)

Inv monitoring: Swan-Ganz monitoring now discouraged because of increase in morbidity and mortality (Jama 2001;286:309), use only when cardiac output and/or wedge data will change rx; in and out as quickly as possible (Ann IM 1985;103:445) since cmplc are pulmonary infarction, pulmonary artery rupture, knotting, endocardial thrombosis (50%), subsequent endocarditis (8%) (Nejm 1984;311:1152)

Urine: Proteinuria, why? (Nejm 1982;306:1031)

Echocardiogram: EF < 50% in systolic dysfunction, > 50% in diastolic dysfunction often seen in elderly

Xray: Chest shows redistribution of blood to apices on upright, perihilar "haze," Kerley B lines, increased heart size, pleural effusions R > L (Nejm 1983;308:696) possibly because thoracic duct provides a "pop-off valve" to L pulmonary vasculature, ie, better lymphatic drainage (J. Sutherland 6/95)

Rx (Nejm 1996;335:490; Ann IM 1994;121:363): Acutely:

- O_2 at 2-3 L/min (Ann IM 1989;111:777) w CPAP (Nejm 1991;325:1825)

- Dobutamine iv acutely best choice immediately post-MI, better than digoxin or diuretics, no arrhythmias, short half-life (Nejm 1980;303:846)

- Nitrates, eg, nitroprusside iv or nitroglycerine iv drip; help even if severe aortic stenosis? (Nejm 2003;348:1735,1756)

- Nesiritide iv (Jama 2002;287;1531,1578; Nejm 2000;343:246), natriuretic peptide drip helpful

  Chronically: See medication section p 51 for dosing (Med Let 1999;41:12; Nejm 1998;339:1848). Generally use ACEIs and other vasodilators, diuretics, + digitalis (Nejm 1993;329:1)

- Exercise training helps (Jama 2000;283:3095; Circ 1999;99:1173; Ann IM 1996;125:1051)

- Avoid NSAIDs, especially if hyponatremia (Nejm 1984;310:347), and calcium-channel blockers (Nejm 1996;335:1107)

- ACEIs alone increase survival from 50% to 73% at 6 mo (Jama 1995;273:1450; Med Let 1994;36:69); to doses of enalapril 20 mg qd, or lisinopril 30 mg qd, or captopril 150 mg qd; may need to decrease diuretic doses to avoid hypotension; less effective in blacks (Nejm 2001;344:1351). Or ARBs (Nejm 2003; 349:1893), like losartan (Cozaar) 12.5-50 mg po qd or valsartan 80 mg qd-160 bid if cough or angioedema prevent ACEI use, but combined use w ACEI no benefit, and ARBs are 5× as expensive as ACEIs.

- β-Blockers (Med Let 2000;42:54) to reduce sympathetic tone, improve survival even in severe CHF if pt can tolerate (Nejm

2001;344:1651,1659,1711; Jama 2003;289:712, 2000;283:1295; Lancet 1999;353:9)

- Metoprolol 12.5-25 mg of CR/XL type or in tid doses titrated up to 100-200 mg po qd, or
- Bisoprolol (Zebeta) 1.25-10 mg po qd, or
- Carvedilol (Coreg) 3.125-25 mg po bid
- Spironolactone (Med Let 1999;41:81) 12.5-25 mg po qd, if creatinine < 2.5 mg %, used w ACEI and digoxin improves survival and hospitalization by 30% (Nejm 1999;341:709,753) but also quadruples the rate of hyperkalemia hospitalizations and deaths (Nejm 2004;351:543)
- Diuretics like thiazides, furosemide, and occasionally metolazone (Zaroxolyn), always use with ACEIs; beware decreased po absorption with increased CHF (Ann IM 1985;102:314); transient CHF worsening for 20 min via renin-angiotensin system (Ann IM 1985;103:1)
- Nitrates, eg, nitroprusside acutely, or TNG paste 1-5 in. q 3-6 hr, or isosorbide up to 40 mg po t-qid also clearly shown to prolong life
- Inotropes like digitalis glycosides, especially if S_3 gallop (Ann IM 1984;101:113; Nejm 1982;306:699) and/or EF < 35% (Nejm 1993;329:1), decreases admission for CHF but doesn't decrease mortality (Nejm 1997;336:525) and in fact incr mortality in women (Nejm 2002;347:1403), a poor derivative study (Jama 2003;289:730) suggests levels in high therapeutic range may harm; amrinone ok acutely but not useful chronically po (Lancet 1994;344:493 vs ACP J Club 1995;122:33)
- Vasodilators such as hydralazine especially w nitrates when ACEI intolerant, eg, questionable drug company study of nitrates/hydralazine in blacks (Nejm 2004;351:2049)
- Experimental: co-enzyme Q10 (Clin Investig 1993;71:S134) 50 mg po b-tid, increases mitochondrial ATPase and decreases CHF cmplc; vasopressin antagonists like tolvaptan (Jama 2004; 291:1963,2017)

if IVCD (QRS > 0.12-0.15 sec), atrio-biventricular pacing improves sx and function (Jama 2003;289:730; Nejm 2004;350:2140, 2002;346:1845, 2001;344:873) but many being done w/o prolongation of life

of first fatal Vtach w single-lead ICD shock only, in pts w EF < 35% improves mortality (NNT-5 = 14) (Nejm 2005;352:225,285)

Surgical: Heart transplant, 3500/yr in U.S., 65% 5-yr survival (Jama 1998;280:1692)

of Cheyne-Stokes breathing: O_2 or CPAP improves survival (Nejm 1999;341:985), which also improves CHF in silent sleep apnea (Nejm 2003;348:1233)

2.3   Arrhythmias

Paroxysmal Supraventricular Tachycardias

Cause: Aberrant conduction pathways with different conduction rates within the AV node **(av nodal reentrant tachycardia)** (AVNRT) or outside the AV node **(av rentrant tachycardia, Wolff-Parksinson-White syndrome)** (AVRT, WPW) (p 99), allowing setup of circus movement continous stimulation when the aberrant or usual pathway conducts retrograde; or ectopic irritable atrial focus **(paroxysmal atrial tachycardia)** (PAT), often associated with digoxin toxicity especially if manifest w associated block, eg, 2:1 or 3:1

Epidem: AVNRT and AVRT of about equal prevalence and each represents about 45% of all PSVTs; PAT constitutes 9%, and rare other syndromes like **permanent junctional reentrant tachycardia** (PJRT), the last 1%.

Pathophys: Reentrant tachycardias occur with things that increase excitability, decrease refractory period, and increase conduction velocity

A. Normal Sinus Rhythm

B. Atrial Tachycardia

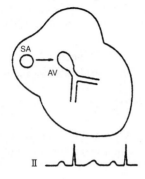

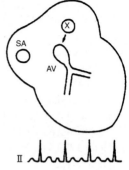

C. AV Nodal Reentrant Tachycardia

D. Bypass Tract Tachycardia

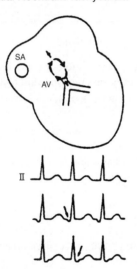

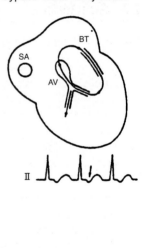

Figure 2.2   Circus tachycardias. Reproduced from Goldberger and Goldberger, Fig. 12-4, Clinical Electrocardiography, 5th ed; St. Louis: Mosby 1994, p159, with permission from Elsevier.

Sx: Paroxysmal episodes of palpitations often associated with dizziness, nausea; precipitated by caffeine, alcohol, nicotine, hyperthyroid states, ephedrine in diet supplements, etc; often relieved by Valsalva maneuver by patient. Neck pounding in AVNRT types but not accessory pathway (WPW or AVRT) SVT because nearly coincident atrial and ventricular contraction in former cause cannon waves in neck that can be felt (Nejm 1992;327:772).

Si: Rapid tachycardia 150-210/min

Crs: Recurrent from teenage years on

Cmplc: Rare permanent junctional reentrant tachycardia variant associated with myocardopathy if stays in arrhythmia a long time, reversible if rx'd.

Post PAT T-wave inversions may last days-weeks (Nejm 1995;332:161)

Lab: EKG shows SVT w narrow complexes; AVNRT usually has no apparent P waves, AVRT has P waves closer to the last QRS than the next one, and PAT and PJRT have P waves closer to the next QRS and beyond the T wave. PSVT is very regular, even when aberrant and wide, unlike Vtach; QRS aberrancy always < 0.14 sec whereas Vtach often (> 50%) > 0.14 sec, axis is −30° to +120° unlike the LAD with Vtach 60% of time (J. Love 9/85) (see Brugada criteria p 105).

Rx: Carotid sinus pressure

Adenosine 6-12 mg iv, gone in 10 sec, potentiated by dipyridamole and carbamazepine, inhibited by theophyllines (Med Let 1990;32:63); or verapamil 5-10 mg iv; perhaps propranolol iv 1-5 mg

Electrical cardioversion with sync if meds fail or if unstable, ok to do even if digoxin on board as long as levels therapeutic and not toxic, and K^+ ok (Ann IM 1981;95:676); in resistant cases, implanted atrial burst pacers (Ann IM 1987;107:144) or catheter ablation of atrial slow pathway works 95% of the time (Med Let 1996;38:40, Nejm 1994;330:1481)

For chronic prevention: Avoid stimulants; β-blockers; maybe verapamil or digoxin, though both can worsen some cases

Atrial Fibrillation (AF), Flutter (AFlut) and Related Tachycardias [including wandering atrial pacemaker (WAP), multifocal atrial tachycardia (MFAT), and sick sinus syndrome (SSS)

Nejm 2004;351:2408 (AF); 1990;322:1713 (MFAT); Mod Concepts Cardiovasc Dis 1980;49:61,67 (SSS)

Cause: Associated with normal variations, idiopathic, CHF, rheumatic heart disease, atrial dilatation (eg, in mitral stensosis or regurgitation), pericarditis, COPD especially with hypoxia and bronchodilators, ASHD; w hyperthyroidism especially in the elderly as measured by low TSH, which has a 30% 10-yr incidence in contrast to 10% 10-yr incidence w normal TSH (Nejm 1994;331: 1252) and w toxic multinodular goiter; w alcoholic myocardiopathy

Aflut and MFAT often (60%) from pulmonary disease, including pulmonary emboli

Epidem: Common; supraventricular prematures are not associated with ASHD or sudden death (Ann IM 1969;70:1159)

Pathophys:

Sx: Polyuria, palpitations, faintness

Si:

Crs:

Cmplc: Chronic AFib causes embolic CVA in 20% if recent CHF, HT, or previous embolus (Ann IM 1992;116:1) but < 1%/yr if none of those and no increase in LA size or LV dyskinesis on echo (Ann IM 1992;116:6); likewise, others find rate only 1.3% after 15 yr where no other disease and < age 60 (Nejm 1987;317:699); embolic CVA increased 5× in ASHD type compared to age-matched controls, 17× in rheumatic (Neurol 1978;28:973)

in SSS, 16% develop arterial emboli (Nejm 1976;295:190)

r/o hyperthyroidism, silent mitral stenosis, alcoholic myocardiopathy, and pulmonary embolism

Lab:

Chem: TSH

Noninv: EKG: Sick sinus syndrome is diagnosed by SVTs alternating w some heart block, and suggested by P < 90 after 1-2 mg atropine, or asystole > 3 sec after carotid sinus massage

MFAT, P > 100, and ≥ 3 different PR intervals and P-wave morphologies; looks superficially like AF but digoxin won't help it; WAP is same thing but rate < 100

Holter monitoring to find, when intermittent; or better, event monitor (Ann IM 1996;124:16)

Echo, TEE is 99% specific, 100% sens for LA thrombus (Ann IM 1995;123:817)

Rx: (Med Let 1991;33:55): All but β-blockers may prolong or cause ventricular arrhythmias (Ann IM 1992;117:141)

• Afib: Perioperative prevention post-CABG w amiodarone (Nejm 1997;337:1785)

Rate control: iv diltiazem, β-blocker like esmolol, or digoxin but latter's rate is easily overridden by catechol/exercise stimulation (Ann IM 1991;114:573). Outcome of stroke and mortality as good or better than attempts to cardiovert (Nejm 2002;347:1825,1834,1883) but no estimates of morbidity outcomes like dyspnea or decreased exercise capacity.

Conversion: Especially if LA size is < 50 mm, use cardioversion; embolic risk post-conversion in 1st 48 hr is ≤ 1% but if > 48 hr is 5-7% (Ann IM 1997;126:65), but if unknown onset and TEE negative, can start warfarin × 4 wk and procede w immediate cardioversion w/o increased embolic risk (Nejm 2001;344:1411)

Medical conversion w:

- Amiodarone 30 mg/kg po ×1 converts 87% (NNT = 2) (Am J Cardiol 2000;85:462; Ann IM 1992;116:1017);
- Propafenone (Rythmol) 450 mg if < 70 kg, 600 mg if > 70 kg po, converts 95% within 6 hr safely (Ann IM 1997; 126:621); or
- Flecainide 200 mg po if < 70 kg, 300 mg if > 70 kg; or
- Ibutilide (Corvert) 1 mg iv over 10 min, repeat ×1 (Nejm 2004;351:2384); or
- Dofetilide 500 mg po bid (Med Let 2000;42:41) perhaps;
- Digoxin alone is no better than placebo (Ann IM 1987; 106:503).

Electrical cardioversion with sync and w transthoracic (AP better than anterior-lateral: Lancet 2003;138:61) or esophageal-transthoracic paddles (R. Fletcher 1/00) if unstable or eventually if meds fail, ok to do even if dig on board as long as levels therapeutic and not toxic, and K^+ ok (Ann IM 1981;95:676); start at 300 J, not lower (Am J Cardiol 2000; 86:348)

Maintenance rx: Amiodarone 200 mg po qd (Arch IM 1998;158:1669; Ann IM 1992;116:1017) cheapest and best (Nejm 2005;352:1861); sotalol or other β-blocker; verapamil; or digoxin, which controls resting but not exercise rate; quinidine? (Nejm 1998;338:37) po, which holds in NSR better but death rate is 3× placebo (Circ 1990;82:1106), or procainamide; possibly dofetilide, esp in CHF (Med Let 2000; 42:41; Nejm 1999;341:857,910); or flecainide but tricky (p 56)

Anticoagulate chronic (Ann IM 2004;141:745, 1999;131:688; Jama 1999;281:182) or intermittent Afib with warfarin to INR > 2 but < 3.5 best balances risk and benefits (Lancet 1996;348:633; Nejm 1996;335:540,587, 1995;333:5), which reduces risk of CVA from 7% to 1-2% at any age at least up to age 85 (NNT-1.5 = 25) (Circ 1991;84:527; Nejm 1990;

323:1505). Annual bleeding risk ~2.5% (Ann IM 1992; 116:6); chronic Afib anticoagulation benefit very small (NNT = 200) (Ann IM 1999;131:492) to nonexistent (Ann IM 1994;121: 41,54) if very low risk: age < 60 yr, no h/o TIA, no valve disease, normal echo, and no hypertension. Use ASA if can't use warfarin (Ann IM 1999;131:492; Nejm 1990;323: 1505) or pt is low risk (Jama 2001;285:2864). Warfarin to INR < 2 is no better than ASA (Nejm 2003;349:1019).

Catheter isolation/ablation of ectopic foci, which are often found in pulmonary veins (Nejm 1998;339:659) or the left atrium. 90% successful and may be 1st choice rx (Jama 2005;293:2634), rarely need chronic antiarrythmics and increases Ef by 20% and thus improves CHF (Nejm 2004;351:2373).

Ablation of AV node w permanent pacer (Nejm 2001;344:1043)

Combined atrial defibrillator/pacer devices (Nejm 2002;346:2062)

- Aflut: Carotid sinus pressure trial, then rx as Afib since > 50% go on to Afib and embolic risk is as great (Ann IM 2004;140:265)
- MFAT: Rx the primary disease, usually COPD or sepsis; verapamil iv with pretreatment with iv $CaCl_2$ (Ann IM 1987; 107:623) or po for chronic; Mg iv, especially if low; β-blockers if no COPD; catheter ablation? (Circ 2002;106:649)
- SSS: Permanent pacer preferably w atrial pacing to reduce emboli (Lancet 1994;344:1523), anticoagulation, then meds to control tachycardias

Wolff-Parkinson-White (WPW) Syndrome

Mod Concepts Cardiovasc Dis 1989;58:43

Cause: Aberrant conduction pathways around the AV node; sometimes are inherited as autosomal dominant single amino acid substitution in a protein kinase gene on chromosome 7 (Nejm 2001; 344:1823), and sometimes are developmental (Nejm 1987; 317:65)

Epidem: Common

Pathophys: Circus movements set up between the atria and ventricle via the aberrant pathway antegrade and/or retrograde, causing the recurrent tachycardias

Sx: Recurrent tachycardias, feel like "butterflies" in the chest. Often precipitated by alcohol, coffee, smoking, and other stimulants.

Si: When asx, none; when in PAT, pulse = 180; or less commonly in Afib, pulse is irregular and fast

Crs (Ann IM 1992;116:456): Recurrent tachycardias over years in $\frac{1}{2}$ found in asx phase; rarely limiting or fatal, 0/20 deaths in Manitoba heart study; disappears over several years in many cases

Cmplc: Sudden death; fatigue

Lab:

Noninv: EKG has a short PR interval (< 0.12 sec, usually < 0.10 sec) with delta wave; type A, most common, has large R in V_1 from an accessory pathway in left lateral atrium (Am J Cardiol 1987;59:1093)

r/o **Lown-Ganong-Levine Syndrome,** similar but no delta wave, ie, no antegrade conduction; Fabry's disease (Nejm 1973;289:357) (See Figure 2.3)

Rx: of PSVT (p 4); Cath lab ablation of accessory pathway if sx, 93% effective contrasts w 33% cure on medical rx (Nejm 2003; 349:1803)

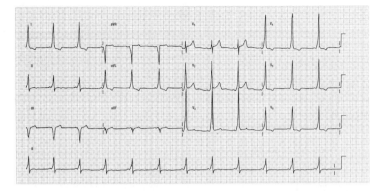

Figure 2.3 WPW EKG. Reproduced with permission from Garcia T, Holtz N. The 12 Lead EKG, The Art of Interpretation. Sudbury, MA: Jones & Bartlett, 2001, p124.

Bradyarrhythmias and Heart Blocks

Nejm 2000;342:703

Cause: Digoxin, ASHD, congenital, granulomatous disease, metastatic calcification (Nejm 1971;284:1252)

Epidem: Rarely associated w HLA-B27 and aortic insufficiency (Ann IM 1997;127:621)

Pathophys: Congenital is associated w maternal autoantibody disease (eg, SLE, Sjögren's), w anti-SSA (Ro antibodies) (Ann IM 1994; 13:544)

Sx: 1st-degree heart block usually causes no sx
2nd-degree heart block may cause dizziness or dyspnea
3rd-degree heart block may cause syncope, especially on
standing

Si: 1st-degree heart block = PR > 0.22 sec
2nd-degree heart block = some unconducted P waves
3rd-degree heart block = no relationship between P waves
and QRS

Crs: 1st-degree heart block usually benign if not associated with organic disease (Nejm 1986;315:1183)

Cmplc: r/o Lyme disease if from endemic area, even if no other sx, w serology, rx with antibiotics and temporary not permanent pacer (Ann IM 1989;110:339)

Athletes' arrhythmias (Sports Med 1998;25:139), eg, 1st- and 2nd-degree (Mobitz I) heart blocks, sinus bradycardia, junctional rythmns; all from increased vagal tone, all go away w exercise and deconditioning

Lab:

Noninv: EKG; Holter monitoring may miss a majority of intermittent heart blocks (Nejm 1989;321:1703)

Mobitz I (Wenkebach) heart block: Intranodal; progressively increase PR, then dropped beat w progressively shortening R-R interval; usually in AV node, especially w digoxin or inferior MI/ischemia, but can occur in SA node (detect by closer and closer R-R intervals), or in distal system if BBB conduction pattern

Mobitz II heart block: Infranodal; fixed PR and dropped beats; R-R intervals of drop are exactly 2× the normal R-R interval, unlike Mobitz I; if several in a row, may have distal escape rhythm; usually going to need permanent pacing; r/o hyperkalemia and rarely meds (procainamide, quinidine, amiodareone) as causes

Rx: 1st degree may not need rx; 2nd and 3rd degree: isoproterenol iv or sl, atropine iv, theophylline 100 mg/min iv up to 250 mg (Ann IM 1995;123:509), or external pacer, until can get transvenous pacemaker

Transvenous pacemaker: Temporary first, then permanent unless inferior MI, which will usually reverse spontaneously. Prophylactic pacers in bifascicular blocks only if 2 or more syncopes, and even then questionable (Nejm 1982;307:137,180). Placement with EKG guidance, sample leads (Nejm 1972;287:651). Coronary sinus placement ok for temporary; tip is seen posteriorly on lateral chest xray.

Permanent pacemaker (rv-Jama 2002;287:1848; Ann IM 2001;134:1130; Nejm 1996;334:89; Mod Concepts Cardiovasc Dis 1991;60:31): Dual-chamber "physiologic" types more expensive, use when need atrial kick (Ann IM 1986;105:264), mainly in pts w sick sinus syndrome (Nejm 2002;346:1854; 1998;338:1097); use may decrease later Afib incidence (Nejm 2000;342:1385)

Table 2.2   Pacer Nomenclature

Chamber Paced	Chamber Sensed	Sensing Mode of Response
Ventricle	V	Triggered
Atrium	A	Inhibited
Dual	D	D
	0 (none)	0 (none)

R is added to designation if rate adaptive capability is present.

Thus a VVI pacer paces the ventricle and senses ventricular beats by inhibiting the next paced beat

Ventricular pacer cmplc: "Pacer syndrome," coincident atrial and ventricular contractions from retrograde atrial activation cause low cardiac output sx (Ann IM 1985;103:420), tachyarrhythmias due to "endless loop" of PVC causing a retrograde P that is sensed, causing a V pace, causing a retrograde P which is sensed, etc; can occur with any sensing pacer. Microwave or cellular phone interference is minimal unless phone is put over pacer (Nejm 1997;336:1473).

Premature Ventricular Contractions, Ventricular Tach, and Sudden Death

Cause: Idiopathic, scar from myocardiopathy (Nejm 1988;318:129) including alcoholic "holiday heart" (Ann IM 1983;98:135), or MI with reentry, CHF, mitral prolapse syndrome, torsades de pointes (p 109)

In children, young adults (Ann IM 2004;141:829; Nejm 1996;334:1039) and athletes (Jama 1996;276:199) most common causes are IHSS (36%), anomalous coronary arteries (13%), and cardiomyopathies; also congenital heart disease esp tetralogy of Fallot and pulmonic stenosis, long QT syndrome, mitral valve prolapse, cocaine, Marfan's w aortic dissection, Kawasaki's induced coronary aneurysms; rarely Vfib induced by "commotio cordis" blow to chest, eg, baseball, hockey puck, or lacross ball, at ascent of T wave (Jama 2002;287:1142; Nejm 1998;338:1805)

Epidem: Increased with tobacco, caffeine (not so: Ann IM 1991;114:147), carbon monoxide levels > 100 ppm (Ann IM 1990;113:343), alcohol (Nejm 1979;301:1049,1060), and subtle ST-T wave electrical alternans (Nejm 1994;330:235). Decreased 50% w weekly fish consumption (Jama 1998;279:23).

Pathophys: Increased sympathetic tone? (Nejm 1991;325:618)

Sx: Syncope that may progress to sudden death

Si: VT is mildly irregular by EKG, unlike very regular PSVT and Aflut with 2:1 block

Crs: of sudden death: 47% 2-yr mortality after first episode; 86% if no MI, 16% if transmural MI (J. Love 2/86; Nejm 1982; 306:1341, 1975;293:259)

If asx, prognosis very good even if complex arrhythmias or VT (Nejm 1985;312:193) even in pts w CHF (Circ 2000;101:40)

of PVCs in asx men: 2× incidence of later MI or other cardiac event (Ann IM 1992;117:990) but frequent PVCs during or immediately after exercise predict double that rate (10% 5-yr mortality: Nejm 2003;348:781)

Cmplc: r/o digoxin toxicity; mitral valve prolapse (p 128); "slow ventricular tachycardia" is a benign regular accelerated idioventricular rhythm < 100/min and asx, seen often in inferior MI;

Lab:

Noninv: EKG

VT: Unlike SVT with aberrancy, Vtach QRSs are wide (85% > 0.14 sec; 0% false positives, 30% false negatives: J. Love 7/86), and are not as regular; however, 5% are ≤ 11 sec because they originate close to the conduction system (Ann IM 1991;114:460)

Brugada criteria (98% overall sensitivity) indicating Vtach rather than SVT w aberrancy (Circ 1991;83:1649):

1. No precordial RS complex, all pos or all neg, ie, monomorphic Rs or QSs (20% sens), or
2. Beginning of any precordial R to S nadir > 0.10 sec (52% sens), or
3. AV dissociation present, or
4. V_{1-6} criteria
   a. RBBB pattern, R/S < 1 and/or Q in V_6 and some positive R forces in V_1; or
   b. LBBB pattern + Q in V_6; and R in $V_{1 \text{ or } 2}$ > 0.04, or beginning of R to S nadir in V_1 or V_2 > 0.06, or notching of S down stroke in V_1 or V_2.

   Holter monitoring w exercise (Nejm 1993;329:445)

Rx: See algorithm for pts w ventricular arrythmias (Jama 1999;281:176)

Field defibrillation with external automatic defibrillator by BCLS personnel increases number who are alive at hospital discharge from 20% to 30% (Seattle: Nejm 1988;319:661), 4% to 5.2% (Ontario: Jama 1999;281:1175), or as high as 75% if provided within 3 min (Nejm 2000;343:1206,1210,1259), eg, by bystanders using EADs in airports, 10/18 neurologically intact 1 yr later (Nejm 2002;347:1242); in elderly > age 70 yr CPR success so low not worth it? (Ann IM 1989;111:199 vs Jama 1990;264:2109). If field trial unsuccessful, not worth continuing in ER (Nejm 1991;325:1393). Antiarrhythmic drug-induced type has the highest incidence within the 1st 3 d, so start drug rx in hospital (Nejm 1988;319:257).

Acutely: If sustained, maybe 1st chest thump; then cardioversion with 200-360 J; amiodarone, procainamide, MgSO4, lidocaine, or sotalol

Chronic (Nejm 1994;331:785; Ann IM 1991;114:499): No clear evidence yet that rx increases survival but β-blockers, esp sotalol, and amiodarone used (Nejm 1998;338:35; Ann IM 1994;121:529); huge natural variability day to day and month to month (Nejm 1985;313:1444)

After sudden death episode, immediate angiography (Nejm 1997;336:1629); try stopping all drugs; then:

- Implantable defibrillator (Nejm 2000;133:901; Med Let 2002;44:99), 1st choice over antiarrhythmics in post–sudden death survivors (Nejm 1997;337:1577; Circ 1995;91:2195); in post-MI pts w EF < 35-40% and documented asx runs of Vtach, this approach decreases the 30% 2-yr mortality by 50-75% (Nejm 1999;341:1882, 1996;335:1933), or from 20% to 14% 20-mo mortality in pts w EF < 30% (Nejm 2002; 346:877) or in any asx pt w EF < 35% using single-lead shock-only ICD, NNT-5 = 14 (Nejm 2005;352:225); cost $30,000

- Antiarrhythmics, debatably (Nejm 1999;341:1882) like β-blockers even if CHF, RAD, DM, elevated lipids (Ann IM 1995;123:358), eg, metoprolol bid (Nejm 1992;327:987), or sotalol (Nejm 1994;331:31), or amiodarone if CHF present? (Nejm 1995;333:77 vs Nejm 2005;352:225)

When to let drive car? No consensus but most states require 6-12 mo asx (Ann IM 1991;115:560), but most pts on rx resume sooner and accident rate lower than general population (Nejm 2001;345:391).

Surgical aneurysectomy rarely

Long QT Syndrome

Nejm 2004;350;1013; 2004;351:1053,1089; 2000;343:352

Cause: Primary types: Most are autosomal dominant; 4 mutations affect cardiac ion channels (Nejm 1998;339:960); some are autosomal recessive (Romano-Ward syndrome: Nejm 1997;336:1562), or with associated deafness (Jervell and Lange-Nielsen syndromes); or sporadic

Secondary type: From quinidine, procainamide, disopyramide (IA antiarrhythmics), sotalol and indapamide (Lozol) especially if used together, amiodarone, diltiazem, verapamil; hypokalemia, hypocalcemia, and hypomagnesemia; arsenic poisoning; nonsedating antihistamines like astemizole (FDA Bull 1992;22:2); macrolides (p 525), moxifoxacin, or ketoconazole-like antibiotics (Jama 1996;275:1339), ciprofloxacin, all protease inhibitors, all antiretrovirals; phenothiazines especially thioridazine (Mellaril) and haloperidol (Haldol) (Ann IM 1993;119:391), tricyclics, lithium, SSRIs, and atypical antipsychotics (p 940) especially clozapine and ziprasidone (Geodon), perhaps methadone in high doses (Ann IM 2002;137:501); tamoxifen; CVAs and other CNS trauma; alcoholism; abnormal liver function tests; liquid protein diet (Ann IM 1985;102:121); anorexia nervosa; vagotomy or endarterectomy; acute MI, myocarditis; mitral valve prolapse; pheochromocytoma

Epidem:

Pathophys: Abnormal K^+ outward or Na^+/Ca^{2+} inward repolarizing currents making susceptible to β-adrenergic-induced instability (Ann IM 1995;122:701; Nejm 1995;333:384). Secondary causes can bring out a primary type. Perhaps due to defective *ras* gene proteins, which normally modulate K pumps in cell membrane (Sci 1991;252:704).

Sx: Often precipitated by fever. Syncope (63%) and sudden death (5%), often swimming (Nejm 1999;341:1121) by hx in autosomal dominant type; deafness in autosomal recessive type. SIDS in children (Nejm 2000;343:262).

Si: Torsades de pointes ventricular tachycardia

Crs: Up to 80% sudden death mortality by age 40 in men w QTc > 500 msec (Nejm 2003;348:1866), reducible to 6% with β-blocker rx?

Cmplc: Sudden death
r/o pheochromocytoma, which can produce the syndrome

Lab:

Chem: PCR analysis to find gene defect in pt and family (Nejm 1999;341:1121)

Noninv: EKG may show torsades de pointes Vtach; between attacks of Vtach, shows QTc > 0.44 sec; in pts w positive family hx, specif 87% in men and 64% in women, sens 95% in men and 100% in women; > 0.47 sec, in men is 100% specif but only 60% sens, in women 98% specif and 90% sens. Holter monitoring for arrhythmia detection.

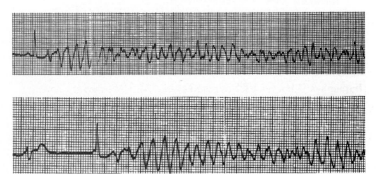

Figure 2.4 Torsades de pointes. Reproduced with permission from Garcia T, Miller G. Arrythmia recognition; the art of interpretation. Sudbury MA: Jones & Bartlett, 2004, p417.

Rx: If sx or documented Vtach by Holter monitoring, stop all drugs and be sure potassium is ok; 1st choice rx = β-blockers (Circ 2000;101: 616), especially propranolol, though not fully protective especially in some genotypes (Jama 2004;292:1341); also used but now less often are phenytoin (Dilantin)/tocainide; pacemaker; left-sided cervicothoracic sympathectomy; automatic defibrillator

of torsades de pointes: 1st choice $MgSO_4$ iv even if not low (Med Let 1991;33:55; Circ 1988;77:392); fix K^+; defibrillate; iv isoproterenol if not congenital type and if no ischemic heart disease; overdrive pacer (Ann IM 1983;99:651)

2.4 Hypertension

Essential Hypertension

Cause: Low calcium, and/or potassium intakes? (Ann IM 1985;103: 825; Sci 1984;224:1392). Genetic by defective angiotensin gene on chromosome 1 (Nejm 1994;330:1629); elevated insulin levels? (Arch IM 1992;152:1649); possibly chronic low level lead exposure (Jama 2003;289:1523; Nejm 2003;348:277; Am J Pub Hlth 1999;89:330).

Epidem: Increased prevalence in blacks; in sleep apnea, especially in older men, is this cause or effect? (Nejm 2000;342:1377); with > 2 drinks of alcohol qd (Ann IM 1986;105:124); with insulin resistance (Nejm 1991;324:723)

Both systolic and diastolic pressures are significant in the elderly (Ann IM 1989;110:901).

Pathophys: Renally secreted prostaglandins protect; renin-aldosterone-angiotensin worsen. Elevated ADH does not increase BP. Calcium and sodium intakes modulate BP via parathyroid hormones and the renin-angiotensin system (Ann IM 1987;107:919), but long-held postulates that HT prevalence in populations is proportionate to their average Na intake are much debated (Sci 1998;281:898,933). Alcohol induces via CRH release (Nejm 1995;332:1733).

Sx: None usually; occasionally epistaxis, headache. Home BPs correlate w control and cmplc better than office values (Jama 2004;291:1342) but leads to undertreatment (Jama 2004;291:955) by RCT

Si: Correct BP-taking technique (Jama 1995;273:1211); mild HT if diastolics 90-105 mm Hg and/or systolics 140-160; moderate, diastolics 105-120 and/or systolics > 160; severe, systolic ≥ 210, diastolics 120+. Use correct cuff size; systolic false increase in elderly due to lead pipe arteries, tell by "Osler's maneuver" (feel artery when occluded above by BP cuff: Nejm 1985;312:1548); r/o white-coat HT present in 20% (Jama 1997;278:1065).

Crs: In elderly, LVH decreases over 6 mo and function improves if rx'd with verapamil, atenolol, or thiazides (Jama 1998;279:778; Nejm 1990;3322:1350) or better w ACEIs as 1st choice, then calcium-channel blockers, then β-blockers and diuretics (Jama 1996;275:1507). Rx of isolated systolic HT (> 160) reduces CVAs by ⅓ (NNT-5 = 33) (Jama 1991;265:3255), stroke mortality by 36%, and cardiac mortality by 25% (Ann IM 1994;121:355), as does rx of systolic and diastolic HT up to age 85 yr (NNT-1 = 75 in preventing death) (Lancet 1995;345:825, 1991;338:1281).

Isolated moderate systolic HT still associated w increased cardiovascular risks of 1.5× (Nejm 1993;329:1912)

Cmplc: Hypertensive crisis (Nejm 1995;332:1029): Papilledema, obtundation and seizures, renal failure; encephalopathy with stroke

Chronic renal failure

Cardiovascular events increase proportionate to systolic and diastolic BP even at 130+/80+ (Nejm 2001;345:1291,1337) including LVH, which, when present, increases risk of MI, CVA, Vtach, death, and sudden death 3-4× more than HT alone (Nejm 1992;327:998, 1987;317:787; Ann IM 1986;105:173); CHF has bad prognosis, 25-30% 5-yr survival (Jama 1996;275:1557)

Diabetes via hypertension-induced insulin resistance (Nejm 1987;317:350)

r/o secondary types of HT (Nejm 1992;327:543): sleep apnea (present in 30%!?) (Nejm 2000;342:1377; Ann IM 1994;120:382, 1985;103:190), alcohol and other drug/medicine use, primary renal disease, renovascular causes including coarctation of the aorta (check coincident radial and femoral pulses, rarely need check temporal and radial in proximal type: Nejm 1973; 288:899), pheochromocytoma, Cushing's, Conn's, toxemia of pregnancy and BCPs, lead-induced renal disease (most "essential hypertensives with creatinine > 1.5 mg %"?: Nejm 1983;309:17), acromegaly

Lab: Routine initial w/u: Urine analysis, K^+, BUN/creatinine, EKG (3-8% sens) or echo (100% sens, ? specif) for LVH; lead level if creatinine > 1.5 mg %, treatable w chelation (Nejm 2003; 348:275)

Urine: microalbumin/creat ratios as predictive of cmplc and survival as in diabetes (Ann IM 2003;139:901)

Noninv: Ambulatory monitoring of questionable value (Ann IM 1993;119:867,889)

Rx: Nondrug regimens (BMJ 1994;309:436; Ann IM 1985; 102:359)

- Increase K^+ intake, natural or supplemental (J Hypertens 1991;9:465; Ann IM 1991;115:753; Nejm 1987;316:235, 1985;312:746,785), especially if on a diuretic to avoid paradoxical elevation of BP from hypokalemia (Ann IM 1991; 115:77)
- Lose weight if obese (Ann IM 2001;134:1), better than Na restriction because fewer adverse sx (Ann IM 1998;128:81); helps in the elderly as well (Jama 1998;279:839)
- Regular aerobic exercise (Nejm 1995;333:1462), although benefit debatable (Jama 1991;266:2098)

- Decrease alcohol (Ann IM 1986;105:124)
- Increase fruit/vegetable fiber and decrease saturated-to-polyunsaturated fat ratio (Nejm 2000;344:3,53, 1997;336:1117)
- Lessen sodium intake to < 3 gm Na qd helps (Ann IM 2001;135:1019,1084), in elderly as well (Arch IM 2001;161:685; Nejm 2001;344:3,53)
- Increase calcium intake, eg, 1 gm po qd at least if deficient (Jama 1996;275:1016) but the effect, though positive, is inconsequential (Ann IM 1996;124:825)
- Perhaps supplemental Mg^{++}
- Avoid or stop NSAIDs (Jama 1994;272:781; Ann IM 1994;121:289), especially indomethacin (Indocin), piroxicam (Feldene), and ibuprofen (Ann IM 1987;107:628)
- Behavior modification of minimal help (Ann IM 1993;118:964)

Drug regimens (p 56; Med Let 2004;46:45): "Go low, go slow" drug rx should follow several mo attempt at nondrug rx if diastolic 90-100 (Ann IM 1992;116:686) but drug rx clearly helpful if persists (Arch IM 1997;157:638).

Stepped care (start with one drug and maximize dose; then add 2nd and later a 3rd from different drug groups sequentially); one drug alone controls 50-66%, two drugs control 90%. Thiazide diuretics and/or β-blockers are the only 2 types shown to help in long-term trials (Arch IM 1997;157:2413, Jama 1997;278:1745).

If appear resistant, first r/o pseudoresistance with home BPs and an echo for LVH (Ann IM 1990;112:278). Overtreatment below diastolic of 85 increases cardiac events and no help for CNS events (Jama 1991;265:489), debatable (Nejm 1992;326:251).

1st: Thiazides usually 1st choice (ALLHAT: Ann IM 2004;141:39; Jama 2002;288:2981,3039) especially in elderly > 60 yr (Jama 2004;292:2849, 1998;279:1903), and even in diabetics (Jama 1996;276:1886); in mild hypertension, old reports that may increase mortality perhaps from hypokalemia, hypomagnesemia, or hyperlipidemia (MRFIT: Jama 1997:277:582, 1983;249:366); erectile dysfunction more common than with ACEIs or β-blockers (Ann IM 1991;114:613); eg, hydrochlorothiazide 25 mg po qd, or w K^+ sparer like amiloride 5-10 mg po qd, better than β-blocker in elderly (BMJ 1992;304:405) or as Dyazide (hydrochlorothiazide 25 mg + triamterene 50 mg) avoids all the MRFIT mortality risks (Ann IM 1995;122:223; Nejm 1994; 330:1852)

1st: β-Blockers; all about same (Med Let 1982;24:44); no significant side effects (DBCT: Am J Med 2000;108:359) although may slightly increase subsequent type 2 diabetes (Nejm 2000; 342:905)

2nd: ACE inhibitors: May best preserve renal function even w early renal failure, eg, enalapril 5 mg po qd-qid (NNT = 4) (BMJ 1994;309:833). Angiotensin II receptor blockers (ARBs) equally good (Nejm 2001;345:851,861,870,910) alone though more expensive, or used w ACEIs (Bmj 2000;321:1440). Mild (< 30%) increase in creatinine w ACEIs or ARBs ok as long as plateau and eventually decrease to baseline (Nejm 2002;347:1256)

3rd: Calcium-channel blockers, long-acting types only, eg, diltiazem SR 60-180 bid (Ann IM 1987;107:150) or long-acting dihydropyridine types like nifedipine (Ann IM 1986; 105:714) but do increase cardiovasc mortality over other combinations (Jama 2004;292:2849)

4th: Direct vasodilators like hydralazine or minoxidil; or andrenergic inhibitors like clonidine, α-methyldopa; or α receptor blockers like prazosin 2-10 mg po bid, or doxazocin but less good than thiazides (Jama 2000;283:1967)

In pregnancy, propranolol ok (Nejm 1981;305:1323); so are hydralazine, α-methyldopa, clonidine; avoid teratogenic ACEIs

In elderly age 65-80, thiazides best monotherapy choice (Jama 1998;279:1903); rx w thiazide or β-blockers clearly helpful so long as no other complicating contraindications, NNT-5 = 18 to prevent MI/CVA (Jama 1994;272:1932); or a dihydropyridine calcium-channel blocker

Rx of isolated systolic HT (Jama 2002;288;1491, 2000;284:465) > 160 to < 160 or decrease by at least 20 mm halves rate of CHF development (NNT-4.5 = 15), MIs, and CVAs over age 60; losartan plus thiazide better than atenolol as measured by mortality, CVAs, etc. Over 80 yr, esp if frail, rx may do more harm than good (ACP J Club 1999;131:29; Lancet 1991;338:1281).

In diabetes, diastolic goal should be 80 mm Hg rather than 85-90 as in other HT pts (Lancet 1998;351:1755; ACP J Club 1998;129:59)

of HT crisis (Nejm 1990;323:1178; Med Let 1989;31:32):

1st: Nitroprusside drip, or fenolopam (Nejm 2001;345:1548; Med Let 1998;40:57) 0.05-0.15 μgm/kg/min drip

2nd: Propranolol 1-3 mg bolus q 5-10 min iv or other β-blocker best; labetalol 20-80 mg over 20 sec up to 300 mg q 10 min iv; diazoxide 50-150 mg iv q 5 min with propranolol 3 mg/hr and/or diuretic; hydralazine 10-20 mg iv × 1; nicardipine iv drip

Then, po nifedipine, clonidine, captopril, etc

Nifedipine 10 mg sl with pinholed capsule used in the past but no studies show helpful benefits and definite substantial complications (Jama 1996;276:1328)

Renovascular Hypertension

Nejm 2001;344:431

Cause: Atherosclerosis of renal arteries w renal artery stenosis (90%), renal artery fibromuscular hyperplasia (10%) (Nejm 2004;350:1862), coarctation of aorta, other intrinsic renal disease

Epidem: 0.2-4% of all hypertensives

Pathophys: Decreased flow to the renal juxtaglomerular apparatus causes renin production leading to angiotensin II (8-peptide), which causes arterial constriction, which increases aldosterone

Sx: None usually, unless hypertension severe; then headache, CHF sx, epistaxis

Si: Coarctation lacks coincident radial and femoral pulses, rarely need to check temporal and radial in proximal type (Nejm 1973;288:899)

Hemorrhages and exudates in fundi; 30% of patients with them have renovascular hypertension (Nejm 1979;301:1273)

Abdominal bruit present in 60% (40% false neg), but 28% of all hypertensives have, so specif ≤ 35% (65% false pos) (Nejm 1967;276:1175); others find higher specificity (90%), and if restrict to continuous bruits, sens = 40%, specif = 99% (Jama 1995;274:1299)

Crs:

Cmplc: Like essential hypertension

Lab (Ann IM 1992;117:845):

Chem: Peripheral plasma renin (50-80% sens, 85% specif) with coincident urine Na^+, most useful if low since can then stop w/u; or renin levels before and after po captopril challenge show an increase to above 12 μgm/L/hr; if creatinine < 1.5 mg %, sens ≥ 75%, specif ≥ 90%. Uric acid elevated (Ann IM 1980; 93:817). Hypokalemia; urinary K^+ < 60 mEq/24 hr after 3 d of 4+ gm Na diet (G. Aagaard, 1969).

Xray: Renal scan (scintigraphy) before and after captopril 50 mg po shows decreased flow in affected kidney, 90% sens/specif (Ann IM 1992;117:845; Jama 1992;268:3353) vs 72% sens, 90% specif (Ann IM 1998;129:705)

Duplex ultrasound if hard-to-control HT and azotemia and/or peripheral vascular disease, 98% sens/specif (Ann IM 1995;122:883); can also use to calculate a renal artery resistance index to decide between angioplastic or surgical repair (Nejm 2001;344:410)

Angiography, digital subtraction type, is the gold standard, whereas MRA and CTA are < 65% sens, 84-92% specif (Ann IM 2004;141:674 vs 730)

Rx: Medical rx as good or better than angioplasty or perhaps even surgery (Nejm 2000;342:1007) when cause is atherosclerosis, unlike fibromuscular hyperplasia. ACEIs 1st choice, to BP < 140/90 (Jama 2002;288:2421).

Percutaneous transluminal angioplasty (Nejm 1997;336:459) w stenting

Surgical correction even in face of diminished renal function may help both BP and function (Nejm 1984;311:1070). In coarctation, pretreat with propranolol to prevent post-op hypertension (Nejm 1985;312:1224).

Pheochromocytoma

Ann IM 2001;134:315; Nejm 1992;327:1009

Cause: Neoplasia of adrenal or extraadrenal autonomic ganglia; genetic transmission often as an autosomal dominant

Epidem: 75% are isolated cases; 25% are associated with autosomal dominant detectable oncogenetic defects (Nejm 2002;346:1459, 1486) causing MEN type IIa (Sipple's syndrome) (Nejm 1996; 335:943; Jama 1995;274:1149), which includes medullary carcinoma of the thyroid, bilateral pheochromocytomas, parathyroid adenomas (10%), and mucosal neuromas (10%); rarely are associated with MEA type IIb (pheochromocytoma, gi ganglioneuromatosis, and Marfanoid habitus), or von Recklinghausen's disease, or von Hippel-Lindau disease (retinal angiomas, CNS hemangiomas, renal cysts, and cancer) where 19% have pheo (Nejm 1993;329:1530)

Pathophys: Epinephrine and norepinephrine are released, as well as precursors in malignant types. Rule of 10s: 10% are familial; 10% are bilateral; 10% are extra-adrenal (D. Oppenheim 2/91).

Sx: Pheo triad: paroxysmal (lasts minutes to hours; in 50%) palpitations, perspiration, and pain (headache, chest, and abdominal); 55/76 pheo's had at least $^2/_3$; 3/76 had none. Weight loss, anxiety, tremor, diarrhea (Nejm 1975;293:155), nausea and vomiting, weakness. Only 9% have no sx at all.

Si: Orthostatic systolic BP drop (already maximally constricted); hypertension (60% chronically; 40% have only with attacks); circumoral pallor

Crs:

Cmplc: Myocarditis and cardiomyopathy, diabetes, CVA, malignant degeneration in 10%
    r/o baroreflex failure w episodic hypertensive spells if h/o neck surgery (Nejm 1993;329:1449,1494)

Lab:

Chem: Plasma free metanephrines—99% sens, 89% specif (Jama 2002;287:1427)—and normetanephrins 1st choice. Plasma catechols > 2000 pgm/cc, supine 30 min after needle placed; best test, 5-10% false negatives, no false positives. Clonidine suppression test if plasma catechols 1000-2000 pgm/cc: 0.3 mg po with plasma norepinephrine level before and at 3 hr; all normals suppress to < 300 pgm/cc (Nejm 1981; 305:623).

    24-hr urine metanephrines, 5% false pos, 2% false neg, 50% pos predictive value, or as metnephrine/creatinine ratio > 0.354 is even better (Ann IM 1996;125:300)

Table 2.3   Sensitivity and Specificity of Biochemical Tests for Diagnosis of Pheochromocytoma

Biochemical Test	Sensitivity (%)	Specificity (%)	Sensitivity at 100% Specificity
Plasma metanephrine level	99	89	82
Plasma catecholamine level	85	80	38
Urinary catecholamine level	83	88	64
Urinary metanephrine level	76	94	53
Urinary vanillylmandelic acid level	63	94	43

The sensitivities of tests of plasma metanephrines or plasma and urinary catecholamines were determined, respectively, as the percentage of patients with pheochromocytoma who had positive test results for normetanephrine or metanephrine or for norepinephrine or epinephrine. The specificities of tests of plasma metanephrines or plasma and urinary catecholamines were determined as the percentage of patients without pheochromocytoma who had negative test results for both normetanephrine and metanephrine or for both norepinephrine and epinephrine. The sensitivities and specificities of tests of urinary metanephrines reflect tests of urinary total metanephrines (that is, the combined sum of free plus conjugated normetanephrine and metanephrine). The sensitivities at 100% specificity indicate the percentage of patients with pheochromocytoma in whom test results are so high that they unequivocally confirm the presence of a pheochromocytoma. These sensitivities were determined by increasing the upper reference limits for each test to levels at which no patient without pheochromocytoma had a positive test result. Sensitivity was determined for tests in 151 patients, and specificity was determined for tests in 349 patients. Reproduced with Permission from Pacak K, et al. Recent Advances in Genetics, Diagnosis, Localization, and Treatment of Pheochromocytoma. Ann Int Med 2001;134:318

VMA, 20-60% false neg; catechols, especially free norepinephrines, 80-100% sens, 98% specif (Nejm 1988; 319:136)

Xray: CT of adrenals picks up if > 1 cc in size (92% sens, 80% specif) MRI may better distinguish malignant from benign pheos

Rx: Volume replete the usually huge deficits, eg, 10+ L
Meds:

- Phentolamine 5 mg iv gives a short effect
- Nitroprusside drip for rapid control or during surgery
- Phenoxybenzamine 40-100 mg po qd, beware of lowered insulin requirements
- Prazocin 2-5 mg po bid, then propranolol
- Metyrosine 0.25-1 gm po in qid doses (Med Let 1980;22:28)
    Surgical removal under a blockade, eg, with phenoxybenzamine or prazosin and with huge volume replacement
    of malignant pheo: Combination chemotherapy (Ann IM 1988;109:267)

2.5   Endo/Peri/Myocarditis

Endocarditis, Subacute and Acute Bacterial

Nejm 2001;345:1318

Cause: *Strep. viridans;* pneumococcus; *Staph. aureus* (usually acute bacterial endocarditis); coag-negative staph; enterococcus; nonenterococcal group D strep often initially misidentified as enterococcus; and rarely anaerobes, fungi, gram negatives, lactobacillus, psittacosis organism (Nejm 1992;326:1192), and other unusual organisms (Nejm 1992;326:1215) like *Bartonella sp.* (Ann IM 1996;125:646)

Epidem: 4000-8000 cases/yr in U.S.; 75% in pts w abnormal or prosthetic valves. Increased in patients with mitral valve prolapse syndrome, congenital (VSD, PDA, tetralogy of Fallot) heart disease especially aortic stenosis both repaired and unrepaired (1.5-20% at 30 yr) (Jama 1998;279:599), rheumatic heart disease even when given SBE prophylaxis before dental work and surgical procedures (Jama 1983;250:2318), HIV disease, hemodialysis, diabetes, and poor dental hygiene

Pathophys: < 5% are right-sided; higher in iv drug users. Renal damage: diffuse vasculitis, focal "embolic" glomerulonephritis, and renal infarction.

Sx: Fever (98%), hematuria (29%), weight loss

Si: Murmur (85% at presentation, 99% eventually; 66% in right-sided type); splenomegaly and/or infarction (25-50%); mucosal petechiae and splinter hemorrhages in nails (29%); clubbing (13%); Roth spots in fundi (2%); Osler's nodes in finger tips

Crs: 100% die without rx; 80% 10-yr survival w rx (Ann IM 1992;117:567)

Cmplc: CHF (25%) due to chordae rupture and myocarditis; peripheral systemic arterial emboli, mostly with *Strep. viridans* type (Ann IM 1991;114:635); pulmonary emboli (60% in right-sided type); CNS including TIA, CVA, mycotic aneurysm, abscess, encephalopathy, and bacterial as well as aseptic meningitis); renal failure

r/o acute rheumatic fever, collagen vascular disease, acute glomerulonephritis, marantic endocarditis. And **atrial myxoma** (Nejm 1995;333:1610): Rare; occasionally familial; left/right = 4:1; pedunculated lesion causes sx when plugs or extends through AV valve making it stenotic or insufficient; sudden CHF sx, cachexia, anemia, fever; murmur can be unusual, variable, or mimic MS or MR; may have the clinical picture of SBE; cmplc: peripheral emboli, complete stenosis of AV valve, FUO; find w echo (Nejm 1970;282:1022), ESR markedly elevated; rx w surgical removal.

Lab:

Bact: Blood cultures (Ann IM 1993;119:270), 10 cc ×3 adequate unless given antibiotics in past 2 wk, then should do ×5 (Ann IM 1987;106:246); positive in 80%; if negative, r/o murantic (thrombotic type seen in cancer patients), brucella, anaerobes, rickettsial Q fever, and fungi like histo and aspergilla; if *Strep. faecalis* (an enterococcus) reported by the lab, r/o *Strep. bovis,* often so misidentified, associated with colon cancer (Nejm 1973;289:1400), and very sensitive to penicillin

Hem: Crit < 38% (50%); ESR up (80%)

Noninv: Echocardiograms (Nejm 2001;345:1318): transthoracic 80% positive, 20% false negative; transesophageal echo 90±% sens and specif (Nejm 1991;324:795, 1990;323:165)

Serol: RA titer positive (50%) (Ann IM 1968;68:746); low C_3 complement

Urine: rbc's (95%: K. Holmes, 1971; 29%: L. Weinstein, 1987)

Rx: Prophylaxis (p 609)

Therapeutic antibiotics (Jama 1995;274:1706): For *Strep. viridans* and *bovis,* penicillin or ceftriaxone or vancomycin iv × 4 wk or penicillin iv + aminoglycoside × 2 wk; for *Staph. aureus,* nafcillin or oxacillin or cefazolin or vancomycin + debatably 3-5 d gentamicin (Ann IM 1996;125:969 vs Ann IM 1982;97:496); for *Staph. albus,* gentamicin + rifampin + vancomycin (Ann IM 1983;98:447); for *Enterococcus faecalis,* penicillin or ampicillin/vancomycin + aminoglycoside × 4 wk unless sx > 3 mo or on mitral valve, in which case rx for 6 wk (Ann IM 1984;100:816)

Surgical interventions rarely needed except for valve ruptures and infections of implanted valves (Ann IM 1982;96:650) but over time (10 yr) 25% of mitral and 60% of aortic valves need surgery (Ann IM 1992;117:567)

Pericarditis

Nejm 2004;351:2195; Jama 2003;289:1150

Cause: Acute: 90% are idiopathic; also uremic, bacterial from a subdiaphragmatic abscess (Nejm 1967;276:1247), post-MI, viral especially coxsackie, postsepticemic (Ann IM 1973;79:194), mycoplasma (Ann IM 1977;86:544), or malignancy invading pericardium

Chronic: Tuberculosis, sarcoid

Epidem: Coxsackie viral type probably is the most common cause and occurs in late summer and fall like other enteroviruses

Pathophys: The stiffening causes restriction of ventricular diastolic filling; increased heart rate must compensate for decreased stroke volume; can tolerate 1-3 L if slowly accumulates, only 300-400 cc if rapid accumulation

Paradoxical pulse if constrictive (exaggeration > 10 mm Hg of normal drop of systolic BP with inspiration) due to impaired venous return and normal increased pulmonary vascular volume w inspiration (Mod Concepts Cardiovasc Dis 1978;47:109,115)

Sx: Dyspnea; chest pain, often pleuritic and better when sits up

Si: Ascites, poor heart sounds, no PMI, tachycardia; pleural effusions on left more often and larger than on right, unlike CHF (Nejm 1983;308:696)

In constrictive pericarditis: Increased CVP with Kussmaul's si, r/o RV infarction; rapid Y descent and rebound, r/o infiltrating myocardiopathy, eg, amyloid. Paradoxical pulse > 10 mm Hg, r/o asthma, RV myocardial infarction (Nejm 1983;309:551).

Crs:

Cmplc: Pericardial tamponade

Lab:

Noninv: EKG ST elevation and/or PR depressions in limb and precordial leads, which exclude early repolarization; early repolarization usually has precordial lead (ST's) or limb (PR's) involvement only; T's invert only after ST's back to normal. May show electrical alternans, ie, alternate QRSs have higher and lower voltages.

Echo shows pericardial fluid and and may show tamponade hemodynamics

Xray: Chest shows large heart, "boot-shaped." CT may show calcifications in 27% of constrictive types, usually chronic, $^2/_3$ w/o a dx, occasionally is tbc (Ann IM 2000;132:444)

Rx: ASA, ibuprofen, or other NSAID rx, avoiding indomethacin and/or steroids especially if ASHD and recent MI (Circ 1996;94:2341), and colchicine 0.6 mg po bid

If constrictive, tap under echo or EKG guidance; pulmonary edema can develop if tap too much too fast, leading to an overload of a deconditioned heart (Nejm 1983;309:595); if constrictive and chronic, surgical pericardectomy

Myocarditis/Dilated Cardiomyopathies

Nejm 2000;343:1388; 1994;331:1564

Cause:

- Arrythmias: Ectopic atrial and permanent junctional reentrant tachycardias, reversible cardiomyopathy if ablate focus (R. Fletcher 1/00)
- Collagen vascular: SLE, polyarteritis nodosa, endocardial fibroelastosis (occasionally seen in children due to a treatable inherited carnitine deficiency: Nejm 1981;305:385), sarcoid, carcinoid (last 2 may be restrictive and/or congestive)
- Deficiencies: Hypophosphatemia from antacid binding, reversible (Ann IM 1978;89:867); thiamine (beriberi), selenium, carnitine
- Endocrine: Thyrotoxicosis (Nejm 1982;307:1165) and hypothyroidism; pheochromocytoma (Nejm 1987;316:793); homocystinuria (p 317), hypocalcemia
- Lymphocytic myocarditis (Nejm 1997;336:1860)
- Idiopathic ($< 50\%$)
- Infectious from any severe bacteremia, eg, meningococcal, diphtheria, mycoplasma (Ann IM 1977;86:544); viral includ-

ing CMV, influenza, echo, coxsackie B, yellow fever, mumps, polio, rubella, HIV (Nejm 1998;339:1093); parasites including toxoplasma, Chagas' disease

- Ischemic
- Genetic neurologic/myopathic (30%): Friedreich's ataxia; dyskalemic myopathies; muscular dystrophies including limb girdle, Emery-Dreifuss (Ann IM 1993;119:900), and myotonic; Refsum's disease; familial sarcomere protein gene mutations (Nejm 2000;343:1688) and other autosomal dominant genetic causes affecting cellular function (Nejm 1999;341:1715, 1996;335:1224)
- Peripartum (Nejm 2001;344;1567, 1629): Onset 1 mo prior or up to 6 mo postpartum w variable outcomes but usually some residual dysfunction
- Toxic agents: Alcohol (Ann IM 1974;80:293; Nejm 1972;287:677), daunorubicin (Daunomycin) (p 443) and bleomycin, cobalt in beer (Ann IM 1969;70:277), arsenic (p 26); lead, cocaine, mercury, carbon monoxide, phenothiazines; most reversible except chemotherapy drugs

Epidem: Idiopathic type prevalence = 36/100,000 (Circ 1989;80:564): blacks/whites = 2.5/1; males/females = 25/1

Pathophys: Dilation of both ventricles; mural thrombi

Sx: CHF sx's; muscle weakness in alcoholic type since 83% have skeletal myopathy as well (Ann IM 1994;120:529)

Si: Afib and other supraventricular arrhythmias; S_3 gallop (Ann IM 1969;71:545); CHF si's

Crs (Nejm 2000;342:1077): Often chronic and indolent; in alcoholic type, it can rapidly resolve with abstinence. Postpartum type has best prognosis (90% 5-yr survival); idiopathic, ischemic, daunorubicin, and infiltratives types = 50% 5-yr mortality; HIV type = 25% 3-yr mortality

Cmplc: Systemic emboli from mural thrombi and Afib

r/o hypertrophic (IHSS); "hibernating myocardium," ie, ischemic myocardopathy reversible w revascularization (Nejm 1998;339:173); **restrictive myocardiopathies** (Nejm 1997; 336:267): amyloid, hemachromatosis, familial, idiopathic, endomyocardial fibrosis, eosinophilic cardiomyopathy, sarcoid, Gaucher's, Fabry's, and Hurler's disease; and **"stress stunning,"** transient myocardopthy seen in grieving widows w dramatic T-wave changes (Nejm 2005;352:534)

Lab:

> *Noninv:* EKG may show Afib (20%), cloven T waves especially in alcoholic type (Ann IM 1969;71:545), arrhythmias, blocks, Q waves, or LVH. Echocardiogram most helpful, EF < 45%.
>
> *Path:* Endocardial bx (Nejm 1982;307:732) in peripartum and all types to dx infiltrative disease; not helpful in dilated types, IHSS, Wilson's disease, etc (complete list: Ann IM 1982;97: 885; Nejm 1983;308:12); but does not correlate well with clinical findings or prognosis (Nejm 1985;312:885)

Rx: Anticoagulate acutely and chronically; prednisone rx even when inflammatory by bx is no help (Nejm 1989;321:1061) or even w additional immunosuppressive drugs (Nejm 1995;333:269); perhaps human growth hormone 4 IU sc qod (Nejm 1996;334:809, 856); transplantation

> of CHF: vasodilators
>
> of ventricular arrythmias: Improve EF w digoxin, ACEIs, β-blockers, amiodarone (Mayo Clin Proc 1998;73:430), implantable cardioverter/defibrillator prolongs life in non-ischemic type (Nejm 2004;350:2152)

Hypertrophic Cardiomyopathy (Idiopathic Hypertrophic Subaortic Stenosis)

Nejm 2004;350:1320; Jama 2002;287:1308

Cause: Genetic, over 10 different mutations can cause, one on chromosome 14 (Nejm 1992;326:1108, 1989;321:1372), autosomal dominant with nearly complete penetrance when measure thickness of interventricular septum (Ann IM 1986;105:610)

Epidem: Prevalence = 1/500; male/female = 4:1 in sporadic type, but equal in genetic type (E. Braunwald, 1978); higher incidence in Fabry's disease (Nejm 1982;307:926)

Pathophys: 50% due to mutations in the myosin heavy-chain gene (Nejm 1992;326:1108, 1991;325:1753). Abnormal intraventricular septum produces dynamic aortic root obstruction and subaortic stenosis; mitral regurgitation is due to anterior mitral leaflet being distorted by the septum; obstruction is worsened by diuresis and vasodilators, and increases in contractility, eg, by digoxin, PVCs, catechols, and exercise. Reentrant PVCs because of different refractory periods in different muscle groups (Nejm 1980;302:97). Increased calcium channels increase the muscle sensitivity and contraction strength (Nejm 1989;320:755). Myocardial bridging of epicardial coronary arteries also occurs (Nejm 1998;339:1201) and causes myocardial ischemia/infarcts and coronary microvascular dysfunction (Nejm 2003;349:1027).

Sx: Onset age 15-46 yr, positive family hx in $\frac{1}{3}$ (E. Braunwald, 1978); syncope (3/18), dyspnea (13/18), chest pain (7/18), angina that starts when exercise stopped, palpitations

Si: LVH by palpation and double PMI, with diphasic arterial systolic peak murmur
   Aortic murmur without radiation into neck (Nejm 1988;318:1575), decreases with leg elevation and squatting, which increase venous return; worse with isoproterenol, exercise, standing, amyl nitrite inhalation, alcohol ingestion, and Valsalva maneuver

Crs: Two types: slowly progressive and generally benign (Jama 1999;281:650; Nejm 1989;320:749); and "malignant," with premature death in young adulthood w myosin heavy-chain mutation (Nejm 1992;326:1108). Outlet obstruction makes prognosis worse (Nejm 2003;348:295).

Cmplc: Sudden death by Vtach/Vfib (Nejm 1988;318:1255) correlates w LV wall thickness (Nejm 2000;342:1778); Afib in 20-
25%; endocarditis

r/o **"athlete's heart"** w LV wall thickness always
< 16 mm, rarely > 13 mm (Nejm 1991;324:295), which overlaps
w IHSS in men but not in women (Jama 1996;276:210); and
glycogen storage disease hypertrophic cardiomyopathy (Nejm
2005;352:362)

r/o causes of sudden death in athletes (Nejm 1998;339:364):
cardiomyopathy (22%), ASCVD 15%), anomalous coronary
artery (12%), IHSS (2%) (see screening cardiac exam p 926)

Lab:

Noninv: EKG shows LVH, big Qs in V_{1-2} (hypertrophied septum)
Holter monitoring for malignant PVCs. Nonspecific
EKG changes occur in affected children before echo changes
(Nejm 1991;325:1753).

Echo shows hypertrophied septum and LV wall and systolic anterior motion of mitral valve; Doppler shows subvalvular gradient

Path: Endocardial bx shows chaotic muscular disorder (Nejm
1977;296:135). Genetic PCR studies of peripheral lymphocytes can detect in presymptomatic stage (Nejm
1991;325:1753).

Xray: Chest shows LVH

Rx (Jama 2002;287:1308): Avoid competitive sports
Avoid digoxin, diuretics, catechols, alcohol (Nejm
1996;335:938), nitrates and other vasodilators
Implantable cardiovertor defibrillator (ICD) (Nejm
2000;342:365,422) to prevent Vtach/sudden death; cardioverts
11%/yr when used as secondary (after VT) and 5% as primary
prevention in high-risk pts
Antiarrythmic rx, not justified in asymptomatic pts by efficacy trials

Iatrogenic anteroseptal MI effective (Njem 2002;347:1326) but often causes complete heart block, 50% need pacer

Surgical myotomies when resting obstruction > 75 mm or class II sx despite medical rx; 80% success (Ann IM 1972;77:515); dual-chamber pacing; and angiographic septal ablation?

of CHF: Neg inotropes like β-blockers, verapamil (Mod Concepts Cardiovasc Dis 1990;59:1; Ann IM 1982;96:670), disopyramide (Norpace: Nejm 1982;307:997) 150-200 mg po qid

of Afib: Amiodarone and warfarin anticoagulation

2.6   Valvular Heart Disease

Mitral Valve Prolapse Syndrome

Nejm 1989;320:1234; Ann IM 1989;111:305

Cause: Genetic, autosomal dominant; decreased penetrance in males; less frequent over age 50 yr

Epidem: Associated with various inherited connective tissue diseases, including Ehler-Danlos syndrome, Marfan's, osteogenesis imperfecta, pseudoxanthoma elasticum (Nejm 1982;307:369), and von Willebrand's disease (Nejm 1981;305:131). Prevalence < 2.5% in adults (Framingham: Nejm 1999;341:1,8).

Pathophys: Abnormal cordae and valve, not papillary muscle. Atrial muscle in valve may also produce electrical atrial and ventricular bypass tracts and reentrant arrhythmias (Nejm 1982;307:369).

Sx: Palpitations (premature junctional beats, PACs, PVCs), anxiety often leads to discovery although no more prevalent in anxious pts than in normals

Si: Midsystolic click (92%), late systolic murmur (85%) that moves toward S$_1$ with standing or other decrease in venous return. Tricuspid prolapse may occur too (6/13: Nejm 1972;287:1218).

Crs: Same as matched controls at Mayo (Nejm 1985;313:1305); 90% 10-yr survival, < 10% get major cmplc

Cmplc: Sudden death rarely (2.5% at Mayo?: Nejm 1985;313:1305); PVCs associated with sx, present in 16% of children with Barlow's on ETT (J Peds 1984;105:885); endocarditis (1% at Mayo-Nejm 1985;313:1305; 3%: Nejm 1989;320:1031); CVA/TIAs (Nejm 1980;302:139) vs no incr rates (Nejm 1999;341:8); Graves' disease (Nejm 1981;305:497); valvular insufficiency requiring surgery in 6% (Nejm 1989;320:1031)

r/o benign MVP w insignificant mitral regurgitation = $^2/_3$ of all w MVP (Nejm 1989;320:1031)

Lab:

Noninv: EKG normal in 76%; may show "inferior ischemia" or PVCs

Echocardiogram

Rx: SBE prophylaxis when mitral regurgitation present (ie, a murmur)

Propranolol or other β-blocker rarely needed

Surgical valve replacement occasionally (< 5%) necessary if severe mitral regurgitation, esp in men > 60 yr

Valvular Heart Disease

Nejm 1997;336:32

Including aortic stenosis (AS), aortic insufficiency (AI), mitral stenosis (MS), mitral regurgitation (MR) (Nejm 2001;345:740), tricuspid stenosis (TS), and tricuspid insufficiency (TI)

Cause: Many are rheumatic (p 1082)

Epidem: AS most common in elderly now; MS/MI in females age 20-40; TS/TI always accompanies mitral or aortic disease but occurs in only 2-4% of patients with rheumatic heart disease (RHD)

Pathophys: Rheumatic pancarditis causes chordae fibrosis and shortening, and valvular vegetations at points of trauma. MS always present in RHD to some degree; hemoptysis in MS is due to shunts from pulmonary veins to bronchial veins. 70% of all patients with chronic MR in the 1960s was due to RHD, while 30% was due to chordae rupture from MI, endocarditis, and trauma. Severe AI alone rarely is due to RHD; usually from trauma, syphilis, dissecting aneurysm, endocarditis, SLE, RA, ankylosing spondylitis. AS now rarely (10%) is due to RHD; most is calcific aortic stenosis on bicuspid or previously normal valves.

Sx: MS: Exertional dyspnea, orthopnea, hemoptysis
MR: Exertional dyspnea, orthopnea
AS: Angina, CHF, syncope
AI: Gradual CHF sx

Si: MS: Afib; mid-diastolic murmur with presystolic accentuation even in Afib (Nejm 1971;285:1284); opening snap; loud S_1
MR: Loud systolic murmur, radiates to axilla
AS: CHF, loud systolic murmur radiates into carotids and left shoulder (uniquely); worsens with amyl nitrite inhalation in contrast to MR and VSD
AI: Early diastolic murmur; this typical murmur is present in 73% (sens), and is heard only 8% of the time in patients who lack AI (92% specif-Ann IM 1986;104:599). Austin-Flint murmur of functional MS narrowed by AI regurgitant jet. Very soft S_1 as mitral valve floats closed from the AI and indicating urgent need for surgery.

Crs: MS: Slow progression
MR: Even if asx, if severe, has a 40% 5-yr mortality (Nejm 2005;352:875)
AS: If heavily calcified, < 0.02 cm² but asx, 80% 4-yr mortality (Nejm 2000;343:611,652); after angina, 50% survive 5 yr; after syncope, 50% survive 3 yr; after CHF, 50% survive 2 yr

Cmplc: MS: CHF, SBE, emboli
AS: Angina, sudden death, CHF, gi angiodysplasia with gi bleed disappears after valve replacement (Ann IM 1986;105:54).

After onset of any of the 3 sx, mortality is 75% at 3 yr unless valve replaced (Mayo Cl Proc 1987;62:986).

Lab:

Cardiac cath: MS significant valve diameter < 1.2 cm$_2$, no sx if > 2.5 cm^2 (L. Cobb, 1971). AS critical if < 0.07 cm^2/M^2 (Nejm 1997;336:32).

Noninv: 2-D echo and Doppler for valves, chamber sizes, and estimates of valve diameters or regurgitation amounts; in AI, $> 90\%$ sens/specif (Ann IM 1986;104:599)

Xray: Chest: in MS, shows large left atrium, pulmonary artery, and right ventricle, and may show valvular calcifications; in AS, may show 4-chamber enlargement, valvular calcifications usually only with significant disease

Rx: MR: Repair before EF $< 60\%$ or end diastolic ventricular dimension < 45 mm; if due to full flail leaflet, repair sooner rather than later since prognosis w/o repair poor (Nejm 1996; 335:1417)

MS: May do closed commissurotomy or percutaneous catheter commissurotomy via interatrial septum (Nejm 1994;331:961), which may diminish embolization if done early (Ann IM 1998;128:885); valve replacement if calcifications/clot, porcine (Nejm 1981;304:258) or bovine pericardium w higher structural failure rates vs mechanical w higher bleeding cmplc (Nejm 1993;328:1289). Control Afib w digoxin or β-blocker; anticoagulate w warfarin especially if Afib, concomitant AI, or clot by echo (Ann IM 1998;128:885)

AI: Nifedipine po long term reduces/delays LV dysfunction development and consequent valve replacement (Nejm 1994;331:689,736). Repair before EF $< 55\%$ or end diastolic ventricular dimension < 55 mm.

AS: Valve replacement if angina, CHF, or syncope; even in elderly pts if healthy (Nejm 1988;319:169; Ann IM 1989;110:421), and perhaps before sx develop of CHF: Anticoagulate if platelet survival < 3 d (Nejm 1974;290:537) or evidence of emboli; rheumatic fever penicillin prophylaxis; SBE prophylaxis

Surgical: Valve choices (Nejm 1996;335:407); w mechanical valve replacement, ideal protime INR is 3-4 or 3-5 for maximal benefit/risk ratio (Nejm 1995;333:11); w bioprosthetic valves, warfarin to INR = 2-3 × 3 mo, then just ASA unless other embolic risk factors like Afib, dyskinetic segment, etc; in pregnancy after valve replacement, warfarin is teratogenic in 1st trimester (25%) so heparin is used but is less than adequate anticoagulation (Nejm 1986;315:1390) and usually combined w ASA (for normal and abnormal heart sounds w various valves, see table in Nejm 1996;335:410)

2.7 Congenital Heart Disease

Atrial Septal Defects: Primum and Secundum Types

Nejm 2000;342:256

Cause: Congenital malformations

Epidem:

Primum: 1-2% of all CHD; most common type of CHD in Down's syndrome (25%)

Secundum: 10-15% of all CHD; associated w anomalous pulmonary venous return

Pathophys:

Primum: AV canal defects including low ASD, high VSD, cleft mitral and/or tricuspid valves, or even a common AV valve

Secundum: Mid or upper ASD allows left to right shunt; many are functional patent foramen ovales, ie, only open if sudden increase in right-sided pressures

Sx:

   Primum: Dyspnea, fatigue, pulmonary infections, and CHF in infancy in complete form, later in incomplete types

   Secundum: Rarely any in infancy or childhood; later dyspnea w CHF and pulmonary HT, palpitations if arrhythmias

Si:

   Primum: Cyanosis mild or absent. Harsh systolic murmur, apical, pansystolic from MR (33%), TI or VSD (75%). P_2 increased; splitting present; CHF; RVH.

   Secundum: Mild systolic murmur (pulmonic) at upper-left sternal border; mid-diastolic rumble at lower-left sternal border from high flow. S_2 wide and fixed; RVH.

Crs:

   Primum: Complete types cause CHF in infancy and death in 1-2 yr if not repaired; incomplete types get sx later, but survive less well than secundum types

   Secundum: Occasionally CHF sx in 2nd-3rd decade; or may be asx throughout adult life, but overall decrease in life expectancy

Cmplc:

   Primum: CHF, pulmonary hypertension, supraventricular arrhythmias (Aflut or Afib) especially if surgically closed after age 40 (Nejm 1999;340:839), SBE rarely, increased incidence of rheumatic fever; r/o partial anomalous pulmonary venous return

   Secundum: CHF and pulmonary HT late; strokes, multiple in patent foramen oval pts, esp in underwater divers (Ann IM 2001;134:21)

Lab: *Noninv:* Primum: EKG: left axis, pRBBB, RVH and LVH, counterclockwise rotation

   Secundum: EKG axis normal or RAD, partial and full RBBB, RVH and strain; clockwise rotation

Echo: diagnostically abnormal in 90% (Ann IM
1976;84:246) w Doppler, in 100% w TEE

Xray:

Primum: Chest shows small aortic knob; RVH and increased pulmonary flow. If MR, then large left atrium and LV.
Angiography shows "gooseneck deformity" of LV outflow
tract; serated mitral valve leaf; rest depends on particular
variant.

Secundum: Chest shows small aortic knob; RHV + increased pulmonary flow; no LA enlargement unlike patent ductus or VSD

Rx:

Primum: Surgical early if sx; can't if fixed pulmonary hypertension. Open repair or pulmonary artery banding in infants
with severe sx. Operative mortality: 40% if complete, 15% if
partial. Do it at age 5+ ideally. Cmplc: complete heart
block.

Secundum: Open repair with bypass at age 5+ if shunt > 1.5
ratio, > 95% 10-yr survival even in adults > 40 yr (Nejm
1995;333:469); can't if significant right-to-left shunt.
Operative mortality = 1-5%, 50% if right-to-left shunt,
15-20% if CHF or pulmonary HT. Cmplc: return of shunt,
and can never be sure it isn't anomalous pulmonary veins or
sinus venosum. In adults w small patent foramen ovale, warfarin may be a reasonable alternative to surgery.

Ventricular Septal Defect

Ann IM 2001;135:812; Nejm 2000;342:256

Cause: Congenital malformation

Epidem: 20% of all CHD; associated with triad of 3rd-degree heart
block, ventricular septal defects, and corrected transposition

Pathophys: Causes a left-to-right shunt, which in end-stage disease
reverses to a right-to-left shunt (Eisenmenger's syndrome) with
clubbing and cyanosis

Size of defect is crucial to sx, location unimportant. At birth, high hematocrit keeps PA pressure up and thus low shunt flow and minimal murmur; with dropping crit postpartum these appear (Nejm 1982;306:502).

Sx: Usually asx; can develop dyspnea, fatigue, and pulmonary infections

Si: Loud, harsh pansystolic murmur at lower-left sternal border, widely transmitted over precordium. Apical diastolic rumble if large shunt; loud P_2 if pulmonary HT.

Crs: Spontaneous closure in $\frac{1}{3}$ in childhood; life expectancy > 65 yr if shunt $< 2:1$

Cmplc: SBE (5-30% lifetime risk), CHF, pulmonary HT; with Eisenmenger's, $\frac{2}{3}$ die in pregnancy (Nejm 1981;304:1215)

Lab:
>   *Noninv:* EKG normal unless huge left-to-right shunt causing LVH; RVH suggests fixed pulmonary hypertension
>   Echo w Doppler

Xray: Chest usually normal; larger defects cause LVH and prominent pulmonary vasculature and a large left atrium; small aortic knob

Rx: SBE prophylaxis (p 609)
Surgical: Indications: L-to-R shunt $> 2:1$ or CHF; PA banding in infants; optimal age for final repair is 5 yr; contraindicated if R-to-L shunt. Operative mortality: 1-5%, increases to 15% if pulmonary HT ($> 70\%$ of systemic pressures); banding mortality 25%. Surgical cmplc: complete heart block (rare), aortic insufficiency (rare).

Patent Ductus Arteriosus

Nejm 2000;342:256

Cause: Persistence of patent ductus postpartum

Epidem: 10% of all CHD; female/male = 3:1; increased incidence in RDS infants rx'd w fluids, furosemide (prostaglandin E effect: Nejm 1983;308:743)

Pathophys: Left-to-right shunt, which in end-stage disease reverses to a right-to-left shunt (Eisenmenger's syndrome) with clubbing and cyanosis

Persistence of normal fetal channel between left pulmonary artery and aorta just distal to left subclavian artery

Sx: Usually asx; can develop dyspnea, fatigue, and pulmonary infections

Si: "Machinery" murmur maximum at left base; r/o coronary AV fistula, ruptured sinus of Valsalva; bounding pulses indicate wide pulse pressure; pink fingers, blue toes with Eisenmenger's

Crs: Case report of patient who lived to age 90 (Nejm 1969;280:146); $^2/_3$ die by age 60

Cmplc: SBE, CHF, pulmonary hypertension; with Eisenmenger's, $^2/_3$ die in pregnancy (Nejm 1981;304:1215)

r/o coarctation of aorta

Lab:

Noninv: EKG normal; occasionally LVH; if has RVH, suggests fixed pulmonary hypertension

Xray: Chest normal with small PDA; w larger PDA, LVH, enlarged aortic knob with dilatation of the proximal relative to the distal aorta, and large LA with prominent pulmonary vasculature

Rx: Indomethacin iv in neonates (Nejm 1981;305:67,97; Med Let 1981; 23:95); prophylactically if < 1 kg (Nejm 1982;306:506) although 18-mo survival w/o neurologic impairment not improved (Nejm 2001;344:1966). Or ibuprofen iv q 24 hr ×3 to premies < 30 wk gestation successfully prevents as well w less renal failure but not available (Nejm 2000;343:674,728; Jama 1996; 275:539)

SBE prophylaxis (p 609)

Surgical: For lesion persistence or CHF; division and closure; optimal age for final repair: age 2-12 yr; contraindications: bacterial infection of PDA; operative mortality: 0.5-10%; cmplc: recurrent laryngeal nerve injury (rare), reopening of ductus after ligation, or mycotic aneurysm (rare)

Aortic Stenosis

Nejm 2000;342:256

Cause: Congenital malformations

Epidem: 3% of all CHD; occasionally associated with a syndrome of retardation, hypercalcemia, facial distortions, and supravalvular aortic stenosis

Pathophys: Anatomic obstruction at supravalvular, valvular, or infravalvular (p 125) areas; bicupid valve is most common type, present in 2-3%

Sx: Often asx; or occasionally only mild fatigue and exertional dyspnea; angina and/or syncope are ominous; CHF late; dysphagia (Nejm 1967;276:832)

Si: BP normal; narrow pulse pressure; loud ejection murmur maximum at base; no MR unlike in IHSS; ejection click (split 1st heart sound); CHF si's

Crs: Like acquired AS (p 129)

Cmplc: Ischemia, Vtach/Vfib, CHF, SBE, heart blocks (Ann IM 1977;87:275); reversible acquired von Willebrand's syndrome (Nejm 2003;349:343)
r/o bicuspid aortic valve (1-2% of U.S. population)

Lab:
Noninv: EKG is normal; or LVH and strain; 2-D echo

Xray: Chest shows LVH, dilatation of ascending aorta

Rx: SBE prophylaxis (p 609)
Surgical: if valve area < 0.7 cm^2/M^2; open valve replacement with bypass; operative mortality $= 1$-5% for commissurotomy, 10% for subvalvular type; cmplc: aortic insufficiency, SBE, 13% incidence over 25 yr (Jama 1998;279:599)

Pulmonic Stenosis

Nejm 2000;342:256

Cause: Congenital malformations

Epidem: 5% of all CHD

Pathophys: RV outflow (10%), valvular (90%), or infundibular (rare alone)

Sx: Often asx; or occasionally only mild fatigue and exertional dyspnea; cyanosis and CHF in severe cases

Si: P_2 diminished; loud ejection murmur at upper-left sternal border neck and back; CHF including hepatomegaly in children; ejection click, decreases with inspiration

Crs: Very stable (Nejm 1972;287:1159, 1196)

Cmplc: SBE, CHF

Lab:
> *Noninv:* EKG is normal, or LVH + strain; P pulmonale
> Echocardiogram

Xray: Chest shows PA dilatation, RVH, diminished pulmonary vasculature

Rx: SBE prophylaxis (p 609)
Surgical if gradient > 60 mm or area < 0.7 cm^2/M^2; operation type either open commissurotomy with bypass, which has a high incidence of valve incompetence post-op, or percutaneous balloon valvuloplasty in children and adults (Nejm 1996;335:21, 1982;307:540); operative mortality: 1-5%; cmplc: pulmonic insufficiency (13%), which usually disappears w time

Tetralogy of Fallot

Nejm 2000;342:334

Cause: Congenital malformation

Epidem: 10% of all CHD; 50-70% of cyanotic CHD; 85% of adult cyanotics

Pathophys: VSD and pulmonic stenosis of varying positions and severities, and dextroaorta with right-sided aortic arch (25%)

Sx: Cyanosis onset after age 3 mo unless total pulmonary atresia present; dyspnea; squatting relieves sx

Si: Cyanosis, clubbing; P_2 decreased; loud systolic along left sternal border; absent in severe cases

Crs:

Cmplc: Hypoxic spells (paroxysmal dyspnea with marked cyanosis leading to unconsciousness); brain abscess; paradoxical embolism; relative anemia; SBE; CHF (rare); pneumonia; gout; hemoptysis; pulmonary artery dissection; sudden death from ventricular arrythmias even after repair

Lab:
  Noninv: EKG shows right axis, RVH + strain; in acyanotic form, LVH
  Echocardiogram

Xray: Chest shows small heart, "boot-shaped," diminished pulmonary vasculature; right-sided aortic arch (25%)

Rx: Preventive: SBE prophylaxis (p 609)
  Surgical: "Open" total correction, patch VSD, resect pulmonary infundibulum, incise pulmonary valve (for age 3-5 yr); mortality < 3% in children and < 10% in adults, good (> 86%) 30-yr survival if survive the surgery (Mayo-Nejm 1993;329:593); cmplc: heart block (rare) and pulmonary insufficiency

Coarctation of the Aorta

Nejm 2000;342:256

Cause: Congenital malformations

Epidem: 5% of all CHD; male/female = 4:1

Pathophys: Associated with PDA often, and bicuspid aortic valve (70-90%). Hypertension is renal via angiotensin (Nejm 1976;295:145).

Sx: Rarely sx (CHF, leg pains, headache) in childhood; CHF in 3rd-4th decades

Si: Hypertension in arms, normal or low BP in legs; decreased/delayed femoral pulses; systolic murmur (75%) in upper-left back or pulmonic areas

Crs:

Cmplc: SBE on bicuspid aortic valve; intracranial bleeding; hypertensive encephalopathy; ruptured/dissected aorta; hypertensive cardiovascular disease

Lab:
> *Noninv:* EKG normal, or LVH; if RVH, suggests PDA beyond the coarc ("fetal type")

Xray: Chest, normal heart, and pulmonary vasculature; coarctation visible on plain chest occasionally; rib notching in older patients

Rx: Surgical resection of coarcted segment and end-to-end aortic anastomosis ideally done at age 5-15 yr; operative mortalities > 20% in infancy, < 1% age 5-15 yr, 10% over age 30; cmplc: spinal cord ischemia (rare); acute necrotizing arteritis of mesenteric vessels (rare); hypertension post-op in most pts

CONGENITAL HEART DISEASE; MISCELLANEOUS SYNDROMES

Ebstein's Anomaly

Nejm 2000;342:336
> Low tricuspid valve ("atrialization of RV"); ASD with right-to-left shunt, cyanosis, and clubbing; PAT and other arrhythmias; exertional dyspnea; lucent lung fields; pRBBB, WPW type B (20%), P pulmonale, SBE diathesis, but no RVH unlike tetralogy

Eisenmenger's Syndrome

Nejm 2000;342:339; Ann IM 1998;128:745

Pathophys: Left-to-right shunting from ASD, VSD, or PDA,

Sx: Dizziness

Si: Clubbing, cyanosis, RVH, pulmonary insufficiency murmur (Graham-Steell)

Crs: 45% 25-yr survival; worsened by higher altitudes

Cmplc: Thromboembolism (PE, CVA); high mortality w surgery or pregnancy; gout; gall stones; renal failure

Lab: Echo, Holter monitor for arrythmias

Rx: Phlebotomy to keep crit < 60%; heart-lung transplant if medical management failing

Holt-Oram Syndrome

Nejm 1994;330:885

Abnormal gene on chromosome 12, autosomal dominant; 1/100,000 births; ASD and/or VSD; radius, thumb, or shoulder girdle bony changes

Kartagener's Syndrome

Autosomal recessive; ciliary microtubular defect, also immobilizes sperm (Ann IM 1980;92:520; Nejm 1979;300:53); bronchiectasis; sinusitis; MS, ASD, and situs inversus totalis

Pectus Excavatum

Diminished cardiac output at maximal exercise even with moderate pectus; restrictive lung disease and pulmonary hypertension w severe disease; surgically correctible (Nejm 1972;287:207)

Transposition of Great Vessels

Nejm 2000;342:337

Anomalous origins of aorta from RV and PA from LV, w VSD, ASD, and PDA allowing communication

Rx: Postpartum, stat prostaglandin E to keep PDA open + creation of ASD by balloon catheterization; eventually surgically switch aorta and PA

Table 2.4   Differential Dx of Congenital Heart Disease

	Xray	EKG	Differential Dx
Cyanotic	Decreased pulmonary vasculature	RVH	Severe PS with VSD (tetrology or ASD) Severe pulmonary vasculature obstruction (Eisenmenger's physiology) with ASD, VSD, ductus, etc
		LVH	Tricuspid atresia
		Concentric ventricular hypertrophy	Truncus with hypoplastic PA
	Decreased pulmonary vascularity with huge RA	RAH and pRBBB	Ebstein's
	Increased pulmonary vascularity	RVH	Postductal coarctation Complete transposition of pulmonary veins
		Combined ventricular hypertrophy	Transposition of great vessels, or Single ventricle, or Truncus
Acyanotic	Normal pulmonary vasculature	RVH LVH Normal	PS or MS MR, AS, AI, coarctation Mild forms of all of above
	Increased pulmonary vasculature	RVH	ASD, secundum type, or Incomplete transposition of pulmonary veins, or All L-to-R shunts with increased RV pressures
		LVH	VSD, small to moderate, or PDA, small to moderate, or ASD, primum type, or AV fistula including aorta/pulmonary fenestration
		Normal	Mild forms of all of above

(Mod Concepts Cardiovasc Dis 1986;55:20; Nejm 1981;305:1235)

2.8 Peripheral Vascular Disease

Abdominal Aortic Aneurysm

Nejm 2003;348:1894

Cause: Unknown mix of genetic, mechanical, and other factors

Epidem: 15,000 deaths/yr in U.S., 6% prevalence at age 80 yr in men, 4.5% at age 90 in women; 18% incidence in brothers > 60 yr of affected pts (Ann IM 1998;130:637)

Pathophys: Spontaneous rupture at 5-7 cm diameter

Sx: Age > 55 yr; pain, usually in back, can be buttock or testicular; rarely can be colicky; may dissect down to give perianal hematoma (Nejm 1969;280:548)

Si: Pulsating abdominal mass; shock

Crs: If > 5 cm diameter by ultrasound, 3-12% (Nejm 1993;328:1167) vs 25% (Nejm 1989;321:1009,1040) rupture in 5 yr; if < 5 cm diameter only 5% rupture in 8 yr (Nejm 1989;321:1009). After rupture, 62% die before getting to hospital, 30% in hospital, and < 8% survive.

Cmplc: Rupture into bowel, peritoneal cavity, vena cava, retroperitoneum; disseminated intravascular coagulopathy (Nejm 1971;285:185). **cholesterol emboli,** sometimes precipitated by warfarin in 3-12 wk, presents with livedo reticularis without hypotension (the usual cause), pain, worsening renal failure; no rx possible, dx w bx's of skin, kidney, etc (Nejm 1993;329:38). Increased morbidity and mortality from other ASCVD (Ann IM 2001;134:182).

Lab:

Urine: Microscopic hematuria sometimes

Xray: KUB shows calcification in aorta; with rupture, bilateral loss of psoas shadow; lateral abdomen may show aneurysm in calcified aorta > 5 cm

Ultrasound: 100% sens and easy way to follow
CT of abdomen

Rx: Prevent by screening w abdominal exam (90% sens, 65-85% specif in thin pts > 50: Arch IM 2000;160:833) and/or ultrasound in males > 65 yr (ACP J Club 2003;138:66; P. Frame, Ann IM 1993;119:411; Can Med Assoc J 1991;145:783); do surgery if ≥ 5.5 cm, no surgery if ≤ 4 cm; 4-5.5 cm (maybe slightly less in women), follow q 3-6 mo (Nejm 2002;346:1437,1445; Lancet 1998;352:1649,1656)

Surgical excision and Dacron replacement for > 5.5 cm; can do only if renal vessels spared; mortality < 5% if done electively, 50% if done emergently; cmplc: spinal cord infarct and paraplegia (rare: Nejm 1969;281:422). In fragile pts and perhaps others, endovascular stent possible (Nejm 2004;351:1607,1677, 1997;336:13) but very expensive, many studies on it are doing it on small aneurysms < 5.5 cm

Acute Aortic Dissection

Jama 2000;283:897; Nejm 1997;336:1876

Cause: Atherosclerotic; traumatic usually at ligamentum arteriosum in chest (Nejm 1970;282:1186); Marfan's syndrome (medial cystic necrosis of aorta), or Ehler-Danlos syndrome

Epidem: 1.5× as common as ruptured abdominal aortic aneurysm. Increased incidence w hypertension, Marfan's syndrome (medial cystic necrosis of aorta), and Ehler-Danlos syndrome. No increase in syphilitic, rheumatoid, or atherosclerotic (?) aortitis.

Pathophys: Medial rupture of vasovasorum causes a dissecting hematoma that ruptures back into lumen, usually—though not always—distally creating a double-barreled lumen. Lathyrism is an experimental duplication by feeding sweet peas to rats, thereby creating defective collagen formation.

Stanford classification: type A = ascending aorta involved; type B = no involvement of ascending aorta, descending only

Sx: Pain (95%), thoracic, abdominal or in back; often migrating

Si: BPs in legs and arms unequal; asymmetric pulses (15%), aortic insufficiency murmur (32%)

Crs: Mortality 1%/hour, 50% overall in type A with ascending aorta involvement, 5% overall for type B

Cmplc: Organ ischemia due to vessel occlusion

r/o aneurysm of thoracic aorta (Jama 1998;280:1926) especially in elderly women; rx by aggressively treating HT, or if partial rupture or ≥ 6cm w surgery or endovascular stent (Nejm 1994;331:1729)

Lab:

Chem: Smooth muscle myosin heavy-chain protein elevation > 25 μgm/L within 3 yr of onset of sx, > 90% sens and specif for proximal dissection (Ann IM 2000;133:537)

Noninv: Transesophageal echo (TEE) (97% sens, 77% specif); also very accurate for traumatic aortic rupture (Nejm 1995;332:356); or, less good, transthoracic echo (57% sens, 83% specif) (Nejm 1993;328:1,35)

Xray (Nejm 1993;328:1,35):

Plain chest xray may show aortic knob widening

CT of chest w contrast (94% sens, 87% specif)

MRI (98% sens, 98% specif)

Aortogram to define point of origin, aortic insufficiency, and any vessel compromise but MRI + TEE may obviate need for this

Rx: 1st: Nitroprusside 25-50 μgm/min w β-blockers (Med Let 1987;29:18) such as propranolol 0.05-0.15 mg/kg iv q 4-6 hr

2nd: Trimethaphan (Arfonad) 1-2 mg/min iv

Surgical for all type A (ascending aorta involvement) and many type B; > 20% mortality

Stent grafts possible for both types A and B (Nejm 1999; 340:1539,1546,1585)

Deep Venous Thrombophlebitis

Nejm 2004;351:268

Cause: Venous stasis and intimal injury; coagulation abnormalities; iv's are an occasional cause; $^2/_3$ due to particulates in iv, $^1/_3$ chemical and/or needle irritation, < 1% bacterial (Nejm 1985;312:78); trauma pts have a 60% incidence, 18% is proximal DVT (Nejm 1994;331:1601). Usually lower extremities; upper-extremity DVT has similar causes though less common (Ann IM 1997;126:707).

Malignancies (Jama 2005;293:715) increase risk especially in 1st 6 mo of dx, hematologic, lung and gi

Inherited/acquired protein deficiencies (Nejm 2001; 344:1222); one of these deficiencies is present in 31% of outpatients with lower-extremity DVT and 9% of pts w upper-extremity DVT (Ann IM 1997;126:707); a h/o DVT in the family or at a young age does not increase the likelihood (Nejm 1990;323:1512)

- Factor V (Leiden) mutation (Ann IM 1998;128:15, 1997;127:895; Nejm 1997;336:399) in 25-40% of pts w idiopathic DVT (Nejm 1999;340:901), a heterozygous single amino acid point mutation causing resistance to protein C. 3-5% prevalence in U.S. Caucasian population (Jama 1997; 277:1305); one study finds increased DVT risk only if assoc w 20210A mutation (Nejm 1999;341:801). Heterozygotes' risk of thromboembolic cmplc increased ×3, homozygotes ×18 (Ann IM 2004;140:330). Also associated w increased fetal loss, miscarriage, and stillbirth in both heterozygotes and homozygotes (Ann IM 1999;130:736), and perhaps w a slight increase in CVAs (Ann IM 1996;125:264 vs Ann IM 1997;127:895). Screening of asx population is not worth anticoagulation risks since annual incidence of DVT < 1% (Ann IM 2001;135: 322, 367, 1997;127:895), nor is screening prior to joint replacement indicated since no increased risk (Ann IM 1998; 128:270).

- Prothrombin gene position 20210 mutation of G to A; most common abnormality after factor V (Leiden) (Ann IM 1998;129:89; Blood 1996;88:3698), present in 5% w idiopathic DVT (Nejm 1999;340:901)
- Protein C deficiency or resistance: Normally inactive protein C circulates in blood, is activated by clot on endothelium, and that activated form breaks down activated factors V_a and VIII_a. Deficiency is autosomal dominant, vitamin K dependent (Nejm 1986;314:1298); but many with heterozygous protein C deficiency have no thrombosis, so there may be some other associated defect in some (Nejm 1987;317:991). Homozygous protein C deficiency causes neonatal purpura fulminans (Nejm 1991;325:1565).
- Protein S deficiency (Ann IM 1998;128:8): A protein C cofactor, also autosomal dominant (Ann IM 1993;119:779) and vitamin K dependent, associated with nephrotic syndrome (Ann IM 1987;106:677; 1987;107:42); 1.5-7% prevalence in pts w DVT. Homozygous state causes neonatal purpura fulminans; 50% of affected pts will have sx by age 30. Can also occur as an acquired autoimmune deficiency (Nejm 1993;328:1753).
- Antithrombin III deficiency: autosomal dominant (Ann IM 1992;116:754)

   Antiphospholipid antibodies like lupus anticoagulant, or anticardiolipin antibodies (Nejm 2002;346:752) often in SLE, ITP, or **primary antiphospholipid syndrome** (Ann IM 1996;125:747, 1992;117:303,997, 1992;116:293) w elevated PTT, present in 5% of pts w idiopathic DVT (Nejm 1999; 340:901), manifest by arterial thrombi and DVTs, rx'd w warfarin to INR > 3 (Nejm 1995;332:993,1025), and thrombocytopenia rx'd w steroids and/or danazole (Ann IM 1994;121:767)

   Idiopathic factor VIII levels > 243 IU/100 cc (Nejm 2000;343:457)

   Homocystinemia (p 317) (Nejm 1996;334:759; Ann IM 1995;123:746)

Epidem: Associated w occult cancers (15%), may be either superficial migratory or DVT type (Ann IM 1982;96:556); cancer present in 10% w one identifiable episode, > 20% w more than one idiopathic episode (Nejm 1992;327:1128). Increased incidence (Nejm 2001;344:1222) w pregnancy, BCP use (Nejm 2001;344:1527), ERT, elevated factor VIII levels.

Pathophys: See above

Sx: None; or calf pain; unlateral edema

Si: None; or Homan's sign, or increased calf diameter

Crs (Arch IM 2000;160:769; Ann IM 1996;125:1): 75% 5-yr survival, 25% recurrence over 5 yr, 30% in men and 8% in women excluding genetic predispositions (Nejm 2004;350:2558)

Cmplc: Pulmonary embolus (14%), but incidence decreases to < 0.4% w and after rx (Jama 1998;279:458); in idiopathic upper-extremity DVT, PE rate is 26% (Ann IM 1999;131:510)

Chronic postphlebitic syndrome (edema, pain, stasis dermatitis, ulcers) in 50% after 2 yr, incidence can be decreased by half w post-episode use of below-the-knee compression stockings × 2 yr (Ann IM 2004;141:249,314) vs 2-3 wk (Lancet 1997;349:759)

Thrombotic skin necrosis, especially of penis with protein C deficiency and warfarin rx; rx with vitamin K, avoid by using heparin rx (Sci Am Text Med 1984)

r/o superficial phlebitis rx'd w local heat and NSAIDs

r/o occult cancer w H + P, chest xray, and standard labs; don't pursue further unless abnormalities found there (Nejm 1998;338:1169; Ann IM 1996;125:785) vs more extensive non-inv studies (Nejm 1998;338:1221)

Lab (Ann IM 1998;128:663):

Hem: D-Dimer (fibrin split products) by ELISA methods > 500 ngm/cc 96% sens, 77-82% specif for proximal DVT (Ann IM 2004;140:589), but lower specif when prevalence higher, eg, w carrier (Ann IM 1999;131:417; Circ 1995;91:2184); and higher sens (>99.5%) in moderate- and low-risk pts (Ann IM 2003;138:987; Nejm 2003;349:1227); but lower sens w latex agglutination 5 min bedside tests (SimpliRED et al.) (Ann EM 2000;35:121)

Thrombosis panels can be done while anticoagulated for all but protein C and S, and antithrombin III

Noninv: Beware that many noninv labs and xray depts call the femoral vein "the superficial femoral vein" when it really is a deep vein (Jama 1995;274:1296); all detect above-the-knee DVT; below-the-knee DVT not significant unless extends above, hence do at least one follow-up test 5-7 d later if first neg

Ultrasound (Ann IM 1998;129:1049), simple compressibility of groin and popliteal space (Ann IM 1998;128:1), or duplex: noncompressibility with probe (91% sens, 99% specif-Nejm 1989;320:342), all in pts w sx. If ultrasound negative, ok to withold heparin in pts w sx since < 1% false neg tests (counting calf DVT as positive) (Ann IM 2004; 140:985); repeat q 4-7 d if high risk

Xray: MRI > 90% sens and specif (Ann IM 2002;136:89); venogram, but induces DVT 2% of the time

Rx: Prevention:

- Avoid estrogen as BCPs or ERT; although in factor V Leiden, incidence of thromboembolism < 2% (Ann IM 2001;135:322)

- LMW heparin, unfractionated bid, or LMW (Circ 2004;110:874; Am J Med 1999;106:660; Nejm 1993;329:1370) like enoxaparin 30-40 mg qd; graduated compression stockings in neurosurg pts (Nejm 1998;339:80), (NNT = 3-5) in hip replacement pts (Jama 1994;271:1780), but regular heparin and warfarin are also effective; use throughout pregnancy if h/o DVT, 3 miscarriages, or even one stillbirth (Nejm 2001;344:1222)

- Pneumatic calf compression post-op probably as good as above (Med Let 1985;27:45)
- Elastic compression stockings for pts > 56 yr on 8+ hr economy-class air flights decrease incidence from 12% to 0% (NNT = 9) (Lancet 2001;357:1485)
- ASA qd helps some (Lancet 2000;355:1295)
- Experimental: Prophylaxis w desirudin (Revasc; recombinant hirudin) (Nejm 1997;337:1329,1383) or w polysaccharide (Nejm 2001;344:619), ? more effective than LMWH

Therapy:

- Heparin iv × 5 d, LMW heparin better than unfractionated heparin for acute DVT (ACP J Club 2005;142:71; Nejm 2001;344:626; Ann IM 2001;134:191) because faster thrombus regression and less frequent thrombocytopenia (Nejm 2001;344:673), and allow home rx: enoxaparin (Lovenox) 1mg/kg sc qd or bid (Nejm 1996;334:677; Ann IM 1996;124:619), or others (p 52)
- Plus warfarin (p 52) started on day 1 (Nejm 1992;327:1485); overlap heparin and warfarin w adequately prolonged INR (> 2) at least 2 d before stopping to avoid hypercoag state (Nejm 1996;335:1822); continue warfarin × 6 mo (Nejm 1999;340:901,955, 1995;332:1661) vs 3 mo (Nejm 2001; 345:165) if no specific cause, × 1-2 mo if transient specific cause, and lifelong if recurrent idiopathic type (Nejm 1995; 332:1710) after 2nd episode does prevent recurrence but w 10% bleeding risk (Nejm 1997;336:393). D-Dimer < 250 μgm/cc after cessation of warfarin indicates very low risk of recurrence (Jama 2003;290:1071). Long-term anticoag to INR = 1.5-2.0 protects w less bleeding risk? (yes: Nejm 2003;348:1425,1478 vs no: Nejm 2003;349:631,702).

   if due to antithrombin III deficiency, anticoagulate after first episode to INR = 3-4

   if due to antiphospholipid syndrome, standard AC to INR = 2-3 adequate (Nejm 2003;349:1133)

- IVC filter to reduce pulmonary embolus rate from 4% to 1.5%, but subsequent recurrent DVT is 20+% vs 11%, and short- and long-term mortality are the same (Nejm 1998;338:409)

    of post-phlebitic syndrome (pain, stasis changes, edema): BK compression stockings (30-40 mm @ ankle) (Ann IM 2004;141:249) forever

Peripheral Vascular Occlusion and Ischemia

Nejm 2001;344:1608, 1991;325:577

Cause: ASCVD causes thrombotic type and incidence is increased by HT, DM, hyperlipidemia, and smoking; embolic from post-MI (10%), mural thrombus, Afib (75%), and valvular heart disease (15%)

Epidem: 30% of patients with premature (age < 50 yr) peripheral and CNS thromboembolic vascular disease are heterozygotes for homocystinuria (p 317) variants (Nejm 1985;313:709)

Pathophys:

Sx: Cold, pale extremity; decreased sensation and motor strength; pain usually, but not always, worse with elevation; claudication, progresses to rest pain (r/o spinal stenosis in elderly)

    Embolic incidence to femoral (34%), brain (20%), popliteal (14%), iliac (13%), viscera (10%), aorta (9%), axillary (5%)

Si: Pale with elevation > 1 min, then dependent rubor (reactive erythema) when first put down (Mod Concepts Cardiovasc Dis 1976;45:91); diminished or absent pulses; mottled skin; ischemic ulcers; gangrene

Crs: Sx progress over 6 yr though pt may decrease activity level to control them (Jama 2004;292:453). In embolic, without rx, extremity loss is axillary 10%, popliteal 12%, femoral 40%, aorta 80%

Cmplc: Gangrene of extremities
    r/o venous occlusion

r/o abdominal aortic aneurysm with **cholesterol emboli,** sometimes precipitated by warfarin in 3-12 wk (Circ 1967; 35:946), angiography, or surgical aortic manipulation; presents with blue toes and livedo reticularis without hypotension (the usual cause) or pain; may see emboli in retinal vessels, elevated amylase/lipase, low complement, worsening renal failure, no rx possible, dx w bx's of skin, kidney, etc (Nejm 1993;329:38)

r/o **thromboangiitis obliterans (Buerger's Disease)** (Nejm 2000;343:864): rare (in U.S.) disease of young male smokers, due to endarteritis obliterans of vasa vasora, presents w claudication especially of instep and has a positive Allen's si (with posterior occlusion of radial and ulnar arteries and the rapid release of one leads to rapid filling on that side alone, and is delayed several seconds on other) and superficial thrombophlebitis (40%); treat by stopping smoking, vasodilators, and hyperbaric oxygen to rx ulcers (Nejm 1998;339:672)

Lab:

Noninv: Ankle-brachial index (ABI) < 0.5 suggestive of significant disease (Ann IM 2002;136:873); even < 0.9 being used as sens and specific marker of peripheral vascular disease in some studies (sponsored by Plavix) (Jama 2004;292;453). Doppler studies for segmental systolic BPs and Doppler wave forms (Nejm 1983;309:841).

Xray: Duplex ultrasonography (Brit J Surg 1996;83:404)
Angiography only if plan to do surgery as you would if embolic

Rx (Med Let 2004;46:13): Stop cigarettes; control BP, DM, and cholesterol/lipids

Weight loss; exercise program of walking to pain within 5 min and continuing as tolerated, then rest and resume to > 30 min walking time at least tiw for at least 6 mo helps (Nejm 2002;347:1941; Jama 1995;274:975); β-blockers may, but don't usually, worsen sx (Arch IM 1991;151:1769) unless coincident nifedipine use (BMJ 1991;303:1100); ASA 325 mg po qd (Lancet 1992;340:143)

Medications:

- Antiplatelet rx w ASA 1 po qd, clopidrogel (Plavix), and/or ticlopidine (Ticlid) 250 mg po bid, which decreases claudication and need for bypass surgery, and increases graft patency post-op (Nejm 1997;337:1726)
- Cilostazol (Pletal) (Med Let 1999;41:44) 50-100 mg po bid; platelet inhibitor and vasodilator; half-life increased by erythromycin, ketoconazole, diltiazem, omeprazole, grapefruit; adverse effects: headache, diarrhea, dizziness, worse CHF
- Pentoxifylline (Trental) 400 mg po tid for claudication (Can Med Assoc J 1996;155:1053; Ann IM 1985;102:126)
- Heparin sc qd helps modestly (Am J Med 1999;107;234)
- Ginko (Am J Med 2000;108:276) 120-160 mg po qd
    Bypass surgery if ulcers or intolerable pain
  of acute thrombotic or embolic occlusion: Embolectomy within 6 hr with Fogarty catheter; or thrombolysis iv × 2+ d w indwelling catheter using urokinase for acute (< 2 wk) or chronic obstruction, w f/u angioplasty, helps 50-80% (Nejm 1998;338:1105 vs 1148; Ann IM 1994;120:40); anticoagulation with heparin then warfarin

Subclavian Steal Syndrome

Jama 1972;222:1139; Nejm 1967;276:711

Cause: Atherosclerosis of subclavian artery

Epidem:

Pathophys: Steal syndrome due to retrograde vertebral arterial flow to arm, which, with exercise, siphons ("steals") blood from cerebral circulation

Sx: Precipitated by arm exercise (20%), head turning to side, standing. Dizziness (11/13); transient blurred vision (6/13); syncope (4/13); aphasia (4/13); dysarthria (3/13); dementia (6/13).

Si: Diminished capillary filling with arm elevation; diminished pulse in arm (13/15); left arm to right arm BP differences of > 20 mm Hg (11/13); bruit in 8/9 incomplete blocks, 1/6 complete blocks; lateralizing motor or sensory changes (4/13)

Crs:

Cmplc: CVA

Lab:

Noninv: Doppler analysis as good as angiography; 30-msec delay in pulse measurable

Xray: Angiography; MRA or duplex scanning of neck to detect retrograde vertebral flow

Rx: Surgical reconstruction; carotid vertebral bypass when on left; vertebral artery ligation especially when on left; on right can precipitate a carotid steal; a minor procedure. Contraindications: vertebral thrombosis, high technical risk, hemodynamically insignificant risk. Morbidity/mortality: 1/13 post-op mortality; 2/13 have residuum from pre-op stroke. Cmplc: contralateral steal syndrome, especially if repair a total occlusion and a partial occlusion exists on other side (Nejm 1967;277:64).

2.9 Miscellaneous

Cardiac Exam

Auscultatory BP gap: Loss of Korotkoff sounds between systolic and diastolic pressures; in HT pts correlates w ASHD (Ann IM 1996;124:877)

Ejection clicks: Systolic click as blood enters a dilated pulmonary artery or aorta, seen with ASD, PDA, mild pulmonic stenosis or aortic stenosis, bicuspid aortic valve

Gallops (Nejm 1968;278:753):

S_3 (Nejm 1992;327:458), ventricular gallop: Idiopathically normal in people age < 35 yr (Nejm 1983;308:498); any LV dilatation, not hypertrophy, due to early LV filling with high atrial filling pressure pushing forward flow, eg, in CHF (overly compliant ventricle), and mitral regurgitation (abnormally high, early AV flow)

S_4, atrial gallop: Due to any LV hypertrophy (diminished compliance) with slowed diastolic filling and significant atrial push, eg, in hypertension, aortic stenosis, post-MI where there is an "indurated" noncompliant wall

Heart sounds, timing of: w JVP and EKG: c wave is not due to carotid artery (starts sooner in patients with LBBB: Nejm 1971;284:1309)

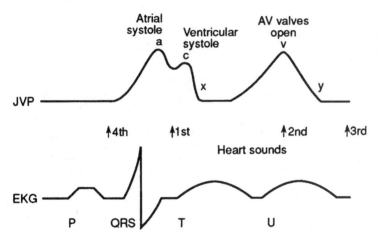

Figure 2.5 Timing of heart sounds.

Hepatojugular reflux: 10-30 sec midabdomen compression causes increased JVP, which falls immediately with release; correlates with PCWP ≥ 15 mm Hg (Ann IM 1988;109:456), 10% false pos and neg, false positives from isolated right ventricular disease

JVP clinical estimate: Of cm above angle of Louis (manubrial-sternal junction), which is 5 cm above LA; upper limit of normal = 7-9 cm; at 45° angle, JVP only visible if > 7cm (Jama 1996;275:630)

LVH: By xray > 1.5 cm behind inferior vena cava on lateral, 2 cm up from diaphragm by PE, apical pulse sustained throughout systole

LV enlargement without LVH by PE: Apical impulse > 3 cm^2 in left lateral decubitus position is reliable (> 90% sens/specif-Ann IM 1983;99:628; 100% sens 30% specif-Jama 1993;270:1943) for LV dilatation, much better than position relative to sternum or mid-clavicular line supine; but dullness > 10.5 cm from midsternum has 90% sens, 30% specif (Jama 1993;270:1943)

Maneuvers during cardiac exam: To bring out and suppress various heart sounds (Nejm 1988;318:1572; for sens/specif-Ann IM 1983;99:346):

- Valsalva maneuver, squatting, inspiration, and leg raising increase venous return and thus right-sided murmurs and decr IHSS murmur
- Squatting to standing decreases venous return and hence diminishes right-sided murmurs and increases IHSS
- Hand grip or, even more so, bilateral arm BP cuffs at 20 mm above systolic pressure for 20 sec (Ann IM 1986;105:368) increase peripheral vascular resistance and hence left-sided regurgitant murmurs like MR, AI, and VSD
- Amyl nitrite inhalation (reduces peripheral vascular resistance) decreases mitral regurge, AI, and VSD murmurs (Mod Concepts Cardiovasc Dis 1975;44:23) but reflex tachycardia may mask
- Carvallo's maneuver (deep inspiration) in 80%, and by hepato-jugular reflux in 66% (Ann IM 1984;101:781), to emphasize tricuspid regurgitation
- Respiratory variations of heart sounds (Mod Concepts Cardiovasc Dis 1981;50:37)

Murmur mimics: Austin-Flint murmur is a "murmur of mitral stenosis" caused by aortic insufficiency; Graham-Steell murmur is a "murmur of AI" caused by mitral stenosis-induced pulmonic insufficiency

Palpitations

Nejm 1998;338:1369

Cause: SVT (Afib, AVNRT, AVRT), Vtach, PVCs, anxiety/panic disorder

W/u: H + P, EKG, Holter or event monitor, ? electrophysiologic testing

Rx: β-Blockers for nonspecific rx

Pediatric murmurs, benign: (p 905)

Pericardial rubs: 18% monophasic, 24% diphasic, 58% triphasic (atrial systole, ventricular systole, and protodiastolic components), 22% palpable (Nejm 1968;278:1204)

Pericardial tamponade (Nejm 2003;349:684): JVP increased, BP decreased, distant heart sounds, paradoxical pulse (r/o severe asthma, PE, severe hemorrhagic shock), Swan-Ganz numbers show equal pressures, ie, RAP = RVDP = PADP = PCWP, often electrical alternans. 7% may have both tamponade and visceral pericardial constriction, so tap alone not enough (Nejm 2004;350:469).

   r/o acute RV infarct w functional pericardial tamponade from acute RV dilatation (J. Love 3/95; Nejm 1983;309:39, 551)

Split heart sound: Differential dx:
   1st sound, split: RBBB (r/o click)
   2nd sound, wide or fixed split: RBBB, pulmonary stenosis, pulmonary hypertension, ASD; rarely VSD, PVCs, mitral regurge (Mod Concepts Cardiovasc Dis 1977;46:7)
   2nd sound, paradoxical split: LBBB, aortic stenosis, WPW syndrome type B, patent ductus arteriosus, IHSS

Central venous catheters: Insertion technique w diagrams, infection prevention (Nejm 2003;348:1123). Swan-Ganz use is associated w severity-adjusted increased morbidity + mortality or at least no benefit and use should be curtailed (Nejm 2003;348:5; Jama 2003;290:2713); maybe use in hypotension to manage iv nitroprusside and/or pressors like dobutamine and dopamine especially in R ventricular infarct patients with hypotension

Syncope

Nejm 2005;352:1004, 2002;347:878,931; Am J Med 2001;111:177; ACP J Club 2002;136:77; Nejm 2000;343:1856; Ann IM 1997;126:989, 1997;127:76

Unknown/Idiopathic (14-36%)

Cardiac (9-11%); 10% risk of sudden death within 6 mo
- Arrhythmic (70%), eg, long QT, SVT, Vtach, heart block
- Acute coronary syndrome (1%)
- Aortic stenosis (1%)
- Pulmonary embolus (1%)
- IHSS (< 1%)

Noncardiac (70-90%)
- Carotid hypersensitivity (1%)
- Neurologic (5%)
- Psychiatric (2%)
- Other (1%)
- Vasovagal (21-37%) (Ann IM 2000;133:714); including reflux and pharyngeal stimulation (Ann IM 1992;116:575); good prognosis
- Orthostatic/postural hypotension (24%): (in elderly: Nejm 1989;321:952) rx (p 753). Testing: Supine BP after 2 min, then standing BP after 1 min; positive if P increases by > 30/min, and or systolic BP decreases by > 20 mm Hg (Jama 1999;281:1022)

Reflex vasodilatation: psychiatric, carotid sinus pressure, swallow and micturition syncope, inferior MI. Or neurally mediated hypotension (Jama 1995;274:961); in that case, strong ventricular contractions may cause via C-fiber–induced peripheral vasodilatation (Ann IM 1991;115:871); bring out with tilt table and isoproterenol infusion; but such maneuvers cause syncope in patients with no h/o blackouts almost as often (Ann IM 1992;116:358), although if bradycardia and hypotension occur quickly on tilt table alone, dx may be more secure (Nejm 1993;328:1117). Associated w chronic fatigue syndrome: pacer rx no help (Nejm 1993;328:1085); rx by avoiding diuretics, vasodilators, and tricyclics, increase salt intake; try fludrocortisone (Florinef), β-blockers, anticholinergics like disopyramide (Norpace) (Jama 1995; 274:961), or SSRIs like paroxetine 20 mg qd (J Am Coll Cardiol 1999;33:1227).

Decreased venous return: Blood loss, 3rd spacing, micturition, cough/exertion, syncope, venous pooling from varicosities; postprandial splanchnic blood pooling probably is most common cause of orthostatic hypotension in elderly (Ann IM 1995;122:286); caffeine no help

Decreased peripheral resistance: Arteriovenous malformation, heat

Circulating vasodilator: Carcinoid, mastocytosis

Renin excess and aldosterone deficiency states

Autonomic neuropathy (p 753 for w/u and rx)

Miscellaneous: Deconditioning, starvation, pulmonary embolus, pheochromocytoma, CNS tumor, marijuana, sepsis, billowing mitral valve, Addison's disease

Rx for all: Increase fluids, salt, isometrics w sx; midodrine 2.5-10 mg po tid, fludrocortisone 0.1-0.2 mg po qd, β-blockers, SSRIs, pacing

Wide pulse pressure: Differential dx: thyrotoxicosis, aortic insufficiency, calcific arteriosclerosis, arteriovenous shunt

Perioperative Risk Assessment

Point systems: 4 extant systems (Am Col Cardiol: Nejm 1997;337:1132; Detski/ACP: Ann IM 1997;127:309,313; Goldman: Nejm 1977;297:845; and a Canadian system based on anginal severity); all use mix of similar pt characteristics and operative risk categorization, and perform comparably but identify only $^2/_3$ of the risk (Ann IM 2000;133:356; 384)

Table 2.5   Goldman Criteria

Condition	Points
Age > 70 yr	5
MI within 6 mo	10
S_3 or JVD	11
Significant valvular AS	3
Rhythm other than NSR or PACs	7
> 5 PVCs/min documented any time in past	7
Generally poor health, eg, $pO_2 < 60$, creatinine > 3 mg %, $pCO_2 > 50$, abnormal PFTs, $K < 3.0$ mEq/L, $HCO_3 < 20$, BUN > 50	3
Intraperitoneal or thoracic, or aortic operation	3
Emergency operation	3

Table 2.6   Risks

Points	Class	Surgical Risk of Nonfatal Cardiac Cmplc (%)	Surgical Risk of Cardiac Death
0-5	I	0.7	0.2
6-12	II	5	2
13-25	III	11	2
26+	IV	22	56

Prophylactic peri-op β-blockers (Nejm 1999;341:1789) markedly reduce peri-op cardiac risk if ≥ 1 risk factors present (Ann IM 2003;138:506); or atenolol 10 mg iv pre- and post-op +

50 mg po bid until hospital discharge, decreases cardiac morbidity/mortality by 11% over 2 yr (Nejm 1996;335:1713,1761)

Stable angina by itself not a risk. Risk of post-MI cardiac cmplc of surgery is 5.8-30% at 0-3 mo, 2.3-15% at 3-6 mo, 1.5-5% at 6 mo and beyond (Anesthesiol 1983;59:499; Jama 1972;220:1451). W/u beyond chest xray and EKG (eg, ETT, dobutamine stress echo [Jama 2001;285:1865]) needed only if functional status unclear or high risk as defined by points, eg, > 20 (Ann IM 1997;127:311; Nejm 1995;333:1750). No benefit in fixing stable CAD before major vascular surgery (VA: Nejm 2004;351:2795).

Pulmonary evaluation (Nejm 1999;340:937): Maximize COPD/asthma states w antibiotics if infected, steroids, and pre-op training for post-op incentive spirometry; PFTs controversial. Also maximize post-op pain control.

Geriatric surgical cardiac risk (Ann IM 1985;103:832): Pts classified as low risk can be given a 2-min ETT supine to raise pulse > 99; pts unable to do so suffer a 20% severe cardiac cmplc rate, whereas pts able to do so have only a 1.5% severe cardiac cmplc rate

2.10 EKG Reading

General

- Always use limb leads rather than V leads for measurements where possible
- Peri-infarction block not a clinically useful concept
- Q waves < 0.04 sec wide or < $\frac{1}{3}$ R height are insignificant (eg, septal) except in the face of LBBB
- Pediatric differences: Big R in V_1 + RAD in infants; former may persist to age 5, latter gone in 2-3 yr. Anterior T inversions out to V_4 may last into early teen years.
- Interval calculation:
  PR = beginning of P to beginning of QRS

QRS = beginning of QRS to J point where QRS joins ST segment

QT = beginning of QRS to end of T; upper limit of normal (see Figure 2.6) = QT/$\sqrt{\text{previous R-R}}$ (Heart 1920;7: 353), or quickly calculated by being normal if < ½ R-R interval

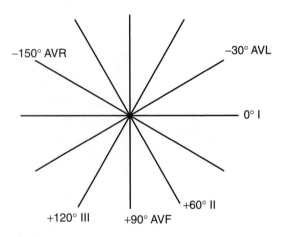

Figure 2.6   Axis calculation.

Table 2.7   Normal Q-T Intervals and Their Upper Limits of Normal

Heart Rate/Min	Normal Q-T Intervals		Upper Limits of Normal Q-T Intervals	
	Men and Children (sec)	Women (sec)	Men and Children (sec)	Women (sec)
40.0	0.449	0.461	0.491	0.503
43.0	0.438	0.450	0.479	0.491
46.0	0.426	0.438	0.466	0.478
48.0	0.420	0.432	0.460	0.471
50.0	0.414	0.425	0.453	0.464
52.0	0.407	0.418	0.445	0.456
54.5	0.400	0.411	0.438	0.449
57.0	0.393	0.404	0.430	0.441
60.0	0.386	0.396	0.422	0.432
63.0	0.378	0.388	0.413	0.423
66.5	0.370	0.380	0.404	0.414
70.5	0.361	0.371	0.395	0.405
75.0	0.352	0.362	0.384	0.394
80.0	0.342	0.352	0.374	0.384
86.0	0.332	0.341	0.363	0.372
92.5	0.321	0.330	0.351	0.360
100.0	0.310	0.318	0.338	0.347
109.0	0.297	0.305	0.325	0.333
120.0	0.283	0.291	0.310	0.317
133.0	0.268	0.276	0.294	0.301
150.0	0.252	0.258	0.275	0.282
172.0	0.234	0.240	0.255	0.262

Reproduced with permission from Chung EK. Chung's Pocket Guide to EKG Diagnosis. Malden MA: Blackwell Sci., 1996, p267.

CARDIOLOGY

Table 2.8   EKG Interpretation

EKG Segment	Dx	Criteria/Abnormalities
• P waves	RAE	P > 2.5 mm high in II, III, aVF, or V$_1$; or > 1.5 mm in V$_2$
	LAE (+/or conduction delay)	P ≥ 0.12 sec in II, III, or aVF (volume only, eg, mitral stenosis), or P > 1 mm^2 negative area in V$_1$ (33% false neg; mitral re-gurg volume and/or pressure can cause: Circ 1969;39: 339; Am J Cardiol 1977;39:967)
PR interval: Short	LGL, Fabry's disease	< 0.12 sec with no delta wave
	WPW	< 0.12 sec with delta wave present
Long	1st-degree heart block	> 0.20, or > 0.22 sec if rate slow (< 60)
Elevated	Pericarditis (p 121)	In both limb and precordial leads, usually associated w ST elevations (Nejm 1976;295:523)
• QRS		
Axis deviation and hemiblocks	LAD + LAHB	Axis ≤45° (? ≤30°) and small Q$_1$ and/or small R$_{III}$; but no LBBB
	RAD + LPHB	Axis > 105°, > 90° if age > 50 yr, and R$_1$ +/or Q$_{III}$ but don't call if RVH
	Bifasicular block	Either of above + RBBB
Wide QRS	pRBBB	QRS < 0.10, S$_I$, S$_{II}$, S$_{III}$ + RSR' in V$_1$ or aVR
	Osborn waves	Terminal QRS widening in hypothermia (p 21)
	RBBB	QRS ≥ 10 sec and (almost always), S$_I$, S$_{II}$, S$_{III}$, and RSR' in V$_1$, or other evidence of forces to R shoulder like terminal R in aVR or terminal S in V$_6$
	IVCD	QRS > 0.10 but < 0.12 sec without above pattern and with an aVL septal Q and/or a V$_1$ septal R
	pLBBB	Like IVCD but without aVL septal Q or V$_1$ septal R

LBBB	QRS > 0.12 sec, big slurred R_I and QS in V_1; rarely benign (Ann IM 1969;70:269); if new, 50% 10-yr mortality (Ann IM 1979;90:303)
Low voltage	1st one then other over time (slowed not fully blocked) Voltage < 10 mm in all leads; or overall voltage of QRS in I + II + III < 15 mV (Chung)
Bilateral BBB	
Myxedema, COPD, amyloid, obesity, MI damage, pericardial effusion	
Ventricular hypertrophies	Single precordial S or R > 25 mm (relatively nonspecific criterion); or $S_{V_2} + R_{V_6}$ or $S_{V_1} + R_{V_5}$ > 35 mm (good); or $R_{avL} \geq 1$ mm (better criterion), or $R_{avL} + S_{V_3}$ > 28 mm (J Am Coll Cardiol 1985;6:572) (better); or $R_I + S_{III}$ > 23 mm (best)
LVH; when prolonged ventricular activation time (first 0.04 sec) and LVS, increased ASHD; 60% 12-yr, 50% males >45 yr 2-yr mortality (Am Hrt J 1949;38:273)	Can't read in LBBB
RVH (Am Hrt J 1970;72:813)	
R > S in V_1	R_{V_1} > S + T inverted in V_1; or R_{V_1} > 7 mm; or $S_{V_{5-6}}$ > 7 mm; or $R_{V_1} + S_{V_5}$ > 10.5 mm; or, w RBBB, R_{V_1} > 10 mm
RVH and strain	Above + inverted Ts and/or depressed STs in V_{1-3}
RBBB	See above criteria
WPW type A	Short PR and delta wave
Direct posterior MI	Initial R_{V_1} > 0.04 sec wide + Ts upright in V_1
Dextrocardia	Increasing R voltage right precordial leads R_{V_1} to R_{V_6}
Anterior MI, r/o COPD and poor lead placement	Poor R-wave progression, ie, R < S still in V_4
MI patterns: All w initial ST elevations, then T inversions + Qs if transmural,	
Anterior septal MI	Qs in V_{2-3}

Table 2.8	continued	
EKG Segment	Dx	Criteria/Abnormalities
r/o LBBB, WPW, cardiomyopathy	Anterior MI	Loss of R force across precordium or Q waves in V_{3-4}
	Anterior lateral MI	Qs in V_{5-6}
	High lateral MI	Qs in I, avL, V_6
	Inferior wall MI	Qs in at least two of II, III, or avF
MIs w LBBB (Am Hrt J 1988;116:23); all w about 25% sensitivity, > 90% specificity)	Septal MI	LBBB + new "septal" Q in avL or R in V_1; really is RV forces seen through infarct "window" of septum; or LBBB + Q wave in ≥ 2 leads V_{3-5}; or LBBB + late notching of S in ≥ 2 leads V_{3-5}
	Any area MI	LBBB + evolving ST-T changes; or (Nejm 1996;334:481) on initial EKG, ≥ 1 mm ST elevations concordant w QRS, ≥ 1 mm ST depressions in V_1, V_2, or V_3, ≥ 5 mm ST elevations opposite direction from QRS in any lead; or upright T V_5 or V_6
Pulm embolus patterns		$S_1Q_3T_3$, very specific but only w massive emboli (Am J EM 1997; 15:310); anterior T-wave inversions (68% sensitivity) (Chest 1998;113:850); or ≥ 3 of the following (70% sensitivity) (Am J Cardiol 1994;73:298): RBBB or pRBBB, S in I and avL ≥ 15 mm, poor R progression, Q in III and F not II, RAD > 90°, voltage < 5 mm in limb leads, T inversions in II + F or V_1-V_4
Poor R-wave progression (clockwise rotation)	Lead misplacement, COPD, non-specific anterior MI indicator	R < S still in V_4
Counterclockwise rotation	Normal variant, RVH, posterior MI	R > S in V_1

- **ST segments**

Depressions	Significant (2+ vessels w > 50% occlusions) ischemia	ETT induced > 1 mm at 0.08+ sec past J point and horizontal or downsloping; greater likelihood w increased depression, as move from upsloping to downsloping, and w pretest likelihood (Nejm 1979;300:1354)
	LV strain; subendocardial ischemia/infarct, dig effect	Depressions w or w/o partial T inversions
Elevations (Nejm 2003;349:2128)	Reciprocal changes of MI	Elevations > depressions
	Acute injury	Reciprocal changes often also present
	Pericarditis	Reciprocal changes not present; always involve limb and precordial leads, axis 0°–+30° (Nejm 1976;295:523), Ts don't invert until STs normal; PR depressions
	LV aneurysm	Persistent elevations after transmural MI
	Early repolarization variants	Young pt, upward coving, usually precordial leads, axis 0°–+30° (Nejm 1976;295:523), no evolution; a normal variant
	Prinzmetal angina	Chest pain; neg enzymes; transient

- **QT intervals**

Short (< 0.20 sec)	Hypercalcemia	ST segment really short, not the T-wave portion
	Dig effect	
Long (see p 107)	Hypocalcemia	ST segment long w normally shaped Ts though may be inverted
	Hypokalemia, quinidine, phenothiazines, MI, CVA, myotonic dystrophy, myxedema	QT long w flat Ts; U waves; w or w/o ST depressions
	Hypothermia	Osborn waves (p 21)

Table 2.8 continued

EKG Segment	Dx	Criteria/Abnormalities
• T waves		
Peaked	Hyperkalemia	> 10 mm high (evolve to wide QRS, and later sine wave pattern), narrow
	Hyperacute MI	> 10 mm high, wider
Inversions	LV strain, subendocardial ischemia	Inverted asymmetrically
	LVI	Inversions w/o ST depressions
	RV strain	Isolated to V$_{1-3}$
	Old MI and/or IMMI or BBB	Inverted symmetrically and > 5 mm
	Juvenile pattern	Under age 12 and inverted V$_{1-4}$
	Hyperventilation; gi disease like cholecystitis (Ann IM 1992;116: 218), may elevate STs as well	Inverted asymmetrically and reversion to normal w atropine or isoproterenol
	Subarachnoid bleed	Symmetric, deep inversions across precordium

ASMI = anterior septal MI; ETT = exercise tolerance test; IMMI = intramural MI; IVCD = intraventricular conduction delay; IWMI = inferior wall MI; LAD = left axis deviation; LAE = left atrial enlargement; LAHB = left anterior hemiblock; LGL = Lown-Ganong-Levine syndrome; LPHB = left posterior hemiblock; LVH = left ventricular hypertrophy; LVI = left ventricular ischemia; LVS = left ventricular strain; pLBBB = partial left bundle branch block; pRBBB = partial right bundle branch block; RAD = right axis deviation; RAE = right atrial enlargement; RVH = right ventricular hypertrophy; SEI = subendocardial ischemia; WPW = Wolff-Parkinson-White

Chapter 3

Dermatology

D. K. Onion and E. Sahn

3.1 Dermatologic Medications

Antifungal Agents

Med Let 1997;39:63

Topicals

- Butenafine (Mentax) cream qd × 4 wk for T. pedis, 80% cure
- Ciclopirox (Loprox) 1% lotion/cream bid for tinea, $27/15 gm
- Clotrimazole (Lotrimin) topical × 2-4 wk; used vs monilia and tinea; OTC, inexpensive
- Econazole (Spectazole) cream, for tinea, $12/15 gm
- Haloprogin (Halotex) (Med Let 1988;30:99) topical; used vs tinea, 5% absorbed; $12/15 gm
- Ketoconazole (Nizoral) cream, $15/15 gm; shampoo (Med Let 1994;36:68) $16/4 oz
- Miconazole (Monostat) topical × 2-4 wk; used vs tinea and monilia; $2/15 oz generic, OTC (Micatin)
- Naftifine (Naftin) topical; used vs non-monilial dermatophytes; $17/15 gm gel
- Nystatin (Mycostatin) topical; used vs monilia
- Selenium sulfide (Med Let 1994;36:68) 1% OTC or prescription 2.5% shampoo; for tinea versicolor and dandruff by decreasing spore spread; $2.70/4 oz generic
- Sertaconazole (Ertaczo) (Med Let 2004;46:50) 2% cream bid for T. pedis; 4× cost of generics and OTC types

- Sulconazole (Exelderm) cream vs tinea; $10/15 gm
- Terbinafine (Lamisil) cream or spray vs tinea bid × 1-2 wk; $28/15 gm, OTC
- Terconazole (Terazole) topical; similar to ketoconazole for vaginal candidiasis
- Tolnaftate (Tinactin) topical × 2-4 wk; used vs tinea, 70+% effective; OTC, cheapest and most cost-effective (Jama 1994;272:1922)
- Undecylenic acid (Cruex, Desenex) creams

Oral/Systemic

- Fluconazole (Diflucan) (J Am Acad Derm 1994;30:684; Ann IM 1990;113:183); 50-400 mg po qd, eg, 150 mg po × 1 for vaginal candidiasis (Med Let 1994;36:81); vs candida, dermatophytes, and T. versicolor; none of H_2 blocker interference or testosterone problems of ketoconazole
- Griseofulvin (Fulvicin) 250 mg po bid × 4 wk ($22) for skin, × 6-8 wk for foot skin, 500 mg po bid × 6+ mo for fingernails and × 12 mo for toenails ($710); best absorption with a fatty meal, used vs monilia and tinea, prevents infection of newly formed skin; drug of choice in children w T. capitis; adverse effects: gi intolerance, SLE, sleepiness and headache resolve with continued use.
- Itraconazole (Sporonox) (J Am Acad Derm 1994;30:684; Med Let 1993;35:7) 100-200 mg po qd × 3-4 mo for onychomycosis (Med Let 1996;38:5); or pulsed doses of 200 mg po bid 1/4 wk × 3-4 mo; 100 mg po qd × 2-4 wk for tinea corporis; vs candida, dermatophytes, and T. versicolor but cmplc's don't justify use usually; also used vs histo, blasto, invasive aspergillosis; 80-90% effective, but amphotericin still better if life-threatening; needs gastric acid to be absorbed, less toxic than ketoconazole but adverse reactions (Med Let 1996;38:72) include increased toxicity of cytochrome C-metabolized drugs like erythromycin, benzodiazepines, cisapride, nonsedating antihistamines, as well as hepatotoxicity and CHF; $5/d for 100 mg qd

- Ketoconazole (Nizoral) topical $12/15 oz; 200-400 mg po qd ($2-4/d); more toxic than griseofulvin; vs candida, dermatophytes, and T. versicolor; adverse effects: nausea and vomiting, hepatitis (can be fatal) so monitor LFTs q 2 wk, Antabuse-like effect, need gastric acid to absorb, antitestosterone synthesis causes impotence and gynecomastia (Nejm 1987;317:812); decreased levels with rifampin (Nejm 1984;311:1681), INH, anticholinergics, and H_2 blockers; increases effects/levels of warfarin, cyclosporin A, oral hypoglycemics, and phenytoin
- Terbinafine (Lamisil) (Med Let 1996;38:72) 250 mg po qd × 6 wk for fingernails (90% cure), × 12 wk for toenails (40-80% cure), or pulsed rx w 500 mg qd 1/4 wk × 3 mo slightly less effective; adverse reactions: headache, gi, taste changes; occasional rash and hepatitis (follow LFTs); rare pancytopenias, red eye and anaphylaxis; $5/d

Antiviral Agents

- Valcyclovir 2 gm po q 12 hr × 2 doses for HSV of lip; or other regimens (p 691)
- Cimetidine 300 mg po tid × 8 wk for warts in children (Arch Derm 1996;132:680; J Am Acad Derm 1994;28:794)
- Imiquimod (Aldara) topically tiw × 3-4 mo; for common and venereal warts and molluscum; avoid in pregnancy; cost $100/mo
- Interferon-α2b used vs warts locally by injections (Med Let 1988;30:70)

Topical Steroids

Most come in 15, 30, 45, 60, 120, and 240 gm tubes, or for solutions 20 or 60 cc

Adverse effects: local skin atrophy especially on face and especially with intralesion injections, but never occurs with simple hydrocortisone; hypopigmentation and telangiectases; adrenal suppression may occur when rx lasts over 2 wk, especially with occlusive dressings

Table 3.1   Topical Corticosteroids Ranked by Potency

	Generic Name	Brand Name
I. High Potency[1]		
	Clobetasol propionate cream, ointment, gel, or emollient, 0.05%	Temovate
	Foam, 0.05%	Olux
	Betamethasone dipropionate cream or ointment, 0.05%	Diprolene
	Diflorasone diacetate ointment, 0.05%	Psorcon
	Halobetasol propionate cream or ointment, 0.05%	Ultravete
II. Potent		
	Amcinonide ointment, 0.1%	Cyclocort
	Betamethasone dipropionate cream, 0.05%	Diprolene
	Betamethasone dipropionate ointment, 0.05%	Diprosone
	Desoximetasone cream or ointment, 0.25%, and gel, 0.05%	Topicort
	Diflorasone diacetate ointment, 0.05%	Maxiflor
	Fluocinonide cream, gel, or ointment, 0.05%	Lidex
	Hakinonide cream, 0.1%	Halog
	Mometasone furoate ointment, 0.1%	Elocon
III. Mid-potent		
	Amcinonide cream or lotion, 0.1%	Cyclocort
	Betamethasone dipropionate cream, 0.05%	Diprosone
	Betamethasone valerate ointment, 0.1%	Valisone
	Diflorasone diacetate ointment, 0.05%	Maxiflor
	Fluocinonide cream, 0.05%	Lidex-E
	Fluticasone propionate ointment, 0.005%	Cutivate
	Halcinonide ointment, 0.1%	Halog
	Triamcinolone acetonide ointment, 0.1%	Aristocort A
IV. Mid-potent		
	Betamethasone valerate foam, 0.12%	Luxig
	Fluocinolone acetonide ointment, 0.025%	Synalar
	Flurandrenolide ointment, 0.05%	Cordran
	Hydrocortisone valerate ointment, 0.2%	Westcort
	Hydrocortisone probutate cream, 0.1%	Pandel
	Mometasone furoate cream, 0.1%	Elocon
	Triamcinolone acetonide cream, 0.1%	Kenalog

Table 3.1 (continued)

	Generic Name	Brand Name
V. Mid-potent		
	Betamethasone dipropionate lotion, 0.05%	Diprosone
	Betamethasone valerate cream, 0.1%	Valisone
	Fluocinolone acetonide cream, 0.025%	Synalar
	Flurandrenoilde cream, 0.05%	Cordran
	Fluticasone propionate cream, 0.05%	Cutivate
	Hydrocortisone butyrate cream, ointment, solution, 0.1%	Locoid
	Hydrocortisone valerate cream, 0.2%	Westcort
	Triamcinolone acetonide lotion, 0.1%	Kenalog
VI. Mild		
	Alciometasone dipropionate cream, or ointment, 0.05%	Alcovate
	Betamethasone valerate lotion, 0.05%	Valisone
	Desonide cream, 0.05%	DesOwen Tridesilon
	Flumethasone pivalate cream, 0.03%	Locorten
	Fluocinolone acetonide cream or solution, 0.01%	Synalar
	Triamcinolone acetonide cream, 0.1%	Aristocort A
VII. Mild		
	Topicals with hydrocortisone, dexamethasone, flumethasone, prednisolone, and methylprednisolone	

1. Group I compounds are arranged by potency. Reproduced from Linden KJ, Weinstein GD. Psoriasis current perspectives with emphasis on treatment. Am J Med, 1999;107:599 and modified 2005 with permission from Excerpta Medica Inc.

3.2 Dermatoses

Acne Vulgaris

Cause: Hormonal changes of puberty; bacterial (corynebacterium)?, iodides and bromides

Epidem: Teenagers; XYY genotype may correlate, especially with early age of onset (Ann IM 1970;73:270); associated with seborrheic dermatitis

Pathophys: Hypertrophic sebaceous glands lead to increased sebum production and desquamation, especially with androgen stimulation, w comedone formation; sebum undergoes lypolysis by bacteria, which in turn causes inflammation. Cystic acne is associated with increased androgen levels from partial adrenal 2I-OH deficiency or polycystic ovaries, hence low-dose dexamethasone and/or birth control pills help (Nejm 1983;308:981).

Sx: Acne; iodide and bromide types lack comedones and may be in unusual places

Si: Papules on erythematous base, pustules, comedones, nodules, cysts, scars

Crs:

Cmplc: **Hidradenitis** in axilla or groin, rx with topical and systemic antibiotics, and antibacterial soaps, intralesional steroids; birth control pills occasionally helpful. Avoid I + D; rx severe cases with excision of apocrine gland-bearing skin

　　　r/o **Acne rosacea** (Nejm 2005;352:793), which is central facial; has telangiectases, papules, and pustules without comedones or scarring; rx with dietary vasodilator restriction, topical rx with metronidazole 0.75% cream bid (Med Let 1989;31:75), azelaic acid 15% gel bid, and po tetracycline w strict photo protection

Lab:

Rx (Nejm 2005;352:1463; Jama 2004;292:726):
Mild:
- Avoid facial creams; wash face bid and hair qod
- Topical rx (Med Let 1996;38:53) with:
  Benzoyl peroxide, resorcinol, salicylic acid (Pernox, Xerac, Fostex, Banoxyl, Syntex, Abiotin)

Retinoids; all $35/15 gm:

- Tretinoin (Retin A, Avita) 0.025%, 0.05%, or 0.1% cream or 0.025% or 0.1% gel; adverse effects: burns transiently 1st week, sun sensitivity and thus skin cancer risk, and rarely hepatic dysfunction in case of neuropsych toxicity (Ann IM 1996;124:227)
- Tazarotene (Tazorac) 0.05% or 0.1% cream or gel qd (Med Let 2002;44:52); more effecive and more irritating than the other 2 options
- Adapalene gel (Differin; a retinoid) q hs

Antibiotics:

- Erythromycin 2% soln gel or cream bid, or 2%, 3%, or 5% soln w benzoyl peroxide gel (Benzamycin)
- Clindamycin 1% gel, soln, or lotion (Nejm 1980;302:503); w benzoyl peroxide (BenzaClin, Duac)
- Metronidazole 0.75% gel (Metrogel) $38/30 gm, or 1% cream (Noritate) qd-bid; $50/30 gm
- Azelaic acid (Azelex) 20% cream bid; or as 15% gel (Finacea) (Med Let 2003;45:76) bid esp for rosacea; adv effects: stinging, burning; $43/30 gm

Moderate:

- Oral antibiotics:

  Tetracycline 250-500 mg po bid until better, then qd and taper; because of sunburn, use sunscreen or stop in summer, especially w doxycycline (Nejm 1976;294:43); beware of pregnancy in women since stains infants' teeth

  Clindamycin po as good or better but higher *C. difficile* colitis risk

  Erythromycin also works

  Azithromycin 250 mg po b-tiw or less, expensive

- Antiandrogens:

  Birth control pills, esp those w 50+ μgm of estradiol (p 834) in women; avoid norethindrone- and norgestrel-containing ones, as they have some androgen effect

Spironolactone 50-100 mg po qd

Flutamide 250-500 mg po qd

- Narrow-band blue light (clear light is ineffective) (Med Let 2003;45:50)

Severe/cystic:

- Retinoids:

    Isotretinoin (Accutane) (Med Let 2002;44:82) 1-4 mg/kg po qd × 4 mo after derm consult; $100+/mo; 95% remissions; adverse effects (FDA Bull 13:21): 33% teratogen in 1st trimester (Nejm 1985;313:837), now legally virtually prohibited for potentially pregnant women (Nejm 1989;320:1007); elevated uric acid; regional ileitis; corneal opacities; elevated lipids may cause atherosclerosis (Nejm 1985;313:981); pseudotumor cerebri; hyperostosis, at least at higher doses that are used in ichthyosis (Nejm 1983;308:1012); arthritis and fatigue limit use in athletes (R. Kenney 12/85); possibly depression and suicide

    Acitretin (Soriatane) (Rx Let 1997;4:64) po qd; less long-acting metabolites than isotretinoin but alcohol counteracts this advantage by converting it to those toxic forms

- Low-dose dexamethasone, with or without birth control pills (Nejm 1983;308:981)
- Intralesional steroids
- Cryotherapy

Alopecia Areata

Cause: Probably autoimmune

Epidem: Common; 17/100,000 population

Pathophys: Nonscarring alopecia

Sx: Sudden loss of hair in round or oval patches

Si: Nonscarring patchy hair loss; "exclamation mark" hairs; when regrows, may come in white ("hair turned white overnight")

Crs: Waxes and wanes

Cmplc: r/o other nonscarring alopecia: local active infection, drugs (chronic heparin, colchicine, methotrexate, bc pills, cyclophosphamide), xray rx, hypo- and hyperthyroidism, secondary syphilis (eyebrow and "moth-eaten" occipital hair), tinea capitis, **trichotillomania** (nervous tic in which pt pulls own hair out). These contrast with scarring alopecia: trauma, lichen planus, tertiary syphilis, discoid lupus, postinfectious (deep mycosis, typical and atypical tuberculosis, pyoderma).

Lab: Screen for associated conditions w CBC, TSH/T4, FBS

Rx (Nejm 1999;341:964)

Steroids: Topical clobetasol (Temovate) bid or intralesional triamcinolone

Minoxidil topically as 2% ointment or lotion, or 5% soln, helps 85% within 6 wk (BMJ 1983;287:1015), may only prevent further loss and must be continued forever; adverse effects: minimal systemic absorption and its effects; cost: $2/d for 1 cc bid, OTC less costly

Anthralin (Drithro-creme) 0.1% × 2-4 hr qd

If resistant, 5% minoxidil + 0.5% anthralin (Arch Derm 1990;126:756); or rarely topical immunotherapy like diphenylcyclopropenone (Derm Clinics 1996;14:739)

Capillary Hemangiomas, Sturge-Weber Syndrome, and Port Wine Stains (PWS)

Nejm 1999;341:173

Cause: Congenital

Epidem: PWS: 3/1000 births

Pathophys: CNS, skin, and other organ (eg, liver) hemangiomas

Sx: Skin lesions usually flat though may be rounded; seizures in Sturge-Weber

Si: Thrills and bruits, hemiparesis and/or other neurologic si's

Crs: Capillary ("strawberry") hemangiomas: 25-50% present at birth, rest appear within 2 mo; maximum growth by 6-12 mo; involution begins in 16% at 6 mo, 65% at 12 mo, gone in 98% by age 9 yr

Sturge-Weber and port wine stains gradually darken and thicken until middle age; no involution

Cmplc: CHF; thrombocytopenia (Kasabach-Merritt syndrome) due to platelet trapping; spinal cord mass lesion si's due to hemangioma there, often (20%) with overlying arteriovenous malformation in same dermatome (Nejm 1969;281:1440)

Glaucoma in 45% if both 1st and 2nd branches of Vth cranial (trigeminal) nerve involved in Sturge-Weber syndrome

Lab:

Xray: Skull in Sturge-Weber may show parallel lines of vessel ("tramline") calcification

MRI in Sturge-Weber to find leptomeningeal hemangiomas

Rx: of capillary hemangiomas: Treat symptoms (bleeding, pain, ulceration, or infection). Will usually involute; if life-threatening cmplc or severe deformity of adjacent structures, use intralesional or systemic steroids; pulsed dye laser; or if that fails, interferon-α2a sc qd (Nejm 1992;326:1456).

of PWS: Flashlamp pulsed tunable dye laser rx under age 5 up to early adulthood works in > 95% (Nejm 1998;338:102, 1989;320:416; Med Let 1997;39:10, 1991;33:104)

Dermatitis Herpetiformis

Nejm 1983;308:816

Cause: Genetic association in 90% (HLA B8 and DR_W3: Ann IM 1982;97:105) but not clinically hereditary

Epidem: Associated with Hashimoto's thyroiditis, hypothyroidism, hyperthyroidism, and thyroid nodules in 50% (Ann IM 1985;102:194); pregnancy; hypoparathyroidism

Males > females

Pathophys: IgA deposition at dermal/epidermal junction, because is allergic in etiology (J Am Acad Derm 1992;27:209; Ann IM 1982;97:105)

Sx: Debilitating itch and rash; precipitated by UV, steroids, and infection (Ann IM 1984;100:677)

Si: Umbilicated, grouped vesicles; r/o other viral (*H. simplex, H. zoster,* variola, varicella)

Crs:

Cmplc: Lymphomas
r/o pustular psoriasis, often indistinguishable even histologically (Ann IM 1984;100:677)

Lab:
Path: Small bowel bx shows sprue-like pathology even though asymptomatic; skin bx shows IgA at dermal-epidermal junction

Rx: Gluten-free diet, rice and oats ok (Nejm 1997;337:1884) but takes 2 yr to help
Sulfapyridine 4 gm po qd
Dapsone 100 mg po qd; inhibits polys chemotaxis; adverse effects: G6PD deficiency anemia precipitation, severe peripheral neuropathies

Eczematous Dermatitis

Cause:
- Atopic: Genetic, often autosomal dominant, co-inherited w bronchial hyperresponsiveness and asthma (Nejm 1995;333:894); sometimes associated w interleukin-4 receptor mutation enhancing allergy (Nejm 1997;337:1720,1766)
- Contact: Rhus (poison ivy), mango rind (Nejm 1998;339:235), and gypsy moth caterpillar hairs (find with Scotch tape: Nejm 1982;306:1300); by direct contact
- Neurodermatitis (psychiatrically self-induced)

- Type IV DHS reaction to allergen, eg, latex allergy in gloves, 82% of latex allergies are this, rarely are anaphylactic type I (Ann IM 1995;122:43)

Epidem:

Pathophys:

Sx: Acute: Characterized by weeping vesicles, chronic by pruritus and lichenification

Atopic: h/o stress, allergies, asthma

Contact: h/o contact, especially when wet; burning more than itching; appears within 24 hr of contact, hyperpigmentation may occur later

Neurodermatitis: h/o stress, dependent personality, self-excoriation

Si: Atopic: Medial, infraorbital skin pleat (Morgan-Dennie fold)

Contact: Linear lesions somewhere if caused by Rhus plants

Neurodermatitis: Scratching

Crs: No spread

Cmplc: w atopic: Increased (30% prevalence) staph infections due to absence of antimicrobial peptides (Nejm 2002;347:1151)

r/o **"ID" reaction** (autosensitization), which may follow any rash, especially chronic ones of lower extremities like stasis dermatitis

Lab:

Serol: in atopics, IgE elevated ≥ 95 IU and/or ≥ 3 pos RAST tests to common allergens (Nejm 1997;337:1720) often

Rx: Preventive:

- Avoid vaccinations and herpes infections in atopic dermatitis
- Lactobacillus po qd 1 mo pre- and 6 mo postpartum decreases eczema incidence in infants by 50% at age 2 (Lancet 2001;357:1076)

of disease:

- Wet soaks with Domeboro's soln, etc, 10-20 min qid

- Topical steroids immediately after soaks, then emollients, eg, Eucerin, Lubriderm, petrolatum, Crisco, mineral oil
- Antihistamines po, especially hydroxyzine, which can be taken in high doses but may be sedating; antipain meds, since itching is a form of pain
- Doxepin (TCA) 5% topical cream helps though is absorbed (Med Let 1994;36:99)
- Steroids, topically with occlusion; avoid systemic because of rebound
- Tar preparations occasionally help
- Crushed plantain (Nejm 1980;303:583; Shakespeare's Romeo and Juliet 1.2.52-53) for poison ivy
- Tacrolimus (Protopic) 0.03% or 0.1% ointment bid helps (related to cyclosporine) (Med Let 2001;43:33; Nejm 1997;337:816); no skin atrophy if used on face or neck; cmplc: burning sensation, photosensitivity, possible immunosuppression, skin malignancies and lymphomas (black box warning), eczema herpeticum, acute facial flushing w alcohol use (Nejm 2001;351:2740); 30 gm of 0.1% = $60
- Pimecrolimus (Elidel) (Med Let 2002;44:48) 1% topical crm bid; similar to tacrolimus but less potential immunosuppresion; a macrolide that suppresses T-cell cytokines; $50/30 gm

Neurofibromatosis of Von Recklinghausen (Neurofibromatosis Type I)

Jama 1997;278:51; J Am Acad Derm 1993;29:376; Ann IM 1990;113:39; Nejm 1991;324:1283

Cause: Genetic, autosomal dominant or sporadic mutations in germline cells (Nejm 1994;331:1403); mutation on long arm of chromosome 17

Epidem: Incidence: 1/3000-3500 births

Pathophys:

Sx: Onset by age 5, variable depending on site of lesions

Si: Café-au-lait spots (90%); 6 spots, > 1.5 cm in adults, or > 0.5 cm in prepubertal patients (Peds 1992;90:924; J Peds 1990;116:845) are diagnostic; axillary or inguinal "freckles" (Crowe sign) are the same thing; "coast of California" smooth edges unlike "coast of Maine" edges of **Albright's syndrome** (bone cysts and fibrous dysplasia, precocious puberty; rx'd with testolactone: Nejm 1986;315:1115)

Neurofibromas: Soft skin nodules; plexiform neurofibromas are subcutaneous nodules along nerve course; also present internally, especially in bone and CNS

Lisch nodules, dome-shaped pigmented hamartomas on iris; present in 100% by age 20 yr (Nejm 1991;324:1264)

Crs: Variable

Cmplc:

- Pheochromocytomas (in < 1%; 10% of pheos have neurofibromatosis)
- Renal artery stenosis and hypertension
- Bony, especially vertebral, and joint complaints
- Optic pathway gliomas
- CNS lesions, some cause retardation; mass effect, especially at foramen magnum; lesions of 8th cranial nerve often, also of 5th and 11th. Acoustic neuromas are from central type II neurofibromatosis, a distinct and separate genetic abnormality (p 231)
- Sarcomatous degeneration into neurofibrosarcomas in 5-10% (Nejm 1967;277:1363)
- Spinal nerve compression at neural foramina especially in chest
- Pulmonary
- Chronic myelogenous leukemia in children (Nejm 1997;336:1713)

Lab:

Rx: Monitor for cmplc's
Surgical excision of individual neurofibromas

Pseudoxanthoma Elasticum

J Am Acad Derm 1994;30:103; Nejm 1993;329:1237

Cause: Genetic; autosomal recessive, 2 types; less common autosomal dominant, 2 types

Epidem: Rare; women ≥ men

Pathophys: Premature degeneration and calcification of elastic fibers. Angioid streaks are tears in Bruch's membrane, which look like brown jagged streaks radiating from the optic disc (picture: Nejm 1997;337:829).

Sx: Onset of sx between age 20-50 yr usually, though may be present at birth

Si: 60% have all 3
- Skin changes: Yellow papules/plaques on flexor skin; small soft papules parallel to skin folds, looks like leather, may coalesce on exposed and unexposed areas unlike senile elastosis; r/o multiple myeloma and biliary cirrhosis
- Eye changes: Angioid streaking (r/o Paget's, sickle cell disease), may lead to some visual loss; chorioretinitis and hemorrhages may look like dark stippling of fundus
- CV changes: Premature atherosclerosis especially of medium vessels leads to MIs; Hypertension in adolescence due to renal artery stenosis

Crs:

Cmplc: gi bleeding (10%), especially common in pregnancy (Grönblad-Strandberg syndrome)

Lab:
> *Path:* Skin bx shows diagnostic granular accumulations of basophilic material with calcium in middle and lower dermis, stains like elastic tissue but is periodic like collagen, especially in scars (Nejm 1987;317:347)

Xray: Calcified falx cerebri

Rx: Symptomatic only

DERMATOLOGY

Psoriasis

Nejm 2005;352:1899, 1995;332:581

Cause: Probably polygenetic; 91% of patients have positive family history; associated with HLA antigens on chromosome 6

Epidem: Worst in winter, probably from dryness and lack of sunlight; 1-2% of U.S. population, rare in U.S. blacks

Pathophys: Invasion of dermis and epidermis by T cells results in abnormal control of epidermal cell division or differentiation; $5\times$ normal number of cells are synthesizing DNA. Cells migrate through epidermis too fast; hence is an epidermal hyperplastic condition that never becomes neoplastic. Psoriatic arthritis when involves synovium. In exfoliative stage, can lose protein and produce negative nitrogen balance. Perhaps trauma causes initial elbow/knee changes.

Sx: Onset usually under age 30 yr; doubt dx if onset over age 60 yr

Precipitated by stress (emotional, alcoholic binge, postinfection, drug reaction especially propranolol, chloroquine, NSAIDs, and lithium)

Arthritis quite common, often w little or no rash, asymmetric like ankylosing spondylitis

Si: Papulosquamous rash; papule with scale, which, when picked, leads to punctate bleeding (inter-rete ridge capillary); occasional pustular variant. Elbow, knee, scalp, gluteal cleft, flexor surfaces are initial distribution often; nail pitting; Koebner's phenomenon: rash appears at site of scratch or trauma 2-3 wk later.

Crs:

Cmplc: Gout; exfoliative dermatitis (r/o mycosis fungoides if > age 45 yr); pustular exacerbation with fever, inflammation, pain, hypocalcemia/ hypoparathyroidism

r/o **guttate psoriasis:** Small droplet-sized lesions erupt over 1 wk poststrep infection, positive throat culture and ASO titer up

(Arch Derm 1992;128:39), or with perianal strep in children
(Ped Derm 1990;7:97) and spontaneously resolve over
2 mo

Lab:

> *Path:* Skin bx shows acanthosis (increased epidermal thickness);
> retention of nuclei; rete ridges deeper, bigger, and some
> fused; interridge capillaries tortuous and close to surface and
> so bleed when scale picked (Auspitz sign). Feulgen stain
> shows mitochondria, ribosomes, and DNA in stratum
> corneum.

> *Chem:* Uric acid increased (due to increased cell turnover?)

Xray: Hands look like RA except no osteoporosis; whittled-down tufts
like scleroderma, "pencil in cup" dip.

Rx: of scalp: Steroids (DermaSmooth 0.01% hs, or other fluoci-
nolone), salicylic acid solutions, tar shampoos, mineral oil
of other areas:

- Sunlight or other broad-band UVB source, short of burn,
  which will cause flare
- Steroids topically (avoid systemic po steroids, which can precipitate pustular psoriasis) for small areas, with occlusive plastic dressings; or injections, eg, dilute (1:3) triamcinolone with
  lidocaine; adverse effects: widespread use leads to systemic absorption and adrenal suppression; can precipitate exfoliative
  erythroderm; skin atrophy; rebound much more likely than
  with anthralin
- Anthralin paste, 0.1%, 0.2%, or 0.4%, to rash qd for 10 min to
  1 hr, then removal with mineral oil, bath, and extensive hydrophilic ointment; or Z-tar emulsion topically × 1 hr, then
  shower, follow with UV; avoid groin; stains hair, skin
- Calcipotriene (Dovonex) (Med Let 1994;36:70) ointment
  0.005% bid; a vitamin D analog, as good as topical steroids, although tachyphylaxis potential unknown; often used w potent
  or superpotent topical steroid (KOO regimen) initially then

taper steroid; adverse effects: hypercalcemia at high doses because it is a vitamin D analog; $120/10 gm; or similar

- Tazarotene gel (Tazorac; topical retinoid) (Med Let 1997;39:105) 0.05% or 0.1% qd to < 20% of body surface (< 40 gm/wk); for stable plaque type psoriasis; avoid in pregnancy; $2/gm

2nd-line meds, usually used w dermatologic collaboration:

- Methotrexate 2.5-5 mg q 12 hr × 3 doses q 1 wk, but check current guidelines (Arch IM 1990;150:889) w 1 mg folate po qd; 10% get liver disease (Am J Med 1991;90:711); as effective as psoralen (Nejm 2003;349:658)
- Cyclosporine works, though nephrotoxic (J Am Acad Derm 1995;32:78; Nejm 1991;324:1277)
- Psoralen or methoxsalen po with UV-A (PUVA) highly effective, used tiw × 10 wk helps 85% then maintenance q 1-4 wk, but increases incidence of squamous cell cancer × 3 (Nejm 1984;310:1156) including male genitals unless protected (Nejm 1990;322:1093) and melanoma risk w 10-yr lag (Nejm 1997;336:1041)
- Acitretin (Soriatane) (Med Let 1997;39:106) 25-50 mg po qd w food; adverse effects: teratogenic for 3 yr after stop, elevated LFTs can revert on rx, various anterior eye changes, all worse w alcohol, pseudotumor cerebri esp w tetracycline; $7/pill
- Hydroxyurea (J Am Acad Derm 1991;25:522)
- Immune suppression (Nejm 2001;345:248,284): w monoclonal antibodies of CD4 and CD8 T cells w TNF antagonists like infliximab, etanercept, alefacept (Amevive) (Med Let 2003;45:31) 7.5-15 mg iv/im q 1 wk × 12; adverse effects: chills w infusion, cost $8400/12 wk; and efalizumab (Raptiva) (Nejm 2003;349:2004,2014; Jama 2003;290:3073; Med Let 2003;45:97) 1-2 mg/kg/wk sc, esp for severe plaque disease

of arthritis: (p 1075) (Arch Rheum 1996;132:215)

Tuberous Sclerosis (Adenoma Sebaceum)

Arch Derm 1994;130:348

Cause: Genetic; autosomal dominant in 25%, sporadic in 75% (Arch Derm 1995;131:1460)

Epidem: 1/10,000 population

Pathophys: Large hamartomas of brain, skin, et al. White spots due to decreased synthesis of melanin, but since there is a normal number of melanocytes, they are not vitiligo.

Sx: Epilepsy, mental retardation in some

Si: Peri/subungual fibromas especially of toenail; angiofibromas of face (adenoma sebaceum), may look like acne without blackheads; hypopigmented macular patches ("ash leaf" macules or "white confetti") on the legs, best seen under Wood's light (Nejm 1998;338:1887), especially at birth, are first si; collagenoma of lower-back skin looks like pig skin; fibrous plaques on forehead; mulberry tumors in fundus; pitted tooth enamel

Crs: Variable

Cmplc: Seizures (75%); renal failure due to angioleiomyoma and angiomyolipomas on ultrasound and CT (Nejm 1998;338:1886); honeycomb lung; rhabdomyosarcoma of heart (Nejm 1967;276:957); hamartomas throughout body

Lab:

Xray: MRI/CT of head shows calcified tumors or gliomas, subependymal tubers (Nejm 1998;338:1886)

Rx: Monitor for cmplc

Urticaria/Erythema Multiforme

Nejm 2002;346:175, 1995;332:1767, 1994;331:1272 (drug induced)

Cause & Pathophys: Idiopathic (80%)
Direct histamine release by opiates, NSAIDs, IVP dye (steroids protect), thiamine, curare, dextrans, some antibiotics

Immunologic:

- C′ activation by cryoglobulins (IgG or cold agglutinins produced by tumors, multiple myeloma, SLE, arteritis, etc), or by B_1C globulin damage (snake venom, DIC). Angioneurotic edema is C′ mediated but is not urticaria.
- Antibodies vs mast cells; or, in chronic urticaria, their IgE receptors (Nejm 1993;328:1599)
- Mast cells as "innocent bystanders," eg, SLE, serum sickness, viral (especially coxsackie) infections or post *H. simplex* with antigens in all lesions (Ann IM 1984;101:48), leukemias and other malignancies, drugs (especially sulfas, seizure meds, allopurinol, NSAIDs), parasites, hepatitis B, perhaps mononucleosis plus ampicillin; nearly all recurrent erythema multiforme and most primary episodes are due to H. simplex, but a few of the latter are due to mycoplasma and drugs (E. Ringle 1990)
- Mast cell fixed antibody (IgE), eg, to fish, bee sting, penicillin
- Type IV (DHS) immune reaction leads to vasculitis

Physical/"neurogenic":

- Cold urticaria (test with ice cube), perhaps IgE attaches to a cold-dependent skin antigen and releases platelet-activating factor (Nejm 1985;313:405, 1985;305:1074)
- Local heat urticaria
- Systemic heat urticaria, cholinergic; seen when core body temperature is elevated, starts around hair follicles; seen in runners, tennis players, etc
- Light/solar
- Stress
- Dermatographia

Associated diseases: Urticaria pigmentosa occasionally (p 189) and anaphylaxis (p 23)

Epidem: 25% of adult population has had chronic urticaria for wks-mos

Sx: Urticaria (hives), mucosal angioedema with all but physical types; abdominal pain (gi histamine release)

Si: Target skin lesions of erythema multiforme, raised urticarial lesions et al; bilateral symmetry always suggests drug-induced first

Crs: Except in vasculitis, immunologic, and physical types, most lesions last < 24 hr

Cmplc: Epidermal detachment of mucous membranes, locally in Stevens-Johnson syndrome w 5% mortality, or extensively in toxic epidermal necrolysis (p 205) w 30% mortality (Nejm 1995;333:1660) (r/o systemic diseases like SLE, dermatomyositis, scarlet fever [p 365])

Lab:

   Path: Skin bx at site of recent urticaria to r/o vasculitis

Rx: Avoid ACEIs and NSAIDs

   Ephedrine 2% spray for angioedema

   H_1 receptor antagonist antihistamines like loratidine (Claritine) 10 mg po qd (p 238); also cyproheptadine (Periactin); doxepin (Sinequan) 10-25 mg po bid (Nejm 1985;313:405); hydroxyzine (Atarax, Vistaril)

   H_2 blockers like cimetidine sometimes also helpful
   Steroids
   of vasculitis: Steroids
   of mast cell types: Ketotifen 2 mg po bid, stabilizes mast cells (Ann IM 1986;104:507); acyclovir for at least, recurrent erythema multiforme

Urticaria Pigmentosa, Mastocystosis

Nejm 1992;326:639

Cause:

Epidem: Fairly common

Pathophys: Abnormal mast cell proliferation, either neoplastic or reactive to soluble mast cell growth factor (Nejm 1993;328:1302), especially in skin and gi tract; intermittent chemical or mechanical irritation leads to release of histamine, prostaglandin D_2, et al. (Ped Derm 1986;3:265)

Sx: Episodic attacks of flushing, itching, palpitations, headaches, orthostatic sx, hyperventilation, abdominal cramping; attacks may be precipitated by alcohol, narcotics, and aspirin; freckles all over body, if rubbed cause urticaria (urticaria pigmentosa) (J Invest Derm 1991;96:325)

Si: Orthostatic BP changes

Crs: Usually benign in children; may be severe in adults (J Intern Med 1996;239:157)

Cmplc:

Lab:

> *Chem:* 24-hr urine especially after attack, for histamine metabolites (N-methylimidazole acetic acid, N-methylhistamine) and prostaglandin levels
>
> *Path:* Skin bx shows 4+ mast cells in skin lesions

Rx: Acute: Adrenalin

Chronic: Prevent with:

- Avoidance of narcotics, alcohol, dextromethorphan cough medications, and aspirin
- Chlorpheniramine 8 mg po qid or other antihistamine (Med Let 1989;31:43)
- Cimetidine 300 mg qid po or other H_2 blocker
- Na cromolyn 100 mg po (not inhalation) qid (Nejm 1979;301:465) for gi sx
- Ketotifen 2 mg po bid stabilizes mast cells (Ann IM 1986;104:507)
- PUVA rx (psoralens and UVA)

of mast cell tumor load: Interferon-α2b causes dramatic regression (Nejm 1992;326:619)

3.3 Infectious Dermatitis

Candidiasis (Moniliasis, Local) (Including Vaginal)

Nejm 1997;337:1896 (vaginal); Ann IM 1984;101:390

Cause: *Candida albicans*, or rarely *C. tropicalis* (Ann IM 1979;91:539) or *C. glabrata*

Epidem: Associated with diabetes, cancer, blood dyscrasias, multiple antibiotic use, steroids, TPN, thymoma with myositis (Jama 1972;222:1619), various endocrine conditions, eg, birth control use, hypoparathyroidism, hypothyroidism, and hypoadrenalism. One form is due to an inherited defect in suppressor T cells (Nejm 1979;300:164).

Pathophys: Normal flora, opportunistic invasion

Sx: Vaginitis, dyspareunia, vulvar rash, oral mucous membranes as thrush that scrapes off, conjunctivitis or uveitis, nails, perianal (diaper rash), rectum, other skin folds

Si: Inflammatory reactions; skin lesions have whitish central lesion with satellite pustules

Crs:

Cmplc: r/o associated conditions listed above; trichomonal (p 643) and bacterial (p 550) vaginosis

Lab:

Bact: Pseudohyphae (40%) on 10% KOH exam of skin scrapings or vaginal discharge; culture on rice/Tween agar shows distinctive pseudohyphae and condiospores; vaginal pH = 4-4.5

Rx   (for vaginal regimens and costs: Med Let 2001;43:3): All vaginal rx costs $10-30/course

TOPICAL (all > 80% effective)

1st:

- Miconazole (Monistat) 2% cream bid to skin; or vaginally bid, or 100 mg qd × 7 d, or DS × 3 d, or 1200 mg × 1

- Clotrimazole (Lotrimin) 10 mg troches sl work for oral thrush (Nejm 1978;299:1201); or 5 gm of 1% cream or 100-200 mg tab vaginally qd × 7 d, 2 tab qd × 3 d, or 500 mg once
- Butoconazole (Femstat, Mycelex) 2% cream 5 gm qd × 3-6 d (Med Let 1986;28:68), or as Gynazole 5 gm × 1 ($28)
- Terconazole (Terazol) 0.4% or 0.8% cream or 80 mg vag tab qd × 3-7 d
- Tioconazole (Vagistat) 6.5% cream, 4.6 gm hs × 1

2nd: Nystatin 100,000 U topically qd-qid × 14 d; 50% effective for vaginal candidiasis

ORAL/SYSTEMIC (all >80% effective):

- Fluconazole (Diflucan) 150 mg po × 1, or q 3 d × 3; 80+% effective; best for vaginitis, as good as or better than other regimens (Med Let 1994;36:81); adverse effects: headache; $12; 150 mg po q 1 wk to prevent recurrent vaginitis (Nejm 2004;351:876, 1997;337:1896) 90% effective at 6 mo, 40% remain clear 6 mo after stop
- Ketoconazole (Nizoral) 200 mg po qd vs mucocutaneous type; for vaginitis 400 po qd × 5 d, or qd × 14 d, then 100 mg po qd prophylaxis works for frequent recurrences (Nejm 1986; 315:1455)
- Itraconazole (Sporonox) 200 mg po × 3 d (Antimicrob Agents Chemother 1993;37:89)
- Nystatin 5 million U po tid × 1-2 wk to clear gi tract or biw for chronic prevention of especially recurrent vaginal candidiasis

Tinea Capitis, Corporis, Pedis, and Cruris: Onychomycosis, Ringworm, Athlete's Foot

Cause: Dermatophytes, *Trichophyton spp.* most commonly; also *Microsporum, Epidermophyton*

Epidem: Perhaps genetic susceptibility; worldwide; increased in Cushing's patients. Tinea corporis seen in children with puppy or kitten; *T. capitis* especially common in black children.

Pathophys:

Sx: Annular, red, scaly, pruritic rash; on foot arch can form vesicles like "big dyshydrotic eczema"

Si: Scaling rash on head, body, groin, between toes; annular w scale on outside of ring, ringworm appearance often; distorted white flaking nails w onychomycosis. Wood's lamp illumination shows yellow-green fluorescence w *Microsporum spp.* In beard, can look like antibiotic unresponsive folliculitis that has no scale and is KOH neg.

Crs:

Cmplc: Secondary bacterial infections; kerion of scalp, inflammation that can lead to severe scarring

r/o other causes of similar round lesions like granuloma annulare (p 215), which has no scale and is KOH neg, and pityriasis rosea (p 206), which has scale around the inside of the ring; pustular psoriasis when on soles and/or palms; in groin, **erythrasma,** a diphtheroid skin infection that fluoresces coral red in Wood's lamp light, rx w topical or oral erythromycin

Lab:

Bact: KOH prep shows branching hyphae. Culture on Sabouraud's media.

Rx (Med Let 1993;35:77)
TOPICAL:

- Ciclopirox (Penlac nail lacquer) (Med Let 2000;42:51) qd to nails, wash off weekly, 10% effective initially and $\frac{1}{2}$ of those relapse within 3 mo, $180/yr
- Clotrimazole (Lotrimin) OTC, may be more effective than tolnaftate, covers candida (Med Let 1976;18:101), inexpensive
- Tolnaftate (Tinactin); doesn't work in scalp, hair, nails, palms, and soles

- Haloprogen (Halotex); expensive, absorbed (5%) (Med Let 1988;30:99), etc (p 169)
- Selenium sulfide shampoo 2.5% (Selsun) to decrease spore count and intrafamilial spread

    Oral (ACP J Club 2002;135:97; J Am Brd Fam Pract 2000;13:268): (Use only for nails, topical resistant skin infections, or in immunocompromised; E. Ringle rx's only w pos KOH and doesn't rx toe nails because of resistance and drug toxicity)

    1st: Terbinefin (Lamisil) (p 169) for nails, 250 mg po qd × 12+ wk, < 70% effective; $650/3 mo; pulsed rx w 500 mg qd 1/4 wk × 3-4 mo slightly less effective

    2nd: Itraconazole 100 mg po qd × 2-4 wk for T. corporis; 200 mg po qd × 3-6 mo for nails, $1200/3 mo (Med Let 1996;38:5), or pulsed doses of 200 mg po bid 1/4 wk × 3-4 mo

    3rd: Griseofulvin 250 mg po bid × 4 wk for skin, × 6-8 wk for T. pedis, 500 mg po bid × 6+ mo for fingernails, × 12+ mo for toenails, $750; in children w T. capitis, 15 mg/kg qd × 8 wk; best absorption with a fatty meal, eg, whole milk or ice cream

Tinea Versicolor

Cause: *Pityrosporum ovale*

Epidem: Common, 20% adults have; often appears at puberty

Pathophys: A very superficial infection

Sx: Scaly areas of skin especially on shoulders, chest, and arms that are dark in winter, pale (don't tan) in summer

Si: Macular and punctate lesions often coalesce into confluent, scaly patches. Woods lamp fluorescence not clinically useful.

Crs:

Cmplc:

Lab:

> *Bact:* Skin scraping with KOH shows "spaghetti and meatballs" (short hyphae and spores)

Rx:

- Selenium 2.5% (Selsun) shampoo qd, leave on 20 min, × 14 d; often recurs
- Ketoconazole 2% shampoo 5 min/day × 3 d (J Am Acad Derm 1998;39:944)
- Fluconazole (Diflucan) 50 mg po qd × 2 wk ($61) or 400 mg po × 1 ($25); 75% cure at 6 wk (Acta Derm Venereol 1992;72:74)
- Itraconazole (Sporonox) 100 mg po qd × 15 d ($74) (Clin Experim Dermatol 1990;15:101), or 200 mg po × 5 d ($50) (J Am Acad Derm 1990;23:551)
- Ketaconazole (Nizoral) 200 mg po qd × 5 d ($11), or 400 mg po × 1 ($9), repeating in 1 wk or monthly at 200 mg po qd × 2 (DICP 1991;25:395)

Venereal (Genital) Warts

Cause: Human papillomavirus (p 793)

Epidem: Venereal spread and highly infective; incidence ~40% in college women w resolution and reinfection common (Nejm 1998;338:423); prevalence higher in HIV-pos women (Nejm 1997;337:1343). Cause of laryngeal papillomas from aspiration at delivery (Nejm 1983;308:1261).

Pathophys: Virus present in normal as well as wart skin (Nejm 1985;313:784)

Sx: 1-6 mo incubation; pain at site

Si: Warts on genitalia; in male partners, often flat and hard to see (Nejm 1987;317:916)

Crs:

Cmplc: Cervical carcinoma (p 793) (Lancet 2000;355:2189,2194), especially types 16 and 18, intraepithelial neoplasia often within 2 yr of contagion (Nejm 1992;327:1272) and eventual cervical cancer in an unknown but significant number (Nejm 1999; 341:1633); also associated with vaginal, endometrial, vulvar

(Nejm 1986;315:1052), anal SIL and cancer rates higher in gay males esp if HIV pos than cx rates in women (Ann IM 2003;138:453; Nejm 1997;337:1350), laryngeal, and conjunctival (Nejm 1989;320:1442) cancers

    r/o molluscum contagiosum (p 217)

Lab:

Rx: Preventive: Male circumcision halves rates (Nejm 2002;342:1105); barrier method birth control

    Vaccination w PPV 16 at 0, 2, and 6 mo in sexually active women appears to be 100% effective (Nejm 2002;347:1645, 1703)

    of disease (Med Let 1999;41:90): Treat pt and partner; stain area w acetic acid 1st to bring out latent warts for rx, especially in men; all work for common warts rx too.

- Trichloroacetic acid topically, ok in pregnancy
- Electrodessication, ok in pregnancy
- Liquid N_2, ok in pregnancy
- Imiguimod (Aldara) (p 171) topically tiw × 3-4 mo; avoid in pregnancy
- Podophyllin soln, leave on 8 hr 1st time, 24 hr subsequently, or as gel (Condylox); avoid in pregnancy because of fetal damage and even death with only 1-2 cc; use cryotherapy instead
- Interferon injections tiw × 3 wk (Ann IM 1988;108:675; Nejm 1986;315:1059); qd × 1 mo then tiw × 6 mo helps for respiratory papillomas (Nejm 1991;325:613), consider doing this if surgery required on papillomas q 3 mo

3.4 Skin Cancers

Basal Cell Carcinomas

Nejm 1992;327:1649

Cause: Idiopathic; actinic

Epidem: Older patients but rapidly incr in younger pts (Jama 2005;294:681) associated with sun UVB exposure and light complexion; arsenical rx and arsenical keratoses of palm; >> 500,000/yr in U.S., increasing rapidly; > 4× as common as squamous cell Ca

Pathophys:

Sx:

Si: Exposed areas; telangiectasias, pearly raised borders, no increased keratin; may be a pit if marked stromal reaction; central ulceration occasionally; occasionally pigmentation, often stippled

Cmplc: Slight increase in risk of other cancers (5-20%) (Ann IM 1996;125:815); in those dx'd < age 60 yr, risk increased for testicular, breast, and non-Hodgkin's lymphoma

r/o **congenital basal cell nevus syndrome** (Nejm 1986; 314:700); genetic, autosomal dominant; in young patients w pitted palms, large head with frontal bossing and wide eyes, who have multiple basal cell carcinomas; cmplc: jaw cysts, ovarian fibromas, medulloblastoma; rx w topical 5-FU and tretinoin (J Am Acad Derm 1992;27:842)

Lab:
Path: Excisional biopsy

Rx:

- Excision
- Electrodesiccation and curettage, least traumatic but avoid around eyes, ears, nose, scalp, or if > 2 cm or recurrent
- Radiation w 3000-6000 rad total dose @ 300 qd, 89% successful, or w radium needles also possible; avoid in basal cell nevus syndrome since can be carcinogenic
- Cryotherapy
- 5-FU topically on penis or if multiple lesions, usually is only palliative

Refer for Mohs' microsurgery or for surgical excision if aggressive histopathology, recurrent, > 2 cm, or involves ears, temples, midface triangle, or scalp

DERMATOLOGY

Squamous Cell Carcinoma

Nejm 2001;344:975; 1992;327:1649

Cause: Neoplasia from sun exposure directly (eg, Canadian fishermen: Nejm 1975;293:411) or medical PUVA, eg, for psoriasis; or from actinic keratoses, or other chronic irritation, eg, sites of chronic osteomyelitis drainage that have an especially bad prognosis (Nejm 1980;303:367); or in renal and other transplant pts on chronic immunosupression, possibly from diminished surveillance (Nejm 2003;348:1681, 1995;332:1052)

Epidem: >> 100,000/yr in U.S.; 100-150/100,000/yr, over age 75 incidence is 1000-1500/100,000/yr and increasing rapidly in young (Jama 2005;294:681)

   Associated with UVB sun exposure in whites; arsenical rx with arsenical keratoses of palm; **xeroderma pigmentosa** (autosomal recessive inability to repair UV-damaged DNA: Nejm 1986;314:1423), rx with po isotretinoin (Nejm 1988;318:1633)

Pathophys:

Sx: Skin sore that won't heal

Si: Skin ulceration with varying degrees of subcutaneous and intradermal invasion; scale and erythema; cutaneous horn sometimes, r/o seborrheic and actinic keratosis

Crs: Mortality < 1/500, 1500 deaths/yr in U.S.

Cmplc: 30% increase in risk of nondermal cancers like multiple myeloma, lymphoma, leukemias as well as increase in risk of dermal basal cell carcinomas (Am J Epidem 1995;141:916) as well as worse prognosis when get other cancers (Ann IM 1999;131:655)

   r/o: wart recently treated with podophyllin

   actinic keratosis (senile or solar), "liver spots," actinic lentigines: may be multiple, may progress to squamous cell carcinoma; prevent w sunscreen (Nejm 1993;329:1147). Rx w (Med Let 2004;49:42, 2002;44:57) excision; freezing; topical 5-FU (Effudex) 2% or 5% bid × 2-4 wk, < $75 generic; diclofenac gel bid × 3 mo, 50% cure, $105; aminolevulinic acid (Levulan) + blue light, $110; imiquinod (Aldara) 5% cream b-tid × 8-16 wk, $520; tretinoin (retinoic acid) 0.1% cream qd (Nejm 1992; 326:368); gentle cryotherapy; or laser (Med Let 1997;39:10).

r/o **keratoacanthoma,** looks clinically and pathologically very similar, rx like squamous cell cancer

Lab:

Path: Biopsy, excisional or wedge if dx uncertain; in situ lesions called Bowen's disease

Rx: Prevent w PABA sunscreens; 5-FU 5% cream bid × 4 wk to actinic keratoses, produces inflammation, vesiculation, and reso- lution. β-Carotene does not prevent new tumors (Lancet 1999;354:723; Nejm 1990;323:789) but low-fat diet does dramat- ically (Nejm 1994;330:1272).

Therapeutic (J Am Acad Derm 1993;28:628): Surgical excision or referral for Mohs' micrographic surgery if high risk (> 2 cm; into sc tissue; histopathology > well-differentiated grade I; or involvement of scalp, nose, ears, eyelids, or lips); irra- diation; isotretinoin 0.5 mg/kg bid po × months if resistant (to surgery + radiation) or recurrent extensive disease (Ann IM 1987;107:499)

Malignant Melanoma

Nejm 2003;349:2233, 1991;325:171; Ann IM 1985;102:546; Jama 1984;251:1864

Cause: UV irradiation damage esp in childhood, even in cases of ocular melanoma (Nejm 1985;313:789); high-intensity burns that reach melancocytes worse than chronic sun exposure (Nejm 1999;340:1341)

Congenital nevi: Melanoma occurs w highest frequency in those > 20 cm diameter at birth; most feel risk to some degree even < 2 cm but some say no risk there (Jama 1997;277:1439).

Atypical mole syndrome (AMS) (NIH Consensus Statement 1992;10:1) or older term, dysplastic nevus syndrome (DNS) (Nejm 1985;312:91; Ann IM 1985;102:458: both with pictures); on short arm of chromosome 1 (Nejm 1989;320:1367)

Epidem: 8th most common cancer in U.S. (20th in 1985) (Ann IM 1996;125:369); 1/80 lifetime risk in U.S.

Increased in Celts, especially those with red hair

Congenital nevi occur in ~1% of population, though rarely > 20 cm diameter

AMS can be autosomal dominant or sporadic; 2-5% prevalence; of familial type, 100% will get in lifetime and account for 10% of all melanomas; 18% of sporadic type will get in lifetime and account for 30-50% of all melanomas; increased prevalence in Hodgkin's patients (Ann IM 1985;102:37); but a few atypical nevi do not imply AMS although incidence of melanoma is still higher (Jama 1997;277:1439)

Pathophys:

Sx: Black, blue, or gray lesions increasing in size; pain; pruritus; bleeding; notched borders; asymmetric

Si: Central black (or blue-gray, "hurricane gray") papule or nodule in center of lentigo, dysplastic nevus; disorderly color, surface, and edges; inflamed; occasional satellites; does not dimple if squeezed, unlike dermatofibromas (Nejm 1976;294:1511). Amelanotic melanomas most often on soles.

ABCDE criteria (Jama 2004;292:2771): Asymmetry, Borders irregular, Color variable, Diameter > 6 mm, Evolving over time; each has a sens and specif of 60-90%

Crs:

Stage I: Survival by thickness, < 0.75 mm has a 96% 5-yr survival, > 4 mm has a 47% 5-yr survival

Stage II: Nodal mets, 36% 5-yr survival

Stage III: Distant mets, 5% 5-yr survival

Cmplc: 2nd or 3rd primary melanoma, especially in AMS (DNS) r/o other melanotic lesions, including **tinea nigra palmaris** (Nejm 1970;283:1112), junctional, compound, or dermal nevi that may have halos; **lentigo maligna** (only a few bizarre melanocytes), seen most often in elderly, in sun-exposed areas, good prognosis; **nevus of ota,** benign melanosis of eye and surrounding skin in 1st and 2nd branches of trigeminal nerve, seen in 1/200 Asians, rx w laser (Nejm 1994; 331:1745)

Lab:

Path: Excisional (or incisional or punch if too large; never curette) biopsy; melanoma is staged by thickness of tumor. Reverse transcriptase PCR study of sentinel nodes find tumor in $\frac{1}{2}$ of nodes neg by standard path techniques and recurrence rates are higher in those pts (Jama 1998;280:1410).

Xray: CT and gallium scanning especially good for metastases (Ann IM 1982;97:694)

Rx (Nejm 2004;351:998; NIH Consensus Statement 1992;10:1):

Prevention: Excision of congenital nevi, at least those > 20 cm or those that are changing; and of changing atypical moles; photographs can help to follow both

of lesions: Excision with 1-2+ cm margins (Nejm 2004;350:757,823; Jama 2001;285:1819), though 1-2 mm adequate for diagnostic excisions

of metastatic disease: Follow w hx, PE and chest xray to monitor for mets (Jama 1995;274:1703)

- Interferon-α 2 iv may help (Ann IM 1985;103:32)
- Radiation helps palliate local lesions
- Chemotherapy by isolated perfusion of extremities being tried
- Adoptive immunotherapy with tumor-infiltrating lymphocytes (lymphocyte-activated killer cells) + interleukin-2 helps 5-10% to remission when widely metastatic disease (Nejm 1990;323:570; Med Let 1990;32:85)
- Dacarbazine + tamoxifen (Nejm 1992;327:516)

DERMATOLOGY

Cutaneous T-Cell Lymphomas: Sézary Syndrome, Mycosis Fungoides and Reticulum Cell Lymphoma

Nejm 2004;350:1978; Ann IM 1988;109:372

Cause: Malignancies of T-cell lymphocytes (Ann IM 1974;80:685)

Epidem: Mostly in older (age > 40 yr) pts; associated with industrial solvent exposure in older studies, also chronic contact dermatitis

Pathophys: "Helper" T_4-lymphocyte lymphomas
Sézary syndrome has erythrodermic variants plus circulating malignant T cells

Sx: Erythematous, scaly plaques, nodules, and tumors

Si:
Stage I: Polymorphic indurated papulosquamous rash; polycyclic red-brown scaly plaques (r/o sarcoid, Behçet's syndrome)
Stage II: Generalized erythroderm and cutaneous nodules
Stage III: Organ invasions lead to "-megalys"

Crs:
Stage I: 12+-yr average survival (Arch Derm 1996;132:1309)
Stage II: 5-yr average survival; after ulcerates, 3-5 yr no matter what rx
Stage III: 2.5-yr average survival

Cmplc: Meningeal involvement occasionally occurs with CNS symptoms, even when skin changes are in remission (Ann IM 1975; 82:499)

Lab:

Rx: Topical nitrogen mustard, when disease limited to skin
PUVA in early stages (Arch Derm 1996;76:475)
Systemic rx w chemotherapy drugs and interferon is effective palliation, not curative (Ann IM 1994;121:592)
Irradiation

Extracorporeal photochemotherapy with UVA (Med Let 1988;30:96)

of Sézary syndrome: Etretinate and electron beam rx (J Am Acad Derm 1992;26:960)

3.5 Miscellaneous

Papular/Vesicular Rashes

rv of all bullous diseases: Nejm 1995;333:1475

Dermatitis Herpetiformis (p 178)

Dystrophic Epidermolysis Bullosa

Cause: Autosomal recessive and dominant forms

Si: Severe blistering with minor trauma causing contractures and protein loss; die by age 30 yr in recessive forms

Rx: Phenytoin, formerly thought helpful, but not proven so (Nejm 1992;327:163)

Eczema (p 179)

Gonococcemia (p 555)

Si: A few acral lesions, some hemorrhagic

Pemphigoid, Bullous

Jama 2000;284:350

Pathophys: Anti-basement membrane antibodies, usually IgG, occasionally IgE (Nejm 1978;298:417) and IgA in mucous membrane variant

Sx: Similar to pemphigus but in aged, and usually hemorrhagic; less severe than pemphigus; itchy; tense blisters because epidermis intact above split

Rx: Topical better than systemic steroids esp if severe (Nejm 2002;346:321); immunosuppressants like azathioprine (Arch

Derm 1994;130:753), cyclophosphamide, etc; antibiotics like tetracycline and niacinamide (Arch Derm 1986;122:670) are steroid sparing; oral steroids

Pemphigus Vulgaris

Epidem: Associated with $HLA-DR_W4$ in 91% (Lancet 1979;2:441); paraneoplastic type with lymphoma (Nejm 1990;323:1729)

Pathophys: Antiepithelial ("prickle") cell IgG_4 antibody (Nejm 1989;320:1463, 1989;321:631)

Si: Can push blister fluid into new areas of skin (Nikolsky's sign); normal skin sloughs and forms bullae when rubbed; middle-age onset; scalp, mucosal membranes, and flexor surfaces primarily involved; "baggy blisters" because overlying epidermis is very thin, rarely hemorrhagic

Rx: Steroids, and follow antibody titers; cyclophosphamide; azathioprine; or nicotinamide and tetracycline (J Am Acad Derm 1993;28:998)

Pityriasis Lichenoides et Varioliformis Acuta (PLEVA)

Epidem: Rare, in children

Si: Lichenoid papules with a continuum between the acute vesicles and the chronic scarring (J Am Acad Derm 1990;23:473)

Crs: Self-limited

Lab: *Path:* Biopsy shows vasculitis

Polymorphous Light Eruption

Nejm 2004;350:1111, see Table 3.2

Cause: Light exposure plus something else?

Epidem: Common, onset before age 70, females > males

Sx: Papular or pap/vesicular rash w/ hrs–days of a specific sun exposure

Crs: Days–weeks

Cmplc: r/o cutaneous lupus, rare SLE, drug-induced photosensitivity, rare solar urticaria, photo allergies

Rx: Sunscreens, avoidance; desensitize by gradually increasing doses of light

Scalded Skin Syndrome

J Am Acad Derm 1994;30:319

Cause: Staph toxin in children w 1st impetigo episode

Si: Denudation and epithelial slough

Lab:
Bact: Skin culture neg, staph in nose or impetigo areas
Path: Skin bx to r/o toxic epidermal necrolysis

Rx: Penicillinase-resistant penicillins; topical rx like a burn

Toxic Epidermal Necrolysis (Lyell's Syndrome)

Nejm 1995;333:1600

Cause: Drug-induced in adults, esp sulfas, seizure meds, oxicam NSAIDs, allopurinol, penicillin, ASA

Pathophys: Cleavage at dermal–epidermal junction, extreme variant of Stevens-Johnson syndrome

Crs: 15-20% mortality

Lab:
Path: Skin bx to dx

Rx: Burn unit; steroids

Papulosquamous Rashes

Ichthyosis

Cause: Familial, some autosomal and some sex-linked recessives (Nejm 1972;286:821)

Sx: Childhood onset

Si: Fine scales; if recent onset r/o Hodgkin's

DERMATOLOGY

Rx: Hydrophilic ointment with wraps q 3 d; or propylene glycol and water q 1 wk

Leprosy (p 585)

Si: Psoriaform rash with marked decrease in sensation

Lichen Planus

Si: "Polygonal, pruritic (often very), purple papules"; flexor surfaces, especially wrist and mucous membranes; linear configuration often; reticular pattern beneath (use mineral oil); looks white in blacks; "mother of pearl" in mouth; scarring alopecia; r/o leukoplakia and monilia

Rx: Topical steroids with occlusion for skin, systemic steroids for alopecia; PUVA; in mouth, cyclosporine rinse, but costs $70/day (Nejm 1990;323:290)

Mycosis Fungoides (p 202)

Pityriasis Rosea

Cause: Probably viral

Si: Ovoid lesions w central clearing and scale on *inside* of ring ("trailing scale"), in lines of cleavage; vest distribution; white raised papular lesions in blacks; r/o tinea corporis and other pap-squam etiologies, especially syphilis

Crs: Recurs occasionally

Lab: *Serol:* VDRL or RPR to r/o syphilis

Psoriasis (p 184)

Seborrheic Dermatitis/Dandruff

Cause: *Pityrosporum ovale* is a commensal yeast that causes dandruff

Epidem: Common

Si: Red color to skin, looks like acne rosacea but concentrated in nasolabial folds; cradle cap in infants

Rx (Med Let 1994;36:68): Sebulex/Selsun (selenium) shampoos biw 1% OTC and 2.5%, cost: $2.76/4 oz; or similar-priced OTC pyrithione zinc (Head + Shoulders). Alternate same with sebutone (tar); topical steroids hs, foams (Olux, Luxiq) elegant but costly; topical ketoconazole (Nizoral) cream or 2% by rx or 1% OTC shampoo biw, cost: $16/4 oz.

Secondary Syphilis (p 593)

Si: Rash on soles and palms; lymphadenopathy; red papules with scale; not pruritic

Purpuric Rashes

Allergic Vasculitis

Cause: Any vasculitis (Nejm 1997;337:1512), including giant cell, Takayasu's, polyarteritis, Wegener's, paraneoplastic, inflammatory bowel disease, and immune complex types (anaphylactoid Henoch-Schönlein purpura, cryoglobininemia, SLE, RA, Sjögren's, Goodpastures, Behcet's, scleroderma, and drug or viral induced, a continuum from urticaria to erythema multiforme (p 187)

Si: Bilaterally symmetric, palpable (r/o DIC), hematuria- and guaiac-pos stools, hemorrhagic bullae

Bacteremia

Cause: Meningococcus, staph, pseudomonas, GC, SBE

Si: Rash often asymmetric, not palpable; or may present as vasculitis with symmetric palpable purpura

ITP (p 482)

Si: Splenomegaly, decreased platelets, never palpable

DERMATOLOGY

Rickettsial Diseases: Spotted Fever, Typhus, Etc (p 603)

Si: Early lesions may blanche; palms and soles; palpable

Scurvy (p 319)

Cause: Vitamin C deficiency, seen in elderly on poor diets

Si: Purpura never palpable, corkscrew hairs, perifollicular hemorrhage especially on knees; hyperkeratotic papules

Rx: Vitamin C

Other Causes

Leukemias, TTP, thrombocytosis, myelofibrosis

PREGNANCY RASHES

Arch Derm 1994;130:734

Pruritic Urticarial Papules and Plaques of Pregnancy (PUPPP)

J Am Acad Derm 1984;10:473

Sx: In primigravida, 3rd trimester; very pruritic

Si: Papules and plaques begin in the striae on abdomen

Crs: Goes away w delivery

Rx: Antihistamines, cimetidine, steroids

Papular Dermatitis of Pregnancy

Existence debated

Crs: Increased fetal mortality reported (12%) without rx (J Am Acad Derm 1982;6:977)

Lab:
    Chem: Increased HCG (r/o mole) in urine
    Path: Biopsy is nonspecific

Rx: Cortisone 40 mg po qd produces total remission

Pemphigoid Gestationis

Jama 2000;284:350

Previously dermatitis or herpes gestationis

Si: Vesicles and bullae with onset any time during pregnancy; may flare at delivery

Crs: Recurs in subsequent pregnancies

Cmplc: Premature delivery sometimes

Lab:

Path: Biopsy shows specific subepidermal vesicles with polys early, then eosinophiles; C_3 deposition on epidermal basement membrane from low-titer pemphigoid type IgG autoantibodies

Rx: Systemic steroids

Melasma

Si: Pigmented diffuse facial "tanning" common in pregnancy or with bcp use

Rx: Stop bcp's; daily sunscreen (SPF 30+); hydrocortisone cream; Retin A cream; benzoyl peroxide cream, hydroquinone 2-4% bid

PHOTOSENSITIVITY, ACUTE AND CHRONIC CAUSES

See the following tables that present the types and characteristics of acute photosensitivity (Table 3.2), and the types and characteristics of chronic photosensitivity (Table 3.3).

DERMATOLOGY

Table 3.2 Types and Characteristics of Acute Photosensitivity

Type	Prevalence	Affected Persons Approximate Sex Ratio (F:M)	Age	Presentation	Management
Polymorphous light eruption	Very common	3:1	20–40 yr	Papular or papulovesicular eruption within hours or days after exposure to sun, lasting for days to a week or more	Topical or oral corticosteroids for acute rash; sunscreens, sun avoidance, or desensitization for prevention
Subacute cutaneous lupus erythematosus	Common	2:1	20–40 yr	Annular, polycyclic, or psoriasiform eruption within days after exposure to sun, lasting for weeks	Topical or oral corticosteroids for acute rash; sunscreens, sun avoidance, and antimalarial drugs for prevention
Drug-induced phototoxicity	Uncommon	1:1	Any age	Exaggerated sunburn hours to days after exposure to sun, lasting for days to a week or more	Cessation of suspected medications; use oatmeal baths and moisturizers
Solar urticaria	Rare	1:1	20–40 yr	Pruritus and urticaria within minutes of exposure to sun, lasting for hours	Antihistamines and desensitization with phototherapy
Photoallergy (usually caused by sunscreens)	Rare	1:1	Any age	Eczema on exposed areas	Cessation of topical agents; patch test and avoidance of detected allergens

Table 3.3 Types and Characteristics of Chronic Photosensitivity

Type	Prevalence	Affected Persons Sex	Age	Presentation	Management
Chronic actinic dermatitis	Rare	Males	> 60 yr	Eczema on exposed areas year-round or mainly in the summer	Sun avoidance; desensitization with phototherapy or immunosuppressive agents
Actinic prurigo	Rare	Males and females in approximately equal numbers	Any age	Intensely pruritic papules and nodules, often with cheilitis and scarring	Sun avoidance; desensitization with phototherapy
Photoexacerbated atopic eczema	Rare	Females	Any age	Eczema on exposed areas, history of flexural eczema and possibly hay fever and asthma	Sun avoidance; desensitization with phototherapy
Porphyria cutanea tarda	Rare	More males than females	Adults	Erosions and bullae after minor trauma, mainly on dorsal hands and forearms	Measurement of urinary porphyrins; venesection and chloroquine
Systemic lupus erythematosus and dermatomyositis	Rare	More females than males	Adults	Minor photosensitivity, prominent systemic symptoms, and other cutaneous features	Sun avoidance; corticosteroids and antimalarial drugs

DERMATOLOGY

LOCAL LESIONS AND MISCELLANEOUS

Amyloidosis

Si: Waxy papule, rubbed causes purpura (weak capillaries), "pinch purpura"

Baldness, Male Pattern (Androgenic Alopecia)

Med Let 1998;40:25

Rx   (Nejm 1999;341:964): Minoxidil (Rogaine extra strength) 2% or 5% OTC, must maintain rx to keep effect; adverse effects: dizziness; $30/mo

   Finasteride (Propecia) 1 mg po qd; takes 6-12 mo to work, must maintain dose to keep effect; adverse effects: may reversibly decrease libido, decrease PSA levels; $50/mo

Burns, Thermal

rv of rx: Nejm 1996:335:1581 iv fluids to keep urine output $> \frac{1}{2}$ cc/kg/hr, > 1 cc/kg/hr in children. Survival (Nejm 1998;338:362) based on age, extent, and whether concomitant inhalation injury.

Café-au-Lait Spots

Cause: Albright's disease, "coast of Maine" irregular edges, or neurofibromatosis "coast of California" smooth edges

Rx: Med Let 1997;39:10

Clubbing

Ann IM 1994;120:238

Causes: SBE, IBD, lung cancer, abscesses, bronchiectasis, benign familial

Si (Jama 2001;286:341):

- Loss of angle (Lovibond's) between base of nail and dorsal finger surface, hence positive Schamroth sign (no space when dorsal distal phalanges juxtaposed)
- Thickness of distal phalanx at nail bed > thickness at dip joint
- Soft nail bed

Xray: Phalanges and distal arm and leg have periosteal elevations

Decubitus Ulcers (Pressure Sores)

Jama 2003;289:223, 1995;273:865; Ann IM 1981;94:661

Cause: Immobility

Epidem: 18% prevalence in bedridden

Si: Stage I: Persistent redness
Stage II: Partial-thickness abrasion, blister, or ulcer
Stage III: Full-thickness ulcer into subcut tissue, not fascia; w/o undermining
Stage IV: Extensive and/or invasion of fascia, joint, tendon; or undermining

Crs: Follow the area (length × width); stage II, 75% heal in 60 d; stage III, 17% heal in 60 d

Rx   (Med Let 1990;32:17): Prevent w alternating pressure mattress, air mattress (Jama 1993;269:1139), egg crate foam mattress 6.5 in. thick (Lancet 1994;343:568), turning; vitamin C_2 50 mg bid po

Debridement of all eschar and dead tissue (except dry, stable, healing eschar, as long as checked daily): Use topical lidocaine gel in gauze as preparation to debride; use enzymatic rx like Granulex (trypsin), or sharp surgery; hydrocolloid dressings like Duoderm (autolytic)

DERMATOLOGY

Table 3.4   Commonly Used Treatments for Pressure Sores

Type	Examples
Debridement of Eschar	
Sharp surgical	Scoring or excision of eschar
Gauze dressings	Normal saline/disinfectant wet-to-dry gauze; not very practical; very labor intensive
Enzymatic products	Elase (fibrinolysin and DNAase), Santyl (collagenase), Granulex (trypsin), Panafil (papain), Accuzyme
Irrigation	Whirlpool, low-pressure water pick
Protective Dressings (Autolytic)	
Permeable	OpCit, Tegaderm
Hydrocolloid	DuoDERM, Comfeel, Tegasorb, Ultec
Petroleum gauze	Vaseline, Xeroform
Collagen	Medifil Kollagen, more expensive but no better than hydrocolloid (J Am Ger Soc 2003;51:147)
Antimicrobial Dressings	
Disinfectant solutions (dry the wound; use not more than 2 wk)	Acetic acid, hydrogen peroxide, sodium hypochlorite (Dakin's), povidone iodine (Betadine), chloramine-T (Chlorazene), silver sulfadiazine (Silvadene) cheapest but must change q 24 hr; Acticoat absorbent sheets $14 for 6×6 in but last 2-7 d; also Actisorb, Aquacel, Af rope, Contreet, or SilverCel, each w differing rates of Ag release and absorptive capacities
Topical antibiotics if not improving	Mupirocin (Bactroban), metronidazole (Flagyl)
Hypertonic antimicrobials	Hypertonic saline, sucrose (granulated sugar), NaCl gauze, (Mesalt)
Cavity Filling	
Gauze dressings	Normal saline gauze, hypertonic saline gauze (Mesalt)
Hydrocolloids	DuoDERM Hydroactive Gel
Alginates (rope format)	AlgiDERM, DermaSORB, Sorbsan

Erythema Nodosum

Epidem: Associated w drugs, esp bcp's, sarcoid, tuberculosis, ulcerative colitis, regional enteritis, lymphogranuloma venereum, chancroid, cat scratch fever, histoplasmosis, coccidioidomycosis, drug eruptions, diphtheria, strep infections, rheumatic fever, SLE

Si: Very tender nodules, usually on anterior shin, without scarring

Rx: Bed rest, elevation; NSAIDs; colchicine; and, if severe, oral steroids

Granuloma Annulare

Cause: Idiopathic

Epidem: In children often

Sx: Acral (arms, legs)

Si: Raised edges of a rounded lesion, centrally cleared, no scales and KOH neg

Crs: Go away in mos to years

Cmplc: r/o tinea corporis, which has a scale; sarcoid

Rx: Intralesional steroids

Hirsutism/Hypertrichosis (p 842)

Hyperpigmentation

Cause: Postinflammatory, especially in blacks

Rx: Tretinoin 0.1% cream (Retin A, retinoic acid) qd × 40 wk over entire area, not just the spots (Nejm 1993;328:1438); sunscreen (SPF 40-50)

Impetigo

Cause: Staph or strep superficial stratum granulosum (epidermal) infection

Si: Bullae, usually rupture

Cmplc: AGN

r/o ecthyma contagiosum or orf infection from sheep, where skin is invaded a little more deeply and requires longer conservative rx (Cleve Clin J Med 1991;58:531)

Lab: Culture to r/o MRSA

Rx: Antistaph penicillin or topical mupiricin (Bactroban); wet compresses × 20 min bid

Insect Bites

Rx: Prevent w 25% DEET-containing insect repellants; 5 hr avg protection; others don't work (Nejm 2002;347:13); lower % in children to minimize absorption

Keloid

Rx: Prevent recurrence w imiquimod (Aldara) cream post-op hs × 8 wk

Inject with triamcinolone q 1 mo, causes flattening; topical Retin A; expensive Silastic gel sheeting

Laceration

Nejm 1997;337:1140

Cause: Trauma

Cmplc: r/o nerve, tendon, joint involvement that may need OR

Rx: Clean, debride, suture choices (Nejm 1997;337:1144), or use octylcyanoacrylates when available

Leukoplakia

Si: On mucosal surfaces

Cmplc: Oral squamous cell cancers

Lab: *Path:* Biopsy shows nuclei and plasma cells in stratum corneum

Rx: 13-*cis*-Retinoic acid 1-2 mg/kg qd (Nejm 1986;315:1501); resection does not diminish the 25% oral carcinoma rate (Nejm 2002;350:1405)

Lichen Sclerosis of Vulva

Cause: Perhaps due to decreased testosterone levels

Rx: Strong topical steroids (J Reprod Med 1993;38:25; Brit J Derm 1991;124:461)

Testosterone 2% topically bid (Nejm 1984;310:488), but causes masculinizing side effects (Obgyn 1997;89:297)

Molluscum Contagiosum

Cause: Molluscum contagiosum virus

Epidem: Can be venereally spread

Sx: Inguinal papules, anywhere in children

Si: Umbilicated inguinal, 1-4 mm, round, raised lesions

Rx: Excise, freeze, burn; or, in children, less traumatically w cantharidin 0.7% applied w toothpick, cover w tape, wash off in 4 hr; imiquimod (Aldara) (p 171) qd under bandage; curette after topical 4% lidocaine

Orf Ulcers

Nejm 1997;337:1131

Cause: Parapox virus

Epidem: Contact w sheep in which is a common cause of skin lesions

Palm and/or Sole Rashes

Cause: Coxsackie A, hand-foot-mouth disease; dyshydrotic eczema (almost never contact); endocarditis; erythema multiforme; Kawasaki's disease (p 887); atypical measles in patients previously vaccinated (Ann IM 1979;90:873-887); neisserial gonorrhea and meningococcus; psoriasis especially pustular; rat bite fever;

Reiter's; Rocky Mountain spotted fever; secondary syphilis; tinea pedis

Pruritus

Differential dx:
- Metabolic: Gallbladder/pancreatic disease, uremia, hypo- or hyperthyroidism, polycythemia vera, lymphoma/leukemia, abdominal cancer, iron deficiency, diabetes
- Skin lesions
- Psychiatric delusions of parasites
- Real parasites, eg, hookworm, scabies, lice
- Dry skin (xerodermatitis)

Sarcoid

Si: Violet indurated plaque that blanches (p 1117)

Spider Bites, Brown Recluse (Necrotic Arachnidism)

Nejm 2005;352:700

Cause: Bite of any of several *Loxosceles sp.* spiders

Epidem: Southwest and lower Mississippi Valley

Crs: (Nejm 1998;339:379): Minimal inflammation in first 24 hr then severe inflammation and necrosis over 1 wk that may need surgical debridement. Many heal w/o drastic results.

Lab: Culture to r/o community-acquired MRSA

Rx: Supportive care, perhaps w Dapsone started in first 24 hr may prevent necrosis

Stasis (Venous Insufficiency) Ulcers

Ann IM 2003;138:326

Cause: Venous insufficiency

Si: Medial > lateral changes and ulcers in lower extremity, especially over malleoli

Cmplc: r/o arterial ulcers (lateral, no P's, diminished ankle/brachial index)

Rx: Prevent w Ace wraps, elastic stockings w pressures > 35 mm Hg at ankle, elevation

Treat w stoma adhesive qd; Banoxyl, perhaps pentoxifylline (ACP J Club 2001;134:14); if < 6 mo old and < 5 cm^2 area, healing w q 1 wk Zn oxide (Unna) boot likely within 6 mo (Am J Med 2000;109:15)

ASA 300 mg po qd by DBCT

Surgical skin grafts

Sunburn

Med Let 1999;41:43

Cause: UV or sun at 290-320 nm (UVB) or 320-340 nm (UVA II) wavelength; over 100 drugs can increase sensitivity (Med Let 1995;37:35)

Cmplc: Photoaging, actinic damage including keratoses, squamous cell carcinoma, basal cell carcinoma, melanomas; r/o polymorphous light eruption (p 204)

Rx: Prevent w sunblock SPF 15-30, eg, Uval, Solbar, benzones (Med Let 1993;35:54)

Tattoo

Removal best by Q-switch lasers at wavelength of pigments (Med Let 2003;45:95)

Telangiectasias

Cause: Idiopathic; alcoholic spider angiomata; aluminum workers in vest pattern (Nejm 1980;303:1278); **Osler-Weber-Rendu Syndrome** w autosomal dominant telangiectasias of brain, skin, gi tract, liver (Nejm 2000;343:931), etc

Rx: SBE prophylaxis if possible pulmonary AVMs; support group (800-448-6389); various laser rx's possible (Med Let 1991;33:104); ε-aminocaproic acid rx may decrease bleeding in Osler-Weber-Rendu (Nejm 1994;330:1789)

Vitiligo

Jama 2005;293:730

Cause: Genetic; chemical leukoderma, Addison's, Graves', pernicious anemia, tinea versicolor, tuberous sclerosis (present at birth); autoimmune autoantibodies to melanocytes in SLE, Graves' disease, Hashimoto's, diabetes, alopecia areata, rheumatoid arthritis; albinism (genetic, associated with actinic keratoses, cancers, nystagmus)

Rx: Often used in combinations
1st: Narrowband (311 nm) UVB, safe in adults and children; no significant adverse effects
2nd: Topical immunomodulators administered chronically
- Tacrolimus
- Pimecrolimus
- Steroids like Clobetasol but skin atrophy a problem
- Topical vitamin D_3 as calcipotriol
3rd: Surgical grafts, malanocyte cultures

Wrinkles

Cause: Smoking and sun exposure both cause independently (Ann IM 1991;114:840) by decreasing skin collagen

Rx: Laser (Med Let 1997;37:10); topical tretinoins (Nejm 1997;337:1419) by increasing thickness of stratum corneum; injections of collagen (Zyplast, Zyderm, Cosmoderm, et al.) And hyaluronic acid gel (Hyalaform, Restylane) work for 6+ mo (Med Let 2004;46:19)

Chapter 4
Ear, Nose, and Throat

D. K. Onion

4.1 Ear

Otitis Externa (Bacterial, Allergic, Seborrheic, Fungal [Otomycosis], Rarely Viral)

Cause:

Bacterial: Staph, *Pseudomonas*
Fungal: *Aspergillus niger*
Viral: Herpes simplex and zoster

Epidem: Bacterial: Most common type of otitis externa

Pathophys: Bacterial: Local furunculosis, which then becomes more diffuse

Sx:

Allergic: 1^+ pain; 3^+ itching
Seborrheic: 1^+ pain; 1^+ itching
Bacterial: 3^+ pain, especially w movement of pinna
Fungal: 1^+ pain; 3^+ itching
Viral: 1^+ pain w herpes simplex; 3^+ pain w herpes zoster

Si:

Bacterial: Pain w tragal pressure and pinna traction; erythema and edema of external ear canal
Allergic: Acute: weeping small vesicles. Chronic: fissures and scales.

221

Seborrheic: Greasy scales, dandruff
Fungal: Looks like wet newspaper; black discharge is diagnostic
Viral: Vessels in ear may rupture or form hemorrhagic bullae

Crs:

Cmplc: Bacterial: Malignant otitis externa, a severe perichondritis, now only a problem in pts w resistant organisms or diminished resistance, eg, diabetes, cancer, or AIDS

    r/o: acute mastoiditis

Lab:

    Bact: Culture if drainage

Rx: Avoid water in all types

    Allergic: Antihistamines; topical steroids

    Seborrheic: Keep hair away from ears; topical steroids

    Bacterial/fungal: Clean out well

Domeboro's soln, or 9:1 alcohol/vinegar soln gtts, to acidify area, which prevents pseudomonas growth, w wick (eg, "Pope's otowick," a commercial sponge material) if necessary to get into canal

    Topical antibiotics and steroids (Cortisporin or Cipro HC) gtts t-qid, or ofloxacin (Floxin) gtts bid

    Glycerine to decrease swelling by hydroscopic action (VoSol)

    Systemic antibiotics, eg, penicillin, dicloxacillin, cephalothin, or ciprofloxacin especially if *P. aeruginosa* (Nejm 1991;324:392) and if sensitive; malignant external OM, rx w ceftazidime (Rev Inf Dis 1990;12:173)

    Viral: Sedation; occasionally local antibiotics; ? acyclovir

Otitis Media

Nejm 1995;332:1560; Am J Pub Hlth 1977;67:472

Cause: Acute: 75% are bacterial (Jama 1994;273:1598): H. flu (25%), 40% are β-lactamase pos, if associated w conjunctivitis then 70% are H. flu non-β-lactamase types; pneumococcus (35%);

Moraxella (*Branhamella*) *catarrhalis* (25%); other strep; viral (30%: Clin Ped 1972;11:204), although more (40%) may be viral induced (Nejm 1999;340:260), RSV, parainfluenza, and influenza

Chronic: Above plus staph, proteus, pseudomonas

Serous type (chronic OM w effusion): Fluid secretion without culturable organisms usually, although $1/3$ may have organisms (Jama 1998;279:296)

Significant genetic predisposition by twin studies (Jama 1999;282:2125,2167)

Epidem: Some viral infections predispose, eg, RSV, influenza, and adeno (Nejm 1982;306:1377)

Serous OM often follows infectious resolution

Pathophys: Rhinitis and sinusitis spread along eustachian tube. Cmplc's from juxtaposition of several structures, eg, meninges, facial nerve, oval and round windows, semicircular canals, and lateral sinus. Allergic/atopic individuals have much higher persistent rates (D. Hurst, Otolaryngol-Head Neck Surg 2000;123:533; Laryngoscope 1999;109:471).

Sx: Pain, severe and deep, unbothered by external ear manipulation, may improve suddenly w spontaneous drainage; sense of fullness; diminished hearing acuity

Si: Decreased hearing; inflamed drum often bulging; loss of light reflex, poor air movement and pain w pneumatic otoscopy

Crs: Acute usually improves within 48 hr of starting antibiotics, and clears in < 2 wk.

Serous OM is persistent OM w effusion that lasts > 3 mo w hearing loss.

Cmplc:

- Ossicle necrosis, especially of incus
- Chronic otitis with granulomas and polyps
- Mastoiditis leading to "erect ear" si, loss of post-auricular crease

- Meningitis and encephalitis
- Lateral sinus thrombosis with undulating fever and rigors, rx by tying jugular vein to stop spread
- Facial nerve paralysis, in chronic OM rx with surgical decompression
- Labyrinthitis, extension of infection through windows leading to vertigo, rx by destroying labyrinth
- Lateral semicircular canal involvement causes vertigo
- Chronic serous otitis
- Hearing acuity decrease with chronic involvement, but no diminished intellectual/verbal abilities if delay tubes (Nejm 1985;312:1529)

Lab: Tympanometry to evaluate middle ear effusions (Nejm 1982;307:1074); not helpful < age 6 mo

See tympanogram interpretation chart, Figure 4.1.)

Xray: CT of mastoids show haziness early, sclerosis and erosion later

Rx: Prevention:
- Pneumococcal vaccine conjugated @ 2, 4, 6, and 12 mo age, decreases overall incidence by 6%, vaccine type pneumococcal episodes by 20% (NNT-2 = 5) (Nejm 2001;344:403)
- Prophylactic antibiotics, rarely used now: sulfisoxazole, or amoxicillin, or Tm/S all at half rx doses as single hs dose × 3 mo or with URIs (Med Let 1983;25:102); as good as tubes
- Influenza vaccines do not decrease incidence (Jama 2003;290:1608)

of acute OM (see management flowchart: Nejm 1995;332:1560): 1st, antibiotics: amoxicillin 40 mg/kg/d, or 60-90 mg/kg/d if pcn-resistant pneumococcus possible; 2nd, amoxicillin/clavulinic acid (Augmentin); 3rd, Tm/S (8/40 kg/24 hr) in 2 doses; 4th, erythromycin + sulfa (Pediazole); 5th, cefaclor, et al. Or, if won't take po, ceftriaxone 50 mg/kg im up to 1 gm × 1, may dilute w lidocaine to decrease pain (Rx Let 1998;5:10). 5 d rx may be enough over age 2. Could give rx and tell to fill if not better on Tylenol in 48 hr since only ~1/7 cases, over age 2 and otherwise low risk, will need antibiotics and benefit at 2 wk no different than placebo (BMJ 2000;320:350); an especially good strategy if TM not bulging since most of these are viral (Nejm 2002 347:1169).

of serous OM: Antibiotics may help clear (~¹/₃ over 1 mo after 2 wk rx) but many will clear spontaneously (Nejm 1987;316:432); steroids × 7-14 d with antibiotics (Arch Otolaryngol Head Neck Surg 1991;117:984)

Decongestants and antihistamines no help in acute or serous (BMJ 1983;287:654; Nejm 1983;308:297) though many practitioners still feel they help

Surgical: Tubes help hearing acuity, but not verbal/intellectual losses (Nejm 2001;344:1179, 1985;312:1529); polyp and granulation tissue removal; prosthetic replacement for ossicle necrosis. Mastoiditis can be rx'd with simple mastoidectomy, mastoid tympanoplasty, or radical mastoidectomy if advanced. Adenoidectomy may help serous OM esp w tubes (Nejm 2001;344:1188, 1987;317:1444; Jama 1999;282:945 vs 987).

Cholesteatoma

Cause: Epidermal proliferation, though not a true neoplasia

Epidem:

Pathophys: Keratin layering arising in external canal or TM results in TM perforation (usually high on drum, unlike OM), middle ear invasion

Sx: Conductive hearing loss; foul otorrhea several times a month; ear pain

Si: Pearl white growth seen through the drum, or, more often, within marginal perforations often in attic, posterior/superior area (pars flaccida) or filling whole canal; foul otorrhea

Crs: Progressive

Acoustic–Impedance

Type **Earscan Graph**

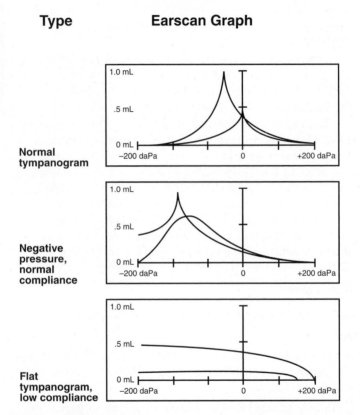

Normal tympanogram

Negative pressure, normal compliance

Flat tympanogram, low compliance

Figure 4.1 Tympanogram interpretation. Reproduced with permission from Micro Audiometrics Corp. *(Continues)*

Acoustic–Impedance

Type **Earscan Graph**

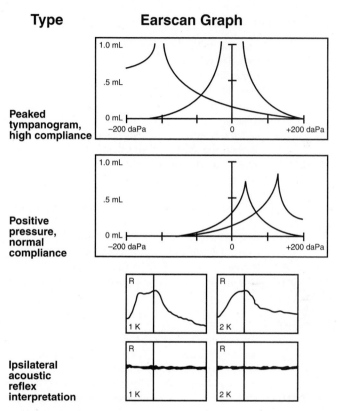

Peaked tympanogram, high compliance

Positive pressure, normal compliance

Ipsilateral acoustic reflex interpretation

Figure 4.1 *(Continues)*

Interpretation

Test Values		Condition
MEP:	0 to -100 daPa (negative value dependent upon examiner criteria)	
PV:	<2.0 mL in young children <2.5 mL in older children and adults	Normal tympanic membrane and
COMP:	>0.2 mL or <1.5 mL	middle ear system.
		Eustachian tube dysfunctio middle ear effusion may be present.
MEP:	-100 daPa or greater (neg. value may vary)	(Rounded tympanograms indicate a higher
PV:	Normal	probability of effusion.)
COMP:	>0.2 mL	
MEP:	?	
PV:	Normal when tympanic membrane intact >2.5 mL when tympanic membrane not intact	Middle ear effusion, or thickened tympanic membrane, or perforation, or
COMP:	<0.2 mL	patent ventilating tube.

Figure 4.1   Tympanogram interpretation. *(Continues)*

Interpretation

Test Values		Condition
MEP:	Normal	Flaccid tympanic membrane, or ossicular discontinuity.
PV:	Normal	
COMP:	>1.5 mL	
MEP:	Negative	Eustacian tube dysfunction and flaccid tympanic membrane, or ossicular discontinuity.
PV:	Normal	
COMP:	>1.5 mL	
MEP:	>0 daPa	High positive middle ear pressure with or without effusion.
PV:	Normal	
COMP:	Normal	
Reflex:	Present	Middle ear function completely normal.
Tympanogram:	Normal	
Reflex:	Absent	Consider adhesions, or ossicular fixation, or sensorineural hearing loss.
Tympanogram:	Abnormal	

MEP: middle ear pressure	daPa: decapascals (approximately equivalent to millimeters of water pressure, mm H_2O)
PV: physical volume	
COMP: compliance	
	mL: milliliter (equivalent to cubic centimeter, cc)

Figure 4.1 *(Continues)*

Cmplc: Brain abscess; facial paralysis; labyrinthine fistula

Lab:

Xray: CT shows erosion of adjacent bone

Rx: Surgery

Meniere's Disease

Cause: Idiopathic

Epidem: Onset usually in 5th decade

Pathophys: Endolymphatic hydrops in scala media causes increased pressure in scala media. Probably due to diminished resorption causing organ of corti damage and semicircular canal involvement.

Attack probably represents an endolymphatic rupture with mixing of endo- and perilymph; endolymph has an intracellular ionic content

Sx:
- Sensorineural hearing loss first; fluctuating ascending low-frequency loss early, then permanent high-frequency loss later
- Episodic tinnitus
- Episodic vertigo, violent, lasts an average $^1\!/_2$-2 hr only (10 min-24 hr min/max); 1-4 attacks/mo; unilateral in 85%

Si: Decreased auditory discrimination, in contrast to conductive losses; recruitment

Crs:

Cmplc: Complete hearing loss in affected ear

Lab: Audiometry shows sensorineural loss without air-bone gap. Recruitment of sound so that loudness increases abruptly with slight increase in decibel level, ie, abnormally loud above the pt's abnormally high threshold; this is the distinguishing feature between cochlear (Meniere's, presbycusis) and retrocochlear disease

Rx: Salt, caffeine, and alcohol restriction
Medications:

- Benzodiazepines in low dose, tapered to minimally effective dose, like diazepam (Valium) 2 mg po tid (never more) initially, then tapered over 1-2 wk to 2 mg qd; or lorazepam (Ativan) 1 mg sl/po
- Antihistamines (Benadryl)
- Antivertigo drugs (scopolamine, meclizine [Antivert], dimenhydrinate [Dramamine], phenothiazines)
- Diuretics prophylactically, eg, thiazides
- Streptomycin, perhaps, 2-3 gm im qd to produce bilateral nerve damage in 10-20 d, unused now

Surgical: Rarely need; labyrinthectomy through middle ear if hearing already gone there; endolymphatic saccule to subarachnoid space shunt; sacculotomy; 8th nerve section

Cerebellar-Pontine Angle Tumors

Nejm 1991;324:1555

Cause: Acoustic neuroma (AN); rarely neurofibromatosis type 2, bilateral acoustic neuromas (Jama 1997;278:51; Nejm 1988;318:684), autosomal dominant on chromosome 22; meningioma; metastatic cancer from lung, breast, prostate, kidney

Epidem: AN is most common; meningioma 2nd most common; and metastatic disease 3rd most common

Pathophys: ANs arise in vestibular portion of 8th nerve and gradually compress cranial nerves VIII and VII, then cerebellum, then IX, X, and XI

Sx:

- Hearing loss unilaterally, sensorineural, usually 1st sx
- Vertigo, mild, slowly progressive, unilateral
- Tinnitus, often unilateral
- Facial palsies

- Dysphagia
- Facial numbness

Si: Sensorineural hearing loss; ataxia, peripheral (eg, fingers), uncrossed; sensory deficits in cranial nerves, eg, distal VII (taste), and V (pin and touch); caloric testing shows no response on affected side (95%)

Crs: Neurofibromatosis type 2 onset in teens and 20s

Cmplc: Neurofibromatosis type 2 is associated with meningiomas and gliomas

Lab:

CSF: Shows elevated protein (67% of those with sx); present earlier in perilymph tap, if done

Noninv: Brainstem auditory evoked responses 100% positive (Nejm 1984;310:1740)

Xray: MRI with contrast; CT with contrast

Rx: Surgical, stereotatic radiosurgery vs microsurgery (Nejm 1998;339:1426); in elderly, first follow with q 6 mo CT or MRI to be sure progressing

Sensorineural Hearing Loss (Deafness)

Nejm 1993;329:1092

Cause:

- Cochlear types include presbycusis in old age, high-frequency losses worst; Meniere's disease, unilateral in 85%; ototoxic drugs, eg, streptomycin, gentamicin, which can be unilateral; and exposure to loud noise, eg, rock and roll music (Nejm 1970;282:467); autoimmune inner ear disease (Jama 2003;290:1875, 1994;272:611) w sudden (days) unilateral or bilateral loss due to anticochlear antibodies
- Neural (retrocochlear), often unilateral; include most commonly viral, like measles, mumps, and adenovirus infections; neuroma, vascular occlusion, hypercoagulopathy, meningitis,

syphilis, multiple sclerosis, collagen vascular diseases, trauma (often with vertigo) (Nejm 1982;306:1029), and cerebellar-pontine angle tumors

- Congenital genetic syndromes; syndromic-like maternally inherited diabetes and deafness (Ann IM 2001;134:721); and nonsyndromic, 50% of which are autosomal recessive mutations of one of 28 genes (Nejm 2002;346:243)

Epidem: Prevalence increased by smoking (Jama 1998;279:1715)

Pathophys:

Si & Sx: Diminished discrimination, poor verbal skills in children, Weber test goes to unaffected side, positive Rinné, no recruitment (except in Meniere's and presbycusis); if loss > 40 db at 2000 cps in best ear in elderly, it causes significant dysfunction and is markedly improved by hearing aid (Ann IM 1990;113:188)

Crs:

Cmplc: r/o conductive loss from wax impaction, or otosclerosis in the elderly especially if > 40 dB loss at speech frequencies (2-3000 Hz)

Lab: Audiometry shows no air–bone gap and diminished discrimination

Rx: Prednisone 60 mg po qd for acute idiopathic sudden unilateral loss w ENT f/u because of recurrence when taper steroids, reduces permanent loss by 50% (Jama 2003;289:1976, 2003;290:1875)

Hearing aid amplification (Med Let 1998;40:62) w conventional analog aid (Chrystal Ear mail-order cheap version = $300, up to $1000); 3 types: linear peak clipper not as good as compression limiter or wide dynamic range compressor by DBCT (Jama 2000;284:1806). Programmable (to pt's frequency loss) digital hearing aids ($2900).

Rarely in the profoundly deaf, cochlear implant hearing aids, $20,000 (Jama 1995;274:1955; Nejm 1993;328:233, 281); cmplc: 30× increase in meningitis (Nejm 2003;349:435)

4.2 Nose/Throat

Hereditary Angioneurotic Edema

Ann IM 1976;84:580

Cause: Genetic, autosomal dominant, or rarely acquired, C'_{1a} esterase inhibitor deficiency (Ann IM 2000;132:144)

Epidem: Most Western races

Pathophys: C'_{1a} esterase inhibitor inactivates clotting factors XII and XI, the latter build up and release kallikreins/kinins causing pain, shock, etc (Nejm 1983;308:1050)

Sx: Onset not until age 20-50 yr; frequently precipitated by trauma, psychologic stress, or pharyngitis; abdominal pain often leads to surgery

Si: Edema of skin, upper gi and respiratory tracts, recurrent, acute, nonpitting, nonpruritic, circumscribed, transient, involves localized areas

Crs:

Cmplc: Laryngeal edema causing asphyxia (26% patients die this way)
r/o:
- ACE inhibitor drug reaction angioedema (Jama 1997;278:232; Ann IM 1992;117:234)
- much more common benign, **acquired angioedema** = 90% of pts with above sx; rx with prednisone 60 mg qd × 1 wk, then qod and decrease to 5-10 mg qod; plus hydroxyzine 25 mg tid helps decrease frequency and severity (Ann IM 1991;114:133); or, if no response, tranexamic acid (ϵ-aminocaproic acid-like drug) up to 1 gm po tid (Am J Med 1999;106:650)
- "pseudo-angioedema" associated with lymphoma and colon cancer
- uvular edema of Franklin's disease (p 507)

Lab:

Immunol: Screen for C_4; if decreased look for serum ϵ_2-globulin inhibitor of C'_{1a} (present in 90%; 10% have inactive, non-functioning C'_{1a} esterase inhibitor)

Rx: Preventively screen family
for prophylaxis:

- Tranexamic acid 1 gm po tid (Am J Med 1998;106:650)
- Androgens like danazol 200 mg tid, prevents attacks, little virilization (Ann IM 1980;93:809; $1/pill); stanozol 0.5 mg b-qid effective, cheaper; oxymethalone 5-10 mg qd, can use 4 d pre-op
- Steroids, like prednisone 60 mg qd × 1 wk, then qod and decrease to 5-10 mg qod; plus
- Hydroxyzine 25 mg tid helps decrease frequency and severity (Ann IM 1991;114:133)

for acute life-threatening attack or its prophylaxis: C'_{1a} inhibitor from vapor-heated pooled plasma concentrate (Nejm 1996;334:1630); + supportive care

Acute Epiglottitis (Bacterial Supraglottitis)

Jama 1994;272:1358 (adults); Nejm 1986;314:1133 (adults)

Cause: H. flu, type B, is predominant organism in children and adults; staph, pneumo, rarely other strep

Epidem: Primarily in children age 1-5 yr, but now more commonly in adults, eg, President George Washington; > 10/million adults/yr
Incidence 1.8 cases/100,000 population/yr in adults, 0.6/100,000 population in children;
Male/female = 1.8:1 in adults

Pathophys: Obstruction of upper airway by edematous epiglottis

Sx: Extremely sore throat (95%), more than dysphagia (94%), plus respiratory distress often over 6-24 hr

Si: Epiglottis and/or other supraglottic structures inflamed and edematous by direct or indirect laryngoscopy (safe to do in adults, not in children), need to sit erect (21%), muffled voice (54%), fever (50%), drooling (40%), stridor (15%); pharynx often (50%) normal

Airway intervention needed in 42% w stridor, 47% w need to sit erect

Crs: Sore throat × 2-4 d, dysphagia and respiratory distress 6-24 hr

Cmplc: Sudden, unpredictable airway obstruction, 7% mortality without prophylactic airway; decreases to 1% with airway prophylactically placed

r/o angioneurotic edema, foreign body

Lab:

Bact: Blood culture

Xray: Lateral soft-tissue film of neck shows narrowed glottis, 20% false neg, not as good as indirect laryngoscopy

Rx: Prevent w H. flu vaccination

Appropriate antibiotic, usually 2nd- or 3rd-generation cephalosporin like cefuroxime, or ampicillin plus chloramphenicol; no evidence that steroids help but most clinicians believe they do

Early prophylactic nasotracheal intubation in OR under anesthesia, especially in children where should not wait for stridor to intubate

Allergic Rhinitis

Jama 1997;278:1849; Nejm 1991;325:860

Cause: Allergens including grass, tree, and ragweed pollens; dust; animal dander; fungal allergens like thermophilic actinomycetes in car air conditioners (Nejm 1984;311:1119)

Epidem: Airborne; prevalence 5-20%, increased to 30% if atopic; peak incidence in childhood and adolescence

Pathophys: IgE produced, attaches to mast cells, and releases mediators when antigen presents; basophils probably responsible for "late" (hours later) exacerbations (Nejm 1985;313:65); but not all w measurable IgE have the clinical syndrome; precipitating antigens most commonly are pollens, animal dander, house mites, insects, mold spores, and food

Sx: Nasal congestion, sneezing, rhinorrhea, pruritus of nose and eyes, sometimes cough, diminished smell

Si: Nasal polyps

Crs: Usually seasonal; recurrence rate of polyps high

Cmplc: r/o **atrophic rhinitis** caused by *T. pallidum*, which somehow impairs cilial action; has a bad smell, crusted discharge, and positive STS; aspirin (COX-1) NSAID-leukotriene–sensitive syndrome, associated w asthma (Nejm 2002;347:1493, 1524)

Lab:

Bact: Nasal smear shows eosinophils

Hem: Eosinophil count increases (66%)

Immunol (Ann IM 2004;140:278): Usually done if no initial response to symptomatic rx

- Phadiatop in vitro test for common IgE types
- Individual in vitro RAST tests, ~$7/antigen, qualitative not quantitative; done by putting antigen on filter paper, adding pt serum, washing, then adding hot anti-IgE, washing again, then counts made
- Skin testing

Rx: Avoid antigens by using electrostatic precipitators and covering and washing bedding

Humidified heat 30 min q 2 hr to raise nose temperature > 43°C cures coryza (Proc Natl Acad Sci 1982;79:4766); no—new studies disprove (Jama 1994;271:1109,1112)

1st-choice medications:

- Decongestants like pseudoephedrine or phenylpropanolamine; topical decongestants are better than systemic, but can lead to **rhinitis medicamentosa** if used > 7 d; rx w steroid nose spray to get off, and systemic absorption increases CVA risk (Med Let 2000;42:113)
- Antihistamines (H_1 blockers) (Nejm 2004;351:2203; Med Let 1994;36:78) like diphenhydramine (Benadryl), triprolidine (w pseudoephedrine = Actifed) or chlorpheniramine (w pseudoephedrine = Sudafed) 4 mg qid (cheap); but more driving impairment than a blood alcohol level of 0.1% (Ann IM 2000;132:354); possibly azelastin (Astelin) (Med Let 1997;39:45) ππ sprays bilat bid, an H_1 blocker w systemic absorption, $50/mo

2nd-:

- Nonsedating-type antihistamines (Nejm 2004;351:2203); metabolism is inhibited by grapefruit juice (Med Let 2001;43:35); have no anticholinergic side effects; all $2-2.50/d until available generically and/or OTC
  - Cetirizine (Zyrtec) (Med Let 1996;38:21,95) 5-10 mg po qd
  - Desloratadine (Clarinex) (Med Let 2002;44:27) 5 mg po qd; derivative of loratidine to preserve Schering market share when patent expired in 2003; similar action and adverse effects
  - Fexofenadine (Allegra) 60 mg po q 12 hr; absorption decreased 70% w any fruit juice
  - Loratadine (Claritin) 10 mg po qd; cmplc: fulminant hepatic necrosis rarely (Ann IM 1996;125:738); $30/mo generic, $17/mo OTC
- LRAs like montelukast (Singulair) (Med Let 2003;45:21) 10 mg po qd; less good than nasal steroids; $90/mo
- Na cromolyn 4% intranasal spray q 3-4 hr (Med Let 1991;33:115). Ophthalmic cromolyn helps if eye sx prominent.

3rd-: Topical steroids (Med Let 1999;40:16) like beclomethasone (Vancenase AQ2, Beconase AQ3) nasal spray π̈ bid ($25/mo); flunisolide (Nasalide) spray π̈ bid ($43/mo); budesonide (Rhinocort) π̈ bid ($43/mo) (Med Let 1994;36:63); fluticasone (Flonase) π̈ bid (Med Let 1995;37:5), $46/mo; triam-cinolone, mometasone, ~$45/mo

4th-: Steroids po × 3 wk, then continue at 5 mg qd × 2-3 mo

5th-: Skin test and desensitize next year; efficacy, at least for grass pollens, clear (Nejm 1999;341:468,522), give × 3 yr, benefits last > 3 yr after cessation

Experimental: Recombinant monoclonal anti-IgE antibody (omalizumab) (Jama 2001;286:2956) 50-300 mg sc q 3-4 wk

Sinusitis

ACP position ppr: Ann IM 2001;134:495; Jama 1997;278:1850; Nejm 2004;351:902

Cause: *Pneumococcus*, H. flu, *Moraxella catarrhalis*, strep, staph, occasionally anaerobes (Nejm 1974;290:735,1351). Cystic fibrosis or heterozygous gene carrier (Jama 2000;284:1814).

Epidem: Associated with rhinitis (90%), dental caries (10%); occurs at any age > 2 yr

Pathophys: Edema around sinus ostia blocks drainage; all sinuses drain to medial meatus, except ethmoidals to superior meatus, sphenoid occasionally to sphenoethmoid area, and lacrimal duct to inferior meatus

Sx: Dull headache; local pain off and on, a maxillary "toothache"; worse when leaning over; purulent nasal discharge; sx are unresponsive to decongestants; loss of smell and taste

Si: Rhinitis, postnasal discharge, pus on middle turbinate, loss of sinus transillumination (for frontals, light below medial supraorbital ridge; for maxillaries, light downward on mid-inferior orbital rim and look inside mouth at palate: Nejm 1992;326:319)

Crs: Either acute ethmoidal or frontal sinusitis is an acute emergency requiring hospitalization, iv antibiotics, and consideration of surgical drainage

Cmplc: Orbital cellulitis, epi/subdural abscess, cavernous sinus thrombosis, osteomyelitis, asthma exacerbation

Lab:

Bact: Culture of nasopharynx correlates with sinus aspiration culture very poorly (30%: Nejm 1981;304:751)

Xray: Not routine, may get if chronic or recurrent; plain films show opacity (85% specificity), air fluid levels (80% specif), or > 6 mm mucosal thickening (Jama 1995;273:1015); if normal the dx is untenable; CT scans, 4 slice, especially for sphenoidal and ethmoids

Rx: Nasal local decongestants like epinephrine gtts 0.5-2%, or phenylephrine 0.25% in saline nasally qid for < 7 d *and* nasal steroids bid (Jama 2001;286:3097) alone or w antibiotics; rx to maxillary sinus usually clears other

Antibiotics (Jama 2001;286:1849):

1st: Amoxicillin × 10 d first in children (Nejm 1992;326:319) and adults (BMJ 1996;313:325; Nejm 1981;304:750), or erythromycin, or erythro/sulfa (Pediazole), or Tm/S; except for ethmoidal and sphenoidal, when should start with a penicillinase-resistant penicillin like amox/clavulinic acid (Augmentin) high-dose SR or ES, or 2nd-generation fluoroquinolone

2nd: Cefopodixime, cefaclor tid, cefuroxime bid, Tm/S × 3 d bid as good as 10 d (Jama 1995;273:1015), azithromycin, clarithromycin, quinolone

Surgical functional endoscopic sinus surgery for drainage if worsening despite medical rx; rarely enteronasal anterostomy (Caldwell-Luc procedure)

4.3 ENT Cancers

Laryngeal Carcinoma

Nejm 2001;345:1890

Cause: Chronic irritation causing neoplasia, esp from smoking (90%) and drinking alcohol

Epidem: 10,000 new pts/yr in U.S.; male/female ratio = 10-20:1; peak incidence age 45-65 yr

Pathophys: 75% involve true cords (glottic); important since true cord itself has poor lymphatic drainage, hence few metastases; subglottic and supraglottic areas are "silent," ie, sx appear late

Cigarette and alcohol-induced mutations in p53 gene, inactivation of which often induces cancer (Nejm 1995;332:712)

Sx: Glottic type: Hoarseness

Supraglottic type: Ear pain, throat lump, dysphagia, aspiration, muffled "hot potato" voice

Si: Tumor on laryngoscopy in all (supraglottic, glottic, and subglottic)

Crs: Supraglottic and subglottic have very poor prognosis even with all forms of rx. Glottic is "a good cancer to have" since early sx and few mets.

Cmplc: Aspiration, pneumonia, weight loss from dysphagia, airway obstruction

Lab:

Path: Bx shows squamous cell carcinoma; occult tumor cells invisible at margins and/or nodes, detectable by PCR assay (Nejm 1995;332:429)

Rx: Prevent by stopping smoking. Even after dx, stopping will double cure rates and survival for all head and neck cancers (Nejm 1993;328:159); isotretinoin prevents the frequent occurrence (30%) of 2nd primary cancers (Nejm 1993;328:15; 1990;323:795)

Radiation, as long as isolated to one cord and not spread to other or ventricle, 90% cure of glottic; possibly hyperfractionated type (Nejm 1998;338:1798). Even in advanced disease, combined w concomitant chemoRx, results in 75% 2-yr sparing of laryingectomy (Nejm 2003;349:2091).

Surgery w laser, or transoral rx of in situ/early lesions; chordectomy; conservative laryngectomy procedures; conservative neck dissections when in piriform area or when neck nodes present

Surgery + post-op radiation yield 40% 5-yr survival plus modest additional recurrence/survival benefit from cisplatin chemoRx, but complc from cisplatin substantial (Nejm 2004; 350:1937,1945)

Nasopharyngeal and Maxillary Sinus Cancer

Nejm 2001;345:1890

Cause: Neoplasia

Epidem: Nasopharyngeal: Most common cancer in Asians; chemical and fume exposures and associated w HLA-A2 locus (Nejm 1976;295:1101), w human papillomavirus 16 (Nejm 2001; 344:1125), and w EBV (Nejm 2001;345:1877, 1995;333:693)

Pathophys: Cigarette and alcohol-induced mutations in p53 gene, inactivation of which often induces cancer (Nejm 1995;332:712)

Early mets

Sx: Bloody nasal discharge

Nasopharyngeal: Nontender neck mass (1st sx in 30%), unilaterally blocked ear

Maxillary sinus: Loosening of teeth or dentures, malocclusion, and recurrent idiopathic epistaxis

Si: Serosanguineous, unilateral nasal discharge

Nasopharyngeal: Nontender neck mass usually in posterior triangle, unilateral serous otitis ("any adult w persistent serous otitis has a nasopharyngeal cancer until proven otherwise")

Maxillary sinus: Gingivolabial fold loss

Crs: Maxillary sinus: Pain, proptosis, neural involvement

Cmplc:

Lab:

> *Path:* Bx shows squamous cell carcinoma. In nasopharyngeal, fine-needle aspiration of primary or metastasis shows EBV by PCR most of the time, plasma viral load present 90% of the time and level correlates w prognosis (Nejm 2004;350:2461)

Xray: CT of maxillary sinus shows increased density or bony destruction w expansion of maxillary sinus

Rx: Prevent by stopping smoking; stopping will double cure rates and survival for all head and neck cancers (Nejm 1993;328:159). Isotretinoin prevents the frequent occurrence (30%) of 2nd primary cancers (Nejm 1993;328:15, 1990;323:795).

Nasopharyngeal:

> 1st: Radiation of primary and mets; possibly hyperfractionated type (Nejm 1998;338:1798)
>
> 2nd: Surgery of primary and mets
>
> 3rd: ChemoRx w cisplatinum + 5-FU (Nejm 1992;327:1115)

Maxillary sinus:

> 1st: Surgery and/or radiation; possibly hyperfractionated type (Nejm 1998;338:1798)
>
> 2nd: ChemoRx w cisplatinum + 5-FU (Nejm 1992;327:1115)

Squamous Cell Cancer of Tongue and Tonsil

Nejm 2001;345:1890

Cause: Neoplasia; ? from chronic irritation

Epidem: Always associated with:

- Smoking (increases relative risk × 27: Nejm 1995;332:712)
- Alcohol use (the two together increase the risk × 20: Arch Otolaryng 1983;109:746)
- Poor oral hygiene
- Snuff dipping in Southern women (Nejm 1981;304:745)
- Betel nut chewing

Pathophys: Cigarette and alcohol-induced mutations in p53 gene, inactivation of which often induces cancer (Nejm 1995;332:712)

Sx: Oral-pharyngeal lesion, bleeding, or mass; neck mass; pain, local or referred to ear (otalgia)

Si: Hard, nontender mass, may ulcerate

Crs: Treatments cure ~30%

Cmplc: Local and/or rarely distant metastases

Lab:

> *Path:* Bx any lesion > 14 d old without known cause (Nejm 1976;294:109); occult tumor cells invisible at margins and/or nodes detectable by PCR assay (Nejm 1995;332:429)

Rx: Prevent by stopping smoking; stopping will double cure rates and survival for all head and neck cancers (Nejm 1993;328:159); and/or w isotretinoin (13-*cis*-retinoic acid) po at high dose × 3 mo, then low-dose maintenance to pts w leukoplakia; works but may not be worth it (Nejm 1993;328:15), but may be able to predict malignant conversion by DNA content analysis (Nejm 2001; 344:1270,1323)

> Surgical excision combined w radiation (hyperfractionated type: Nejm 1998;339:1798), and chemotherapy w cisplatinum + 5-FU (Nejm 1992;327:115), modestly improves survival

4.4 Miscellaneous

Aphthous Stomatitis

Cause: Unknown, viral vs immunologic, possibly stress related

Sx: Painful ulcers, r/o Behçets' syndrome (p 1088), herpes simplex, coxsackie infections (eg, herpangina, hand-foot-mouth disease) (p 684)

Rx:

- Amlexanox (Aphthasol) cream qid, decreases inflammation and speeds healing × 1 d; $20/5 gm
- Phenelzine (MAOI) b-qid (letter: Nejm 1984;311:1442)

- Na cromolyn decreases pain (Ann IM 1978;89:228)
- Tetracycline mouth washes, 125 mg/5 cc tid rinse and swallow
- Thalidomide (Nejm 1997;336:1487; Med Let 1998;40:103) 50-200 mg po qd × 2-4+ wk; esp in AIDS pts; cmplc: teratogenicity, rash, somnolence, HIV proliferation; $0.75/50 mg

Cerumen (Ear Wax)

Loosen w Ceruminex or Colace liquid (not syrup)

Epistaxis (Nosebleed)

Wm Maxwell 1/98

Rx: Prevent w short-term topical Premarin cream bid
1st: Pack nose w cotton strips soaked w topical anesthesia + vasoconstrictor (4% cocaine does both)
2nd: Cauterize w silver nitrate or electric cautery
3rd: Pack, leave anterior packs in place 3 d, posteriors 5 d, w
- Vaseline strip gauze anteriorly, or Merocel pack, or Gelfoam
- Balloon pack (Nozstop, etc), in anterior nose and in nasopharynx
- Posterior pack or Foley catheter

Refer to ENT if bleeding persists for internal maxillary artery ligation

Periodontal Disease

rv-Nejm 1990;322:373 Acute periodontitis and necrotizing gingivitis are caused by a spirochete very similar to *T. pallidum* (Nejm 1991;325:539)

Phonation, Abnormal Causes

- Hollow voice from recurrent laryngeal nerve paralysis: Air escape, requires multiple breaths to say what should be able to say in one breath
  - Left recurrent nerve causes: Cancer of lung (70%), aortic aneurysm, mitral stenosis (rare)
  - Right recurrent causes: Thyroid and other neck pathology

- Hoarseness from laryngeal cancer, benign polyps and nodules, or laryngitis (whispers)

Temporomandibular Joint Syndrome

Many are psychiatric in origin via anxiety (Nejm 1978; 299:123) and bruxism; others feel dental malocclusion is primary etiology. Orthodontic evaluation, surgery only as a last resort.

Tinnitus

Nejm 2002;347:906

Cause:
- Presbycusis most commonly in the elderly; audiogram will show significant loss at 4000 cps
- Idiopathic type common
- Acoustic trauma
- Drugs: aspirin, digitalis, streptomycin, gentamicin and other aminoglycosides, quinidine, quinine
- Diseases: Meniere's

Epidem: Males > females, increases w age; whites > blacks

Sx: Ringing, buzzing, hissing, whistle, "cricket-like," humming sounds

Si: Conductive hearing loss findings by Rinné and Webber tests

Cmplc: r/o real noise from bruits, murmurs, stapedial or tensor tympani muscles, et al.

Lab: Audiometry

Rx: Avoid noise trauma; hearing aids; masking; tricyclic antidepressants

Xerostomia, Postirradiation

Rx w pilocarpine 5-10 mg po tid (Med Let 1994;36:76)

Chapter 5

Endocrinology/Metabolism

D. K. Onion

5.1 Adrenal Disorders

Cushing's Syndrome

Nejm 1995;332:791, 1994;331:629 (NIH—children)

Cause (Nejm 1991;325:899):

- Cushing's disease from chromophobe or basophilic micro- or macroadenoma of pituitary
- Ectopic ACTH production by oat cell or other (ovary, pancreas, carcinoid) cancer; occasionally ACTH-producing carcinoid tumors, especially of lung (Ann IM 1992;117:209)
- Adrenal: Bilateral nodular hyperplasia or unilateral adrenal adenoma (15%) (ACTH receptor genetic defects: Nejm 1998;339:27); rare primary pigmented nodular hyperplasia (Ann IM 1999;131:585) associated w MEA and cardiac myomas; or carcinoma (<1% adults, 4% of children w Cushing's—NIH)

Epidem:

Pathophys: Glucocorticoids cause connective tissue dissolution, have an anti-vitamin D effect, cause proteolysis of muscle, lymphocyte/monocyte inhibition (Nejm 1975;292:236), increased acid/pepsin secretion, increased gluconeogenesis, and decreased glucose uptake. Aldosterone and androgens elevated too when ACTH is the mechanism.

Sx: Muscle weakness, obesity/weight gain; growth retardation in children; easy bruising

Si: Muscle weakness; ecchymoses; moon face, buffalo hump; abdominal striae; truncal fat; osteoporosis and fractures; increased number and severity of infections; peptic ulcers; diabetes, nonketotic, insulin resistant; psychoses; virilization; hypertension (47% in children), and edema

Crs: Excellent prognosis unless cancer or ectopic ACTH (usually cancer) (Nejm 1971;285:243)

Cmplc: See si above

Lab (Ann IM 2003;138:980):

Chem: Serum cortisol, normal level is 10-25 μgm %
(= 280-700 nM/L) in am, dropping to < 7 μgm % in pm; after 1 mg dexamethasone at 11 pm, 8-am cortisol is < 5 in normal; if > 10, r/o Cushing's (100% sens, 90% specif-Ann IM 1990;112:738); false positives with phenytoin (Dilantin). Late-night salivary cortisol levels ≥ 70 nM/L. If studies indeterminant, then give 0.5 mg dexamethasone q 6 hr × 48 hr and measure cortisol; or get 24-hr urinary free cortisol (6% false neg, fewer false pos) and/or 24-hr urine cortisols × 3 ≥ 100 μgm/ 24 hr

If above tests are abnormal, then high-dose tests are done to differentiate cause: eg, baseline 8-am cortisol, 8 mg dexamethasone that night at 11 pm, then 8-am cortisol. Pituitary Cushing's pts, unlike adrenal tumors or ectopic ACTH production types, suppress value to < 50% of baseline value (92% sens, 100% specif-Ann IM 1986;104:180, 68% sens in children; also see Nejm 1994;330:1295 for various tests' sens/specif)

CRH test: ACTH and cortisol increased after CRH given if pituitary tumor, not if ectopic ACTH or adrenal tumor (Ann IM 1985;102:344); 80% sens in children

Petrosal venous sampling for ACTH levels, simultaneous bilaterally reliably lateralize pituitary tumor (Nejm 1985;312:100)

Xray: CT, 60% false neg rate due to small size of adenomas
MRI with gadolinium enhancement, 71% sens (52% sens in children), 87% specif; but 10% of the normal adult population have a lesion (Ann IM 1994;120:817)

Rx: 1st: Surgical transsphenoidal microadenomectomy, 90% success-ful (Nejm 1984;310:889 vs 76%: Ann IM 1988;109:487); bi-lateral adrenalectomy

2nd: Irradiation of pituitary, 83% successful in pts who fail surgery (Nejm 1997;336:172)

3rd: Aminoglutethimide, mitotane, metyrapone, and trilostane (Med Let 1985;27:87); bromocriptine; ketoconazole for its antisteroid synthesis effect (Nejm 1987;317:812)

Conn's Syndrome

Nejm 1998;339:1828, 1994;331:250

Cause: Bilateral adrenal hyperplasia; or unilateral adrenal adenoma secreting aldosterone

Epidem: 1-2% of all hypertensive patients

Pathophys: Increased aldosterone production causes Na retention and K loss, leading to hypervolemia of 2-3 L, hypertension; H+ loss causing metabolic alkalosis. Is there an anterior pituitary "aldosterone-stimulating factor"? (Nejm 1984;311:120)

Sx: Fatigue, weakness, tetany

Si: Hypertension; Trousseau's si, due to alkalosis; little edema, unlike secondary causes of increased aldosterone; proximal myopathy

Crs:

Cmplc: r/o **Liddle's Syndrome,** an aldosterone-like effect caused by an autosomal dominantly inherited renal tubular defect (Nejm 1999;340:1177, 1994;330:178); **Bartter's Syndrome** (Nejm 2004;350:1314, 1999;340:1180) and **licorice ingestion** (Nejm 1991;325:1223), both of which cause a normotensive hy-peraldosteronism by peripheral angiotensin resistance and/or prostaglandin induction; secondary causes of hyperaldosteronism

Rare unilateral adenoma or cancer of adrenal (Ann IM 1984; 101:316)

Lab: *Chem:* Aldosterone levels elevated; $K^+ < 3.7$ mEq/L (80% sens) esp suspicious if Na high or high normal; urine $K^+ > 30$ mEq/24 hr; metabolic alkalosis w elevated HCO_3

Renin levels low, but elevated in secondary types of hyperaldosteronism

Adrenal vein sampling for lateralized aldosterone and cortisol levels

Saline infusion test: 2 L NS iv over 4 hr decreases serum aldosterone to < 10 ng % in normal pts

Captopril test: 25 mg po $\times$ 1 decreases serum aldosterone levels to $< 50\%$ at 2 hr in normal pts

Xray: CT or MRI

Rx: Spironolactone 100 mg qid + antihypertensives (Ann IM 1999; 1341:105)

Surgical adrenalectomy when unilateral lesion, though BP cured by this is only 35% (Ann IM 1995;122:877)

Addison's Disease (Primary Adrenal Insufficiency)

Nejm 1996;335:1206

Cause: Idiopathic autoimmune; metastatic cancer; infection, especially tuberculosis, and meningococcemia with Friderichsen-Waterhouse syndrome; stress in patient chronically suppressed with steroids; HIV in AIDS pts (Ann IM 1997; 127:1103)

Epidem: Peak incidence age 20-40 yr. Associated with HLA-B8 and DR 3/4, and thereby with pernicious anemia, myasthenia gravis, islet cell antibody IDDM, myxedema, vitiligo, alopecia, and primary gonadal failure.

Pathophys: 80% of gland must be destroyed to get sx. ACTH and MSH similar, hence increased pigmentation; both mineralocorticoid and glucocorticoid deficiencies create the si and sx.

Sx: Loss of "sense of well-being"; increased pigmentation, especially of scars, creases, and buccal mucosa; nausea, vomiting, and diarrhea; salt craving and weight loss; galactorrhea, rarely

Si: Hypotension, postural first and later even supine; cachexia; hyperpigmentation, vitiligo, longitudinal nail pigment streaks (Nejm 1969;281:1056); diminished axillary and pubic hair

Crs: 40% eventually develop other glandular failure (especially thyroid, gonadal)

Cmplc: r/o **hyporeninemic hypoaldosteronism** with hyperkalemia and metabolic acidosis seen in AODM and primary renal disease

r/o **adrenoleukodystrophy** in boys, a sex-linked abnormality of fatty acid metabolism (Nejm 1990;322:13); **autoimmune polyendocrinoptahy candidiasis/ectodermal dystrophy** (Nejm 1990; 322:1829): 80% are hypoparathyroid, 70% are hypoadrenal, 60% of women with it are hypogonadal compared to 15% of men; by age 20, 100% have had significant candidal infections

Lab: *Chem:* Na low, HCO_3 low; K elevated; ACTH elevated; 8-am cortisol $<$ 3 μgm is diagnostic, $<$ 15 μgm % when under stress, if $>$ 20 μgm % then dx is unlikely (D. Spratt 1/94). Beware decreased cortisol-binding proteins falsely lowering values in acute illness, measure free cortisol instead? (Nejm 2004;350:1629).

Cosyntropin screening test of adrenal reserve (Ann IM 2003;139:194), perhaps if am ACTH/cortisol ratio ambiguous but not very specific or sens (ACP J Club 2004;140:18): get fasting blood cortisol, then give 250 μgm cosyntropin (ACTH analog) iv and draw repeat cortisol 30 min later (or im and 60 min later); a normal pt's levels increase $>$ 6 μgm % to over 20 μgm % if adequate adrenal reserve (Nejm 1976;295:30)

Hem: CBC may show eosinophilia

Rx (Nejm 2003;348:727):

Glucocorticoids like cortisol 25-30 mg po qd in am to mimic early-am peaks; steroid equivalents in order of diminishing mineralocorticoid component: hydrocortisone 20 mg, prednisone 5 mg, methylprednisolone 4 mg, dexa-methasone 0.75 mg. Cover w stress doses as below when stressed.

Mineralocorticoid, eg, fludrocortisone (Fluorinef) 100-300 μgm qd; adjust dose by renin level, which should be normal if adequate replacement; can cause significant supine hypertension over years (Nejm 1979;301:68)

Androgens can help reestablish sense of well-being and sexuality, especially in females, eg dihydroepiandrosterone (DHEA) 50 mg po qd (Nejm 1999;341:1013)

In steroid-induced adrenal suppression (Nejm 1997;337:1285), slow tapering of steroids (Nejm 1976;295:30) should be done to allow recovery of pituitary/adrenal axis, decrease to a physiologic level of 20 mg hydrocortisone or other steroid equivalent q am, then taper q 4 wk to 10 mg qd by 2.5-mg increments; when 8-am plasma cortisol before pills > 10 μgm %, can stop and expect baseline adrenal function to be ok; still must supplement with stress doses of steroids, eg, 50 mg hydrocortisone or equivalent bid for minor and 100 mg tid for major illnesses (Jama 2002;287:236). When cosyntropin test is normal, no longer need such supplementation (Nejm 1976;295:30).

Adrenal Genital Syndromes

Nejm 2004;350:367, 2003;349:776; Ann IM 2002;136:320 (21-OH deficiency)

Cause: Genetic enzyme deficiencies; all autosomal recessive. In 21-OH, defect is in CYP21 gene for a microsomal cytochrome P450 enzyme (Nejm 1991;324:145)

Epidem: Classic 21β-OH deficiency occurs in 1/16,000; atypical milder forms in 2+/1000

Pathophys: See Figure 5.1.

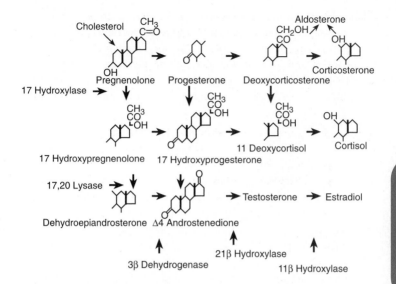

Figure 5.1 Important steroid pathways.

Sx: Usually appears in children; although mild "adult adrenal hyperplasia" may not manifest until adulthood, mainly 21β-OH deficiency, rarely 11β- or 17-OH deficiency, which present with amenorrhea and hypertension

Si: 17-OHase: Hyperaldosteronism, hypogonadism

3βde-OHase: Virilization **(female pseudohermaphroditism),** salt loss, many die at birth

11-OHase: Virilization (female pseudohermaphroditism), hypertension, hypokalemia

21-OHase: Virilization (female pseudohermaphroditism), salt loss may manifest as SIDS in male infants where detected later because ambiguous genitalia not a clue, hyponatremia

Crs: With rx, children grow up short but w normal sexual maturation (Nejm 1978;299:1392)

Cmplc: Iatrogenic Cushing's syndrome; Addisonian crisis; ovarian dermoids; precocious puberty, r/o **Albright's Syndrome:** precocious puberty and other endocrine hyperfunctioning including thyroid, adrenal, and pituitary growth hormone, plus café-au-lait spots (Nejm 1991;325:688), and fibrous dysplasia of the bones (Nejm 2002;347:1670), a somatic mutation that can also cause blindness if sphenoid involvement

Lab: *Chem:* Plasma aldosterone increased in 11β-OH deficiency. In 21-OH deficiency, 17-OH progesterone, androstenedione, and testosterone all elevated.

Urine: 17-Ketosteroid steroids elevated in 11β-OH, 21β-OH, 3βde-OH, and perhaps 17-OH deficiencies. 17-OH steroids elevated in 11β-OH deficiency.

Rx (Jama 1997;227:1077): Prevent w newborn screening?
of disease: Use all 4 (Jama 1997;227:1073):

- Glucocorticoids, like hydrocortisone 25-30 mg/M²/d
- Mineralocorticoids as fludrocortisone (Florinef) 100-300 μgm qd for all ages, or more until reach normal renin levels; may also work prenatally if started within 1 mo of conception to prevent virilization of female infants (Nejm 1990;322:111); these imperfectly decrease feedback production of more precursors
- Flutamide, an antiandrogen, also used to supplement this regimen
- Testolactone, inhibits androgen to estrogen conversion

5.2 Diabetes and Obesity

Diabetes Mellitus

Type 1: Juvenile onset (JODM), usually insulin dependent (IDDM)

Type 2: Adult onset (AODM), usually non–insulin dependent (NIDDM) at least initially

Cause (Nejm 1981;304:1454):

Type 1: Hypoinsulinemia; has an autosomal genetic component; HLA-linked to DQ antigens (Nejm 1990;322:1836); 90% are autoimmune w measurable antibodies to islet cell antigens as early as age 2 (Ann IM 2004;140:882), insulin, glutamic acid decarboxylase, et al. (Nejm 2000;342:301, 1994;331:1428), 10% are not; may be associated with early childhood exposure to cow's milk? (Nejm 1992;327:302,348 vs Jama 1996;276:607; Nejm 1993;329:1853) or cereals (Jama 2003;290:1713,1721,1771) before 3 mo or after 7 mo age. Viral infections like mumps and coxsackie (Nejm 2001;345:1331) induce IDDM, probably through T cells directed against islet antigens (Jama 1997;277:1101).

Type 2: Insulin-resistant (Nejm 1993;329:1988) adult type, substantial genetic/familial component since 90% concordance in identical twins; also associated w glycogen synthetase deficiency (Nejm 1993;328:10), and chromosome 20 gene for glucokinase deficiency (Nejm 1993;328:697)

Epidem: Prevalence of overt disease = 1.5%; 25-50% lifetime risk if live to 80+, depending on ethnicity (Jama 2003;290:1884); 0.3% of all obstetric patients

Type 1 = 10-20% of all diabetics; anti-islet cell antibodies predict onset (Nejm 1990;323:1167). Higher incidence/prevalence in Northern European populations (Nejm 1994;331:1428).

Type 2 = 80% of all diabetics. Increased with parity with a 10-20 yr delay (Nejm 1989;321:1214) and by (Jama 2001;286:1945) hypokalemia, β-blockers, protease inhibitors, atypical antipyretics, iron load (Jama 2004;291:711).

Decreased incidence w ACE inhibitor use (Jama 2001;286:1882), and higher dietary nut intake, including peanut butter (Jama 2002;288:2554)

Pathophys: Theories of neuropathy (Jama 2002;288:2581), retinopathy, and cataract causation: (1) a result of sorbitol accumulation from glucose via aldose reductase (AR)? (Ann IM 1992;117:226); (2) "glycation" of many body proteins like HgbA₁C (Ann IM 1996;124,suppl 1:81); (3) reactive oxygen intermediate theory; or (4) protein kinase C

Microvascular cmplc correlate with renin levels, which decrease with intensive chronic rx (Nejm 1985;312:1412); nephropathy and retinopathy are preceded in IDDM by elevated prorenin levels (Nejm 1990;323:1101)

Infectious cmplc's due to impaired PMNL phagocytosis from high blood sugar levels (Ann IM 1995;123:919)

Insulin increases amino acid uptake, protein synthesis, glucose uptake, free fatty acid (FFA) uptake, glycogen synthetase; decreases lipolysis, glycogenolysis

Muscle and fat tissues metabolize FFA when glucose < 120 mg %. FFAs inhibit glycolysis and hexose monophosphate shunt, hence TPNH and all synthesis and repair; FFAs are metabolized to ketone bodies, causing acidosis, and are converted to triglycerides by the liver and hence may contribute to atherosclerosis.

Glucagon excess may be equally important in pathogenesis

In type 2, genetic peripheral (skeletal muscle) insulin resistance from mitochondrial oxidative phosphorylation dysregulation of intramyocellular fatty acid metabolism and consequent increased insulin levels cause eventual β-cell exhaustion (Nejm 2004;350:664, 1996;334:777; Ann IM 1990;113:905,909); impaired/delayed insulin release to glucose load also allows hepatic gluconeogenesis to persist 1-2 hr, then insulin overshoot occurs (Nejm 1992;326:22). Islet amyloid deposition may also contribute (Nejm 2000;343:411).

In pregnancy, macrosomia due to increased substrate availability and some maternal insulin/antibody complex absorbed by the fetus (Nejm 1990;323:309)

Sx: Polyuria, polydypsia, polyphagia, weight loss

Si: Necrobiosis lipoidica (95%) = pigmented skin plaques with white lipid center, irregular, atrophic; fatty hepatomegaly; retinopathy with hard exudates, microaneurysms and hemorrhages (photos: Nejm 1993;329:320)

Crs: Neuropathies worsen over 5-10 yr when present, in ~50% (Nejm 1995;333:89)

Cmplc (Nejm 1993;328:1676): Acidosis/coma (p 267), and nonketotic, hyperosmolar coma (Nejm 1977;297:1452)

ASCVD rate doubled (Framingham Heart Study) from elevated lipids when HgbA$_1$C levels > 8% (Ann IM 1992;117:42), and perhaps from hypercoagulability induced by high glucose and insulin levels (Jama 2000;283:221); correlates with 5th finger first IP joint hypermobility ("prayer si": Nejm 1981;305:191). Large vessel—not small vessel—disease causes ischemic leg ulcers (Nejm 1984;311:1615).

Eating disorders in 30% of young type 1 women associated w markedly increased microvascular cmplc

Eye: Retinopathy (Nejm 2004;350:48) manifested by microaneurysms, dot hemorrhages, cotton wool exudates, macular edema, and proliferative retinopthy; correlates with poor control; cataracts, associated w doubled mortality rates (Nejm 1985;313:1438)

gi: Nausea and vomiting; diarrhea often from bacterial overgrowth; fecal incontinence

Hypoglycemia at higher, "normal" blood levels in pts who usually run high (Nejm 1988;318:1487); pts report sx with only 15% of episodes (J Intern Med 1990;228:641) but improves as severity and frequency improve though not neuropathic in etiology (Nejm 1993;329:834); driving significantly impaired at 47-65 mg % but pts fail to perceive it 50% of time (Jama 1999;282:750). Autonomic neuropathy and hypoglycemia, like Somogyi effect, due to decreased epinephrine response to hypoglycemia especially during sleep (Nejm 2004;350:2272,

1998;338:1657), r/o "dawn phenomenon" from growth hormone surge (Nejm 1985;312:1473).

Infectious (Nejm 1999;341:1906), including emphysematous pyelonephritis and cholecystitis, necrotizing fasciitis, malignant otitis externa, and mucor infections

"Metabolic syndrome," w HT, obesity, and elevated lipids

Nephropathy ($^1/_3$) and end-stage renal disease (2.5% in 15 yr) (Jama 1997;278:2069); correlate with proteinuria (Nejm 1984;311:89). GFR above normal until macroalbuminuria develops (Nejm 1996;335:1636).

Neuropathies including mononeuritis, eg, of 3rd nerve with pupil sparing unlike internal carotid aneurysm; impotence (60%: Ann IM 1971;75:213); peripheral: sx of numbness daily (25% sens, 95% specif-Diab Med 2000;17:105), stocking/glove, and diminished foot pain and flare contributing to ulcers (Nejm 1988;318:1306); radiculopathy (Ann IM 1977;86:166); decreased visceral pain perception, eg, silent angina and MIs and decreased COPD dyspnea (Nejm 1988;319:1369); autonomic, measure with expiratory-inspiratory respiratory variation in sinus rates, if < 10 suspect it (BMJ 1982;285:559)

Obstetric: Macrosomia; infant respiratory distress syndrome; congenital malformations (Nejm 1981;304:1331 vs 1988;318:671); increased spontaneous abortions if blood sugar elevated (Nejm 1988;319:1617)

Skin ulcers of foot/ankle due to neuropathy w complicating osteomyelitis demonstrable by bone at base w blunt probing (66% sens, 85% specif-Jama 1995;273:721)

Syndrome X (diabetic) (see p 266)

Lab:

Chem (Ann IM 2002;137:263): Fasting blood glucose elevated > 126 mg % (ADA) vs > 140 mg % (Jama 1999;281:1203 vs 1222), or > 200 mg % on 2 hr pc or random BS; FBS > 110 but < 126 mg %, or 2 hr after 75 gm glucose of 140-200

mg % = "impaired glucose tolerance." Home monitoring equipment, or watch-like monitoring wrist band (Glucowatch) (Med Let 2003;45:99; Jama 1999;282:1839). Ob screen for gestational diabetes with 50 gm glucose po at 24-28 wk, get full GTT if 1 hr sugar > 140 mg %.

HgbA$_1$C (glycosylated hemoglobin) > 7.0% (90% specif, 99% sens), usually requires drug rx (Jama 1996;276:1247), increases fast but reflects glucose over past 2 mo; increased by Fe deficiency, decreased by sickle cell disease, not a reliable screen to make dx; get q 3 mo and keep at least < 8% to prevent microvascular cmplc, < 7% dramatically reduces cmplc over 7 yr (Nejm 1993;329:304,977). Avg glucose over past 3 mo = 33 × HgbA$_1$C − 86.

Na$^+$ decreased by increased glucose if not dehydrated; osmoles = 2 × Na + glucose/18; hence blood sugar/40 ≈ Na equivalents

Insulin and/or C-peptide levels abnormally low in type 1, unlike type 2

Lipid profile, get LDL < 100, or screen nonfasting w total and HDL and non-HDL > 160

NonInv: EKG

Path: Liver bx if done shows increased nuclear, decreased cytoplasmic glycogen; vessels show ASCVD; renal bx shows Kimmelstiel-Wilson lesion, glycogen in tubules, thickened basement membrane, which correlates w eye disease (Nejm 1985;312:1282)

Urine: Glucosuria r/o autosomal dominant nephrogenic diabetes (1/500 glycosurics); home monitoring as good as home blood glucose monitoring? (Diab Care 1990;13:1044)

Proteinuria (Nejm 2003;348:2285): Microalbuminuria > 40 mg/24 hr or > 30 μgm/min requires rx; μgm albumin/mg creatinine ratio > 20-300 on spot urine indicates early disease (Nejm 1995;332:1251) but requires f/u 24-hr urine microalbumin for quantitative (Am J Kidn Dis 2002;39:1183)

Rx: Prevent in high-risk pts by improved glucose tolerance (Ann IM 2005;142:323; Nejm 2002;346:393) w diet and daily exercise, NNT-3 = 7; metformin does to a lesser degree, NNT-3 = 13
Stepped care (Ann IM 1998;128:165):

1. Lifestyle changes like diet, exercise, and wt loss
2. po mono rx w sulfonylurea for lean pts, metformin for obese; perhaps disaccharidase inhibitors even at just impaired glucose tolerance stage (NNT-3 = 40; Jama 2003;290:486)
3. Combo rx of 2 + acarbose
4. Combo rx of 2 w insulin
5. Insulin alone
6. Insulin + troglitazone

    Tight control in both types 1 and 2 (Lancet 1999;353:617, 1998;352:837,854), w avg $HgbA_1C \approx 7\%$, at least $< 8.1\%$, to prevent renal failure (Nejm 1995;332:1251) w tid insulin (Diab Care 1996;19:195), improves (Nejm 1993;329:977):

- Motor nerve conduction velocities (Ann IM 1981;94:307)
- Sensory and autonomic neuropathy (Nejm 1990;322:1031) and prevents development of all (NNT-5 = 4 for NCVs, and NNT-5 = 16 for clinical neuropathy: Ann IM 1995;122:561)
- Proteinuria (Nejm 2000;342:381, 1994;330:15)
- Renal failure (Nejm 1991;324:1626)
- Fetal anomalies and death (Nejm 1981;304:1331)
- Retinopathy (Nejm 2000;342:381, 1993;329:304,977)
- Survival post-MI (NNT-2 = 13) (J Am Coll Cardiol;1995;26:57)
- Endogenous insulin secretion if started early in type 1 (Ann IM 1998;128:517)
- Quality of life and cost-benefit ratio (Jama 1998;280:1490)
  ASA 650 mg po qd prevents ASHD cmplc (NNT-5 = 29: Jama 1992;268:1292)

Stop hyperglycemia-producing meds (list: Ann IM 1993;118:536)

Experimental: Monoclonal antibody vs CD3 T cells (Nejm 2002;346:1692); or pancreatic transplants esp if w renal transplant or maybe alone (Jama 2003;290:2817, 2861); or islet cell transplants (Nejm 2004;350:694)

Diet: Mediterranean w olive oil, fruit, vegetables, whole grains, and alcohol qd (Jama 2003;292:1433,1440,1490); total calories more important than ratios. High fiber, 25-50 gm qd, > 50% soluble type, improves glycemic control and lipids (Nejm 2000;342:1392); fenugreek dietary legume supplement; low-glycemic-index foods best (Jama 2002;287:2414); weight loss if overweight as most type 2s are.

Exercise increases receptor sensitivity (Jama 1998;279:669) and glucose uptake, and glycogen synthesis in exercised muscles even in insulin-resistant pts (Nejm 1996;335:1357)

Insulin U-100 sc, human (see Table 5.1). Best regimens (Nejm 1993;329:977): hs NPH, am regular + NPH; or hs NPH, regular before each meal; if giving bid NPH, 2nd dose hs produces much less night-time hypoglycemia (60%) than if given at supper time (Ann IM 2002;136:504); in type 2s, can give 1 dose hs titrated up to get FBS < 110 along w metformin 1000 mg po bid, resulted in best control w least weight gain (Ann IM 1999;130:389)

Avoid leg injection of N with exercise since increases absorption (Nejm 1978;298:79); can even inject through clothing? (Diab Care 1997;20:244). Pumps, external sc, or maybe implanted sc or intraperitoneal (Jama 1996;276:1322): dangerous in patients with autonomic neuropathy, β-blockers, and/or hypoadrenal (Ann IM 1983;99:268) because of impaired glucose and epinephrine production response to hypoglycemia (Nejm 1983; 308:485).

Table 5.1   Insulins

Insulin Type	Onset	Peak	Duration	Comment	Cost/1000 U
Lispro (Humalog), or Aspart (Novolog)	5-15 min	30-90 min	3-6 hr	Helpful in pts w recurrent hypoglycemia; can give ac based on serving size. Ok to mix w Humulins as long as draw up 1st.	$60-70
Regular (Humulin-R, Novolin-R)	30-60 min	2-3 hr	8-10 hr		$25
NPL (neutral protamine lispro)	15 min	2 hr		Plain or as 75%/25% Humalog mix	$65 for mix
Protamine crystalline Aspart	15 min	2 hr		As 70%/30% Novolog mix	$90
NPH (Humulin-N)	2-4 hr	4-10 hr	12-18 hr		$25
Ultra-Lente (Humulin-U) qd hs	1 hr	10-16 hr, minimal	8-24 hr		$25
Glargine (Lantus) qd hs	2-4 hr	None	20 hr	3 aa's altered from human insulin slows release; don't mix w others	$58

(Nejm 2005;352:174)

Table 5.2 Oral Hypoglycemics (Jama 2002;287:360, 373; AnnIM 1999:131:281)

Drug	Dose	Comment
Sulfonylureas: As good as insulin if get glucose control		60-70% successful as single agent at 1st, but 6+% failure rate/yr thereafter; teratogenesis and hypoglycemia of newborn if use in pregnancy
1st generation:		Potentiated by warfarin, can cause hypo Na
• Chlorpropramide (Diabinase)	250-500 mg qd	Renal excretion, multiday half-life; cheap; Antabuse-like effect
• Tolbutamide (Orinase)	500-1000 mg bid	Hepatic metab; 5 hr half-life; $5/mo
2nd generation		
• Glipizide (Glucotrol)	2.5-20 mg bid	Hepatic metab; 2-4 hr half-life; $15+/mo
• Glyburide (Micronase)	2.5-10 mg qd	Hepatic metab; 10 hr half-life; $15+/mo
• Glimepiride (Amaryl) (Med Let 1996;38:47)	4-8 mg qd	Hepatic metab; 9 hr half-life; $20/mo
Meglitinides (non-sulfonylurea secretagogues)		Fast acting so can skip if miss a meal or take if eating irregularly; similar to sulfonylureas, can cause hypoglycemia; can use w metformin; hepatic metab; $80/mo
• Nateglinide (Starlix) (Med Let 2001;43:29)	60-120 mg tid ac	
• Repaglinide (Prandin) (Med Let 1998;4:55,66)	0.5-4 mg po ac (0.5, 1, 2 mg tabs)	$67/mo for 1 mg tid
Biguanides		Won't cause hypoglycemia; decrease hepatic gluconeogenesis, induce wt loss, increase end organ insulin sensitivity
• Metformin (Glucophage) (Nejm 1996;334:574, 1995;333:541; Med Let 1995;37:41)	500-1000 mg hs, bid, or tid up to 2500 mg qd	Alone or w sulfonylurea or insulin (Ann IM 1999;131:182), esp if obese or high triglycerides; cmplc: gi sx, rare lactic acidosis (1/30,000 person-yrs) avoid if creatinine > 1.4 mg %, CHF (Jama 2003;290:81), and/or given angiographic dyes (hold pericath) or abnormal LFT; $47/mo, generic

Table 5.2 (continued)

Drug	Dose	Comment
Disaccharidase Inhibitors		Inhibit pancreatic and brush border enzymes
• Acarbose (Precose) (Med Let 1996;38:9; Diab Care 1997;20: 248; Ann IM 1994; 121:928)	50-200 mg po ac tid	Nonabsorbable oligosaccharide; do not use w metformin; cmplc: hypogly-cemia (rx w glucose not sucrose), flatulence, diarrhea, increase LFT (monitor q 3 mo); $42/mo for 100 mg tid
• Miglitol (Glyset) (Med Let 1999;41:49)	25-100 mg po tid	Similar to acarbose w/o LFT increases; use in type 2 w sulfonylureas; multi-ple drug interactions including w sulfonylureas; $50/mo for 50 mg tid
Thiazolidinediones (Glitazones)		Increase insulin sensitivity; use w insulin or sulfonylureas
• Rosiglitazone (Avandia) (Med Let (1999;41:71); can use w sulfonylureas (Diab Med 2000;17:40)	2-4 mg qd-bid	@ max dose w max metformin only 28% had HgbA$_1$C < 7% (Jama 2000;283; 1695); cmplc: fluid retention, hepato-toxicity including liver failure (Ann IM 2000;132:118,121), get LFT q 2 mo × 1 yr, keep < 3× nl; $75-100/mo
• Pioglitazone (Actos) (Med Let 1999;41:112)	15-45 mg po qd	Increase HDL w/o LDL increase; cmplc: fluid retention, rare hepatitis (Ann IM 2002;136:449), get LFT q 2 mo; $75-100/mo
• Troglitazone (Rezulin)		Pulled from US market in 2000 due to hepatitis
Combination Meds		
• Avandamet (rosiglita-zone + metformin) (Med Let 2002;44:107)	1, 2, and 4 mg/ 500 mg	$112-275/mo
• Glucovance (gly-buride + metformin) (Med Let 2000;42: 105) 1.25/250 mg, 25/ 500 mg, or 5/500 mg		
• Metaglip (metformin + glipizide) (Med Let 2002;44:107)	250/2.5, 500/2.5, 500/5	Cheaper than each separately; $85-100/mo

Rx of cmplc's:

Diarrhea: Cholestyramine, metaclopramide (Reglan), opiates, antibiotics

Foot ulcers/infections (Jama 2005;293:217) w anaerobes and pseudomonas: Screen w monofilament on sole surface of big toe and metatarsal heads; avoid barefoot walking, get good shoes, rx calluses; rx w parenteral imipenem or ticarcillin + clavulinic acid (Timentin), or oral fluoroquinolone + clindamycin po × 10-14 d better than longer rx or more diagnostic testing to r/o osteomyelitis (Jama 1995;273:712); surgical grafting w human skin (Dermagraft) (Diab Care 1996;19:350). Automatic mechanical compression device at least 8 hr/d helps heal faster (Arch Surg 2000;135:1405).

Gastroparesis: Vomiting, poor emptying; rx with small volume, frequent feedings, metoclopramide (Reglan) 10 mg 30 min ac? (Ann IM 1983;98:86)

Hospitalized pt: B-qid BS's plus, if npo, continuous low-dose drip, or low-dose long-acting insulin (N bid, or glargine qd); if taking po, then long-acting plus ac SSI, never just SSI (Arch IM 1997;157:545). Or peri-operative management w $\frac{1}{3}$ normal NPH dose while npo pre-op in am, $\frac{1}{3}$ in recovery with dextrose iv going.

Hyperlipidemia: Aggressive rx for primary prevention of ASHD, increase 2-3× (ACP J Club 2004;140:1); 10-yr incidence in diabetics > 40 yr is around 25%; even fixed-dose atoravastatin 10 mg po qd decreases ASHD (NNT-4 = 32) (Lancet 2004;364:685)

Hypertension: ACE inhibitors 1st choice (Ann IM 2003; 138:587,593; Jama 1997;278:40); tight control decreases morbidity and mortality (Arch IM 2000;160:2447); ok to use thiazides, which are 1st choice in blacks, β-blockers and probably calcium-channel blockers; get pressures to < 140/80 if can

Hypoglycemia: Glucose tabs or gel if on disaccaridase inhibitors, otherwise candy; glucagon im

Impotence (p 1062)

Insulin resistance (Syndrome X) (Nejm 1999;340:1314, 1991;325:938): Insulin resistance, type 2 diabetes, elevated lipids, HT, ASCVD; type A (receptor unresponsive) associated with acanthosis nigrans, polycystic ovary, and obesity; rare autoimmune type B associated with other autoimmune syndromes especially lupus (Ann IM 1985;102:176); rx with U-500 regular insulin (Ann IM 1981;94:653), or insulin-like growth factor in extreme cases (Nejm 1992;327:853)

Ischemic heart disease: Rx risk factors as aggressively as post-MI pts since 7-yr incid > 20% (Nejm 1998;339:229), including aggressive use of β-blockers (Ann IM 1995;123:358); prophylaxis w ASA qd (Am J Med 1998;105:494), and/or 1-2 alcoholic drinks qd (Jama 1999;282:239). CABG results in better survival long term than angioplasty (Nejm 2000;342:989).

Nephropathy/renal failure (Njem 1999;341:1127): Prevent w ACE inhibitor or ARB rx (Nejm 2004;351:1941,1952; Ann IM 1998;128:982), and tight control; BP control; protein and PO_4 restriction (Nejm 1991;324:78); prevents progression of proteinuria to nephropathy (Jama 1994;271:275; Ann IM 1993;118:129) when microalbuminuria > 20-200 mg/24 hr (Ann IM 1993;118:577; BMJ 1992;304:339) and improves lipids (Ann IM 1993;118:246)

Neuropathy:

- TCAs like amitriptyline or desipramine 75-150 mg po qd, both are effective (Nejm 1992;326:1250) and slow progression in pts w established disease but creatinine < 2.5 mg % (Nejm 1993;329:1456,1496)
- Gabapentin (Neurontin) (Jama 1998;280:1831) 300-1200 mg po tid; adverse effects: dizziness, somnolence, confusion

Pregnancy (Nejm 1999;341:1749): Get HgbA$_1$C level < 9% before get pregnant (Nejm 1981;304:1331); IQ of child inversely correlates w 3rd-trimester maternal OH-butyrate levels (Nejm 1991;325:911); keep pc (not ac) blood sugar < 140 mg % using diet and split-dose am and pm NPH/regular insulin, roughly $^2/_3$ dose in am and $^1/_3$ in pm, am dose $^2/_3$ NPH and $^1/_3$ reg, pm dose $^1/_2$ and $^1/_2$ (Nejm 1995;333:1237). *Do not use oral agents*, although glyburide started in 2nd trimester reported to be safe and effective (Nejm 2000;343:1134,1178).

Retinopathy (Nejm 2004;350:48, 1999;341:667): Tight control, regular eye consults for laser rx (Ann IM 1992;117:226, 1992;116:660) and HT control

Diabetic Ketoacidosis

Cause: Insulin-dependent diabetes mellitus

Epidem:

Pathophys:

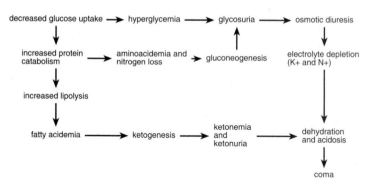

Figure 5.2 Pathogenesis of DKA and coma/shock.

Coma from CSF acidosis, hence rarer in metabolic than respiratory acidosis because CO_2 crosses blood-brain barrier easily; HCO_3 rx may paradoxically induce/worsen coma (F. Plum, Nejm 1967;277:605)

Sx: Malaise, confusion, nausea/vomiting, abdominal pain

Si: Kussmaul's (deep) respirations; stupor/coma; hypotension; dehydration

Crs: Onset over 2-3 d

Cmplc: Cerebral edema leading to coma with 90% mortality 6-10 hr after starting rx especially in children (Nejm 1985;312:1147) w low pCO_2, high BUN, and who get bicarb rx (Nejm 2001;344:264, 302)

r/o hypoglycemia; infection; appendicitis; nonketotic, nonacidotic hyperosmolar coma (Nejm 1977;297:1452) seen in the elderly with NIDDM; causes volume depletion, stupor, and coma

Lab:

Chem: Glucose elevated

Lytes: HCO_3 decreased commensurate with anion gap, but hyperchloremic when not volume depleted (Nejm 1982;307:1603); K low, though may be falsely high in DKA from pH shift of intracellular K to extracellular space (p 1013 for calculation). Osmoles, measured or calculated, may be increased if water depleted; calculated osmoles = glucose/18 + 2 × Na + BUN/2.8 (Ann IM 1989;110:854).

Ketones positive undiluted and to as much as $\frac{1}{8}$ diluted; may be negative if most ketone bodies are metabolized to hydroxybutyrate (measurable too)

Amylase elevated (80%), 65% pancreatic, 35% salivary (Ann IM 1979;91:200)

Rx   (Nejm 1983;309:159): Follow q 1-2 hr glucose, Na, K, HCO_3, ketones, urine output

Insulin, regular, 0.33-0.44 U/kg iv push; then 7 U/hr iv continuous until glucose < 250 mg %; repeat push bolus in 1 hr if glucose not decreased > 10%; then 2-6 U/hr iv continuous (or im, or sc) until glucose < 150 mg %; then routine maintenance. In children, regular insulin 0.1-0.2 U/kg iv push, then 0.1-0.2 U/hr. Fluids: saline, or half-normal saline after 1st L if osmoles elevated (ie, water depleted), with 40 mEq KCl at 1 L/hr until glucose < 250 mg % then change to D_5W or D_5S.

NG tube since many die of emesis and aspiration from gastric atony

HCO_3 iv rx only if HCO_3 < 5 mEq/L or pH < 7.1; gives paradoxical CNS acidosis (Nejm 1971;284:283) and right shift of hemoglobin dissociation curve

PO_4 rx rarely needed? (Nejm 1985;313:447); maybe as K_2PO_4 if low (PO_4 < 0.1-0.5 mg %) to prevent insulin resistance

ENDOCRINOLOGY/ METABOLISM

Obesity

Nejm 1997;337:396

Cause: 70% genetic, including 5% of the morbidly obese w melanocortin-4 receptor gene (MC4R) (Nejm 2003;348:1085,1096,1160) mutations altering alpha MSHormone, and another significant % w leptin receptor gene mutations. Little environmental impact (twin studies: Nejm 1990;322:1477,1483).

Epidem: Prevalence increasing in U.S., ~18% in 1998 (Jama 1999; 282:1519), and varies inversely w breastfeeding duration as infant (Jama 2001;285:2453,2461,2506)

Pathophys: Many theories:

- Brain appetite/satiety center imbalance, "adipostat" set higher (eg, by sedentary lifestyle) or lower (eg, by regular exercise) (Nejm 1995;332:621,673,679)
- Fat tissue regulatory failure, increased numbers of fat cells in utero leads to fat adults (Nejm 1976;295:349)

- Psychiatric
- Cellular sodium pump thermogenesis decreased (in rbc anyway: Nejm 1980;303:1017)
- Lower activity index (Nejm 1988;318:461,467,509)
- Insensitivity of brain to leptin, satiety regulator protein secreted by adipose cells? (Nejm 1996;334:292)
- Ghrelin hormone secretion by stomach/duodenum when dieting is inhibited by gastric bypass procedures (Nejm 2002;346:1623)
- Sleep deprivation decreases leptin and increases ghrelin levels (Ann IM 2004;141:846)

Sx: Frequently pts falsely report more activity and less intake than actually perform, and falsely ascribe inability to lose weight to genetic resistance (Nejm 1992;327:1893)

Si: Triceps skin fold > 23 mm; BP elevated (increased renin and aldosterone: Nejm 1981;304:930); $\geq$ 30 kg/M^2, or 20+% over ideal body wgt (formula for IDBW: men = 106 lb + 6 lb/in. over 5 ft; for women = 100 lb + 5 lb/in. over 5 ft)

Crs: Obesity in adolescence is associated w markedly decreased lifetime comparable to smoking (Ann IM 2003;138:24); also w lower education, incomes, and marriage rates, unlike other chronic disease states; is it genetics, discrimination, or both? (Nejm 1993;329:1008,1076)

Cmplc: Sleep apnea (p 731); osteoarthritis of knees (Ann IM 1988;109:18); gallstones with weight loss (Nejm 1988;319:1567); fatty liver (75%) (Ann IM 2000;132:112); ASHD, diabetes, CHF (incidence increased 5%: Framingham, Nejm 2002;347:305), hypertension, premature death (Jama 1999;282:1523,1530; Ann IM 1985;103:977); increase in almost all cancers, by up to 50%, in severely obese (Nejm 2002;348:1625), including cervical and breast cancers, and less frequent screening for them (Ann IM 2000;132:697)

r/o night eating syndrome (Jama 1999;282:657, 689)

Lab:

Rx: (Ann IM 2005;142:525)

Prevent gallstone formation w ursodeoxycholic acid 300 mg po bid or 600 mg qd, NNT = 4 (Ann IM 1995;122:899); cost $140/mo

Diet:

- 600-800 qd mixed calories; spares muscle and has fewer cmplc than high-protein regimens like arrhythmias with prolonged QT (Ann IM 1985;102:121), or
- Low-carbohydrate (Atkins) diet, < 20-30 gm CHO qd yields better wt loss and lipid effects (Ann IM 2004; 140:769,778,836; Nejm 2003;348:2074,2082,2057).

Exercise program, 45 min at 60-80% maximal pulse 3×/wk helps weight and HDL (Nejm 1991;326:461) no matter the genetic predisposition (Ann IM 1999;130:873)

Medications (Ann IM 2005;142:532; Nejm 2002;346:591): Appetite suppressants (Jama 1996;276:1907):

- SSRIs like fluoxetine (Prozac) 60 mg po qd, or sertraline (Zoloft); but both lose efficancy and wt increases after 6 mo
- Sibutramine (Meridia) (Jama 2003;289:1805, 2001;286:1331; Med Let 1998;40:32) 10-15 mg po qd × 1 mo, then cont × 1 yr if lose ≥ 2 kg in that 1st mo for eventual 8 ± 1 kg avg loss; adverse effects: dry mouth, HA, insomnia, constipation, many drug interactions; $112/30 d
- Ephedra (mahuang)-containing supplements, but many health risks (Nejm 2000;343:1833)
- Zonisamide (Zonegram) 4-500 mg po daily w dietrary counseling can lead to 1 lb/wk losses over 4 mo (Jama 2003;289:1821)
- Herbal *Garcinia sp.* (hydroxycitric acid) no help (Jama 1998;280:1596)
- Gut hormone fragment peptide (ghrelin atagonists) eventually? (Nejm 2003;349:941, 2002;346:1623)

- *NOT* phentermine (Ionamin) + fenfluramine (Pondimin) or dexfenfluramine (Redux), withdrawn because of fatal primary pulmonary HT and cardiac valve abnormalities (Nejm 1998;339:713, 719)

Pancreatic lipase inhibitors:

- Orlistat (Xenical) (J Intern Med 2000;248:245; Med Let 1999;41:55; Jama 1999;281:243,278) 120 mg po tid w meals; adverse effects: fat-soluble vitamin depletion, steatorrhea, possible increase in breast cancer; $120/mo

Other experimental meds: bupropion (Welbutrin) SR, topiramate (Topamax), metformin (Glucophage)

Surgical (Ann IM 2005;142:547; Nejm 2004;351:2683, 2751) gastric bypass, stapling, or plication; at 5 yr, 20% failure, 50% benefit; adverse effects: bacterial overgrowth causing diarrhea and malabsorption, B_{12} and iron commonly (Ann IM 1996; 124:469); fatty liver, cirrhosis, gallstones (Nejm 1974;290:921); immune complex arthritis, rash (Ann IM 1980;93:557), nephritis (Ann IM 1976;84:594); uric acid renal stones (20%) and hyperoxaluria; polyneuropathy, especially position sense, even in stapled patients (Ann IM 1982;96:453); metronidazole (Flagyl) 0.75-2 gm qd po helps all cmplc of blind loop

Surgical liposuction, "tumescent" method w sc lidocaine + epinephrine has cmplc of sudden death (5 cases: Nejm 1999;340:1471)

5.3 Gonadal Disorders

True Hermaphroditism

Cause: Mosaicism; double fertilization? or faulty postconceptual mitosis?

Epidem: Rare; most appear as questionable males at birth and are raised as such

Pathophys: XX/XY mosaics in tissues; both testicular and ovarian tissues develop in same individual

Sx:

Si: Ambiguous but partially virilized external genitalia; hypospadia very common; inguinal hernia (43%); gynecomastia at puberty (80%)

Crs:

Cmplc: r/o **testicular feminization (male pseudohermaphroditism)** (Nejm 2004;350:367); rare, genetic, multiple types; all have XY karyotype and intraabdominal testes; may be due to 5α-reductase deficiency, which converts testosterone to dihydrotestosterone in testicular or sexual end organs; spectrum from female phenotype with uterus and pubertal feminization, to **Reifenstein's Syndrome** (male phenotype with hypospadia and gynecomastia), to normal male with infertility and high testosterone and LH levels from tissue resistance (Nejm 1979;300:223); often raised as girls to puberty then change; buccal smear negative for Barr bodies, XY karyotype; urinary 17-KS and estrogen levels show normal male pattern but low dihydrotestosterone levels postpuberty; rx w vaginal reconstruction, hypospadia repair, etc

Lab:

> *Path:* Wolffian and Müllerian remnants coexist, often unilateral female and other side is male
>
> > Chromosome preps: 80% of patients are chromatin, ie, Barr body positive

Rx: Complicated medically and socially; usually need tertiary care center

Mixed Gonadal Dysgenesis

Cause: Mosaicism (XY and XO) or "silent Y," ie, end-organ resistance; sex-linked recessive

Epidem: Rare

Pathophys: Mutant X or autosomal chromosome operon gene turns off Y (Nejm 1970;283:6); streak gonads

Sx:

Si: Spectrum of female genotype with sterility, to Turner's syndrome (see below), to female with clitoromegaly, to male with hypospadia

Crs:

Cmplc: Gonadal malignancy, especially if Y present (Nejm 1972;287:628)

Lab:
   Path: Chromosome preps show chromatin, ie, Barr body negative

Rx: Estrogens, but increased incidence of endometrial cancer (Nejm 1972;287:628), which cycling w progesterone should prevent
   Surgical removal of any streak gonad in all mosaics

Turner's Syndrome

Nejm 2004;351:1227

Cause: Genetic mutation or transmitted as ? "X-linked or autosomal dominant expressed only in male." No increase w advanced maternal age.

Epidem: Rare, incidence =1/1500-2500 females, prevalence = 50,000-75,000 in U.S.; more common in miscarriage fetuses

Pathophys: Part of mixed gonadal dysgenesis; XO, X with partial X or Y deletion, isochromosome of X or Y, ring chromosome with deletion of X or Y. Lymphatic hypoplasia causes edema.

Sx: Short stature (90% are < 5 ft); primary amenorrhea; multiple moles appear between age 4 and 15 yr

Si: Normal female genitalia; ankle edema; low hairline at base of neck; neck webbing (20%); multiple nevi and nail anomalies; increased carrying angle of elbow, short 4th metacarpal

Crs:

Cmplc: Diabetes mellitus; Hashimoto's thyroiditis in up to 50%; congenital cardiovascular abnormalities, especially coarctation of the aorta (15%) and bicuspid aortic valve; renal and gi congenital abnormalities occasionally; tumors in streak gonads if present; renal HT; scoliosis (10%); OM from malformations of mouth/nose; hypothyroidism (20%); stabismus

Lab: *Path:* Streak gonads w gonadal dysgenesis

Chromosome preps are Barr body negative; get full karyotype to r/o XO-XY mosaicism with increased gonadal cancer incidence

Chem: FSH and LH increased (unlike hypogonadotrophic hypogonadism)

Xray: Prenatal ultrasound may show lymphedema, thickened nuchal fold, cystic hygroma, horseshoe kidney

Knee films show overgrowth of medial tibial condyle

Rx: Growth hormone rx in late childhood (Nejm 1999; 340:502,557); ERT and cycled progresterone in adults; pregnancy possible esp w donated ova

Surgical removal of any streak gonad in all mosaics

Klinefelter's Syndrome

Cause: Genetic; mutation, in case of mosaics, in postconception fetus

Epidem: 1/250 male births (Nejm 1969;280:851); 1/20 aspermic males (Nejm 1969;281:969)

Pathophys: XXY, XXXY in at least some body cells (mosaicism)

Sx: Sexual immaturity, sterility

Si: Aspermic/hypospermic, male phenotype; small testes (< 2.5 cm diameter); gynecomastia; diminished intelligence (IQ); vertical creases on upper lip as age (present in all females without ovaries)

Crs:

Cmplc: Breast cancer incidence is the same as for women (Nejm 1980;303:795)

r/o **"supermale"** = XXYY, XYY; tall, aggressive; have varicose veins; may present looking like Klinefelter's

Lab: *Chem:* FSH and LH elevated (unlike hypogonadotropic hypogonadism)

Path: Testicular bx shows hyalinized tubules with clumped Leydig cells, r/o mumps orchitis

Chromosome preps show buccal Barr body positive (85%); XXY or XXYY by full karyotype, unless missing in a mosaic

Rx: Testosterone 200 mg im in oil q 2-4 wk or pulse

Paternity possible w testicular sperm aspiration and in vitro fertilization (Nejm 1998;338:588)

5.4 Hyperlipidemias

r/o secondary causes (diabetes, hypothyroidism, hepatic and renal disease) first w FBS or HgbA$_1$C, TSH, AST (SGOT)

Alternative nomenclature/classifications of hyperlipemias (Nejm 1999;341:500)

Hypercholesterolemia

Cause: Polygenic and dietary

Epidem: High prevalence in U.S. but decreasing by 10 mg %/10 yr in late 20th century (Nejm 1991;324:941)

Pathophys: Elevated low-density lipoprotein (LDL) cholesterol increases risk of atherosclerotic disease, while high-density lipoprotein (HDL) cholesterol reflects lowered risk because is contained in a transport protein that picks up lipids from the periphery and brings back to the liver for excretion.

Sx & Si: Often none; arcus senilis, xanthomata in 85% of those w LDL receptor defects

Crs: Levels > 210 mg % at age 22 yr associated w higher ASHD rates at age 20 yr (5%), age 25 (10%), age 30 (15%), and years later (Nejm 1993;328:313)

Cmplc: Principally ASHD, eg, angina and MIs; peripheral disease r/o familial type II hypercholesterolemia (p 282); and secondary causes of hypercholesterolemia: myxedema, obstructive liver disease, porphyria, nephrosis (Nejm 1985;312:1544), dysproteinemias

Lab:

Chem: Lipid profile now initial test usually, rather than just total cholesterol, for:

Total cholesterol (mM/L = mg %/40); fasting unnecessary; falsely decreased by acute MI/inflammation

LDL, fasting = total − HDL − TG/5 if TG < 400

HDL, fasting < 40 mg % is itself high risk

Alcohol ingestion (Ann IM 1992;116:881), weight loss (Jama 1995;247:1915) alone or induced w exercise; decreased by uremia, type 2 diabetes, smoking, high-carbohydrate diet (> 60% of calories), and many drugs like β-blockers, anabolic steroids, and progesterones

Rx: Prevention screening and rx (Natl Choles Educ Program: Jama 2001;285:2486): Use diet and exercise first, meds after 3+ mo

1st: LDL rx of all pts ≥ 160 mg % (4.1 mM/I)

- if > 130 mg % (3.4 mM/L), rx pts w 2+ risk factors (smoking, HT, low HDL, family h/o ASCVD before age 55 in men or 65 in women, age > 45 for men or 55 for women)
- if > 100 mg % rx pts w h/o ASHD, peripheral artery disease, carotid disease, or AAA, hence secondary prevention; or if 10-yr ASHD risk > 20% by Framingham tables (see NCEP charts)

2nd: After above accomplished, rx triglycerides > 200 mg % and/or low HDL w nicotinic acid and/or fibrate

Screening and primary prevention drug rx w pravastatin 40 mg po hs in asx men over age 40 w LDL ≥ 150 mg % had improved survival, NNT-5 = 40 (Nejm 1995;333:1301); lovistatin 20-40 mg po qd in pts w avg LDL and total cholesterol but low HDL, men and women up to age 75 had decreased ASHD events, NNT-5 = 50 (Jama 1998;279:1615,1679) but significant limitations (ACP J Club 1998;129:58). Previous increases in violent deaths among men w cholesterol reductions not seen in recent statin primary prophylaxis studies but decrements in attention and psychomotor speed are induced by dietary or statin cholesterol lowering (Am J Med 2000;108:538:547).

Appropriateness in women (clearly not, or barely helpful even in those w CAD: Jama 2004;291:2243), young and old, has been disputed unless h/o ASCVD (Ann IM 2000;132: 769,780,833, 1996;124:518 vs 505; Jama 1995;274:1152); in children who may be harmed by rx (Jama 1995;273:1429,1461 vs Peds 1991;87:943) although statins experimentally used in adolescent boys w heterozygous familial hypercholesterolemia (Jama 1999;282:137); and in elderly, especially women, and in men and women over 70 yr (Jama 1994;272:1335,1372 vs yes for elderly men: Ann IM 1990;113:916). Statins and gemfibrozil cause cancer in animals at levels similar to human blood levels (Jama 1996;275:55).

Secondary prevention is supported by data (Nejm 1997;336:332; Ann IM 1996;124:518 vs 505; Jama 1995;274:1152), by decreasing cholesterol in patients with known CAD, eg, Scandinavian simvastatin study of CAD pts showed 9% absolute risk reduction, NNT-5 = 11 (Lancet 1994;344:1383). In women, MI incidence but not overall death rate reduced (Jama 2004;291:2243).

Exercise, at least walk 2 mi qd or run up to 40 mi q wk helps HDL and ASHD risk in men and women (Nejm 1996;334:1298)

Diet: Helps decrease LDL only if combined w exercise (Nejm 1998;339:12)

- Lose weight
- Low cholesterol < 300 mg qd (Nejm 1993;328:1213)
- Polyunsaturated and monounsaturated fats like olive oil (Nejm 1986;314:745) or canola or soy oil, any of which reduce death in post-MI pts from 5% to 1%/yr (Lancet 1994;343:1454); phyto-estrogens like sitosterol or sitostanol-ester margarine reduce LDL by 10-15% and may improve ASHD (Med Let 1999;41:56; Nejm 1995;333:1308); stearic and oleic, but not palmitic saturated fats are ok (Nejm 1988;318:1244). Transoleic fatty acids just as bad, so margarine no good (Nejm 1990;323:439); partially hydrogenated (trans) fatty acids worsen LDL (Nejm 1999; 340:1933,1994), so liquid oils better than semi-liquid, better than soft, better than stick margerines, and because of better total/HDL ratios, butter not as bad as stick margarine.
- Fish or fish oil pills decrease triglycerides, but elevate LDL (Ann IM 1989;111:900); slow or reverse ASHD progression (Ann IM 1999;130:554), and also help BP (Nejm 1990;322:795)
- Oleic and α-linolenic acid in walnuts (Ann IM 2000;132:538; Nejm 1993;328:603)
- Soy protein 20-40 gm qd (Nejm 1995;333:276)
- Alcoholic drinks 2-4 qd (Nejm 2001;344:549; BMJ 1996;312:731,736)
- Garlic ½-1 clove qd (decreases cholesterol by 9%: Ann IM 1993;119:545) vs no help by double-blind RCT (Arch IM 1998;158:1189; Jama 1998;279:1900)
- Soluble fiber (Nejm 1993;329:21) like psyllium (Metamucil) 4.3 gm pkt in water b-tid (5% cholesterol reduction: Ann IM 1993;119:545; Arch IM 1989;151:1597, 1988;148:292) or oat bran 56 gm qd (Jama 1991;265:1833) or beans 100 gm/d (Med Let 1988;30:111)

Medications (Nejm 1999;341:498; Med Let 2001;43:43): All have a nearly 50% 1-yr cessation rate by pts in practice except HMG-COA reductase drugs (25%) (Nejm 1995;332:1125)

HMG-COA reductase inhibitors (statins) (Med Let 2003;45:17; 2004;46:93); po hs (because cholesterol synthesis occurs mostly at night, all may also stabilize plaques, retard thrombosis (Jama 1998;279:1643), and decrease vascular inflammation (CRP levels: Jama 2001;286:64); and all may slow osteoporosis and fracture rates (Jama 2000;283:3205,3211,3255 vs Ann IM 2003;139:97; Jama 2001;285:1850); cmplc: mild asx hepatitis (1-2%), ? check LFT q 6-12 mo but allow to go up to 3× upper limit of normal; dose-dependent severe rhabdomyolysis/myopathy (Jama 2004;292:2585) heralded by myalgias and increased CPK, more frequently seen w concomitant grapefruit juice, verapamil, erythromycin, ketoconazole, itraconazole, niacin, or gemfibrozil use, can allow asx CPK to increase up to 3× upper normal; also rare peripheral neuropathy, memory loss, sleep disturbance, impotence, gynecomastia, and debatable increase in cancer risk; all cost $60-120/mo for standard dose, cheaper generics coming

- Atorvastatin (Lipitor) (Med Let 1997;39:29; Jama 1995;275:128) 10-80 mg po qd and cheaper 40 mg extended release, being pushed to the 80 mg end by studies showing lower MI rates but no increase in survival (Nejm 2005;352:1425,1483); lowers cholesterol more than others (Nejm 2004;350:1495), also decreases triglycerides by 40%, long half-life, no CNS effect; $70/mo

- Fluvastatin (Lescol) (Arch IM 1991;151:43; Nejm 1988;319:24) 20 (10-40) mg po qd, no CNS effect; $52/mo at 20 mg

- Lovastatin (Mevacor) (primary prevention: Jama 1997;278:313) 20-40 mg po hs; $52/mo

- Pravastatin (Pravachol) 40 mg po hs, worked as primary prevention in Scottish trials (Nejm 1995;333:1301) but cost was $35,000/yr life saved (BMJ 1997;315:1577); no CNS effect; good alternative if intolerant of other statins; $132/mo

- Rosuvastatin (Crestor) (Med Let 2003;45:81) 10+ mg po qd; helps decrease triglycerides and increase HDL like atovavastatin; slow metabolism in some causes myopathy incidence to increase 10× to 5/10,000 pt/yr

- Simvastatin (Zocor) (primary prevention: Jama 1998;279:1615, 1997;278:313) 10-40, occasionally 80 mg po hs; raises HDL and lowers triglycerides as well as atorvastatin; $132/mo

    Cholesterol binders; all can increase triglyercides (L. Keilson):

- Cholestyramine 24 gm qd divided (Ann IM 1990;150:1822)
- Coleserelam (Welcho) (Med Let 2000;42:102) 625 mg tabs, 3-6 po qd or divided; fewer gi side effects and drug interactions, can take w statins; $150/mo
- Cholestipol 5-10 gm b-tid (Nejm 1990;323:1290), alone or w
- Psyllium 2.5 gm po tid decreases lipids more than cholestipol alone, is better tolerated, and costs $1/2$ as much (< $500/yr) (Ann IM 1995;123:493); or

    Cholesterol absorption inhibitors: Ezetimibe (Zetia) (Am J Cardiol 2002;90:1084; ACP J Club 2005;142:16, 2003;139:8) 10 mg po qd, also sold combined w simvastatin 10-80 mg as Vytorin (Med Let 2004;46:73); adverse effects: rare (< 2%) hepatitis, increased myopathy risk when used w statins

    Nicotinic acid (niacin) 100 mg po hs, or 125 mg bid increased gradually over 2 mo to 1 gm qid; or slow-release forms like Niaspan up to 2 gm po hs; or combination w lovistatin (Advicor) 500/10-2 gm/40. Raises HDL the most of all the drugs, helps triglycerides; adverse effects: flushing, which is helped by 300 mg ASA a half-hour before each dose; aggravation of glucose intolerance; hepatotoxicity; rhabdomyolysis sometimes when given w statins.

    Fibrates:

- Gemfibrozil (Lopid) 600 mg bid, similar to clofibrate (Atromid); decreases triglycerides and raises HDL, can decrease recurrent MIs in pts w LDL < 130 but HDL < 40 (Jama

2001;285:1585; Nejm 1999;341:410); adverse effects: gall-stones (Am J Med 2000;108:418), rhabdomyolysis when given w statins though still done cautiously

- Fenofibrate (Tricor) (Med Let 1998;40:68) 67-220 mg po qd, similar to gemfibrozil, used especially for triglyceride elevations; can also cause rhabdomyolysis w statins

Type I Hyperlipidemia

Cause: Genetic or diabetics, autosomal recessive (Nejm 1991;324:1761)

Epidem: Rare except in Quebec French Canadians, 1/40 of whom have the gene; overall the gene prevalence is 1/500 (Nejm 1991;324:1761)

Pathophys: Lipoprotein lipase deficiency causes an increase in chylomicrons, not lysed by heparin (PHLA)

Sx: Recurrent abdominal pain (old surgical scars); early life onset (months old to age 10 yr)

Si: Lipemia retinalis (picture: Nejm 1999;340:1969); hepato-splenomegaly; eruptive xanthomata (pimple-like correlate with chylomicrons)

Crs: Complete reversal with rx

Cmplc: Pancreatitis; possibly ASHD (Nejm 1996;335:848)

Lab: *Chem:* Cholesterol may be increased; total cholesterol/HDL ratio < 4.5. Triglyceride > 1000 mg %, often > 1500 mg %; supranate milky; infranate clear; post-heparin lipolytic activity low

Rx: Diet, low fat (< 20% of calories); stop alcohol; avoid estrogens and cholesterol binders, which worsen
Gemfibrozil or clofibrate, or niacin if sx

Type II Hyperlipidemia (Familial Hypercholesterolemia)

Cause: Genetic, autosomal dominant

Epidem: Common, 1/200 prevalence

Pathophys: Decreased LDL receptors cause increased LDL and some-times VLDL (Nejm 1986;314:879, 1984;311:1658); or, more rarely due to mutations in apolipoprotein B gene, which impair receptor binding (Nejm 1998;338:1577). Apolipoproteins of LDL and HDL correlate better with familial risk than the cholesterol levels in each component (Nejm 1990;322:1494, 1986;315:721). Uremia and β-blockers decrease HDL.

Sx:

Si: Arcus senilis, tendinous xanthomata (80% over age 20 yr have them), tuberous xanthomata in homozygotes, xanthelasmas (only 50% in general population are associated with type II disease, ie, 50% specif)

Crs: Malignant; MIs in pts age 30-40 yr, even in teens in homozygotes

Cmplc: Increased ASHD with MI
             r/o secondary causes of hypercholesterolemia (p 276)

Lab: *Chem:* Cholesterol very high, with high LDL; triglycerides nor-mal in type IIa, slightly elevated in type IIb; supranate and infranate clear in both, PHLA normal in both

Rx: Standard rx of hypercholesterolemia (p 277), statins + resins more effective than either alone; probably safe and helpful in children by age 10 (Jama 2004;292:331,377)
          Liver transplant in severe familial (Ann IM 1988;108:204)

Type III Hyperlipidemia

Cause: Genetic, autosomal dominant

Epidem: 1/500; adults only; males > females; associated with obesity, diabetes, gout

Pathophys: Abnormal apolipoprotein $E_{2/2}$ homozygote, dysfunctional β-lipoprotein causes an increase in VLDL remnants and chylomi-crons plus other undefined factors, possibly obesity and diabetes

Sx: Xanthomas and xantholasmata

Si: Tuberoeruptive and palmar xanthomata (75%); xanthelasmas (25%) (r/o diabetes, type II hyperlipidemia, and normal variant)

Crs: Poor, questionably helped by rx

Cmplc: ASHD with MIs

Lab: *Chem:* Cholesterol may be increased or normal; total cholesterol/HDL ratio < 4.5; triglycerides 400-1000 mg %; supranate milky; infranate cloudy; lipoprotein electrophoresis shows broad β slur; apolipoprotein $E_{2/2}$; PHLA normal
Uric acid elevated (40%)
GTT abnormal (55%)

Rx: Diet to lose weight, stop alcohol, decrease intake to < 300 mg cholesterol qd and fat < 30% of calories
Nicotinic acid 2-3 gm qd works but more side effects than diet alone; or as 2nd choice, clofibrate 2 gm qd (works by increasing cholesterol in bile, hence can cause gallstones) or gemfibrozil

Type IV Hyperlipidemia

Cause: Genetic, autosomal dominant; or alcohol

Epidem: Associated with diabetes (70%), obesity, hyperuricemia; very common

Pathophys: Elevated VLDL; carbohydrate induced, causes liver to make too much triglyceride

Sx: None until MI

Si: None until MI

Crs:

Cmplc: MIs
r/o other causes of increased triglycerides, including drugs (thiazides, bcp's, estrogens, β-blockers, isotretinoin), burns and trauma, sepsis, SLE, MIs, glycogen storage diseases, obesity, alcohol

Lab: *Chem:* Cholesterol increased or normal; total cholesterol/HDL ratio increased; triglycerides 150-1000 mg %; supranate clear; infranate cloudy; PHLA normal; lipoPEP shows increased pre-β-lipoprotein

> Uric acid increased
> GTT abnormal (70%)

Rx: Lose weight; rx diabetes; avoid alcohol, estrogens; diet of cholesterol < 300 mg qd; exercise

> Nicotinic acid (niacin) (p 277)

Type V Hyperlipidemia

Cause: Genetic, autosomal dominant

Epidem: Associated with diabetes, hyperuricemia, alcohol use; rare

Pathophys: Elevated chylomicrons and VLDL; a combination of type I and IV characteristics; fat and carbohydrate induced, ie, type IV with a relative lipoprotein lipase deficiency from increased VLDL synthesis by the liver so that dietary triglycerides more easily overwhelm it

Sx: "Pimples," recurrent abdominal pain

Si: Hepatosplenomegaly, lipemia retinalis (picture: Nejm 1999;340:1969), eruptive xanthomata

Crs:

Cmplc: Pancreatitis, no MIs (debatably: Nejm 1996;335:848)

> r/o other causes of elevated triglycerides, including "metabolic syndrome" (p 266) drugs (poor diabetic control, thiazides, bcp's, estrogens, β-blockers, isotretinoin), burns and trauma, sepsis, SLE, MIs, glycogen storage diseases, obesity, alcohol

Lab: *Chem:* Cholesterol elevated; total cholesterol/HDL ratio increased; triglycerides 1000+ mg %; supranate milky; infranate cloudy; PHLA low

> Uric acid increased
> GTT abnormal (70%)

Rx: Avoid estrogens and cholesterol binders, which increase triglycerides (L. Keilson 5/97)

Decrease dietary fat to < 20% of calories; no alcohol, lose weight

Gemfibrozil, niacin, or clofibrate if pancreatitis or xanthomata

5.5 Parathyroid/Calcium/Magnesium Disorders

Hyperparathyroidism

Jama 2005;293:1772, Nejm 2004;350:1746, 2000;343:1863,

Cause:

- Parathyroid adenoma (90%); vast majority are single, 4% double
- Carcinoma (4%) of parathyroids
- Secondary: Renal failure with autonomous PTH from hypertrophied gland; lithium or thiazide induced

Epidem: Most commonly sporadic nonfamilial; prevalence now dropping, unclear why (Ann IM 1997;126:433)

Sometimes associated with multiple endocrine neoplasia (MEN) syndromes (Nejm 1990;322:723)

- **MEN type I** (95% have elevated PTH: Nejm 1986;314:1287): Hyperparathyroidism; adenomas of pituitary (30%), often prolactin producing; pancreatic adenomas, especially gastrinomas (causing ZE syndrome) or insulin-producing ones (37%). Autosomal dominant from loss of suppressor gene on chromosome 11 (Nejm 1989;321:218).
- **MEN type II:** Hyperparathyroidism, pheochromocytomas, and medullary carcinoma of thyroid

Pathophys: PTH is stimulated by low calcium; increases renal calcitrol (activated, 1.25 OH vitamin D) production (Ann IM 1994;121:633), which in turn increases gi calcium absorption, osteoclastic activity, and renal tubule calcium resorption and

PO$_4$ loss. Relative imbalance of latter can cause stones (Nejm 1980;302:421).

Sx: of hypercalcemia sx (p 291); asx cases found incidently by high calcium level on chem profiles often/usually are stable over many years and can simply be monitored

Si: of hypercalcemia si, esp fatigue and muscular weakness (Ann IM 1975;82:474); palpable neck tumor occasionally

Crs: Carcinoma is invariably fatal

Cmplc: Renal stones in 20% of patients with elevated PTH, 5% of patients with stones have elevated PTH; and eventually, some renal failure

Osteoporosis, esp of distal cortical bone (Colles fx), or even von Recklinghausen's syndrome with generalized decalcification and fractures, brown tumors and bone cysts, and renal stones

r/o hypocalciuric hypercalcemia (p 290), which is not helped by parathyroidectomy

Lab: *Chem:* Serum Ca^{++} > 10.5 mg %, 30% false neg. PTH level high, or PTH/Ca ratios high (PTH abnormally "normal"). Urinary Ca^{++} > 250 mg/24 hr (females), > 300 mg/24 hr (males); 10% false pos, 30% false neg.

Xray: Hands occasionally show punched-out lesions in phalanges, subperiosteal bone resorption distally with unique lacey appearance; dental films may show erosion of lamina dura, but many false pos and neg; clavicle may have distal end resorption

Dexascan shows osteoporosis

Scan w technetium/sestamibi can localize for surgery and distinguish adenoma from hyperplasia (J Nuc Med 1992;33:1801; Arch Surg 1996;131:1074)

Rx: Surgical excision of adenomas, even if asx if young (< 50 yr), if osteoporosis (T score < −2.5), high serum calcium levels (> 12 mg %), urinary Ca > 400 mg/24 hr, and/or renal stones; less urgent if asx and doesn't meet these criteria since no increase in vertebral fractures (Ann IM 1991;114:593); 5% of population have mediastinal and/or paraesophageal parathyroids

Cinacalcet (Sensispar) (Med Let 2004;46:80) 30+ mg po qd; esp for secondary hyperparathyroidism, eg, renal failure and functioning PTH-producing carcinomas; $10/d for 30 mg

Vitamin D 400 IU plus 1-1.5 gm of calcium po qd

Biphosphonates like alendronate

Raloxifene (Evista), a selective estrogen receptor modulator (p 838) perhaps (J Clin Endocrinol Metab 2003;88:1174)

Rx of of hypercalcemia (p 291)

Hypoparathyroidism

Nejm 2000;343:1863

Cause:

- Post-thyroidectomy
- Acquired: Renal failure, hypomagnesemia, alcoholism (by hypomagnesemia or direct suppression of PTH: Nejm 1991;324:721)
- Familial types from genetic hormone defects
- **autoimmune polyendocrinopathy candidiasis/ectodermal dystrophy** (Nejm 1990;322:1829); 80% are hypoparathyroid, 70% are hypoadrenal; 60% of women with it are hypogonadal, 15% of men with it are; by age 20, 100% have had significant candidial infections

Epidem: Associated with Addison's, PA, Hashimoto's, diGeorge syndrome (3rd and 4th pharyngeal pouches)

Pathophys: PTH necessary for osteoclastic response to low calcium, renal tubular calcium resorption and PO_4 excretion, and vitamin D activation

Alkalosis due to blocked PTH stimulation of organic acid production in bones (Ann IM 1972;76:825); monilia infections due to suppressor T-cell defects (Nejm 1979;300:164)

Sx: of hypocalcemia sx: circumoral paresthesias, carpal-pedal spasms, stridor, seizures (brief, mild), bronchospasm, gi cramps, anxiety, cataracts

Si: of hypocalcemia si: tetany (carpal-pedal spasm, Chvostek's si, Trousseau's si); cataracts, vascular corneal opacities (band keratopathy), psychiatric changes, dystonias, and dyskinesias (Nejm 1972;286:762)

Crs:

Cmplc: Pustular psoriasis and dermatitis herpetiformis (Ann IM 1984;100:677)

r/o: **pseudohypoparathyroidism,** which is genetic, sex-linked vs dominant; associated with hypopituitarism, especially types with low TSH and gi lactase deficiency; end-organ (bone and kidney) defect in cyclic AMP protein receptor for PTH as well as other hormones, eg, TSH (Ann IM 1986;105:197); si of hypercalcemia and mental retardation, short stature and phalanges; hypoplastic carious teeth; dx w Ellsworth-Howard test: iv PTH causes no increase in phosphate excretion (< 25 mg/hr) and/or no increase in cAMP excretion (Ann IM 1988;109:800)

r/o **familial hypercalciuric hypocalcemia** from defective calcium-sensing receptor (Nejm 1996;335:1115)

Lab: *Chem:* Hypocalcemia, r/o hypoalbuminemia (p 1135 for correction formulas), lung cancer or its rx, leukemia, ricketts/ osteomalacia, thyrocalcitonin-producing medullary carcinoma of the thyroid?, pancreatitis

Serum PO_4 elevated; metabolic alkalosis
Urine: Hypocalciuria

Xray: Skull films may show basal ganglia calcification (Nejm 1971;285:72)

Rx:

1st: Vitamin D_3 50,000-100,000+ U qd; or 1,25-$(OH)_2$ vitamin D (Rocaltrol), expensive; narrow margins of safety for hypercalcemia

2nd: Calcium po

3rd: Chlorthalidone 50 mg po qd or other thiazide

Hypercalcemia

Nejm 1992;326:1196

Cause/Epidem/Pathophys:

- Hyperparathyroidism (p 286) via renal calcitriol (activated vitamin D) production (Ann IM 1994;121:633,709)
- Cancers, especially lung, breast, and hepatoma (Nejm 1992;327:1663), by:
  1. PTH-like protein secretions, with T-cell leukemias/lymphomas (Nejm 1990;322:1106; Ann IM 1989;111:484)
  2. Secretion of other bone-resorbing substances
  3. Tumor conversion of 25-OH vitamin D to 1,25-OH vitamin D (calcitriol)
  4. Local osteolytic mets
- Sarcoid, Hodgkin's lymphoma, non-Hodgkin's lymphoma, cat scratch disease (Jama 1998;279:532), and tbc, via extrarenal calcitriol (activated vitamin D) production in granulomas (Ann IM 1994;121:633,709)
- Vitamin D intoxication (Nejm 1992;326:1173) including the milk-alkali syndrome (Ann IM 1982;97:242)
- Immobilization
- Thyrotoxicosis
- Thiazides rarely (Nejm 1971;284:828)
- Vitamin A intoxication (Ann IM 1974;80:44)
- Disseminated coccidiomycosis (Nejm 1977;297:431)
- Benign familial hypocalciuric hypercalcemia (autosomal dominant) (Ann IM 1985;102:511)
- Adrenal insufficiency

Sx: Fatigue, weakness, sleepiness, nausea/anorexia, constipation, polyuria/dypsia, and volume depletion

Si: Confusion, delirium, drowsiness, coma

Crs:

Cmplc: Pancreatitis, increased risk of digoxin toxicity

Lab: *Chem:* Calcium elevated (p 1135 for corrections for low proteins) $\geq$ 10.5 mg %; sx usually at 11-12 mg %, really toxic over 14 mg %

Noninv: EKG, Short QT interval w normal T wave, segment from QRS to beginning of T shortened

Xray:

Rx: Acute rx for $Ca^{++} > 13$ mg %, to decrease within hours:
- Normal saline 2.5-4 L/24 hr iv to assure intravascular volume adequately replaced (CVP or Swann monitoring), avoid furosemide (Nejm 1984;310:1718) initially, but often needed after volume replaced to prevent volume overload and accelerate renal calcium clearance
- Pamidronate (Aredia) 60-90 mg iv over 24 hr (Med Let 1992;34:1), or 4-8 mg/hr

    Chronic rx, works over 1-5 d, worth doing even with metastatic cancer since diminishes sx and allows hospital discharge (Ann IM 1990;112:499):
- Biphosphonates, eg, pamidronate (Aredia) 60-90 mg iv infusion over 8-24 hr (Med Let 1992;34:1) or 1200 mg po qd × 5 d
- Steroids (Ann IM 1980;93:269,449) primarily for sarcoid pts, eg, prednisone 20 mg po tid
- Calcitonin 4 U/kg q 6 hr sc or im, relatively weak agent alone
- Indomethacin (rarely helpful if due to cancer)
- Gallium nitrate iv infusion, experimental (Med Let 1991;33:41; Ann IM 1988;108:669) 200 mg/M^2 in 1 L continuous infusion qd × 5 d

Hypomagnesemia

Cause: Gi fluid and electrolyte loss rx'd with Mg-free fluids; malnutrition; fistulae; burns; diuretics; cisplatinum-induced renal disease (Ann IM 1981;95:628)

Epidem: Associated with large gi fluid losses and malnutrition, eg, w ulcerative colitis, regional enteritis, chronic alcoholics, toxemia of pregnancy, primary hypo- or hyperparathyroidism, primary hyperaldosteronism, thyrotoxicosis, RTA, diuretic phase of ATN

Pathophys: Low Mg inhibits PTH secretion, which in turn causes hypocalcemic si and sx (Nejm 1970;282:61). Alcohol inhibits PTH secretion, thus also contributing (Nejm 1991;324:721).

Sx: Cramps

Si: Carpopedal spasm, Chvostek's si, Trousseau's si, delirium, muscle tremor and bizarre movements, convulsions, hypotension

Crs: Ataxias take months to clear

Cmplc: Hypocalcemia; hypo K^+ in cisplatinum type (Ann IM 1981;95:328)

Lab: *Chem:* $Mg^{++} < 1.6$ mEq/L; alkaline phosphatase low
Noninv: EKG shows low-voltage and T-wave abnormalities

Rx: 40-80 mEq $MgSO_4$ (10 cc of 50% hydrated soln) iv in 1 L D_5S or D_5W over 3 hr

Hypermagnesemia

Cause: Renal failure, often parallels K^+ increase. Chronic Mg-containing antacid and laxative use. Enemas, especially in megacolon, with Mg-containing soaps.

Epidem: Less common than hypomagnesemia

Pathophys: Avg qd intake = 20-40 mEq; total body stores = 2000 mEq, half in bones, rest intracellular

Sx: Difficult defecation, urination; nausea; drowsiness at pharmacologic doses only

Si: Depressed DTRs, hypotension (Ann IM 1975;83:657)

Crs:

Cmplc: Heart block, respiratory paralysis

Lab: *Chem:* $Mg^{++} > 2.2$ mEq/L

    Noninv: EKG shows heart block

Rx: Calcium gluconate 5-10 mEq (10-20 cc of 10% soln iv)

5.6 Pituitary Disorders

Acromegaly/Gigantism

Nejm 1991;324:822,1555, 1990;322:966

Cause:

- Micro- or macropituitary adenoma, most commonly producing HGH (15% of all functioning pituitary tumors); of other functioning pituitary tumors, 30% produce gonadotropins, 50% produce prolactin (p 297), 5% produce ACTH (p 247), and 1% produce TSH (D. Oppenheim 9/91)
- Pancreatic islet cell tumor, rarely (Nejm 1985;312:9)
- Growth hormone-releasing hormone production by pulmonary oat cell cancers or pancreatic islet cell tumors; rarely tumors of the hypothalamus, carcinoids, other tumors of endocrine origin, or non-Hodgkin's lymphoma (Nejm 2000;342:1871)

Epidem: Male/female = 1:1; 3-4 cases/1 million/yr incidence; 50-70 cases/1 million prevalence

Pathophys: Excessive HGH causes increased IGF-1 (insulin-like growth factor 1) and stimulates growth, glucose intolerance, sleep apnea, and increased plasma volume, causing hypertension, LVH, decreased systemic vascular resistance, and increased cardiac output ("hyperkinetic heart syndrome": Ann IM 1990;113:921)

Sx: Acral enlargement (big hands and feet) (100%), amenorrhea/impotence (80% of males), headache (60%), osteoarthritis (30%), diplopia (15%), increased sweating, coarsened facial features, big tongue, sleep apnea, and, in children, gigantism

Si: Frontal hyperostosis; lantern jaw; hands with distal spadia; thick skin especially heel pads > 22 mm; bitemporal visual field defects (25%); goiter (25%); aldosterone-induced hypertension (30%) (Nejm 1972;287:795), and LVH that reverses w rx (Ann IM 1992;117:719)

Crs: Years to develop; ask for old photos to compare with present facies

Cmplc: Diabetes mellitus (80%); carpal tunnel syndrome (35%: Ann IM 1973;78:379); osteoarthritis; sleep apnea in most, $^2/_3$ obstructive, $^1/_3$ central (Ann IM 1991;115:527), helped by octreotide rx (Ann IM 1994;121:478); atherosclerotic disease (Ann IM 1974;81:11) like cardiomyopathy and CHF; colonic polyps (46%) and cancer (8%) (Ann IM 1984;101:627), screen for > age 50 yr or when disease present > 10 yr; skin tags, may be a marker

Lab: *Chem:* Somatomedin C (IGF-1) by RIA correlates best with disease activity (Nejm 1979;301:1138)

HGH by RIA; oral GTT may provoke paradoxical HGH rise, HGH 1 hr into GTT < 0.5 ngm/cc is normal without false negatives (N. Elgee 1972)

Diabetic GTT (80%)

Xray: MRI 1st? (Nejm 1991;324:1555), but > 10% false pos in general population (Ann IM 1994;120:817)

CT shows sellar erosion commonly, unlike Cushing's syndrome-producing tumors

Heel pad thickness

Hands show spade-like distal phalangeal tufts, wide cartilages

Rx:

1st: Transsphenoidal surgery

2nd: Radiation by stereotactic proton beam; 50% will become hypopit after 10 yr

3rd: Long-acting somatostatin analog, octreotide 100 μgm sc q 8 hr (Ann IM 1992;117:711), especially helps cardiomyopathy/atherosclerotic disease (Ann IM 1990;113:921) and sleep apnea (Ann IM 1994;121:478); adverse effects: diabetes, gallstones (Ann IM 1990;112:173). Bromocriptine helps ~30% (Nejm 1985;313:1576).

4th: Pegvisomant (Somovert) (Med Let 2003;45:55; Nejm 2000;342:1171) sc daily; HGH receptor antagonist; $50,000-100,000/yr

Table 5.3 Treatment of Various Pituitary Adenomas

Approach	Prolactin-Secreting Tumors	Growth Hormone–Secreting Tumors	ACTH-Secreting Tumors	TSH-Secreting Tumors	Nonfunctioning Tumors
Primary approach	DA: microadenomas, 80–90% response; macroadenomas, 60–75% response	Surgery: microadenomas, 70% response; macro-adenomas, 50% response	Surgery: microadenoma, 80–90% response; macroadenoma, 50% response	Surgery plus irradiation, 67% response	Surgery: improved vision, 70% response
Secondary approach	Surgery: micro-adenomas, 55% response; macro-adenomas, 20% response	Somatostatin analogs, 60% response; DA, 20% response; irradiation, 50% response (by 12 yr)	Irradiation plus cortisol-decreasing drugs	Somatostatin analogs, 75% response	Irradiation
Novel medical developments	Depot long-acting DA, somatostatin receptor subtype-selective analogs	Long-acting somatosta-tins, somatostatin re-ceptor subtype-selective analogs; growth hor-mone receptor or GHRH antagonist		Long-acting somato-statins	Gonadotropin-releasing hormone antagonists

ACTH = adrenocorticotropin hormone; DA = dopamine agonists; GHRH = growth hormone-releasing hormone; TSH = thyroid-stimulating hormone. "Response" refers to normalization of hormone secretion or ablation of tumor mass.
Reproduced with permission from Shimon I, Melmed S. Management of Pituitary Tumors, Ann Intern Med 1998;129:472-483.

Galactorrhea/Amenorrhea Syndrome (Prolactinoma)

Nejm 2003;349:2035

Cause: Abnormal prolongation or initiation of prolactin production
$\frac{1}{3}$ are true primary hyperprolactinemia, over $\frac{1}{2}$ of these are due to micro- or macroadenomas and empty sella syndrome (Ann IM 1986;105:238); the rest are idiopathic, including Argonz-Del Castillo syndrome (spontaneous), and postpregnancy (Chiari-Frommel syndrome)

$\frac{2}{3}$ are secondary types, from hypothyroidism; renal failure; cirrhosis; hypothalamic disease; and medications like reserpine, phenothiazines, verapamil (Ann IM 1981;95:66), metoclopramide (Ann IM 1983;98:86), and cimetidine (Nejm 1982;306:26)

Epidem:

Pathophys: Hypothyroidism causes the syndrome because TRH itself causes prolactin release. Prolactin inhibits LH secretion and peak, thereby inhibiting menses.

Sx: In females, amenorrhea (90%) and infertility; may be masked by bcp use, and therefore present only as galactorrhea; galactorrhea or elicitable lactation

In males, galactorrhea rare, more often impotence and decreased libido (Nejm 1978;299:847); presentation is later, so have higher incidence of hypopituitarism and visual field losses (Ann IM 1986;105:238)

Si: Galactorrhea, ie, any amount of milky substance expressible, no correlation of amount with prolactin level or tumor size

Crs: Usually benign, especially the idiopathic or microadenoma types (Ann IM 1984;100:115), although skeletal and cardiovascular consequences of hypogonadism, if present, must be considered

Cmplc: Panhypopituitarism
Visual field cuts w macroadenoma (> 1 cm) especially during pregnancy, rare w microadenomas (Ann IM 1994;121:473)

Osteoporosis due to low estrogen/androgen levels, reversible with rx (Nejm 1986;315:542)

ASHD from hypogonadism (estrogen lack)

Lab: *Chem:* Prolactin > 100 ngm/cc is likely adenoma, returns to normal w rx; r/o medication causes of moderate elevations (usually < 100 ngm/cc): metoclopramide (Reglan), phenothiazines, butyrophenomes, TCAs, risperidone, MAOIs, verapamil, reserpine, Aldomet

Path: Prolactin-staining microadenoma, but 27% of normals in autopsy series also have? (Nejm 1981;304:156)

Xray: Gadolinium-enhanced MRI (Nejm 1991;324:1555), but 10% false pos in general population (Ann IM 1994;120:817); CT, 15-20% false pos (D. Federman 3/85). Microadenoma ≤ 10 mm diameter, macroadenoma ≥ 10 mm.

Rx: Pregnancy and nursing risks are small with idiopathic or microadenomas

Medical rx w dopamine agonists:

- Bromocriptine (Parlodel) 1.25-20 mg po qd divided, eg, 1.25-2.5 mg po hs with snack × 3-7 d, then 2.5 bid increased to tid gradually; try for higher doses until prolactin level is suppressed to decrease tumor size (Nejm 1985;313:656) in about $^1/_2$; 1st choice if attempting pregnancy, stop as soon as pregnant; adverse effects: hypotension, cost, nausea, peptic ulcer disease, headache, dizziness, Raynaud's at high doses

- Cabergoline (Dostinex) 0.25-1 mg po biw, better tolerated and twice as effective, 83% become normoprolactinemic vs 59% w bromocriptine (Nejm 1994;331:904); can try withdrawing after 3 yr (Nejm 2003;349:2023), 25% recurrence off med

Surgical transsphenoidal resection unreliable but can try if fail medical rx

Growth Hormone Deficiency

Cause: Idiopathic or associated with other pituitary lesions; genetic, autosomal recessive

Epidem: Dwarfism is associated with other pituitary defects in 50% of pts

Pathophys: Growth hormone is responsible for growth stimulation and lipid mobilization/protein sparing. In pygmies and some genetic dwarfs (Nejm 1971;284:809), defect is in end-organ responsiveness from growth hormone receptor deficiency (Nejm 1990;323:1367). Insulin-like growth factor mediates these effects and alone is responsible for most prenatal growth (Nejm 1996;335:1363).

Sx: Dwarfism in children: height impairment is often greater than weight impairment, ie, "pudgy" kids; 50% are < 3rd percentile at 1 yr

Si: In children, short stature, decreased growth velocity, delayed bone age

In adults, osteoporosis, hyperlipidemia, diminished muscle strength and vitality

Crs:

Cmplc: Hypoglycemia often, especially if ACTH deficiency too
r/o growth hormone receptor insensitivity due to mutation, partial or complete (Laron dwarfism) (Nejm 1995;333:1093)

Lab: *Chem:* Hypoglycemia, especially if combined HGH and ACTH deficiencies are present (Nejm 1968;278:57)
HGH (IGF-1) levels low for age, or fail to elevate w stimulation tests (insulin, clonidine, arginine, L-dopa, glucagon) (Nejm 1988;319:201)

Xray: Bone age is younger than chronologic age

Rx (Nejm 1999;341:1206): Replace with recombinant HGH
Children: HGH 0.3 mg/kg/wk im divided into qd doses,

$20,000/yr, or less effective but cheaper GHRH; not for use in short children who are not GH deficient, Turner's syndrome, or chronic renal failure; $5000+/yr (Med Let 1999;41:2) but is being so used (Nejm 1999;340:502,557)

Adults: Use is very controversial (Ann IM 2002;137:190,197,202 vs Ann IM 1996;125:883; Nejm 1989;321:1797), 6-25 μgm/kg; adverse effects: edema, arthralgias; experimentally reverses some somatic aspects of aging in normal patients age > 60 yr (Nejm 1990;323:1), but functional capacities are not improved (Ann IM 1996;124:708); may help some ICU pts (burns, trauma) but worsens others (Nejm 1999;341;785, 837)

Panhypopituitarism

Nejm 1994;330:1651

Cause:

- Neoplasms: Polyendocrine adenomas including FSH-, LH-, and/or TSH-producing ones that rarely secrete intact hormone (Nejm 1991;324:822) unlike (Nejm 1980;302:210) ACTH-, HGH-, and prolactin-producing ones (p 297); craniopharyngiomas; metastases especially from lung; neurofibromas
- Trauma
- Granulomas: Hans-Christian disease, sarcoid (often causes just prolactinemia) (Ann IM 1972;76:545), tuberculosis
- Vascular: Carotid aneurysm, postpartum infarction (Sheehan's syndrome), diabetic vascular disease, prepartum in diabetics (Ann IM 1971;74:357)
- Late cmplc of extracranial head and neck tumor or brain (Nejm 1993;328:87) irradiation
- Congenital

Epidem:

Pathophys: Order of most frequent hormonal defects w pituitary tumor: growth hormone > gonadotropins > TSH > ACTH.

Prolactin may be autonomously produced by some pituitary tumors that cause hypopituitarism.

Sx: Hypogonadism with amenorrhea w or w/o lactation; hypothyroidism; adrenal insufficiency; headaches; bitemporal visual field losses

Si: Findings of above

Crs:

Cmplc: r/o **"Empty Sella Syndrome"** (Ann IM 1986;105:238), an incidental pickup of an enlarged sella on skull xray, usually but not always w normal pituitary function; **Hypothalamic Dysfunction,** seen with weight loss especially in anorexia nervosa

Lab: *Chem:* Serum levels of HGH, T_3T_4, TSH after TRH, testosterone or estradiol, LH, FSH, ACTH, and cortisol all low
Hem: Anemia (Nejm 1971;284:479)

Xray: MRI, or CT if MRI not available, shows pituitary mass; w calcification in craniopharyngioma

Rx (Table 5.3; Nejm 1991;324:1555):

Replacement hormones: L-thyroxine, glucocorticoids, testosterone/estrogen, and recombinant growth hormone (Nejm 1989;321:1797), at least in children and perhaps in adults to preserve bone density (Ann IM 1996;883:932)

Surgical resection via transsphenoidal approach for documented adenomas; cmplc: diabetes insipidus

Bromocriptine (Pergolide) (Nejm 1983;309:704; Ann IM 1982;96:281) for prolactinoma

Radiation in some cases after surgery if residual tumor on MRI

Rx of galactorrhea/amenorrhea prolactinomas (p 297)

5.7 Thyroid Diseases

Hypothyroidism/Myxedema/Cretinism

Clin Ger Med 1995;11:252; Jama 1995;273:808

Cause:
- Immune: Thyroid failure from atrophic or goitrous autoimmune (Hashimoto's) thyroiditis; transient TSH-inhibiting IgG in mother causing cretin children (Nejm 1980;303:739) or nonstimulating TSH receptor-binding IgG antibody (cf Graves' disease: Ann IM 1985;103:26), these thyrotropin (TSH)-blocking antibodies often present in both atrophic and goitrous (Hashimoto's) types (Nejm 1992;326:513)
- Surgical excision
- Radiation: To neck for tumor, lymphoma, etc (Nejm 1991;325:599); or most commonly I^{131} rx (Ann IM 1972;76:721) of hyperthyroidism
- Dietary I_2 deficiency, eg, cretinism in Equador (Nejm 1969;280:296) and China (Nejm 1994;331:1739), or in some patients with possibly underlying subclinical disease
- Lithium rx; acts like I_2 load, causes goiter in 10%, hypothyroidism in 1%
- Rarely secondary hypothryoidism from pituitary or hypothalamic failure, eg, post-brain irradiation (Nejm 1993;328:87)

Epidem: Associated with pernicious anemia and insulin-dependent diabetes through association of those w autoimmune Hashimoto's; phenytoin (Dilantin) and carbamazepine (Tegretol) may precipitate (Ann IM 1983;99:341)

Pathophys: Goiter, caused by edema lymphatic infiltration and hypertrophy

Sx: Hair loss, and coarseness; coarse skin; fatigue; swollen tongue with slurred speech; nonpitting edema; menorrhagia; feel cold; lactation from TRH stimulation of prolactin (Ann IM 1976;84:534);

constipation; muscle cramps; mental dullness. Worsened or precipitated by smoking, which impairs thyroid hormone secretion and peripheral effect (Nejm 1995;333:969).

Si: Goiter; dry skin; hung-up reflexes (r/o hypothermia, β-blockers, pregnancy, procainamide); diminished PMI from pericardial effusion (Nejm 1977;296:1); arthritis with synovial thickening and noninflammatory effusions (Nejm 1970;282:1172)

Crs: Very slowly progressive; insidious; 25% of atrophic type may revert (Nejm 1992;326:513)

Cmplc: Anemias from folate deficiency in 20%, hypoproliferative, Fe-deficient (Ann IM 1968;68:792); bleeding from diminished platelet stickiness (Ann IM 1974;82:342); cerebellar sx (30%); peripheral neuropathies (25%); coma, confusion, psychoses, seizures; hypothermia; hypoventilation, sleep apnea (Ann IM 1984;101:491); ASHD due to lipid as well as homocysteine elevations (Ann IM 2000;132:270, 1999;131:348)

r/o **"Euthyroid-sick Syndrome"**: low $T_3 T_4$, with normal or low TSH in presence of other severe illness (Nejm 1985; 312:546); no specific rx required

Lab: *Chem:* TSH elevated in primary hypothyroidism, the earliest test to become abnormal, may be worth using as a screening test in the elderly (Ann IM 1990;112:840); if on thyroid and indications in doubt, may stop and check TSH, T_4 at 5 wk. Total T_3, free T_4, resin T_3 uptake (a measure of thyroid-binding globulins) all low. In secondary myxedema, TSH stimulation by TRH administration may be slow to respond w delayed peak (Nejm 1985;312:1085).

Cholesterol elevated > 250 mg % in secondary not in primary types ("rapid TSH"); triglycerides elevated

CPK (MM) and liver enzymes often elevated

Xray: Chest may show increased heart size (pericardial effusion)

Rx: L-Thyroxine (Synthroid, Levoxyl, or generic, all the same: Jama 1997;277:1205; Nejm 1994;331:174) 0.1-0.2 mg (100-200 μgm) qd po; 0.1 adequate for ⅔ of pts, 0.125 plenty for most (1.7 μgm/kg) (Ann IM 1986;105:11); monitor sensitive TSH (Ann IM 1990;113:450) to keep ≥ 0.5 mIU/cc so hip fx risk minimized (Ann IM 2001;134:560). Use of T_3 w T_4 replacement no benefit by DBCT (Ann IM 2005;142:412; Jama 2003;290:2952). No benefit from rx of TSH < 10 (Jama 2003;291:228, 239). Beware of concomitant rx w $FeSO_4$, which impairs absorption (Ann IM 1992;117:1010), as do calcium pills like Tums or Os-Cal (Jama 2000;283:2822), phenytoin (Dilantin), carbamazepine (Tegretol), rifampin, cholestyramine, sucralfate, and aluminum hydroxide antacids.

in coma/confusion: 100-500 μgm iv/po qd, usually w concomitant stress steroid doses in case also hypoadrenal

in elderly, go very slowly, eg, ¼ or less these doses, and work up slowly because normal T_3 half-life is several days and may be longer in the elderly, and T_4 half-life is nearly twice that of T_3

in pregnancy, dose requirements may increase; monitor with TSH (Nejm 1990;323:91)

in developing countries, I_2 in oil annually to all w euthyroid goiter? (Nejm 1992;326:236) and/or to pregnant women and babies in areas of endemic cretinism (Nejm 1986;315:791)

Hyperthyroidism, Thyrotoxicosis, and Stimulating Autoimmune Thyroiditis (Graves' Disease)

Nejm 2000;343:1236; Jama 1995;273:808

Cause: Autoimmune stimulating antibody production, occasionally from *Yersinia enterocolitica* infection inducing cross-reacting antibodies (Ann IM 1976;85:735); or exogenous T_3T_4 ingestion; or thyroiditis (p 309); or hot nodule (p 311); or rarely, TSH-producing chorio- or testicular carcinomas, molar pregnancy (Ann IM 1975;83:307), or ovarian cancers, especially struma ovarii with ascites (Ann IM 1970;72:883), and rare pituitary microadenoma (Ann IM 1989;111:827; Nejm 1987;317:12); organic iodine induction possible in any goiter patient (Nejm 1971; 285:523), as can lithium or antiretroviral therapy

Epidem: Graves'-associated positive family hx or at least often abnormal suppression tests in family members; pernicious anemia. Female/male = 4-6:1.

Pathophys: In Graves', IgG thyroid-stimulating immunoglobin (TSI) antibody to TSH receptor (Ann IM 1978;88:379); ophthalmoplegia from immune-mediated periorbital inflammation, and ocular myopathy (Nejm 1993;329:1468)

Toxic si's and sx's from catechol facilitation, eg, lid lag from increased sympathetic tone, and/or primary uncoupling of oxidative phosphorylation

Gynecomastia from increased estradiol (Nejm 1972;286:124)

Sx: Thyrotoxic: Palpitations; weight loss; amenorrhea; hyperactivity; hot, sweaty, smooth skin; prominent essential tremor; decreased libido; frequent often diarrheal stools from steatorrhea, polyphagia of fat, and decreased gi transit time (Ann IM 1973;78:669)

In Graves': Above, plus goiter; diplopia and eye protrusion (proptosis); vitiligo, especially of extremities, often precedes toxicosis by years (Ann IM 1969;71:935)

Si: Thyrotoxic: P > 100 resting; "adrenergic stare" and lid lag; weight loss; apathetic depression, especially in elderly (Ann IM 1970;72:679)

In Graves': Above, plus ophthalmoplegias, especially convergence failure; exophthalmus, cornea > 18 mm from lateral orbital rim, can be unilateral; goiter (97%) diffuse, firm (Ann IM 1968;69:1022); gynecomastia in men frequently; pretibial myxedema and localized dermopathy (picture: Nejm 2005;352:918); onycholysis (nail separation); Plummer's nails (serrated) and clubbing; increased pigmentation (increased ACTH turnover); lymphadenopathy (10%)

Crs: Graves' is cyclic, worse in winter (daylight effects?); usually better in pregnancy from natural immune suppression (Nejm 1985;313:562)

Cmplc: Thyroid storm, especially with surgery or infection (Nejm 1974;291:1396); cardiac (Nejm 1992;327:94) including myocarditis and CHF, Afib, and angina precipitation; myopathies, plain and hypokalemic (Ann IM 1974;81:332), myasthenia syndromes; osteoporosis (Ann IM 2001;134:560, 1999;130:750) increases 3× if TSH < 0.1, reversible w rx ; newborn thyrotoxicosis from TSI at age 7-10 d when mother has been on suppressive medications prepartum, and fetal thyrotoxicosis in mothers with ablated thyroids (Nejm 1985;313:562)

Thoracic inlet obstruction w positive Pemberton si (p 310)

Lab: *Chem:* Total T_4, free T_4, serum thyroglobulin (r/o surreptitious ingestion) all increased; sensitive TSH low; TRH stimulation test w 250 μgm iv, draw TSH at 0 and 30 min, shows no rise, often the only abnormal test, especially in elderly with Afib

Alkaline phosphatase (bony) elevated in > 50% Graves' pts (Ann IM 1979;90:164), parallels thyroid function if no liver disease. Calcium may be increased (in 10-25%), though PTH normal (Ann IM 1976;84:668; Nejm 1976;294:431).

Hem: Atypical lymphs and lymphocytosis

Xray: RAIU elevated and useful to distinguish from I_2-induced and subacute thyroiditis types; usually not necessary, thyroid I^{131} , I^{123}, or technetium scan shows diffusely enhanced uptake

Rx (Nejm 1994;330:1731; Ann IM 1994;121:281): Propranolol 2-10 mg iv, or 20-80 mg po, or atenolol 50-100 mg po qd to control sx; may not fully prevent storm (Nejm 1977;296:263); also will decrease hypercalcemia if symptomatic (Nejm 1976;294:431)

Antithyroid meds (Nejm 2005;352:905): propylthiouracil (PTU) < 100-200 mg po tid, or methimazole (Tapezole) 5-20 mg po qd; block iodination of tyrosine by thyroid peroxidase to T_3T_4; rx × 12-18 mo, then start replacement; PTU preferred in pregnancy and during lactation because methimazole may be teratogenic; 40-50% failure rates, higher if high po iodine intake not controlled (Ann IM 1987;107:510; Nejm 1984;311:426); adverse effects of both: rash, toxic hepatitis, vasculitis (esp w PTU) and agranulocytosis (0.3%) though no point in screening CBCs. Both cost $400/yr.

I^{131} rx may be 1st choice in older pts under β-blocker protection, or used if fail 1 or more PTU courses; use w prednisone 0.5 mg/kg po qd × 1 mo, then 2 mo taper to prevent transient worsening of ophthalmopathy (Nejm 1998;338:73); β-blockade may help sx and won't interfere w I^{131} uptake. 76% become hypothyroid by 11 yr after rx even with most conservative dosing (Nejm 1984; 311:426); ok in premenopausal women as long as not pregnant.

Surgical thyroidectomy may be 1st choice, or if fail 2 or more PTU courses and judged unreliable to return if becomes myxedematous after I^{131}, although > 26% of surgical pts will be hypothyroid at 11 yr (Nejm 1984;311:426)

of storm: 1st β-blockade, volume replacement, and dexamethasone (peripheral T_4 to T_3 conversion blockade); then PTU ~1 gm initial dose po or pr, and possibly SSKI loading dose then 10-15 gtts po qid or lithium 300 mg tid

of ophthalmoplegia: Stop smoking (Ann IM 1998;129:632); steroids as prednisone 0.5 mg/kg po qd for 1 mo then q 3 mo taper, clearly helpful, especially with radioactive iodine rx (Nejm 1989;321:1349); surgery; cyclophosphamide (Ann IM 1979;90:921) or cyclosporine (Nejm 1989;321:1353)

of Graves' in pregnancy: Low-dose PTU ok (Nejm 2005;352:905) but try to keep free T_4 at upper normal and taper off in 3rd trimester if can, β-blockers

of pretibial myxedema: Topical steroids

of pituitary adenoma type: Octreotide (Ann IM 1993; 119:236)

Nonstimulating, Autoimmune Thyroiditis (Including Hashimoto's Thyroiditis)

Nejm 2003;348:2646, 1996;335:99

Cause: Autoimmune

Epidem: Female/male = 6-9:1; usually over age 40 yr. Associated with other autoimmune diseases, including stimulating autoimmune thyroid disease and autoimmune ophthalmoplegia (Ann IM 1978;88: 379); Turner's syndrome; Addison's disease; dermatitis herpetiformis (Ann IM 1985;102:194); postpartum 2 wk-4 mo, perhaps due to peridelivery immunologic changes (Ann IM 1977;87:154).

Pathophys: A chronic destructive autoimmune thyroiditis or, if milder, simply autoimmune goiter-producing disease (silent subacute thyroiditis)

Sx: Hypothyroidism; rarely thyrotoxicosis; goiter; but generally few sx, unlike other thyroiditis; very rarely can be painful (Ann IM 1986;104:355)

Si: As above; nontender gland

Crs: Half proceed on to myxedema over months to years

Cmplc: Myxedema
r/o much rarer Riedel's struma (fibrosis, increasing mass); postpartum thyroiditis, usually transiently toxic then hypothyroid, then return to normal

Lab (Ann IM 1978;88:383):
Chem: TSH elevated as become hypothyroid
Hem: ESR minimally elevated
Path: Thyroid bx shows lymphocytic infiltrate, if done, not necessary
Serol: Elevated antibodies against thyroperoxidase; or antithyroid microsomal antibodies, more specif and more sens (95%) than antithyroglobulin antibodies (60%) (J Lab Clin Med 1979;93:1035)

Xray: Thyroid I^{131}, I^{123}, or technetium scan shows no or patchy uptake; RAIU usually low, often 0

Rx: None, if radioactive iodine uptake is low, until becomes myxedematous; if RAIU is high, may have an organification defect from the autoimmune disease, or may have coincident Graves' and need rx for that (Nejm 1975;293:624)

Subacute Thyroiditis (Giant Cell, De Quervain's, or Pseudotubercular Thyroiditis)

Nejm 2003;348:2650

Cause: Viral?

Epidem: Epidemic pattern. Male/female = 1:4; $^1/_6$ as common as nonstimulating autoimmune thyroid disease; $^1/_8$ as common as stimulating autoimmune thyroid disease. $^1/_3$ of cases follow a URI.

Pathophys:

Sx: Many sx (in contrast to Hashimoto's), including fever, nervousness, tender painful neck

Si: Firm gland, usually tender, although 15% have no goiter or pain (Ann IM 1977;86:24)

Crs: Months 1-2: Hyperthyroid with tender gland
Month 3: Transition with firm nontender gland
Months 4-6: Hypothyroid with firm gland becoming normal
Months 7+: Return to normal function and exam

Cmplc: r/o **acute pyogenic thyroiditis;** hemorrhage into thyroid nodule; amiodarone thyrotoxicosis

Lab:
Hem: ESR 50-80 mm/hr early in course
Serol: Occasionally (20%) positive antithyroid antibodies

Xray: Thyroid I^{131}, I^{123}, or technetium scan shows no uptake; low RAIU

Rx: Palliative, no effect on course, including salicylates; short-term steroids, eg, prednisone 40 mg qd, taper to 20 mg qd over 2 wk; β-blockers when toxic sx, replacement rx when hypo

Multinodular Goiter (Nontoxic and Toxic)

Cause: Nontoxic: Iodine deficiency; lithium, or iodide rx; genetic and/or autoimmune silent subacute thyroiditis (nonstimulating)?
Toxic: Progession from nontoxic

Epidem: Nontoxic: Iodine deficiency especially in Equador (Nejm 1969;280:296)
Toxic: Associated with elderly, CHF, AF, and angina

Pathophys: Nontoxic: Unknown for most common type
Toxic: Autonomous function of 1 or more nodules

Sx: Nontoxic: Goiter
Toxic: CHF sx, angina, palpitations

Si: Nontoxic: Goiter
Toxic: CHF, Afib, apathetic hyperthyroidism of elderly with ptsosis

Crs: Nontoxic: slowly progressive

Cmplc: Both: Tracheal compression (Ann IM 1994;121:757); vague head and neck sx due to thoracic inlet compression manifest by positive Pemberton si = facial and head redness and suffusion w elevations of arms up to ears (Ann IM 1996;125:568)
r/o autoimmune thyroid disease

Lab: *Chem:* Nontoxic: Thyroid function tests normal
Toxic: T_4 increased or normal, r/o benign increase in 15% of sick or psychotic pts; RAIU elevated; TRH/TSH test positive, better than T_3 suppression test; normal = TSH of 2-3 rises to 15+; abnormal = no increase in TSH with TRH stimulation

Xray: Thyroid I^{131} , I^{123}, or technetium scan; in nontoxic, shows large gland w diffuse patchy uptake; in toxic, shows hot nodule(s), rest of gland atrophic and cool

Rx: (Nejm 1998;338:1438): Nontoxic: Thyroid replacement? (p 304), but if any autonomous production, can lead to toxicity, especially in the elderly; I^{131} or surgery especially if compressive sx (Ann IM 1994;1221:757)

Toxic: I^{131} rx; surgery

Thyroid Nodule

Nejm 2004;351:1764

Cause: Neoplastic adenoma; or a nodule of multinodular goiter **(Plummer's Disease)**

Epidem: Present in 4-8% of U.S. adult population by physical exam, < 5% malignant; up to 50% over age 50 yr have one by ultrasound; in 20-30% of irradiated adult population 10-30 yr later, ~10% of which are malignant and $\frac{1}{2}$ of those detectable by physical exam (Ann IM 1981;94:176; Nejm 1976;294:1019). Male/female = 1:4.

Pathophys: Only 5% will be "hot," producing T_3T_4 and toxic sx but that guarantees benign pathology

Sx: Asx

Si: Thyroid nodule

Crs:

Cmplc: Cancer in 5-10% of cold nodules by biopsy studies; increased incidence in the young and males

Lab: *Chem:* TSH to r/o thyrotoxicosis from toxic nodule
Path: Fine-needle aspiration bx first to r/o cancer (Ann IM 1993;118:282); < 1% false positives, others report 80% sens/specif (Am J Med 1994;97:152)

Xray: I^{123} scan useful only if aspiration cytology is suspicious/intermediate because can avoid surgery if nodule is hot (functioning)

Ultrasound especially to guide needle aspiration or f/u of neg nodules

Rx: Medically follow (Ann IM 1998;128:386); if increases in size, do fine-needle bx; if benign, put on suppression rx and watch another year; if increases in size again, surgically excise

of hot nodule: I^{131} rx to control hyperthyroid sx; 25% develop myxedema at 5 yr and 20% stay as big or get bigger (Nejm 1983;309:1473), so may need surgery eventually anyway

Thyroid Papillary Carcinoma

Nejm 1998;338:297; Ann IM 1991;115:133

Cause: Most cases occur as sporadic events in the population; increased incidence from irradiation under age 20, w risk thereafter peaking over 20 yr then declining, eg, 1.7% at 20 yr after radiation rx of Hodgkin's (Nejm 1991;325:599); no increase after I^{131} rx of Graves' disease (Nejm 1980;303:188)

Epidem: 75-90% of all thyroid cancers; mean age at dx is 45 yr. Female/male = 2-3:1.

Pathophys: Local invasion and metastases (primarily lymphatic), less often bloodborne metastases

Sx: Neck mass

Si: Thyroid mass (80%), 40% of the time in an abnormal gland from other thyroid disease

Stage at dx:

47% stage I, small intrathyroid

28% stage II, large intrathyroid

21% stage III, > 4 cm and/or local extranodal invasion

4% stage IV, distant extranodal mets

Crs: Excellent, 90% > 30-yr survival for stages I and II; worse if age > 50 yr, > 4 cm diameter, or local or distant metastases. Patients with positive lymph nodes may have equal survival to those with negative nodes.

Radiation-induced cancers have same course as others (Ann IM 1986;105:405)

Cmplc: r/o follicular and undifferentiated carcinomas, including giant cell, small cell, and medullary carcinoma

Lab: *Chem:* No helpful pre-op tests, post-op is useful to follow thyroglobulin levels (> 10 ngm/cc) as a tumor marker especially of mets

Path: Aspiration biopsy (p 311) and cytology; "rug fringe" effect, ie, papillae, but few mitoses; unlike well-formed follicles of follicular or anaplasia, with giant or small cells of undifferentiated types

Xray: Scan usually cold (Ann IM 1978;88:41)

Rx: Detect in irradiated patients w q 1 yr thyroid physical exam w bx of any nodules; debated if thryoid hormone suppression helps

Surgical thyroidectomy; lobectomy alone is inadequate even for stage I and II disease (4% vs 14% 30-yr recurrence); up to 14% get cmplc of surgery, including hypoparathyroidism and recurrent laryngeal nerve injury. Postsurgical I^{131} rx (Ann IM 1998;129:622) w thyroid hormone suppression.

Chemotherapy possible if metastases with adriamycin (Nejm 1974;290:193), 5-FU, and cisplatin, but none very good

Medullary Carcinoma of Thyroid (Amyloid Struma)

Ann IM 1991;115:140

Cause: Neoplasia

Epidem: May be sporadic, familial, or associated with multiple endocrine neoplasias (MEN) type II A + B (Sipple's syndrome): bilateral pheochromocytomas, gi mucosal neuromas (in 10%: Nejm 1976;295:1287), parathyroid adenomas (10%); inherited with autosomal dominant pattern w RET proto-oncogene (Nejm 2003;349:1517, 1996;335:947; Jama 1995;274:1149)

Pathophys: Neoplasia of parafollicular thyroid cells, multicentric origin (Nejm 1973;289:437); characteristically produce CEA, and/or thyrocalcitonin, and/or serotonin, and other vasoactive substances. RET proto-oncogene type progresses through C-cell hyperplasia to cancer starting at age 3-4 so that by age 20, nearly all have cancer.

Sx: Diarrhea, flushing

Si: Thyroid mass

Crs: Long survival despite anaplastic appearance

Cmplc: Local metastases; pheochromocytoma (30%); secondary Cushing's from ACTH; hyperparathyroidism (Nejm 1968;279:279) in MEN type II

Lab: *Chem:* Thyrocalcitonin elevated by RIA (Nejm 1971;285:1115); CEA elevated

Path: Thyroid bx shows clumps of parafollicular cells surrounded by collagen ("amyloid struma")

Xray: Thyroid scan shows a cold mass, starts in upper poles. Plain films may show calcified metastases that can look like old tbc even with liver mets.

Rx: Prevent cancer deaths in MEN type II families w annual calcitonin stimulation tests (Nejm 1988;318:479)

Surgery with follow-up thyrocalcitonin/CEA levels as markers of residual tumor (Nejm 1974;290:1035)

Chemotherapy w adriamycin (Nejm 1974;290:193)

5.8 Vitamin Disorders

Vitamin A Deficiency

Nejm 1984;310:1023

Cause: Vitamin A deficiency, a fat-soluble vitamin

Epidem: Increased in low-income areas and developing countries

Pathophys: Necessary for visual pigment of eye; other tissue functions not known. Columnar epithelium changes to stratified squamous (keratinization) in trachea, urinary tract, conjunctiva. β-Carotene and other carotenes are precursors.

Sx: Poor growth in children; impaired day and night vision

Si: Keratinization of eye and Bitot spots on sclera (gray plaques); dryness of eyes and skin can be severe (Nejm 1994;330:994)

Crs:

Cmplc: Increased mortality and morbidity from most infections, including measles (Nejm 1990;323:160)

Lab: *Chem:* Low vitamin A levels (1 U = 0.3 μgm)

Rx: Vitamin A; given in small weekly doses reduces overall mortality by 50% in undernourished Indian children (Nejm 1990;323:929) probably by decreasing mortality from respiratory illness; given 10,000 U/lb po q 3 mo, it decreases diarrheal illness in HIV-infected infants (Am J Pub Hlth 1995;85:1076)

Vitamin A Excess

Nejm 1984;310:1023

Cause: Excessive ingestion by vitamin pill users

Epidem:

Pathophys: β-Carotene and other carotenes are precursors; a fat-soluble vitamin

Sx: h/o > 50,000 U (1 U = 0.3 μgm) qd ingestion for 1+ yr. Headache, lethargy, dry skin, sore mouth, fractures, and bone pain.

Si (Nejm 1976;294:805; Ann IM 1974;80:44): Clubbing, fractures (due to abnormal bone growth), desquamative dermatitis, pseudotumor cerebri

Crs:

Cmplc: Cirrhosis (Nejm 1974;291:438); congenital malformations, esp neural tube defects in infants exposed to ≥ 10,000 U/d of vitamin

A (but not β-carotenes), esp in 1st 7 wk of pregnancy (Nejm 1995;333:1369); osteoporosis, hip and other fx from chronic vitamin A intake > 3000 μgm/d (Jama 2002;287:47), or even 1500 μgm/d (Nejm 2003;348:287)

Lab:

Rx: Stop intake

Wernicke's Encephalopathy

Cause: Thiamine (B_1) deficiency + genetic enzyme abnormalities (Nejm 1977;297:1367)

Epidem: Most commonly in alcoholics; also in surgical patients on iv's for weeks without thiamine supplement; rarely, refed starving patients

Pathophys: Unknown (beriberi—see p 317)

Sx:

Si: • Ophthalmoplegia, especially nystagmus (85%) progressing to paralysis of lateral gaze, ie, abducens palsies
• Global confusion
• Ataxia
• Hypothermia

Crs: May recover partially over 1 yr (Nejm 1985;312:16)

Cmplc: Korsakoff's psychosis (80%), confabulating responses

Lab: *Path:* Circummamillary body congestion and hemorrhage at base of brain on postmortem, and along floors of 3rd and 4th ventricles

Rx: Preventively put thiamine in all alcoholic drinks perhaps, especially wine (Nejm 1978;299:285)?
Thiamine 100 mg im, iv (is safe: Jama 1995;274:562) or po qd × 3 d; always give 1st dose before start iv glucose

Beriberi

Cause: Thiamine (B_1) deficiency

Epidem:

Pathophys: Unknown function of thiamine; increased requirement when eating or given glucose; ? in decarboxylation of pyruvate to citric acid cycle; CHF may be due to high cardiac output failure from neuropathic poor vascular tone

Sx: Wet beriberi: Edema
Dry beriberi: "Burning" feet
Infantile beriberi: Nausea and vomiting; dyspnea

Si: Wet beriberi: Edema, elevated CVP
Dry beriberi: Peripheral neuropathy
Infantile beriberi: Cyanosis, tachycardia, seizures, hypotension

Crs: All improve w po or parenteral thiamine

Cmplc: Wernicke's encephalopathy
Wet beriberi: High-output CHF and pulmonary edema
Dry beriberi: Phrenic nerve involvement
Infantile beriberi: CHF and pulmonary edema

Lab:

Xray:

Rx: Thiamine 100 mg po or im qd

Homocystinuria (Homocyst(e)inemia)

Cause: Genetic, autosomal recessive

Epidem: Heterozygote prevalence = 1/70 in general population. Elevations are present in 20-30% of pts with premature (age < 50 yr) ASCVD (Jama 1999;281:1817); overall prevalence similar in over-50 general population and levels correlate w increasing ASCVD risk (Ann IM 1999;131:321,352,363,387). Even secondary elevations w mild folate, pyridoxine, and vitamin B_{12} deficiencies are associated with increased ASCVD, including arteriosclerotic heart (Jama 1996;275:1893; Nejm 1991;424:1149), peripheral, and CNS vascular disease.

in children, mental retardation, 1/200,000-300,000 (Nejm 1999;341:1572)

Pathophys: Accumulation of homocysteine in blood and urine due to blocked conversion of homocysteine to methionine. Vascular disease and emboli due to endothelial cell damage (Nejm 1998;338:1047). Homocystine, the oxidized sulfide of the amino acid homocysteine, is the predominant form in blood and urine (Nejm 1995;333:325).

Sx: of CNS and peripheral thromboembolic arterial and venous vascular disease (Ann IM 1995;123:747); 30% have had by age 20 yr, 60% by age 40 yr (Nejm 1985;313:709). Premature osteoporosis (Nejm 2004;350:2033,2042,2089).

Si: "Marfanoid," arachnodactyly (Nejm 1982;307:781); myocardiopathy with aortic valve disease; mental retardation

Crs:

Cmplc: Lens dislocation, r/o Marfan's syndrome; increase in dementias, DAT and MID (Nejm 2002;346:476)

Lab: *Chem:* Homocysteine level > 10 μM/L (Med Let 2003;45:85); > 15 μM/L in diabetics elevates CAD risk (Ann IM 2004; 140:94)

Rx: Newborn screening

to prevent ASCVD in pts w or in whom mild homocysteinemia may be present (Nejm 1995;332:286), not yet proven in randomized trials:

- Folate (Nejm 1975;292:491) 0.5-5 mg po qd and follow homocysteine levels; 0.14 mg/100 gm cereal grain products now being added in U.S. to prevent neural tube defects but has the added benefit of reducing homocyst(e)ine levels (Nejm 1998;338:1009)

- Betaine (Cystadane) (Med Let 2003;45:85, 1997;39:12) 3-10 gm po bid, < age 3 yr start w 100 μgm/kg qd; a choline derivative, trimethylglycine; may be no better than folate alone; $150/180 gm

    if folate alone doesn't decrease homocysteine levels to normal (Nejm 2001;344:1222):
- Vitamin B_{12} 400 μgm po qd
- Pyridoxine (vitamin B_6) 10 mg po qd

Scurvy

Nejm 1986;314:892

Cause: Vitamin C deficiency

Epidem: Increased incidence in spring because takes 3-4 mo to develop with lack of fruit

Pathophys: Vitamin C part of a coenzyme necessary for hydroxylation of proline; hydroxyproline is essential and unique to collagen, hence results in a primary failure of collagen formation including osteoid, dentine, skin, etc

Sx: Weakness, fatigue, bleeding gums, easy bruising, painful bones (subperiosteal bleeding); postural dizziness; "4 H's" = hemorrhages, hyperkeratosis of hair follicles, hypochondriasis, hematologic anemias of Fe or folate types

Si: Tourniquet test (BP cuff at 80 mm Hg × 5 min) results in petechiae; purpura, impalpable and perifollicular; corkscrew hairs; postural hypotension; poor wound healing; edema

Crs: Resolves with rx

Cmplc: Sjögren's syndrome, reversible (Nejm 1970;282:1120)

Lab: *Chem:* Vitamin C level depressed (normal = 1 mg %)

Xray: Generalized osteoporosis; heavy osteoid lines at epiphyses = cartilaginous zones of provisional calcification; calcified old subperiosteal bleeding sites

Rx: Fruits and/or vitamin C po 60-100 mg qd; for anticancer antioxidant effect w fewest side effects, 100-200 mg qd (Jama 1999;281:1415)

Ricketts (Children) and Osteomalacia (Adults)

Ann IM 1978;89:966

Cause:

- Vitamin D deficiency: Dietary, esp in northern winters (p 41); malabsorption (Am J Med 2000;108:296) including biliary obstruction, steatorrhea, postgastrectomy (in 15%: Ann IM 1971;75:220), post-gastric stapling or bypass, Crohn's disease; relative deficiency, eg, rapid bone formation after parathyroidectomy

- Vitamin D resistance: Hypophosphatasias from phosphate X-linked diabetes, renal tubular acidosis, all Fanconi syndromes including Wilson's, myeloma, old tetracycline, and heavy metals; renal insufficiency and aluminum depositions (Ann IM 1984;101:775) including premies on parenteral feeding (Nejm 1985;312:1337); chronic seizure medications like phenytoin and carbamazepine, via hepatic enzyme inductions (Nejm 1975;292:550, 1972;287:900)

- Calcium-deficient diet in tropical countries? (Nejm 1999;341:563,602)

Epidem: Rare in U.S.

Pathophys: Disease due to failure to calcify new bone matrix
Vitamin D functions:

- Increases gi calcium absorption (Nejm 1969;280:1396)
- Decreases urinary phosphate loss
- Increases reabsorption of bone
- Permissive action on PTH

Sx: Fractures, bone pain

Si: Ricketts includes severe bony distortions, frontal bossing, rickettic rosary (costochondral junctions swollen), long bone bowing

Crs:

Cmplc:

Lab: *Chem:* Ca^{++} low or normal (low in renal insufficiency); PO_4^- low (due to PTH effect on bone and kidney) except in renal failure; alkaline phosphatase increased in all including RTA but not Fanconi and hypo-PO_4 types

Path: Bone bx shows increased number and size of osteoid seams; in children, noncalcification of epiphyseal cartilage

Urine: Ca^{++} low in all with adequate PTH; glucose, amino acids present in RTA and Fanconi

Xray: Wide, thick epiphyseal cartilages in children; pseudocracks (Milkman's fractures) where vessels cross bone. Calcification of tendon insertions and capsules in 60% X-linked hypo-PO_4 ricketts (Nejm 1985;313:1).

Rx: Vitamin D as 25-hydroxy vitamin D 50,000-100,000 U qd; or 125-hydroxy vitamin D (Rocaltrol), expensive and more easily causes hypercalcemia

Perhaps topical precursor to skin with UVB irradiation, gives slower and steadier levels, and is especially good in vitamin D-resistant types (Nejm 1980;303:349)

5.9   Miscellaneous

Asx Adrenal Mass

Found incidentally on CT; work it up only if hypertension, sx of pheochomocytoma, hypo-K^+, cushingoid, or > 5.6 cm (Ann IM 1999;130:759; Nejm 1990;323:1401)

Hypoglycemia, Differential Dx

Nejm 1995;332:1144

Exogenous (Nejm 1992;326:1020, 1977;297:1029):
- Insulin; has lowest plasma C peptide levels
- Sulfonylureas; present in blood and urine

- Other medications (list: Ann IM 1993;118:536)

Fasting (Nejm 1992;326:1020, 1976;294:766):

- Pancreatic functioning tumor
- Nonpancreatic functioning tumor (Nejm 1981;305:1456)
- Liver disease, including:
  Acquired, especially from CHF
  Congenital glycogen storage disease or galactosemia
  Hepatoma
- Alcohol and/or poor nutrition, from decreased gluconeogenesis; eg, in diarrheal disease in children (Nejm 1990;322:1358)
- Endocrine deficiencies, eg, Addison's, hypopituitarism, decreased pancreatic β-cell function
- Normal physiologic responses in women and children (Nejm 1974;291:1275)

Reactive (postprandial); oral GTT no help, get blood glucose prn sx; ≤ 60 mg % is significant (Nejm 1989;321:1421):

- Rapid gastric emptying, rx with anticholinergics
- Fast absorption, rx with phenformin (Nejm 1973;288:1207), although now off the market because caused lactic acidosis
- Prediabetes
- Dumping syndrome
- Leucine sensitivity
- Hereditary fructose intolerance; autosomal recessive (Nejm 1982;307:535)

Hypogonadotropic Hypogonadism (Kallmann's Syndrome)

Cause: Genetic, often X-linked; rarely, if associated w anosmia, secondary in adult men (Nejm 1997;336:410)

Pathophys: GnRH deficiency; aplasia of olefactory tract

Epidem: 1/10,000-60,000

Sx: Sterility in adults; immaturity in adolescents

Si: Hypogonadism, anosmia, cerebellar si's, pes cavus, mental retardation, hearing loss, nystagmus, renal abnormalities, cleft lip, cryptorchidism, sometimes paraplegia

Lab: *Urine:* FSH and LH both low or normal; plasma testosterone < 300 μgm/cc

Rx (Nejm 1985;313:651) (p 844): HCG, pulsatile, alone if onset postpuberty; HCG and FSH if onset before puberty; may help if cryptorchid by causing descent of testes?

Lipodystrophies

Nejm 2004;350:1220

Cause: Acquired types:
- Protease inhibitor rx of HIV disease, local loss on face, arms, legs w buffalo hump and abdominal fat increases
- Autoimmune types assoc w local (face, arms, neck, trunk, sparing legs) adipose loss; or generalized loss
    Inherited autosomal dominant and recessive types

Chapter 6

Gastroenterology

D. K. Onion

6.1 Upper GI Diseases

Gastroesophageal Reflux Disease (GERD)

Nejm 1997;336:924, Jama 1996;276:983, Nejm 1994;331:656; 1992; 326:825

Cause: Mechanical reflux through incompetent sphincter

Epidem: Increased prevalence (Am J Med 1999;106:642) with age, obesity, in women, pregnancy, birth control pill use (progesterone effect: Ann IM 1982;97:93), scleroderma, smokers, drinkers, and those w family hx

Pathophys: Reflux of acid (rarely bile in achlorhydria) through transiently relaxing lower esophageal sphincter, plus inadequately neutralized acid from diminished saliva production; or diminished lower esophageal sphincter (LES) tone, which can be idiopathic, from coffee (Nejm 1980;303:122), lowered intrinsic gastrin levels (Nejm 1973;289:182), or smoking (Nejm 1971; 284:1136)

Hiatus hernia predisposes, present in 70% over age 70 yr. Diaphragmatic crura act as sphincter too (Ann IM 1992; 117:1051).

Sx: Substernal burning radiating upward, especially when recumbent or leaning over, and most often after meals, especially fatty ones

Si: Dental erosions, yellow (dentine) dished-out areas on nonocclusal surfaces (Ann IM 1995;122:809)

Crs: Variable

Cmplc: Stricture, Schatzki's lower esophageal ring; Barrett's esophagus (premalignant dysplasia) and adenocarcinoma (p 328); acid laryngitis, asthma w pulmonary aspirations
   r/o **Rumination Syndrome,** especially in retarded pts (Ann IM 1986;105:573)

Lab: Test only if atypical hx or fails to respond to rx
   Endo: Esophagoscopy, with bx if esophagitis is present in immunocompromised pt; often normal despite reflux sx
   Noninv: Manometry usually shows LES pressure < 10 mm Hg; 24-hr pH probe; continuous ambulatory esophageal pH monitoring is 80-90% sensitive/specific (Jama 1995;274:662). None of these done routinely in clinical practice.

Xray: Ba swallow of debatable help, since sx correlate with reflux, not presence of anatomic hiatus hernia; radiologically induced reflux not clearly correlated with sx

Rx: Achieve ideal body weight; stop smoking and stop other ulcerogens like caffeine, aspirin, and alcohol; elevate the head of the bed; 2-4 hr fast before going to bed; small meals; decrease fat
Medications:

- Antacids to both neutralize acid and increase LES pressure via gastrin (Ann IM 1971;74:223)
- Omeprazole (Prilosec) (Nejm 1990;323:1749) 20 mg po qd-bid, or other proton pump inhibitor (p 334); theoretically could cause B_{12} deficiency long term (Ann IM 1994;120:211), but can be used at doses of 10-20 mg po qd safely at least for 5-6 yr (Ann IM 1994;121:161; GE 1994;106:907, 1994;107:1305). 40 mg po qd × 7 d can be used diagnostically if ablates sx (Am J Med 1999;107:219). But long-term omeprazole in face of chronic *H. pylori* infection causes atrophic gastritis and

presumably increased cancer risk, unlike surgical fundal plication (Nejm 1996;334:1018).

Other options: H$_2$ blockers like cimetidine (Tagamet) 400-800 mg po bid, ranitidine (Zantac) 150 mg po bid then hs, famotidine (Pepcid) 20 mg po bid (Arch IM 1991;151:2394), or nizatidine (Axid) 150 mg po bid

Surgical Nissen (Med Let 2003;45:69) and other fundoplication procedures, probably significant help for severe reflux but no better than medical rx w omeprazole 40 mg bid (Surgery 2001;192:172); can be done laparoscopically; 10-yr data (Jama 2001;285:2331) show inexplicably greater mortality in surgically rather than medically treated pts, and no cancer prevention

Achalasia

Nejm 1997;336:924

Cause:

Epidem: Primary type is most common; secondary is associated with cancer of lung, stomach, and pancreas (Ann IM 1978;89:315). Prevalence = 1/100,000.

Pathophys: Debatable whether spasm leads to achalasia and whether both are part of the same spectrum. Hyperactive esophageal spasm present just in distal (lower) esophageal segment and sphincter (LES) in achalasia, which is hypersensitive to gastrin (Nejm 1973;289:182), while the upper esophageal segment is flaccid; all unlike spasm where entire esophagous involved. Destruction of myenteric plexus by autoantibodies.

Sx: Dysphagia; chest pain; weight loss; sometimes h/o spasm

Si:

Crs:

Cmplc: r/o
- Cardiac pain
- Esophageal cancer since often confused w achalasia, so incidence of cancer is high in 1st yr after diagnosis and overall

incidence is increased × 16 thereafter, but unclear that endoscopic screening improves survival (Jama 1995;274:1359)

- **Esophageal Spasm:** Associated with psychiatric illness in 84% (Nejm 1983;309:1337); solid and liquid dysphagia intermittently, associated with pain; manometry shows increased activity of whole esophagus in uncoordinated contractions, simultaneous contractions on at least 10% of wet swallows (Ann IM 1984;100:242), can precipitate with 5 mg iv edrophonium (Tensilon) (Ann IM 1987;106:593); barium swallow shows uncoordinated contractions; rx w dilatation with mercury bougies, nitrates and nitrites (Nejm 1973;289:23), nifedipine 10 mg t-qid po (Ann IM 1982;96:61), dicyclomine (Bentyl) 20 mg po t-qid pill or liquid, myotomy

Lab: *Noninv:* Manometry shows spasm of LES, failure to relax high resting tone

Xray: Barium swallow shows no peristalsis, spasm of LES, failure of the LES to relax with a swallow, dilated proximal, constricted distal esophageal segments; "rat tail deformity," r/o gastric cancer

Rx   (Gut 1999;44:231; Jama 1998;280:638): Endoscopic dilatation, risk is of perforation; 50+% successful

Botulinum toxin by endoscopic injection of LES, lasts 6+ mo in ⅔ of pts (Nejm 1995;332:774)

Surgical myotomy of LES, 90+% successful; cmplc: reflux and strictures

Esophageal Carcinoma

Nejm 2003;349:2241

Cause:

Epidem: Equal incidence of squamous and adeno types in U.S.; incidence = 4.8/100,000

Squamous cell types associated with smoking, alcohol use and alcoholism, radiation rx w 10-yr lag

Adenocarcinomas associated w smoking as well (but quitting does not decrease risk), radiation rx w a 10-yr lag, and obesity (Ann IM 1999;130:883), reflux sx (7× risk) (Nejm 1999; 340:825) that are also associated w achalasia, webs, and Barrett's esophagus (columnar epithelium-lined lower esophagus) (Nejm 1986;315:362) (30-60× risk); rapidly increasing rates since 1975 may be partly due to increased use of LES relaxing meds (Ann IM 2000;133:165), esp anticholinergics but also nitrates, theophyllins, and other bronchodilators

Pathophys: Rare malignant transformation to adenocarcinoma type in areas of chronic reflux, eg, in Barrett's esophagus, which is also associated with strictures and ulcerations (Ann IM 1982;97:103)

Sx: Dysphagia, weight loss

Si: Positive guaiac stools

Crs: 14% overall 5-yr survival with rx, 95% stage 0, 50-80% stage I, 30-40% stage IIA, 10-30% stage IIB, 10-15% stage III, < 10% w mets (stage IV)

Cmplc: Other upper and lower airway cancers in smokers

Lab: *Endo:* Esophagoscopy usually w gastroscopy and duodenoscopy as well (EGD), and biopsy

Path: Monoclonal antibody staining of lymph nodes predicts survival better than does routine microscopy (Nejm 1997; 337:1188)

Xray: Barium swallow

Rx: Prevent possibly w endoscopy at least once of pts w reflux sx irregardless of Barrett's changes (Ann IM 2003;138:176; Nejm 2002;346:836) and regular f/u endoscopy of dysplasia present; but nothing works well, incidence is low, and there are no clear studies to show that screening works (Jama 2002;287:1972,1982); would have to screen 1400 pts/yr to find 1 cancer if incidence = 20× baseline (Nejm 1999;340:878)

Surgery has < 40% 5-yr survival (Nejm 2002;347:1662), then radiation and chemotherapy w cisplatinum + 5-FU (Nejm 1992;326:1593); or radiation + chemo 1st then surgery (Nejm 1997;337:161, 1996;335:462,509 vs 1998;339:1979) result in 40% 2-yr survival vs 10% for radiation alone, although the complication rate is higher

Peptic Ulcer Disease (Gastric Ulcer [GU], Duodenal Ulcer [DU], Gastritis)

Nejm 2002;347:1175; 1995;333:984

Cause: *Helicobacter pylori* infection (Can Med Assoc J 1994;150: 177,189; Nejm 1989;321:1562, 1987;316:1557,1598; Ann IM 1988;108:70) in GU and DU but not gastritis (Arch IM 1998;158:1427)

Endogenous, nicotine, or NSAID-induced increased acid/pepsin secretion; and/or decreased pancreatic or duodenal HCO_3 secretion (Nejm 1987;316:374); or decrease in other gi defenses

Epidem: Duodenal ulcer, 90% associated w chronic *H. pylori* infection that often begins early in life, occurs in 10% of people, male/female = 4/1. Decreasing prevalence in developed world. *H. pylori* infection runs in families (Nejm 1990;322:359) probably because transmitted in emesis, aerosols, and diarrhea (Jama 1999;282:2240, 2260). Only 15-20% of those chronically infected get DU or GU.

Pathophys: Impaired gi defenses: *H. pylori* infection, organism attaches to blood group O receptors on mucosal cells much like enteropathogenic *E. coli* attaches to bowel wall, tolerates high-acid environment (Sci 1995;267:1621); aspirin and other NSAIDs (Ann IM 1991;114:307) in elderly (Ann IM 1988;109:359), especially if concomitant steroid use (Ann IM 1991;114:735)

Increased acid production in Zollinger-Ellison syndrome (p 344); neurogenically increased secretion, eg, burn or CVA patients (Nejm 1970;282:373); nicotine users (Nejm 1974; 290:469); coffee users, but it's not the caffeine (Nejm 1970;283: 897); TPN pts from the iv amino acids (Nejm 1978;298:27); hypersecretors, who can be divided into hypersecretors and hypergastrin responders (Ann IM 1980;93:540); NSAID and alcohol users (GE 1997;112:683)

Diminished pancreatic secretions: 10% incidence in cystic fibrosis, may be first sx in heterozygote; perhaps w steroids (J Intern Med 1994;236:619; Nejm 1983;309:21)

Sx: Epigastric pain especially 1-2 hr pc and 2 am; gi bleeding, occult, melena or hematemesis

Si: Epigastric tenderness; guaiac-positive stool

Crs: Before *H. pylori* rx, DU recurred in 10% except in smokers, where 72% recur in 1 yr (Nejm 1984;311:689); GU recurred in 50%; take ~8 wk to heal with rx (Ann IM 1985;103:573)

H. pylori may be chronic, recurrent, and resistant to multiple rx attempts (Ann IM 1991;114:662) but 96% don't recur after cleared w antibiotic crs

r/o ZE if does recur, not a smoker, and no *H. pylori*

Cmplc: Persistent bleeding, perforation, obstruction, pain; possibly adenocarcinoma; and non-Hodgkin's gastric mucosa-associated lymphoid tissue (MALT) in pts w *H. pylori* (Nejm 1998;338:804, 1994;330:1267; Jama 1996;275:937), which eradication of *H. pylori* can cure, similar to *Campylobacter*-associated small bowel MALT tumors (p 546)

r/o cancer with all GU, ie, endoscopically document healing; celiac artery compression/obstruction, which gives pc pain (abdominal angina) (Ann IM 1977;86:278); Zollinger-Ellison syndrome (p 376; Nejm 1987;317:1201) if refractory

Lab: Noninvasive tests:

• Stool antigen test (Ann IM 2002;136:280), 94% sens, 97% specif, goes neg within 7 d of successful rx

- Urea breath test (UBT), radioactive-labeled urea broken down to $NH_3 + C^{14}O_2$ in stomach if *H. pylori* present there and $C^{14}O_2$ in breath is measured; is very sens/specif except false negative within 4 wk of po antibiotics (Nejm 1995; 333:984); best for follow-up test of cure, cost $60, 5-10% false neg. ^{13}C-urea blood test, 98% specif, 89% sens (Am J Gastroenterol 1999;94:1522)
- IgG- and IgA-specific antibodies in *H. pylori* type; 75-80% sens/specif overall (Am J Gastroenterol 1999;94:1512), but over age 60 positivity increases to > 50% (Ann IM 1988; 109:11); used to f/u 1 yr after rx, an undetectable level indicates cure (100% sens) but some titer remains in 40% (60% specif) (Jama 1998;280:363)

  Endoscopy (EGD) (Ann IM 2003;139:843):

- Debatably best 1st test rather than empiric trial of H_2 blockers (Lancet 1994;343:811 vs Ann IM 1997;126:280); visible vessel ulcers bleed again within 24 hr 50% of the time
- "CLO test" of biopsy specimens incubated $\times$ 4-24 hr, gel incubation color change system that measures urea splitting by *H. pylori*

Xray: UGIS, but low sens for DU; KUB for subdiaphragmatic air if perforation

Rx (Med Let 1997;39:1; Jama 1996;275:622): Prevent w po vaccine? (Sci 1995;267:1621)

  rx of disease: Stop tobacco, alcohol, NSAIDs, coffee; combined antibiotic + antisecretory rx w/o more w/u is most cost-efficient initial strategy (Ann IM 1995;123:260)

  Medications

1st: Antibiotic rx of *H. pylori* $\times$ 1-2 wk (see Tables 6.1 and 6.2). Only helps if ulcer present (Am J GE 2003;98:2621; Nejm 1999;341:1106); previous metronidazole or macrolide exposure, even yrs earlier, substantially increases *H. pylori* resistance (Ann IM 2003;139:463)

Table 6.1 Medications for *H. Pylori* Rx

Drug	Dose	Cost/Wk
Amoxicillin (not ampicillin)	1 gm po bid or 500 mg qid w meals and hs	Cheap
Bismuth subsalicylate (Pepto-Bismol)	ii tab (120 mg) po qid w meals and hs	$3
Clarithromycin	500 mg po b-tid w meals	$50-$75 (tid)
Metronidazole (Flagyl)	250 mg po qid w meals and hs, or 500 mg bid	$3
Omeprazole (Prilosec)	20 mg po bid ac	$50
Tetracycline (not doxycycline)	500 mg po qid w meals and hs	$3
Levofloxacin 500 mg po qd × 10 d or Rifabutin (Mycobutin) 300 mg po qd	w amox + PPI for f/u rx after failure	?

(Jama 1996;275:624; Med Let 1996;38:51)

Table 6.2 Cure Rates and Costs of Various Combinations to Rx *H. Pylori*

Combination	Cure Rate, 95% CIs	Cost
Bismuth/metronidazole/tetracycline × 1 wk	86-90%	<$10
Bismuth/metronidazole/tetracycline × 2 wk	88-90%	<$10
Bismuth/metronidazole/tetracycline/ omeprazole × 1 wk	94-98%	$60
Bismuth/metronidazole/amoxicillin × 1 wk	75-81%	<$15
Bismuth/metronidazole/amoxicillin × 2 wk	80-86%	<$15
Metronidazole/clarithromycin/omeprazole × 1 wk	87-91%	$200
Amoxicillin/clarithromycin/omeprazole × 1 wk	86-91%	$200
Metronidazole/amoxicillin/omeprazole × 1-2 wk	77-83%	$50-100 (2 wk)
Amoxicillin/clarithromycin/lansoprazole (PrevPac) × 2 wk	84-90%	$200

(Jama 1996;275:624; Med Let 1996;38:51)

2nd: H_2 blocker, histamine antagonists (Nejm 1990;323:1749);
for all, double dose hs as good as normal dose bid; prophylaxis with normal dose qd works for all; only cimetidine and
ranitidine (slightly) alter cytochrome P450 enzyme systems;
cimetidine and ranitidine available as generics and cheap;
action onset takes $\frac{1}{2}$ hr but lasts 6-10 hr (Jama
1996;275:1428); renal excretion, lower dose if creatinine
clearance < 50

- Cimetidine (Tagamet) 300-400 mg po bid or 800 mg hs
  better than split doses, or iv q 6 hr; decrease dose if BUN
  up; adverse effects: antiandrogen (Nejm 1989;321:1012);
  confusion (Med Let 1978;20:77); drug level increases w
  benzodiazepines (Nejm 1980;302:1012; Ann IM 1980;
  93:266); propranolol (Nejm 1981;304:692); and decreased levels with concomitant antacids (Nejm 1982;
  307:400)
- Ranitidine (Zantac) 150 mg po bid or 300 mg hs, 150-300
  mg iv/24 hr continuous drip better than bolus rx (Ann IM
  1990;112:334); less CNS toxic than cimetidine
- Famotidine (Pepcid) 20 mg po bid or 40 mg hs; less CNS
  toxic than cimetidine (others disagree, say all equal: Ann
  IM 1991;114:1027)
- Nizatidine (Axid) 150 mg bid or 300 mg hs

2nd: Proton pump inhibitors (Med Let 2000;42:65); better than
H_2 blockers; some antibacterial action vs *H. pylori*; especially good in reflux esophagitis and ZE ulcers; better healing
of ulcers ($\sim$80%) in face of ongoing NSAID use than H_2
blockers (Nejm 1998;338:719); adverse effects: B_{12} deficiency w long-term use (Ann IM 1994;120:211), nocturnal
erections, gynecomastia, anaphylaxis, and erythema multiforme; increased blood levels of phenytoin (Dilantin),
diazepam, warfarin, digoxin, and disulfiram (Antabuse);
$3-$5/tab

- Esomeprazole (Nexium) (Med Let 2001;43:36) 20-40 mg po qd; S-isomer of omeprazole
- Lansoprazole (Prevacid) (Med Let 1995;37:63) 30 mg po qd, 15 mg po qd as prophylaxis (Ann IM 1996;124:859); $116/mo
- Omeprazole (Prilosec) 20 mg po qd-bid (Nejm 1991;324:965); $125/mo, OTC generic $25/mo
- Rabeprazole (Aciphex) (Med Let 1999;41:110) 20 mg po qd, $111/mo
- Pantoprazole (Protonix) (Med Let 2002;44:41) 40 mg po qd, or 40-80 mg iv, can then drip @ 8 mg/hr if unstable; none of the usual PPI drug interactions and few of the usual adverse effects; $90/mo

3rd: Others

- Antacids, eg, Maalox or Mylanta 30 cc po 1 hr pc and hs (Ann IM 1981;94:214); avoid ones with $CaCO_3$ because of acid rebound (Nejm 1973;288:923) although rapid onset (min) valuable (Jama 1996;275:1428)
- Propantheline (Pro-Banthine) 15 mg ac, works, potentiates cimetidine (Nejm 1977;297:1427)
- Sucralfate (Carafate) (Nejm 1991;325:1017) 1 gm po qid 1 hr ac, benign; binds tetracycline, cimetidine, digoxin, warfarin

Surgical: Vagotomy and pyloroplasty (Nejm 1982;307:519); antrectomy and Billroth II, cmplc: dumping (Ann IM 1974; 80:577), and retained antrum with high gastrin levels, or alkaline gastritis (rx with roux-en-y, helps the bilious emesis: Ann IM 1985;103:178)

Prophylaxis

After an ulcer:

- Stop smoking
- H_2 blocker like cimetidine (Tagamet) 400 mg hs (Nejm 1984;311:689), or ranitidine (Zantac) 150 mg po hs × years (Nejm 1994;330:382,428)

NSAID use:

- Proton pump inhibitor; either omeprazole 20 mg po qd or lansoprazole better than H_2 blocker or misoprostol (Nejm 1998;338:727)
- Misoprostol (Cytotec) (Ann IM 1991;114:307; Med Let 1989;31:21) 100 μgm qid or 200 μgm b-tid (Ann IM 1995;123:344) po prevents NSAID-induced type ulcers debatably (Arch IM 1996;156:2321, 1994;154:2020; Nejm 1992;327:1575 vs Ann IM 1995;123:241 [elderly], 1993;119:257); adverse effects: teratogenic in 1st trimester, causes Möbius's syndrome (Nejm 1998;338:1881) (p 812)

in ICU patients, especially those w respiratory failure or coagulopathy (Nejm 1994;330:377,428):

- Antacids or H_2 blockers like cimetidine 300 mg iv q 6 hr (Ann IM 1987;106:562), or ranitidine 50 mg iv q 8 hr (Nejm 1998;338:791)
- Sucralfate 1 gm q 6 hr (Nejm 1987;317:1376) and although not quite as good as antacids or ranitidine (10% bleed vs 4-6%), less pneumonia in ventilated pts because acid killing of bacteria by stomach is preserved? (Ann IM 1994;120:653 vs Nejm 1998;338:791)

of bleeding (Nejm 1994;331:717): diagnostic endoscopy and endoscopic electrocoagulation and/or injection of visible vessel in ulcer crater decreases recurrent bleeding acutely from 11% to 1% (Ann IM 2003;139:237); and/or acute po omeprazole (Nejm 1997;336:1054); possibly octreotide (Ann IM 1997;127:1062)

of perforation: Antibiotics, NG drainage and recheck in 12 hr is as good as immediate surgery (Nejm 1989;320:970)

of obstruction: Endoscopic balloon dilatation

Carcinoma of Stomach (Stomach Cancer)

Nejm 1995;333:32

Cause: Neoplasia

Epidem: Decreasing incidence in U.S. in past 50 yr, increasing incidence in Japan. Higher incidence in patients with blood type A (pernicious anemia predisposition in the same group).

Correlates w severe *H. pylori* gastritis (Nejm 2001;345:784) and GU but not duodenal disease. Polyps do not predispose, but probably diet constituents of unknown type do (maybe nitrosamines from cured/fermented foods).

Pathophys: *H. pylori* infection clearly increases risk markedly by 3-12× (Sci 1995;267:1621)

Sx: Pain (51%), cachexia and weight loss (62%), hematemesis or melena (20%), dysphagia (26%)

Si: Acanthosis nigrans; when present in pt over age 40, pt has a high chance of having a gi adenocarcinoma; r/o lymphoma, hereditary ataxia telangiectasia, obese patients, children, or diabetics especially insulin-resistant diabetics (Nejm 1978; 298:1164)

Guaiac-positive stools

Crs: Rapidly downhill even with surgery; overall 5-yr survival: 10-15%; with surgery and negative nodes may be as high as 45%; better in Japan

Cmplc: Bleeding. Metastases to lung, especially via lymphatics and may appear as a diffuse pulmonary process; to ovaries, especially if signet ring cell type (Krukenberg's ovarian tumor); to bone, especially vertebrae

r/o gastric lymphoma (MALT: mucosa-associated lymphoid tissue), low-grade B-cell lymphoma associated w *H. pylori* infection and 50% cure rate w antibiotic rx of *H. pylori* (Ann IM 1999;131:88)

Lab: *Endo:* Gastroscopy with 6+ biopsies and brushings (Ann IM 1984;101:550)

Xray: UGIS usually positive; failure of ulcer to project beyond normal margin of stomach suggests is malignant rather than benign

Rx: Prevention in future perhaps by *H. pylori* screening and rx (Jama 2004;291:187,244; Nejm 2001;345:829)

Surgical, perhaps followed by local irradiation and chemoRx (Nejm 2001;345:725)

ChemoRx, palliative only, but multiple drug, eg, 5-FU, adriamycin, mitomycin C

6.2 Pancreatic Diseases

Acute Pancreatitis

Nejm 1999;340:1412, 1994;330:1198

Cause:
- Gallstones (45-75%); in lower common duct (Nejm 1974; 290:484), or biliary sludge, half the time visible on ultrasound, probably the occult cause in $^2/_3$ of idiopathic types (Nejm 1992; 326:589)
- Alcohol (10-35%), possibly from sphincter of Oddi spasm
- Idiopathic (10-30%)
- Hereditary types I and V hyperlipidemia
- Other, rare causes (10%): posterior duodenal ulcer; trauma, accidental or at operation; hyperparathyroidism w calcium stone formation; infectious, eg, mumps, coxsackie, many viruses including HIV as well as ascariasis and clonorchiasis in developing countries; cancer of duodenum, pancreas, or ampulla; choledochal cysts, duodenal diverticula; pancreas divisum; pregnancy; protein starvation (Ann IM 1971;74:270); vasculitis; drugs such as thiazides, steroids, sulfasalazine (Azulfidine) and other sulfas, furosemide, azathioprine (Nejm

1973;289:357); postpump after bypass surgery, probably from the iv CaCl given (Nejm 1991;325:382)

Epidem: Male/female = 2:1; incidence ≈ 400/million/yr, but in AIDS, 5-20/100/yr

Pathophys: Enzyme (trypsin and lipase) activation and retention in pancreatic substance leads to autodigestion. Hypocalcemia from calcium soap formation? (Nejm 1986;315:496) or glucagon-induced? (Nejm 1976;294:512)

Sx: Epigastric abdominal pain relieved by leaning forward, radiates to back/flank; abdominal distention, nausea, and vomiting

Si: Ileus; guarding; fever, or hypothermia sometimes; erythema nodosum–like lesions due to focal fat necrosis; Grey-Turner si = flank ecchymoses w retroperitoneal bleeding

Crs: 50-80% never recur

Table 6.3   Ranson Criteria

| | Risk Factors | |
	If Not Gallstone Induced	If Gallstone Induced
On admission	Age > 55 yr	Age > 70 yr
	WBC > 16,000	WBC > 18,000
	Glucose > 200 mg %	Glucose > 220 mg %
	LDH > 350 IU	LDH > 400 IU
	AST (SGOT) > 250	AST (SGOT) > 250
Within 48 hr of admission	Hct drops > 10 pts	Hct drops > 10 pts
	BUN increased > 5 mg %	BUN increases > 2 mg %
	Ca < 8 mg %	Ca < 8 mg %
	pO_2 < 60 mm Hg	
	Acidotic	Acidotic
	> 6 L volume depleted	> 4 L volume depleted

Risk factors: Mortality < 1% if ≤ 2 risk factors, 16% if 3-4, 100% if 7 or more (Am J Gastroent 1982;77:633)

Cmplc: ARDS; ATN; tetany with hypocalcemia; shock; pancreatic abscess (4%) (Nejm 1972;287:1234); **Pancreatic Pseudocyst** formation, which can result in infection or rupture into peritoneal cavity, spleen, or dissection along body planes (Nejm 1972;287:72); gi bleeding and splenomegaly from splenic vein thrombosis rare (Ann IM 1971;75:903)

Lab: *Chem:* Amylase: serum levels up for 3 d, > 225 IU, 95% sens, 98% specif (Ann IM 1985;102:576); higher in gallstone (often > 1000) than alcoholic type; r/o false neg with elevated triglycerides; false pos with renal failure, macroglobulin binding (Nejm 1967;277:94), and salivary source (Ann IM 1979;91:200)

Lipase stays up longer than amylase, peaks at 4-7 d, correlates with hypertriglyceridemia that follows acute attacks

Isoamylase equally as good as lipase as a confirmation test (Ann IM 1985;102:576)

Glucose may be up from transient glucagon release (Ann IM 1975;83:774)

Calcium reaches nadir at 2 d (Ann IM 1975;83:185)

Alanine aminotransferase (ALT; SGPT) ≥ 3 normal indicates gallstone etiology w 95% certainty (Am J Gastroenterol 1994;89:1863)

Paracentesis fluid has elevated amylase (> 100 U) and polys but no bacteria, helps r/o bowel strangulation

Amylase/creatinine clearance ratio probably not useful

Hem: Crit may be > 60% due to plasma loss; white count may be > 25,000/mm^3

Xray: CT with contrast. Lytic bone lesions (fat necrosis); calcifications in pancreas; gallbladder ultrasound 2-3 wk after acute episode.

Rx: Opiates usually necessary although may worsen

Surgery substantially increases mortality; rarely needed if ERCP available; perhaps debridement late if massive necrosis or infected phlegmon

NG suction or cimetidine to decrease acid stimulation of pancreas via secretin debated, but neither shown to help (Ann IM 1985;103:86); NG tube usually needed for ileus anyway

Antibiotics, eg, imipenem usually used × 2-4 wk, debatable help to prevent secondary bacterial infection of necrotic tissue (GE 2004;126:997 vs Cochrane database rv 2004 (2); CD 002941); more clearly helpful if gallstone induced

ERCP perhaps early (within 24-72 hr) with sphincterotomy only if obstructive jaundice or cholangitis (Nejm 1997;336:237)

Peritoneal lavage no help (Nejm 1985;312:399)

Chronic Pancreatitis and Pancreatic Insufficiency

Nejm 1995;332:1482

Cause: Recurrent acute attacks; chronic alcohol use (70%), damage precedes 1st attack of acute pancreatitis (p 338); surgical resection; cystic fibrosis, sometimes as the only manifestation of a CF gene mutation (Nejm 1998;339:645,653,687); hyperparathyroidism; sclerosing pancreatitis (Nejm 2001;344:732)

Epidem:

Pathophys: Sx from impairment of exocrine and endocrine function; > 90% destruction necessary before exocrine and/or endocrine function is impaired

Sx: Recurrent acute attacks or abdominal pain; steatorrhea; weight loss

Si: Cachexia

Crs: 50% 20-yr mortality

Cmplc: Malabsorption and maldigestion including B_{12} deficiency, vit K deficiency, etc (p 373), diabetes; nightblindness from vit A malabsorption (Nejm 1979;300:942); pancreatic duct obstruction into "chain of lakes"; pseudocyst formation (Nejm 1972;287:72); a small (2-4%) increased incidence of pancreatic carcinoma after

10-20 yr (Nejm 1993;328:1433); biliary obstruction w reversible hepatic fibrosis (Nejm 2001;344:418)

Lab: *Chem:* Amylase and lipase normal or mildly elevated because no more pancreatic tissue to release

Noninv: Maldigestion tests (p 373)

MRCP and endoscopic ultrasound to evaluate duct if not clear on CT

Stool: Qualitative and quantitative elevations of fat by Sudan stains

Xray: Ultrasound, especially for cysts, 85% sens/specif; CT/MRI, especially for tumors and cancer

KUB: Pancreatic calcifications (30%)

Rx: Avoidance of alcohol may prevent recurrent pain but fibrosis can still progress

Pancreatic enzymes 6-12 gm qd po with meals, eg, pancrelipase (Viokase) 6 tab po qid helps pain; microspheres, eg, Creon

Cimetidine 300 mg po $\frac{1}{2}$ hr ac can speed enzyme transit through stomach and thus help po enzymes work better (Nejm 1977;297:854, 1977;299:995)

Surgically or endoscopically drain cysts, sphincterotomies, and pancreaticojejunostomies of pain: Celiac blocks, octreotide 200 mg sc tid

Pancreatic Carcinoma

Nejm 1992;326:455

Cause: Neoplasia

Epidem: Incidence = 9/100,000/yr; increased in smokers, obesity (Jama 2001;286:921,967), gasoline/naphthalene/benzidine workers, pts after partial gastrectomy, and perhaps cholecystectomy pts and diabetics (Jama 2000;283:2552 vs Nejm 1994;331:83)

Pathophys: Si and sx produced by compression of adjacent tissues, especially in head, and invasive replacement of pancreatic tissue

Stage I: Intrapancreatic
Stage II: Adjacent organs without nodes
Stage III: Node involvement
Stage IV: Diffusely metastatic
> 75% are in head of pancreas, rest are in body and tail

Table 6.4   Frequency of Sx and Si in Pancreatic Cancer

	Head (%)	Tail (%)		Head (%)	Tail (%)
Sx					
Weight loss	92	100	Weakness	35	43
Jaundice	90	7	Pruritus	24	0
Pain	90	90	Diarrhea	18	3
Anorexia	62	33	Melena	12	17
Nausea	45	43	Hematemesis	3	17
Vomiting	37	37	Abdominal distention	8	17
Si					
Icterus	87	13	Palpable gallbladder	29	0
Big liver	83	33	Tenderness	26	27
Ascites	14	20	Abdominal	13	23

Crs: 20% 1-yr, 3% 5-yr survival—lowest of all cancers

Cmplc: Diabetes (80%), duodenal obstruction (10%)
r/o ampullary or distal bile duct cancer (Nejm
1999;341:1368), which has a 50% 5-yr survival with resection

Lab: Jaundice w/u
Path: Needle aspiration cytology is 60-90% sensitive but causes
seeding; ultrasonographic endoscopic fine-needle aspiration,
90% sens, 95% specif (Ann IM 2001;134:459)
Serol: Ca 19-9 antibody > 70 U/cc; 70% sens, 87% specific (Ann
IM 1989;110:704); useful to follow post-op like CEA in
colon cancer, not diagnostically, but useful if elevated in a
nonoperative candidate w a mass on CT

Xray: Ultrasound, 36% false neg, usually done first to distinguish obstructive from nonobstructive jaundice, done endoscopically nearly 98% sens (Ann IM 2004;141:753); CT scan 25% false neg (do first: Ann IM 1985;102:212). MRCP if any of the above positive.

Rx: Surgical Whipple procedure or less if stage I, maybe if stage II, not if stage III or IV. This means only 5-10% are eligible; 10% operative mortality; 5-15% 5-yr survival.

  Adjuvant chemoRx post-op w 5-FU (Nejm 2004;350:1200) improves 3-yr survival from 12% to 30% but radiation adjuvant worsens prognosis.

  Palliative biliary and/or gastrojejeunal bypass for younger pts, or ERCP stenting for elderly or sick pts; increase survival from 6 mo to nearly 1 yr in some; chemotherapy w 5-FU + intra- and post-op radiation as adjuvant rx, or gemcitabine (Gemzar) (p 295). Celiac plexus block helps but not superior to standard systemic analgesics (Jama 2004;291:1092).

Pancreatic Islet Cell Neoplasms

Nejm 1987;317:1201 [ZE], 1982;306:580, 1980;302:1344

Cause: Benign or malignant (60% of ZE and insulin types) neoplasia; autosomal dominant (at least with Zollinger-Ellison [ZE] syndrome).

Epidem: 8/100,000 develop either endocrine or exocrine tumor of pancreas

Pathophys: Secretion of active hormone, often of more than one type (Nejm 1988;319:605):

- Gastrin (ZE); 75% are sporadic while 25% are associated with MEN-type parathyroid adenomas (Nejm 1999;341:635), elevated calcium causes further increase in gastrin, multiple primary sites often including duodenum
- Insulin type, which produces a high proportion of proinsulin (Nejm 1970;283:713)

- Vasoactive intestinal peptide (VIP; Ann IM 1979;90:932)
- Glucagon (Nejm 1976;295:242)
- Somatostatin from D-cell tumor causes diabetes (Nejm 1979; 301:285)

Sx & Si: ZE: Acid-peptic sx and diarrhea (fluid and steatorrhea)
Insulin type: Whipple's triad = (1) fainting/seizures, (2) hypo-glycemia to < 50 mg %, and (3) relief with iv glucagon
VIP: Watery diarrhea, hypo K^+, achlorhydria
Glucagon: Weight loss, migratory dermatitis (perioral, hands), stomatitis, anemia, diabetes
Somatostatin: Diabetes, steatorrhea, gallstones, duodenal tumor

Crs: Insulin type can live decades (Ann IM 1984;100:233); VIP types die of hypovolemia without surgical excision of tumor

Cmplc: ZE: Metastases; r/o **Ménétrier's Disease** with big gastric folds and depressed serum proteins (Ann IM 1984;100:565); rx w monoclonal antibodies vs epidermal growth factor receptor (Nejm 2000;343:1697)
VIP: r/o other causes; only 1/87 patients referred for VIP w/u had it; 20 were occult laxative users, 14 irritable bowel, 13 idio-pathic, 9 bile salt use, 5 pancreatic insufficiency, 4 carbohy-drate malabsorption, 2 bacterial overgrowth (GE 1980;78:264)

Lab: *Chem:* HCG levels increased with malignancy in all types of islet cell tumors (Nejm 1977;297:565)
in ZE: Gastrin level up and even higher with secretin or calcium stimulation, unlike retained antrum causes (Ann IM 1989;111:713)
in VIP (Nejm 1983;309:1482): Vasoactive peptide level > 100 pmol/L; hyperchloremic metabolic acidosis; stool measured osmolarity = $2\times$ (stool Na + K), unlike other os-motic (Ann IM 1985;102:773) causes of diarrhea where measured osmoles >> measured Na + K (commercial kits

also available; in latter case, r/o laxative abuse w commmercial laxative screen of blood and urine

in insulin type: Proinsulin $\geq$ 20% total RIA insulin or measured C-peptide (not present in injectable insulin)

Xray: Endoscopic ultrasound (82% sens, 95% specif) better than angiography (Nejm 1992;326:1721)

Labeled octreotide (somatostatin analog) scan for primary and mets since most pts have somatostatin receptors, 70% sens (Ann IM 1996;125:26, Nejm 1990;323:1246), or labeled VIP scans (Nejm 1994;331:1116)

In ZE, UGIS shows large rugae from hyperplasia r/o Ménétrier's

Rx: Chemotherapy for all types: Streptozocin, chlorozotocin, 5-FU, doxorubicin (Nejm 1992;326:519), dacarbazine; ligate hepatic artery first if liver mets present (Ann IM 1994;120:302)

of ZE: Excision works in 93% of sporadic cases, not in MEN-I types (Nejm 1999;341:635); followed by regular gastrin and secretin stimulation tests (Ann IM 1993;119:199); omeprazole 80 mg po qd-bid (Nejm 1984;310:758) or other proton pump inhibitor

of VIP: Streptozocin sc; octreotide sc bid (Med Let 1989;31:66)

of insulin type: Streptozocin with 5-FU; diazoxide and other thiazides; mithromycin (Nejm 1978;299:134)

of glucagon type: Octreotide sc bid (Med Let 1989;31:66)

6.3   Biliary Diseases

Cholecystitis and Biliary Colic

Nejm 1993;328:412

Cause: Cholelithiasis (gallstones), often with secondary bacterial infection with common gi organisms. Possibly biliary sludge (Ann IM 1999;130:301) but also seen reversibly in pregnancy, prolonged starvation/fasting, TPN (100% have sludge at 6 wk), ceftriaxone and octreotide therapy.

Epidem: Female/male = 2/1; stones present in 10% of U.S. adult women, 70% of Southwestern Native American women (Nejm 1970;282:53). Higher incidence of stones with increasing age, multiple pregnancies (Nejm 1980;302:362), during pregnancy but reverting (Ann IM 1993;119:116), hemolytic disease, birth control pill (Nejm 1974;290:15) and marginally w ERT (Ann IM 2001;135:493), alcoholism, cirrhosis (45%), vagotomy, lower exercise levels (Nejm 1999;341:777), obesity especially during weight loss (Ann IM 1999;130:471), ileal disease, elevated triglycerides.

Lower risk w coffee (Jama 1999;281:2106), statin rx (Ann IM 2001;135:493)

Pathophys: Stones are usually mucin protein + cholesterol (75%), less often w bilirubin and calcium (Hepatol 1982;2:879). Cholecystitis is inflammation/infection of gallbladder; colic is caused by an obstructed gallbladder.

Sx: Colic: Steady (thus colic is a misnomer), epigastric or right upper quadrant pain that subsides over several hours, radiates to right scapula; nausea and vomiting, with temporary partial relief after vomiting

Cholecystitis: Persistent steady pain over days, first periumbilical, radiating to right upper quadrant as parietal peritoneum involved

Si: Fever; Murphy's si (tender subcostally on deep inspiration)

Crs (Ann IM 1993;119:606): 10-20% chance of sx with stones over 20-30 yr (Nejm 1982;307:798), 2%/yr × 5 yr then diminishes; after first sx, 50% will recur over 20 yr, 25-50% get complications vs $\frac{1}{3}$ will recur in 2 yr, 70% in 5 yr (Ann IM 1984;101:171)

Cmplc: Pancreatitis; common duct stone with biliary obstruction; **cholangitis,** infection of obstructed biliary collecting system;

GASTROENTEROLOGY

hydrops and/or empyema of gallbladder; perforation and peritonitis; rarely gallstone "ileus," a small bowel obstruction usually at ileocecal valve from stone that has eroded through gallbladder into duodenum or stomach; perhaps gallbladder cancer (Nejm 1979;301:704), though stones may be effect rather than cause

Lab:

Chem: if stones in common duct or severe edema, usual pattern is obstructive LFTs including bilirubin, GGTP, and alkaline phosphatase elevation, usually higher than > AST (SGOT) or ALT (SGPT) elevations, though sometimes reversed

Urine: Urobilinogen elevated if bacterial infection in biliary tree is breaking down bile, eg, recently relieved obstruction, improving hepatitis, or ascending cholangitis

Xray: KUB may show calcified stones (20%); air in duodenal cap next to inflamed gallbladder (sentinel loop); or air in biliary tree, if cholangitis from gas formers or fistula formation; "porcelain gallbladder," ie, wall calcified, associated w cancer of gallbladder ~50% of the time

Gallbladder ultrasound (Ann IM 1988;109:722) 5-10% false neg, 2-6% false pos, 1% indeterminant; sens/specif = 95%

HIDA scan: No visualization of gallbladder indicates cholecystitis, no tracer into duodenum indicates common duct obstruction

Percutaneous cholangiography or ERCP if common duct obstruction

MR cholangiography (GE 1996;110:589)

Rx: Prevention of stones w ursodeoxycholic acid 600 mg po qd in weight loss programs, NNT-4mo=5 (Ann IM 1995;122:899)

of asx stone rarely indicated (Ann IM 1993;119:606,620); but maybe for people away from medical care, typhoid carriers, "porcelain gallbladders" (cancer risk), long-term TPN, and questionably in diabetics due to high operative mortality, especially if nonfunctioning, but not statistically demonstrable (Ann IM 1988;109:913) and in other pts w predictably deteriorating health

of cholecystitis: Cholecystectomy, usually acutely

of symptomatic gallstones: Even though ~30% won't recur (Ann IM 1993;119:606, 620), usually open minilap vs laparoscopic cholecystectomy w ERCP 1st if suspect common duct stones that cannot get laparoscopically; laparoscopic technique shortens stay with less pain (Nejm 1991;324:1075; Med Let 1990;32:115) and lower mortality and being done at higher rate than opens were done (Nejm 1994;330:403; Lancet 1994;343:135); adverse effects: **Post-Cholecystectomy "Cholecystitis" Pain Syndrome** due to obstruction of sphincter of Oddi, can rx w ERCP sphincterotomy (Nejm 1989;320:82) but has a 21% cmplc rate (Nejm 1996;335:909). Rarely lithotripsy plus po rx with ursodeoxycholic acid (Ursodiol) (Ann IM 1994;121:207; Nejm 1990;323:1239).

Primary Biliary Cirrhosis

Nejm 1996;335:1570

Cause: Autoimmunity (Nejm 1974;290:63); associated with HLA-DR$_w$8 (Nejm 1990;322:1842). Impaired hepatic sulfoxidation (Nejm 1988;318:1089).

Epidem: Middle-aged women predominantly; female/male = 10:1; all races; incidence, 10/1 million/yr, 1000× higher in members of affected families

Pathophys: Circulating immune complexes may be picked up by the liver and cause complement fixation and liver damage (Nejm 1979;300:274); damage also due to intracellular toxic bile acid deposition (Nejm 1991;324:1548). Pruritus of this and other causes of cholestasis probably induced via central opioid system (Ann IM 1995;123:161).

Sx: Chronic pruritus, most frequent initial sx along w fatigue, with subsequent insidious onset of jaundice; frequently also picked up by finding asx elevations of alkaline phosphatase. Diarrhea due to fat malabsorption/digestion.

Si: Xanthomata (40%) in late disease; hepatomegaly initially, later small liver; splenomegaly in 35?% at time of dx, more later

Crs: Median survival 13 yr if asx, 7 yr if sx at time of dx; bilirubin levels are a rough predictor of course, consider transplant when become jaundiced

Cmplc: CREST syndrome, scleroderma, Sjögren's, primary hypothyroidism (20%), osteoporosis in most perhaps due to toxic impairment of osteoblast function (Ann IM 1985;103:855) with consequent fractures. No increase in ASHD despite elevated lipids (Ann IM 1975;82:227).

r/o sarcoid overlap disease (Nejm 1983;308:572); cholestatic drug reactions; mechanical obstruction by ultrasound, MRCP, or CT; primary sclerosing cholangitis (p 351)

Lab: *Chem:* Alkaline phos and GGTP elevations >> bilirubin elevation (obstructive picture)

Cholesterol total and HDL elevated (50%), occasionally > 1000 mg %

Path: Liver biopsy shows cirrhosis, elevated copper content, sometimes as high as in Wilson's disease (Ann IM 1972;76:62), bile duct dropout and granulomas (r/o sarcoid, etc: Nejm 1972;287:1284), small cell infiltrates in portal areas; staging predicts crs

Serol: Complement levels depressed (Ann IM 1979;90:72)

Antimitochondrial antibodies elevated in 90-95% (Ann IM 1972;77:533), but may be falsely positive in chronic (> 3 mo) extrahepatic obstruction (Nejm 1972; 286:1400); M_2 fraction has high specif

Rx: Supportive: Cholestyramine or colestipol may help pruritus; vitamin D and calcium to prevent osteoporosis; vitamins K, E, and A

Medical: • Ursodeoxycholic acid (Ursodiol) 13-15 mg/kg qd by
RCT (Nejm 1994;330:1342 vs Lancet 1999;354:1053)
• Methotrexate 5 mg po q 12 hr × 3 q 1 wk (Ann IM
1997;126:682)
Surgical liver transplant (Nejm 1990;322:1419,
1989;320:1709) can produce 70% 5-yr survival

Primary Sclerosing Cholangitis

Nejm 1995;332:924

Cause: Genetic, plus viral precipitation?; HLA-DR$_w$52a present in all,
and HLA-C$_w$7 present in 86% (Nejm 1990;322:1842)

Epidem: Associated with inflammatory bowel disease often (70%),
especially ulcerative colitis, and retroperitoneal/mediastinal fibrosis; highest incidence in young men; 70% males; 70% < age 45 yr

Pathophys: Ongoing inflammation, destruction, and fibrosis of intra-
and extrahepatic bile ducts, possibly from toxic bacterial products
of the gut?

Sx: Insidious ($\geq$ 1 yr) onset, fatigue, pruritus, jaundice; attacks of
RUQ pain and chills

Si: Jaundice, big liver, big spleen (one or more present upon dx in
75%)

Crs: Many fatal within 10 yr w/o early detection and rx, but many
cases much more benign

Cmplc: Cirrhosis and portal hypertension
r/o primary biliary cirrhosis (p 349), chronic active hepatitis
(p 360), and idiopathic biliary ductopenia (Nejm 1997;336:835)

Lab: *Chem:* Alkaline phosphatase $\geq$ 2× normal, ceruloplasmin and
other copper studies elevated (75%), bilirubin elevated in
50%

Noninv: ERCP is diagnostic, showing narrowings and dilatations
of ducts

Path: Liver biopsy shows cholangitis/portal hepatitis, and later periportal hepatic fibrosis with bridging and eventual biliary cirrhosis

Xray: Cholangiograms show strictures, irregular tortuosity of intra- and extrahepatic bile ducts; extrahepatic duct involvement distinguishes from primary biliary cirrhosis

Rx: None short of liver transplant; 70% 1-yr survival with transplant

Antibiotics for acute bouts of pain

Ursodiol (ursodeoxycholic acid) (Nejm 1997;336:691; Hepatol 1992;16:707); plus perhaps immunosuppressants (Ann IM 1999;131:943) like azathioprine, prednisone, and/or methotrexate (GE 1994;106:494 vs Ann IM 1987;106:231), all may help LFTs but no effect on crs

6.4 Hepatic Diseases

Gilbert's Disease (Familial Nonhemolytic Jaundice)

Ann IM 1972;77:527; Nejm 1967;277:1108

Cause: Genetic, autosomal recessive, but positive family hx in 40% because so common; defect is in the promoter region of the gene so less glucuronyl transferase produced, although that made is normal (Nejm 1995;333:1171)

Epidem: Male/female = 2:1; common explanation of mild elevations of unconjugated bilirubin found serendipitously on chem screens. Prevalence = 3-10%

Pathophys: Diminished hepatocyte uptake of circulating unconjugated bilirubin and decreased glucuronyl transferase activity; some studies show 50% decrease in rbc survival but others subsequently show no increased in hemolysis (Ann IM 1975;82:552)

Sx: Jaundice especially with starvation (> 24 hr), infection, alcohol, exercise. Hepatic tenderness often present with onset but probably because it is a nonspecific sx that brings attention to the jaundice.

Si: Scleral icterus in otherwise healthy person

Crs: Benign, does not appear before age 10 yr

Cmplc: None

Lab: *Chem:* Bilirubin = 1-3 mg %, predominantly indirect; unnecessary usually to confirm by checking fasting (< 300 cal/d) levels that rise to 6 mg % over 3 d. Other LFTs normal.
Hem: CBC normal
Path: Liver bx, which should not be done, will be normal

Rx: None (phenobarb has been given for questionable sx of malaise, probably unrelated)

Alcoholic Hepatitis

Nejm 1988;319:1639

Cause: Ethanol and poor nutrition

Epidem: Perhaps an unusual metabolism in predisposed people, hotly debated (Nejm 1976;294:9); but something genetically and metabolically different since twins raised apart and sons of alcoholic fathers raised apart have increased incidence (Science 1984;225:1493)

Pathophys (rv of ethanol metabolism: Nejm 1970;283:24,71): Acute and chronic complications of alcohol occur more often in women than men due not to size differences but to differences in gastric mucosa alcohol dehydrogenase activity (Nejm 1990;322:95)

Sx: Those of hepatitis

Si: Fever; Dupuytren's contractures; parotid enlargement

Crs:

Cmplc: Laënnec's cirrhosis; hepatic failure (p 367)

Lab: *Chem:* AST (SGOT) increased > ALT (SGPT), usually

Hem: Depressed platelets, smaller than average size, indicates direct alcohol suppression of synthesis

Path: Liver bx shows fatty liver infiltration—r/o fatty infiltration of pregnancy (p 827)—and other non-alcoholic steatohepatitises (Nejm 2002;346:1221) w abnormal LFTs as in obesity (Ann IM 2000;132:112), diabetes, tetracycline in high doses, CCl_4, steroid rx, starvation, and hyperlipidemias (Am J Med 1999;107:450; Ann IM 1997;126:136); usually alcoholic hyaline distinguishes it from viral hepatitis

Rx:

- Prednisone 40 mg qd × 28 d, possibly helpful in severe acute alcoholic hepatitis (Ann IM 1990;113:299, 1989;110:685 vs Gut 1995;37:113)
- Pentoxifylline (Trental) (GE 2000;119:1637) 400 mg po tid × 4 wk may be better than prednisone

Autoimmune Hepatitis

Nejm 1996;334:897, 1995;333:958,1004

Cause: Autoimmunity to HLA IB8, IIDR3, and DR52a loci

Epidem: Females >> males; overlap w primary biliary cirrhosis, primary sclerosing cholangitis, chronic hepatitis C (Ann IM 1996;125:588)

Pathophys:

Sx: Malaise, jaundice

Si: Those of chronic liver disease, eg spiders, jaundice, splenomegaly

Crs:

Cmplc: Cirrhosis/liver failure, reversible w rx (Ann IM 1997;127:981)

Lab: *Chem:* ALT (SGPT), AST (SGOT), bilirubin all elevated
Serol: Globulins increased, esp γ globulins; autoantibodies, esp ANA, anti-smooth muscle, and anti-actin antibodies at titers > 1/40 (Nejm 1995;333:958,1004)

Rx: Steroids + azathioprine help > 85%

Hepatitis A (Infectious Hepatitis)

Nejm 1985;313:1059

Cause: Hepatitis A virus, a pico-RNA enterovirus

Epidem: Fecal/oral contact with infected persons for up to 1 yr after clinical disease (Jama 1958;200:365); occasionally parenteral; higher incidence in parents of day-care-center children, children are often asx (Nejm 1980;302:1222)

In developing countries, 3/1000/mo incidence for first-class hotel users, 20/1000/mo for community-living guests; thus is most frequent preventable infection in travelers (Jama 1994; 272:885)

In US incidence has plummeted w childhood immunization in majority of states (Jama 2005;294:194)

Pathophys: Only in humans; because it is an enterovirus, incidence up in late summer and early winter; 45% of adults have had it (Nejm 1976;95:755); increased incidence in gay males (Nejm 1980; 302:438)

Sx: 15-40 d incubation period (Am J Med 5/62)
In children, only 5-15% get sx
Malaise (48% in children/63% in adults), anorexia (41%/42%), abdominal pain (48%/37%), fever and/or chills (41%/32%), jaundice (65%/88%), diarrhea (58%/18%), dark urine (58%/68%), light stools (58%/58%), nausea and vomiting (65%/26%)

Si: Jaundice, though anicteric form also common and more benign

Crs: Benign, 15% morbidity and rare (0.3%) mortality (Ann IM 1998; 128:111); sx peak 2 wk after onset and take about 4 wk to clear; relapse in 6% at 1-3 mo (Ann IM 1987;106:221)

Cmplc: Fulminant hepatitis, relapsing hepatitis, no chronic active hepatitis (Eric Mast, CDC 11/95)

r/o Q fever, mononucleosis, CMV, toxoplasmosis, Fitzhugh-Curtis syndrome, psittacosis, and other viral non-A, non-B hepatitis like **Hepatitis E** infection, an enterovirus that causes only acute hepatitis like hep A (Nejm 2004;351:2367, 1997;336: 795) and that is spread via water sources esp in equatorial areas (Virol 1993;4:273) and in pregnant women who have a 25% mortality (Eric Mast, CDC 11/95); and **Hepatitis G**, rare, benign, blood-borne (Nejm 1997;336: 741,747,795; Ann IM 1997;126: 874), and may impair HIV virulence (Nejm 2001;345: 707, 715,761)

Lab: *Chem:* Typical hepatitis enzyme picture w ALT (SGPT) > AST (SGOT) > LDH > alkaline phos levels

Serol: Hepatitis A IgM antibody present when first sx present (Ann IM 1982;96:193); later IgM goes negative and IgG appears and stays

Rx: Prevent by:
- Avoiding fecal contamination
- Vaccine, inactivated (Havrix, or Vaqta) (Nejm 1997;336:197; Med Let 1995;37:51; Jama 1995;273:906, 1994;272:885; Nejm 1992;327:453) 2-shot (1 cc w 1440 ELU im) series for adults 6-12 mo apart, 3-shot (0.55 cc w 720 ELU im) series for children at 0, 1 mo, and 6-12 mo; 100% effective, no need to screen titers if born after 1945, may be useful post-exposure (80% efficacy) (Lancet 1999;353:1136) but not clearly better than IgG (ACP J Club 1999;131:45), how often to reboost unclear; cost: $55/dose

    Prophylax w IgG 0.02 cc/kg up to 2 cc im if exposed

Hepatitis B

Nejm 1997;337:1733

Cause: Hepatitis B virus

Epidem: Primarily spread venereally or via blood and blood products (transfusion risk = 1/63,000: Nejm 1996;334:1685), fresh, dry, or frozen. Transmitted by mucous membranes but not by urine and feces (Nejm 1969;281:1375); and via eczematous skin (Ann IM 1976;85:573).

Pathophys: Sometimes viral DNA incorporated into liver genome, then less hepatitis, but still can produce hep BsAg, associated with carcinoma more often (Nejm 1986;315:1187)

Sx: 60-160 d incubation period; arthralgias/arthritis (Nejm 1978; 298:185; Ann IM 1971;74:207, 1971;75:29), cryoglobulins (Ann IM 1977;87:287), urticaria and other rashes (Ann IM 1978; 89:34)

Si: Many cases anicteric

Crs: Acute hepatitis leads to:
- Benign crs, recover or have relapsing, or portal mild hepatitis; or
- Acute liver necrosis, all of whom die w/o transplant; or
- Submassive hepatic necrosis (bridging), of whom 60% die or go on to postnecrotic cirrhosis, the balance recover completely; or
- Chronic active hepatitis, usually with a progressive downhill course over 5-10 yr; or
- Asx carrier state in ~90% newborns, 20% school-age children, < 1% young healthy adults (Nejm 1987;316:965)

Cmplc: Hepatoma, 2% after 10 yr (Ann IM 2001;135:759), 10% higher if Hep BeAg present (Nejm 2002;347:168); chronic active hepatitis (10%) (p 360); delta (δ) agent infection **(hepatitis D)**, an RNA viral parasite of hep B virus, only can replicate if hep B around, leads to acute hepatitis itself or severe chronic active hepatitis (Nejm 1987;317:1256); fasting hypoglycemia (Nejm 1972;286:1436); serum sickness (20%), polyarteritis, nephritis especially membranous GN (Nejm 1991;324:1457)

Lab: *Chem:* Typical hepatitis enzyme picture w ALT (SGPT) > AST (SGOT) > LDH > alkaline phos levels; get CPK to r/o myopathy if LDH > AST (SGOT) > ALT (SGPT)

Path: Liver bx

Serol: Core IgM antibody always up by time of 1st sx (Nejm 1978;298:1379); HBsAg (Ann IM 1982;96:193) elevated; e-antigen elevation correlates with infectivity; anti-HBsAg appears shortly after sx develop, but there may be a window of infectivity when HBsAg and antibody are negative but core (c) antibody is positive, which, if IgM, can be distinguished from remote infection where there is attenuation of all but IgG core antibody (S. Sears 11/95)

Rx:

Prevention

- Body fluid precautions, including wearing gloves (Ann IM 1981;95:133)
- Monitor Hep B pos health workers but let work unless surgeons doing high-exposure surgery, then should not work if Hep B e Ag positive or documented transmissions (Nejm 1997;336:178)
- Screen all pregnant women for HBsAg (Ann IM 1987;107:412) so can prophylax and immunize their infants
- Hep B immune globulin (HBIG) prophylaxis 0.05 cc/kg × 2, 30 d apart within 24-72 hr of exposure, $160/dose; for newborns of HBsAg pos mothers 0.5 cc within 12 hr of birth along w vaccine
- Immunization w recombinant vaccine (Nejm 1997;336: 196; Med Let 1985;27:118), lasts > 15 yr (Ann IM 2005; 142:333); cmplc: rare post-vaccine alopecia (Jama 1997; 278:1176), no increase in later MS (Nejm 2001;344:319, 327), perhaps other autoimmune diseases (RA?)

    Adults/children w 20 μgm q 1 mo × 2 then 3rd dose in 6-12 mo like dT, or q 1 yr × 3 doses also works; $100; neither vaccine nor HBIG necessary if anti-HBc present

Newborns, all w 10 μgm at birth, 1 and 6 mo (Jama 1995;274:1201), esp to SE Asian children to prevent 7% incidence of child-to-child transmisssion (Jama 1996;276: 906; Nejm 1989;321:1301); for newborns of HBsAg pos mothers (Med Let 1992;34:69), vaccinate and give HBIG as above. Vaccination has halved Taiwan rate of child-hood hepatoma (Nejm 1997;336:1855).

of chronic disease, to prevent cirrhosis progression and/or hepatoma:

- Lamivudine (3TC) 100+ mg po qd × 1 yr (Nejm 2004;351:1521,1567, 2002;346:1706) resistance develops so multidrug regimens being developed, eg, w pegylated interferon α2b (Ann IM 2005;142:240) or dipivoxil; $160/mo
- Adefovir (Hepsera) (Nejm 2003;348:800,808; Med Let 2002; 44:105) 10 mg po qd if HBsAg positive, for chronic suppression (Nejm 2005;352:2673); use if lamivudine resistance develops (Ann IM 2005;142:821); renal toxicity, resistance develops in 6%; $500/mo
- Interferon-α2b or peginterferon α2a (Nejm 2005;352:2682) × 4-6 mo may permanently help 30-40% if given early on, certainly for chronic δ-agent infection (Nejm 1994;330:88), and for chronic hep B (Nejm 1994;330:137), esp if e-antigen pos (Nejm 1996;334:1422); $2000/mo
- Entecavir
- No steroids (Nejm 1976;294:722)

Hepatitis C

Ann IM 2002;136:747, 2000;132:296; Nejm 2001;345:41

Cause: Hepatitis C RNA virus, several genotypes, 1a and 1b most common in U.S.

Epidem: 1.8% prevalence of antibodies in U.S., 4 million infected (Nejm 1999;341:556), but up to 5% in Africa and Middle East.

Over 50% of cases due to iv drug use; 50-80% of iv drug users contract within 1st yr of use. 97% of post-transfusion hepatitis in U.S. (Nejm 1991;325:1325).

Transfusions incidence = 1/100,000 transfusions using screened blood (Nejm 1996;334:1685), 18/10,000 using unscreened blood (Nejm 1992;327:369)

Post-organ transplant, eg, renal (Nejm 1992;326:454)

Sexual transmission rates are low but real, eg, 2-3% annual incidence in wives of infected hemophiliacs (Ann IM 1994;120:748, 1991;115:764)

Neonatal transmission rate low, 2.5% (Ann IM 1992;117:881,887) to 5% (Nejm 1994;330:744), as is intrafamilial rate (Jama 1995;274:1459)

Chronic carrier state develops in 85+% after acute infection and lasts years even with normal LFTs (Nejm 1992;327:1899); 75-90% with hep C antibody have viremia (Nejm 1990; 323:1107)

Pathophys: No protective antibody response develops

Sx: 2-20 wk incubation, 6-7 wk average; 80% are anicteric

Si:

Crs: 17+ yr after infection, 80+% had fatigue, all had at least mild inflammation on bx, 55% had pos enzymes, but only 2% had cirrhosis (Jama 2000;284:450; Nejm 1999;340:1228); vs 11% of HCV pos army recruits who eventually got liver disease over 45 yr (Ann IM 2000;132:105)

Cmplc: Mixed cryoglobulinemia (p 516)

B-cell non-Hodgkin's lymphoma, reversible w rx of Hep C (Nejm 2002;347:89)

Chronic Hepatitis in 80% over 10+ yr, 20-35% of whom go on to cirrhosis over 20+ yr; hepatocellular carcinoma 1-4%/yr after onset of cirrhosis; get CPK, especially if LDH > AST (SGOT) > ALT (SGPT) to r/o myopathy; liver biopsy (do if sx beyond 6-12 mo or worsening) shows fibrosis with bridging between hepatic lobules but pathologic picture waxes and wanes

Vasculitis of various types

r/o other causes of chronically elevated LFTs:
Hemochromatosis, Wilson's disease, α_1-antitrypsin deficiency (Nejm 1981;304:558), drug-induced hepatitis from various drugs, primary biliary cirrhosis (p 349), alcohol and other toxins, diabetes, myxedema, myopathies

Lab: *Chem:* Elevated LFTs, esp SGPT (ALT), but not 100% sens (Ann IM 1995;123:330)

Serol: Anti hep C virus IgG antibody levels (ELISA) first detectable 10-50 wk after exposure and 4-50 wk after LFT elevations appear; hep C viral RNA titer correlates with infectivity and persistence as chronic hepatitis, tested for by PCR (target amplification) method, or more inconsistent branched-chain DNA (signal amplification) assay (Ann IM 1995;123:321) used primarily to monitor rx

Cryoglobulins in 50%

Rx: Prevent by avoiding high-risk behaviors (iv drugs, sexual promiscuity), taking body fluid precautions, and by screening donors for anti-HCV levels will prevent 60% (Nejm 1990; 323:1107) to 85% of cases; a small % of donors will be infectious but won't yet be antibody positive. Barrier methods of bc probably not necessary in monogamous couples given 1-3% lifetime risk (MMWR 1998;47:1). Prophylaxis with immune globulin is ineffective.

Prevent hepatocellular carcinoma w 45 mg po qd vitamin K_2 (menaquinone), impressively effective in initial Japanese study (Jama 2004;292:358)

of disease (Ann IM 2000;133:665) (elevated ALT, viremia, and cirrhosis on bx): Decreases incidence of hepatoma × 50% (Ann IM 2005;142:105, 1999;131:174); much more effective in the 25% of pts w a susceptibility gene (Nejm 1996;334:77), much less effective in blacks (19%) than whites (52%) (Nejm 2004;350:2265); NIH CDC suggests checking ALT and RNA levels after 6 mo rx and stopping if not markedly improved (Ann IM 1997;127:855,866,918; Hepatol 1996;24:778). Can reverse cirrhotic fibrosis (Ann IM 2000;132:517)

- Interferon-α2a (Roferon-A), or interferon-α2b (Intron-A) or as peginterferon α2b sc tiw × 24-52 wk but 12 wk enough if RNA level goes to 0 at 4 wk w ribavirin (Nejm 2005;352:2609); or better, prolonged-release form, peg-α2a (Peg-Intron or Pegasys) (Jama 2004;292:2839; Nejm 2004;351:438,451; Med Let 2003;45:19) q 1 wk w ribavirin better than regular w ribavirin, 30% eradication in HIV pts rather than < 14%, and 55-65% eradication in immunocompetent pts; $1000/mo; alone × 6 mo in acute disease may prevent chronic Hep C infection (Nejm 2001;345:1452)
- Ribavirin (Med Let 1999;41:53; Am J Med 1999;107:112; Lancet 1998;352:1426) (sold w interferon-α2b as Rebetron; ways to give w peg-α2a available soon) × 6-12 mo depending on Hep C genotype (Ann IM 2004;140:346,370), many side effects and $8000/6 mo, but helps over 50% cost-effectively (Am J Med 2000;108:366)

    other options: Liver transplant; hep A and B vaccination if not immune already, to prevent frequently fatal hepatitis in chronic hepatitis C (Nejm 1998;338:286)

Wilson's Disease

Ann IM 1991;115:720

Cause: Genetic, autosomal recessive, on chromosome 13

Epidem: Onset age 6-50 yr; usually late childhood; hepatitis sx usually appear before age 30, CNS sx usually after 30. Heterozygote (single gene) prevalence = 1/200; disease prevalence = 1/30,000.

Pathophys: A chronic hepatitis. Defective copper (Cu) metabolism/ excretion with deposition in liver and basal ganglia; ceruloplasm binding defect from diminished ceruloplasmin synthesis, a chromosome 13 gene. Either hepatic or neurologic sx may predominate or exist alone.

Sx: Tremulousness (50% at time of dx); abdominal pain (42% at dx); dystonia (36% at dx), especially loss of fine hand motor function, eg, writing, piano playing; excessive salivation and drooling; psychiatric sx; hepatic failure sx

Si: Kaiser-Fleischner ring (68%), brownish opacity around edge of cornea, usually seen by slit lamp only early (Ann IM 1977; 86:285); hepatomegaly (50%); splenomegaly (50%); neurologic si's like resting and intention tremors (50%), dysarthria (50%) and drooling (12%), ataxia (32%), rigidity, and major psychiatric si (12%); blue nail lunulae

Crs: Chronic illness leading to death before age 30 yr if no rx

Cmplc: Portal hypertension, hypersplenism; hemolytic anemia (Ann IM 1970;73:413); proximal tubule Fanconi-like syndrome (Ann IM 1968;68:770)

Lab: *Chem:* Ceruloplasmin < 20 μgm %, 7% false negative, false positive in heterozygotes 10% of the time and in babies < 6 mo old, or with estrogen rx (Ann IM 1977;86:285)

  Uric acid decreased due to poor proximal tubule reabsorption; r/o ASA rx, Fanconi syndrome, and other renal tubular syndromes (Ann IM 1974;80:42)

Hem: Thrombocytopenia (22%)

Path: Liver bx shows chronic hepatitis or biliary cirrhosis (Nejm 1982;306:319) and Cu content > 100 μgm or 3.9 mmol/gm dry liver, false positive in primary biliary cirrhosis and heterozygotes; > 250 μgm/gm dry liver, false positive only in babies < 6 mo old (Nejm 1968;278:352)

Urine: Cu excretion/24 hr > 100 μgm in later stages; aminoaciduria

Rx: Prevent by screening family members w Ceruloplasmin and copper levels, or by PCR analysis (Ann IM 1997;127:21)

of disease:

    1st: D-Penicillamine po daily; probably reasonable to rx asx people; questionable if children can be on it safely (Nejm 1975; 293:1300); adverse effects: rash and renal tubular damage

    2nd: Trientine qd divided between meals; increase q 6 mo to get Cu < 20 μgm % (Nejm 1987;317:209)

    3rd: Zinc po (Ann IM 1983;99:314), which inhibits gi Cu absorption

Hemochromatosis

Nejm 2004;350:2383, 1999;341:1986; Jama 1998;280:172

Cause: Genetic (Ann IM 1999;130:953), most are autosomal recessive HFE gene mutation C282Y on chromosome 6 (Nejm 1999;341:718,755), 50+% manifestation in homozygotes; but a small % are H63D mutations of the same gene (Jama 2001;285:2216)

    Iron overload, eg, in thalassemia major patients (Ann IM 1983;99:450), or dietary overload in African genetically predisposed pts (Nejm 1992;326:95). Heterozygous state may have some reproductive advantage to women by preventing iron deficiency (Nejm 1996;335:1799).

Epidem: Usually in patients > 40 yr old; women usually older than men since menstruation protects (Ann IM 1997;127:105). C282Y gene frequency ≈ 1/15, 1/250 whites are homozygotes (Nejm 2005;352:1769; 1999;341:718,755). Many homozygous pts have asx or unreported complc and go undetected (Nejm 2000;343:1529).

Pathophys: A chronic hepatitis; hemosiderin deposition especially in pancreas, skin, liver, testes, heart, kidneys

Sx: Increased skin pigmentation (iron stimulation of melanin production); weakness/fatigue (70%); abdominal pain (60%); arthritis (1st sx in 40-60%); diabetic sx's

Si: Skin pigmentation (75%), diabetic si's (60%); cardiac failure

Crs: Normal life expectancy with phlebotomies if no cirrhosis (Nejm 1985;313:1256); heterozygotes have mildly elevated iron levels but no iron overload cmplc's (Nejm 1996;335:1799)

Cmplc: Hepatic cirrhosis (60%), hepatoma (10%); pituitary impotence (30%), reversible with rx (Ann IM 1984;101:629); CHF from myocardiopathy with a rapidly downhill course; diabetes, usually insulin dependent

Lab: *Chem:* α-Fetoprotein elevated (r/o hepatoma); hepatitis LFTs
  - Ferritin > 250 μgm/L (women), > 350 μgm/L (men) (99.5% sens, 94% specif) (Ann IM 1998;128:338) or less (Ann IM 2000;133:329); cirrhosis very unlikely unless ferritin > 1000 (7% false neg: Ann IM 2003;138:627)
  - Iron/TIBC % saturations > 60% (Nejm 1982;307:1702) in men, > 50% in women (98% sens, 94% specif) (Ann IM 1998;128:338) or less (Ann IM 2000;133:329)
  - Genetic analysis for C282Y mutation of HFE gene (Ann IM 2000;132:261)

Path: Bx of liver, synovium, marrow, rectal mucosa all show increased iron deposition and, in liver, cirrhosis with periportal concentrations

Rx: Prevent by screening all adults with iron and TIBC for homozygous state by above iron level criteria (Ann IM 1998;128:338); or pt and family members for C282Y mutation of HFE gene, useful and cheap ($95) (Ann IM 2000;132:261)

of disease:

  1st: Phlebotomy of 1 U q 3-7 d to keep ferritin < 50 μgm/L, may take 1+ yr, then 3-4×/yr to keep there; rapid, effective, and safer than deferoxamine (Clem Finch, 1972)

  2nd: Deferoxamine iv or sc (Nejm 1977;297:418); 12-hr sc pump best, especially for iron overload pts, eg, thalassemia major (Ann IM 1983;99:450); adverse effects: deafness and blindness (Nejm 1986;314:869). Or L_1, an iron chelator, oral as effective as parenteral (Clin Pharmacol Ther 1991; 50:294).

Hepatoma and Hepatocellular Carcinoma

Cause: Chronic hepatitis B or hepatitis C (Ann IM 1991;115:644) and many other causes of cirrhosis, including hemachromatosis

Epidem: Increasing incidence associated w hepatitis C in Japan (Nejm 1993;328:1797,1802) and in U.S. 3/100,000 (Ann IM 2003;139:817; Nejm 1999;340:745)

Pathophys: Hepatitis causes hepatoma by viral genome incorporation into liver cell DNA

Sx: Failure to thrive; worsening ascites or liver failure

Si: Abdominal mass; cachexia

Crs: < 5% 5-yr survival (Nejm 1999;340:745)

Cmplc: Polycythemia, gynecomastia due to HCG production, hypercalcemia due to increased PTH (Nejm 1970;282:704), dysfibrinogenemia bleeding, 2nd primary hepatoma in 45% at 3 yr (Nejm 1996;334:1561)

 r/o birth control pill-induced pedunculated liver tumors (Ann IM 1975;83:301), can regress off pill (Ann IM 1977;86:180)

Lab: *Chem:* Alkaline phos elevated more than bilirubin

 α-Fetoprotein/protein ratio increased (a nonfunctioning fibrinogen: Nejm 1978;299:221); 50% false neg, 1% false pos (Nejm 1968;278:984), r/o embryonal cell testicular and gastric cancers (Nejm 1971;285:1058), and low-level elevations in ataxia telangiectasia

Hem: Polycythemia (10%)

Xray: Hepatic mass by ultrasound, CT, or MRI; hot by gallium

Rx: Prevent by screening Hep C and B cirrhotics w α-fetoprotein levels (questionable benefit, 50% specif, 90% sens-Ann IM 2003;139:46), vitamin K_2 (menaquinone) 45 mg po qd (Jama 2004;292:358), and ultrasounds? (Nejm 1991;325:675)

Surgical lobectomy sometimes possible (Nejm 1994;331:1547) followed by interferon rx if Hep C caused (Ann IM 2001;134:963), or total hepatectomy w liver transplant (Ann IM 1998;129:643; Nejm 1996;334:693)

Percutaneous ethanol injection of tumor, or surgical extirpation w f/u vitamin A analog po qd decreases rate of 2nd primary tumors (Nejm 1996;334:1561)

Chemoembolization no help (Nejm 1995;332:1256)

Hepatic Failure: Ascites

Nejm 2004;350:1646

Cause: Multiple etiologies result in end-stage hepatic failure, which has four major complications: ascites, hemorrhage, renal failure, and encephalopathy

Pathophys: Ascites underfill theory is that postsinusoidal block raises portal vein pressure, which causes capsular weeping, which causes decreased blood volume and increased aldosterone and ADH, which causes more extracellular fluid and/or ascites; or underfill may be due to vasodilatation of splanchnic bed (cf pregnancy: Nejm 1988;319:1127) and caused by excess nitric oxide production by endothelial cells (Nejm 1998;339:533). Budd-Chiari hepatic vein occlusion occurs.

Sx: Abdominal swelling/edema

Si: Increased abdominal girth; fluid wave, shifting dullness, spiders, hepatosplenomegally

Crs: 50% 2-yr mortality

Cmplc: Pleural effusions, usually on right side from ascites leakage into chest (Am J Med 1999;107:262)

Spontaneous bacterial peritonitis (Nejm 1999;341:403); present in 20% of those admitted w ascites; dx by peritoneal fluid wbc counts > 250 and cultures; rx w cefotaxime plus iv albumin to prevent hepatorenal syndrome;

r/o **Meig's Syndrome** of ovarian carcinoma and peritoneal mesothelioma

Lab: *Ascitic fluid:* Serum albumin level $\geq$ 1.1 gm % greater than ascitic albumin level (Ann IM 1992;117:215), contrasts with malignant ascites (Am J Med 1984;77:83)

Bact: Ascitic fluid with pH < 7.31 suggests peritonitis; if poly count > 250/mm^3, take cultures in blood culture medium flasks

Chem: Hyponatremia in ascitics from hypovolemia-induced ADH (Ann IM 1982;96:413)

Rx: Prophylaxis of spontaneous bacterial peritionitis in acute vericeal bleed w norfloxacin 400 mg po bid or 400 mg iv qd × 7 d, or w cipro 200 mg iv qd + Augmentin (w variceal bleed); in asx pt w norflox 400 mg po qd + cipro 750 mg po q 1 wk and ss Tm/S 5 d/wk

of nontense ascites: Na restriction, furosemide iv/po, and amiloride or spironolactone up to 400 mg qd to achieve 1 kg/d loss if edema present, 0.3 kg qd if not

of tense ascites:

- 4-6 L paracentesis w or without optional 6-8 gm albumin iv (GE 1996;111:1002; Ann IM 1990;112:889) or dextran (J Clin Gastroenterol 1992;14:31); then repeated outpt taps; or

- Transjugular intrahepatic portosystemic stent (TIPS) shunt placement works like other shunting procedures w a 5% significant bleeding cmplc rate and 25% encephalopathy induction rate; used for both bleeding and intractable ascites (Nejm 1995;332:1192, 1994;330:165,182; Ann IM 1995;122:816; Jama 1995;273:1824); worse than large-volume taps? (GE 2003;124:634, 2002;123:1839 vs Nejm 2000;342:1701 vs 1745); or

- Peritoneal/venous LaVeen shunt (Nejm 1991;325:829; 1989;321:1632); or
- Liver transplant

Hepatic Failure: Hemorrhage

Nejm 2001;345:669, 1993;329:1862

Cause: Multiple etiologies result in end-stage hepatic failure, which has four major complications: ascites, hemorrhage, renal failure, and encephalopathy

Pathophys: Variceal bleeding and/or gastritis/ulcers; depressed prothrombin and fibrinogen; depressed platelets from bleeding and hypersplenism; increased plasminogen activators due to diminished hepatic filtration

Sx: Hematemesis, melena

Si:

Crs: Cause of death in 20% of cirrhotics (Nejm 1966;275:61)

Cmplc:

Lab: *Hem:* Clotting studies, serial hemoglobin/hematocrit

Rx: Preventive maneuvers (Ann IM 1992;117:59; Nejm 1987;317:893):

- Propranolol or other β-blocker to pulse < 60, decreases recurrent bleeding and first bleeds, and increases survival by 5-10% (Nejm 1999;340:1033 vs 988, 1991;324:1532)
- Isosorbide (Isordil) 20-40 mg po bid as good (GE 1993;104:1460), or used w β-blocker is better than scleroRx (Lancet 1996;348:1677; Nejm 1996;334:1624); and then endoscopic ligation (Nejm 2001;345:648)
- Transjugular intrahepatic portosystemic stent (TIPS) shunt placement works like other shunting procedures w a

5% significant bleeding cmplc rate and 25% encephalopathy induction rate; used for both bleeding and intractable ascites (Jama 1995;273:1824; Nejm 1994;330:165,182)

- Surgical shunt for recurrent bleeding, not prophylactically of acute bleeding:
  - Somatostatin analogs like octreotide 25 mg/hr iv continuous drip (Nejm 1995;333:555 vs BMJ 1995;10:310); or valpreotide 50 μgm iv bolus then drip/hr (Nejm 2001; 344:23), prior to endoscopy to help decrease acute bleeding but no increase in survival (ACP J Club 2002;135:93)
  - Endoscopic ligation (Ann IM 1995;123:280; Nejm 1992;326:1527) as good as surgery (which has a 50% survival), better than medical rx after a bleed but not used prophylactically if has never bled (Nejm 1991;324:1779), also better than sclerosis (Ann IM 1993;119:1)
  - Sclerosis of varices directly via gastroscope (Nejm 1987; 316:11); also useful preventively after a bleed (Ann IM 1997;126:849,858)
  - Open esophageal stapling if scleroRx fails (Nejm 1989; 321:857)

Hepatic Failure: Hepatorenal Syndrome

Nejm 2004;350:1651

Cause: Multiple etiologies result in end-stage hepatic failure, which has four major complications: ascites, hemorrhage, renal failure, and encephalopathy

Epidem:

Pathophys: Unknown etiology, but acts like ATN, although ATN is not present in biopsies, and is reversible since can transplant hepatorenal kidneys to other patients (Nejm 1969;280:1367)

Sx: of renal failure (p 1023)

Si:

Crs: 20% of patients with hepatic failure die from renal failure

Cmplc: of renal failure (p 1023)

Lab: *Chem:* Elevated BUN and creatinine; low urinary Na

Rx: Supportive care including dialysis
Midodrine 7.5-12.5 mg po tid w octreotide 100-200 μgm
sc tiw
Terlipressin 0.5-2 mg iv q 4-12 hr
Albumin 1 gm/kg iv day 1 then 20-40 gm iv qd

Hepatic Failure: Hepatic Coma/Encephalopathy

Nejm 1993;329:1862

Cause: Multiple etiologies result in end-stage hepatic failure, which
has four major complications: ascites, hemorrhage, renal failure,
and encephalopathy

Epidem:

Pathophys: Nitrogen-induced types, by blood in gut or protein-
containing food ingestion. Lactulose helps by producing H^+ in
bowel, which traps NH_3, and by causing diarrhea.

Sx: Organic brain syndrome/delirium (p 773)

Si: Spectrum from mild flap (asterixis) to decorticate/decerebrate
coma (Nejm 1968;278:876)

Crs: 33% of pts w hepatic failure die from coma

Cmplc:

Lab: *Chem:* Blood NH_3 elevated, although degree of elevation does
not correlate with severity but may be useful to follow individual
pt. r/o other causes of ammonia elevations like ureterosigmoidos-
tomy or atonic bladder causing UTI and hence systemic NH_3 absorption (Nejm 1981;304:766); or **Orotic Aciduria**, sex-linked
with coma in men and postpartum women who are carriers
(Nejm 1990;322:1641, 1652).

GASTROENTEROLOGY

Rx (Nejm 1997;337:473):

    1st: Lactulose 30-60 gm qd po to produce 2-4 acidic (pH < 6) stools qd helps all types, though more expensive (ADP J Club 2004;141:59); can cause osmotic diarrhea and hypernatremia

    2nd: Antibiotics like
- Neomycin 6 gm qd
- Metronidazole (Flagyl) 800 mg po qd
- Ampicillin
- L-dopa (Ann IM 1975;83:677)

    Others:
- Bromocriptine po hs (Nejm 1977;296:793)
- Flumazenil (Romazicon) iv helps 25%; if oral becomes available, may be useful

Budd-Chiari Syndrome

Nejm 2004;350:578

Cause: Myeloproliferative diseases, especially P. vera, even when not clinically apparent; also PNH, antiphospholipid syndrome, and inherited deficiency of protein C, S, and antithrombin III, factor V Leiden mutation, and prothrombin gene mutation; birth control pill use

Epidem:

Pathophys: Acute or chronic occlusion of hepatic veins

Sx: Abdominal pain, hepatomegally, and ascites in most pts. Nausea, vomiting, and icterus in acute pts.

Si: Spenomegally and varices in chronic pts

Cmplc: r/o tricuspid regurgitation, constrictive pericarditis, and atrial myxoma; cholecystitis

Crs:

Lab: *Chem:* AST and ALT increased markedly; alk phos and bilirubin elevated in some pts

Xray: Ultrasound, MRI, and CT all show the lesion

Rx: Thrombolysis if within 2 wk of onset; angioplasty/stents; TIPS/surgical shunts; liver transplant

6.5   Small Bowel Diseases

Malabsorption

Cause:

Failures of digestion:

- Blind loops, strictures, diverticula, and inadequate mixing syndromes, eg, postsurgery or associated with disorders of motility with secondary bacterial overgrowth causing bile salt breakdown, poor lipase stimulation, and poor absorption especially of fats (Nejm 1967;276:1393)
- Zollinger-Ellison syndrome: High duodenal pH inactivates pancreatic enzymes
- Pancreatic: Either disease destroying > 90% of the organ (Nejm 1972;287:813) like cystic fibrosis, alcoholic pancreatitis, or postgastrectomy lack of cholecystokinin stimulation of pancreas

Inadequate absorption length:

- Gross lesions, eg, > 50% small bowel resection, gastric acid often overwhelms the residual bowel, but can rx with cimetidine (Nejm 1979;300:79)
- Specific lesions, eg, ileal and/or proximal colon resection causing loss of enterohepatic circulation and hence of bile salts, which causes fat malabsorption
- Relative, ie, rapid transport syndromes
- Mesenteric arterial insufficiency
- Lymphatic obstruction impairing fatty acid and triglyceride absorption, as in tumor or Whipple's disease

Enteropathies:

- Inflammatory, like sprue, regional enteritis, tbc, amyloid, sarcoid, milk allergy (Nejm 1967;276:761), giardia, coccidiosis (Nejm 1970;283:1306)
- Biochemical and/or genetic disorders like hypoparathyroidism, defects in carbohydrate, fat, and protein absorption

Sx: Weight loss, steatorrhea (greasy, smelly, floating diarrheal stools), abdominal distention

Si: Cachexia

Crs: Depends on etiology

Cmplc: Tetany from vitamin D deficiency and calcium salt precipitation; bleeding from vitamin K malabsorption; anemia from B_{12} deficiency and bleeding; vitamin E deficiency (Nejm 1983;308:1063) w secondary spinocerebellar dysfunction w progressive ataxia: r/o rare α-tocopherol transfer protein deficiency (Nejm 1995;333: 1313); drug absorption abnormal with malabsorption

Lab (Nejm 1971;285:1358):

Chem: Carotene low (25% false neg), worth doing?
  Specific malabsorption vs maldigestion tests like

- Schilling test (rarely used): First load with im B_{12}, give hot B_{12} po 3 hr later and measure excretion in 24-48-hr urine sample; normal > 15%; then repeat with intrinsic factor to see if corrects
- Gly-1-C^{14}: Give hot cholate po, and if $C^{14}O_2$ in breath in 3 hr, means poor ileal absorption of bile salts or bacteria in small bowel (Nejm 1971;285:656)
- Xylose tolerance test: 25 gm po; with malabsorption, $\geq$ 5 gm in urine in 5 hr; bacterial overgrowth or ascites will cause false pos

Path: Intestinal bx

Stool: Sudan stain for qualitative fat positive; 72-hr stool fat

Rx: Cholestyramine 16 gm po qd for ileal resection diarrhea if mild (< 20 gm fat qd)

Pancreatic enzymes; can enhance absorption with omeprazole rx (Ann IM 1991;114:200)

Vitamins D, E, B$_{12}$, and K

Disaccharidase Deficiencies

Nejm 1984;310:42

Cause: Genetic

Epidem: Lactase deficiency discovered in Holland during World War II when babies with it improved during milk shortages; present in 80% of blacks (Nejm 1975;292:1156), 10% of Caucasians (Nejm 1967;276:1283), 100% of Asians, 25% of U.S. adults, 75% of all other adults (Nejm 1995;333:1)

Sucrase-isomaltase deficiency (Nejm 1987;316:1306) in 0.2% of U.S. population, 10% of Greenland Eskimos

Pathophys: Mucosal cell deficiency of invertases lactase and sucrase-isomaltase. Diarrhea from osmotic effect, bacterial degradation of these sugars to lactic acid, and steatorrhea.

Sx: Osmotic diarrhea; sucrose or milk intolerance causes bloating and cramps; most common cause of recurrent abdominal pain in children (Nejm 1979;300:1449)

Si:

Crs: Decreasing tolerance as patient ages from 1-11 yr (Nejm 1967;276:1283)

Cmplc: r/o milk allergy (p 900)

Lab: *Chem:* Lactose tolerance by breath test; or by giving 50 gm lactose po and do with hourly blood sugars over 3 hr; a normal person should increase blood sugar by 20 mg % if not diabetic

Stool: Elevated lactic acid, lowered pH (test after a milkshake)

Rx: Withhold milk and/or malt and/or sucrose, or prepare food with or add lactase to milk before feeding, although 250 cc (8 oz) milk qd is generally tolerated (Nejm 1995;333:1); yogurt may be tolerated (Nejm 1984;310:42). Baker's yeast po with sucrose decreases sx (Nejm 1987;316:1306).

A-β Lipoproteinemia (Acanthocytosis)

Cause: Genetic; autosomal recessive

Epidem:

Pathophys: Apolipoprotein serine missing; important for LDL and VLDL transport (Nejm 1971;284:813)

Sx: Steatorrhea

Si: Ataxia, hepatomegaly, fatty stools, retinitis pigmentosa (r/o Refsum's disease, toxoplasmosis)

Crs:

Cmplc: Vitamin E deficiency w ataxia from spinocerebellar dysfunction (Nejm 1995;333:1313), areflexia, impaired position and vibratory sense (Nejm 1985;313:32)

Lab: *Chem:* Serum lipoprotein electrophoresis shows absence or decrease in β-lipoprotein; triglycerides low and no increase with fatty meal; cholesterol < 100 mg %
Hem: Spiculated rbc's (acanthocytes)
Path: Small bowel bx shows fatty mucosal infiltration; liver bx shows fatty change

Rx: Vitamin E

Whipple's Disease

Nejm 1992;327:293, 346

Cause: *Tropheryma whippelii,* Whipple's bacillus

Epidem: Males > females; peak incidence in middle age. Incidence = 10/yr worldwide.

Pathophys: Infection of small intestinal mucosal layer causes lymphatic blockage, which in turn causes fatty acid malabsorption, probably at lamina propria level

Sx: Diarrhea, steatorrhea, and malabsorption; postprandial pain; polyserositis including arthritis in 70%, frequently the presenting sx; fever, weight loss; lymphadenopathy; hyperpigmentation of skin; blurred vision from uveitis, may be only sx (Nejm 1995;332:363)

Si: As above

Crs:

Cmplc: Myocarditis and aortic insufficiency (Nejm 1981;305:995); CNS, including gaze paresis, nystagmus, myoclonus, polydipsia, hypersomnolence, all of which may be a continuing problem if primary sx are treated with an antibiotic that doesn't the cross blood–brain barrier (Nejm 1979;300:907)

Lab: *Bact:* Gram-pos bacillus of actinomycetes group; identifiable by PCR; culturable now (Nejm 2000;342:620)
Hem: CBC peripheral smear may show red stippled rbc's (organisms in the red cells) (Nejm 1994;331:1343)
Path: Intestinal bx shows diagnostic changes of enlarged villi; foamy, carbohydrate-filled macrophages staining positive with PAS; and fat in mucosa, lacteals, and lymph nodes (Nejm 1971;285:1470); r/o AIDS or M. *avium* intestinal infection; and, if has noncaseating granulomata, sarcoid

Rx (Nejm 1996;335:26): Procaine penicillin 1.2 million U im qd × 14 d + streptomycin 1 gm im qd × 14 d + Tm/S bid prophylaxis continuously

Celiac Disease (Nontropical Sprue)

Ann IM 2005;142:289; M. Integlia 1/05; Nejm 2002;346:180

Cause: Ingestion of gluten, a protein in rye, barley, wheat (not oats, but often cross-contaminated w others). Genetic component, HLA-DQ2 or -DQ8 linked, which are also diabetes linked.

Epidem: Associated with dermatitis herpetiformis (p 178), Hashimoto's thyroiditis, and insulin-dependent diabetes (Nejm 1983;308:816). Seen in 1/300 Caucasians, 1/100 in Finland (Nejm 2003;348:2517), not blacks or Asians. Timing and dose of gluten exposure at age 4-7 mo may induce the disease.

Pathophys: T-cell and IgA-mediated immune response to gluten in genetically predisposed pts. Wide variety of clinical manifestations, from classic malabsorption, to atypical w fevers and gi sx, to asx.

Iron deficiency occurs from both malabsorption and occult gi bleeding (Nejm 1996;334:1163)

Sx: Onset at any age. Malabsorptive sx including diarrhea, flatulence, weight loss, and fatigue.

Si: Of malabsorption; iron or folate deficiency anemias; osteoporosis and fractures; peripheral neuropathies, ataxia, bad teeth

Crs: Nearly normal prognosis on gluten-free diet

Cmplc: Infertility; malabsorption; ulceration, perforation can cause death even in remission (Nejm 1967;276:996); increased incidence of foregut tumors of esophagus, pharynx and stomach, and lymphomas

r/o IgA deficiency

Lab: *Path:* Endoscopic or videocapsule biopsy of duodenum for dx shows villous atrophy and crypt hyperplasia, which improves on gluten-free diet

Serol: Anti-endomysial antibodies, 90+% sens, 98+% specif; or IgA/IgG tissue transglutaminase antibodies (tTG) (Nejm 2003;348:2517); but do not obviate need for bx (Scand J Gastroenterol 1994;29:148); both falsely neg on diet; anti-gliadin IgA and IgG antibodies too insensitve to use now

Genetic: HLA testing for DQ2 (95% sens, 70% specific) and DQ8; if both tests neg, 99% sens/specif; can do while on diet

Hem: Increased protime; mixed anemias

Chem: Hypocalcemia; incr alk phosphatase

Xray: Small bowel followthrough

Rx: Patient info: www.celiac.com
    Gluten-free and, initially, or later if not improved, lactose-free diet; can resume milk products in 3-6 mo once enteropathy improves; rice, corn (maize), and oats ok (Nejm 1995;333:1033); if fails, consider lactose deficiency or *Giardia* infection coincident with disease; 70% improve in < 14 d

Regional Enteritis (Crohn's Disease and Granulomatous Colitis)

Nejm 2002;347:417

Cause: Genetic component in some types on chromosome 16, impacting macrophages; and another on chromosome 5, affecting cytokine receptors

Epidem: Males = females; increased in Jews, and relatives of patients, smokers (unlike ulcerative colitis)

Pathophys:

Sx: Age of onset = 11-35 yr (75%). Cramps, partly relieved by bowel movement; diarrhea, although constipation may also intermittently predominate and may be bloody, although less often than in ulcerative colitis.

Si: Inflammatory mass. Extraintestinal manifestations: iritis; erythema nodosum; sclerosing cholangitis (p 351); pyoderma gangrenosum; clubbing and arthritis (20%), especially of knee, ankle, PIP joints, and may even develop clear-cut ankylosing spondylitis.

Crs: Teenagers get the most malignant form of ileocolitis; older people more often have a more localized disease

Cmplc: Abscesses; strictures and fistulas; malabsorption; small bowel obstruction; anemias; renal stones, usually oxalate for unclear reasons; gallstones; sclerosing cholangitis (p 351); stress and depression result, do not cause (Ann IM 1991;114:381); rare avascular necrosis of femoral head (Nejm 1993;329:1314)

GASTROENTEROLOGY

In pregnancy, moderate increase in spontaneous abortions; otherwise, healthy babies and no significant increase in risk for mother even if need surgery, steroids, or sulfa (Nejm 1985; 312:1616)

r/o bile salt diarrhea, rx with cholestyramine; *Yersinia* (Nejm 1990;323:113)

Lab: *Path:* Small bowel or colonic bx may show noncaseating granulomas and distorted glandular architecture

Noninv: Endoscopy (colonoscopy) may demonstrate diagnostic findings

Xray: UGIS and small bowel followthrough show segmental involvement ("string sign"). BE shows ileitis with reflux into ileum and/or proximal colon; disease characterized by "stepladder" mucosal edema pattern and longitudinal intramural fistulas (Nejm 1970;283:1080).

Rx (Nejm 1996;334:84, Ann IM 1990;112:50):

Medical rx of acute disease/flare:

- Mesalamine (Asacol) (5-ASA) 800-1600 mg po t-qid
- Steroids like prednisolone 40 mg po qd × 2 wk then taper 5 mg qd over 6 wk (Nejm 1994;331: 842); or budesonide LA (Entocort-CIR) 9 mg po qd × 8 wk (Nejm 1998;339:370) but not quite as effective as po steroids and much more expensive (Med Let 2002;44:6)
- Azathioprine (Imuran) or 6-MP (Ann IM 1995;123:132) adjusted by CBC and platelets, helps heal fistulas over 2-4 mo (Ann IM 1989;111:641; Nejm 1980;302:981), induces/maintains remissions

Others:

- Methotrexate 25 mg im q 1 wk (Nejm 1995;332:292)
- Infliximab (Remicade) (Med Let 1999;41:19; Nejm 1997;337:1029), a monoclonal antibody to TNF-α 5 mg/kg iv infusion at week 0, 2, and 6 helps > 50% within 1 mo when given to pts w refractory fistula producing dis-

ease (Lancet 2002;359:1541), although pts develop anti-bodies to it over time w increasing infusion reactions and decreasing response (Nejm 2004;350:876,934, 2003; 348:601)

- Natalizumhad (Antegren) (Nejm 2003;348:24) 3-6 mg iv × 2; monoclonal antibody vs integrin
- Metronidazole (Flagyl) 250 mg b-qid × 2-4 mo helps peri-anal and colonic disease
- Monoconal antibody to interleukin 2, possibly (Nejm 2004;351:2069)
- Human growth hormone (Nejm 2000;342:1633) 5 mg sc qd × 1 wk, then 1.5 mg sc qd

Medical remission maintenance (steroids not worth the risk: ACP J Club 1999;130:36):

- Immuran/6MP as above, plus
- Methotrexate 15 mg im q 1 wk, esp if induced w mtx (Nejm 2000;342:1627)
- Mesalamine (Pentasa) 500 mg po qid given chronically (GE 1993;104:435), or Asacol 800 mg po tid

Surgical: ~40% require reoperation within 15 yr (Nejm 1981; 304:1586). Big debate about appendectomy performance. Colectomy may cure if isolated there (debated: Nejm 1972; 287:111).

TPN (Nejm 1977;297:1104) or enteral elemental diets are important adjuncts in severe disease

Carcinoid Tumor (Argentaffinoma)

Nejm 1999;340:858

Cause: Neoplasia

Epidem: 1-2/100,000/yr in U.S.

Pathophys: Derived from argentaffin cells in primitive foregut (Ann IM 1972;77:53). Syndrome develops only after metastases. Symptoms related to secreted serotonin (Nejm 1967;277:1103), kallikrein (Ann IM 1969;71:763), gastrin (Nejm 1978;299:1053), histamine, dopamine, substance P, prostaglandins.

Also arises in stomach w ZE or atrophic gastritis and sometimes pernicious anemia due to excessive gastrin stimulation (Nejm 1997;336:866), lungs, ovary, or pancreas (Ann IM 1972; 77:53); or gi tract. Those originating in appendix are rarely malignant and rarely metastasize, while those of small bowel origin become malignant (20%) and many metastasize; rectal ones small and without sx.

Sx: Diarrhea, wheezing/asthma, red/violaceous flushes inducible by alcohol

Si: Right-sided heart murmurs, due to right heart scarring (Nejm 2003;348:1005); fundi during flush show decreased blood flow; plastic induration of penis (Nejm 1973;289:844)

Crs: Very low-grade malignancy, can live years with mets

Cmplc: r/o mastocytosis (p 189)

Lab: *Chem:* 24-hr urine shows 5-HIAA (a serotonin degradation product) elevated, 86% sens, 100% specif (D. Oppenheim, 11/93) but can get false positives with glycerol guiacolate expectorants, bananas, phenothiazines, caffeine, acetaminophen (Tylenol)
Path: Biopsy positive on silver stains
Provocative tests: Epinephrine 0.5-1 mg iv (Ann IM 1971; 74:711); pentagastrin (Nejm 1978;299:1055)

Xray: Scan with labeled octreotide (somatostatin analog) to pick up primary (12/13) and mets (Nejm 1990;323:1246)

Rx: Cimetidine (Tagamet) + diphenhydramine (Benadryl) (or any other H_2 + H_1 blocker combination) decrease flush sx (Nejm 1979;300:236)

Somatostatin analog (octreotide) sc q 8-12 hr controls flushing and diarrhea sx (Med Let 1989;31:66; Nejm 1986;315:663) by blocking somatostatin receptors on the tumor (Nejm 1990; 323:1246)

Streptozocin and 5-FU or cyclophosphamide for malignant types

Surgical rx of appendiceal types: Simple appendectomy if < 2 cm or elderly; right colectomy if > 2 cm irrespective of degree of wall or other invasion (Nejm 1987;317:1699)

of metastatic disease: Hepatic artery occlusion followed by 2-drug chemoRx (Ann IM 1994;120:302); perhaps liver transplant

Small Bowel Ischemia/Infarction

Cause: Thrombosis, embolism, hypotension associated with atherosclerosis, hypercoaguable states

Epidem: Embolic from Afib or MI; thrombosis from atherosclerosis, low-flow hypotensive states, rarely birth control pills (Nejm 1968;279:1213)

Pathophys: Superior mesenteric artery or vein (Nejm 1997;336:567) thrombosis

Sx: Acute: Sudden onset, pain disproportionate to physical findings
Chronic: h/o weight loss, pc abdominal pain for days to weeks; pain, often radiating to back; abdominal distention within 24 hr

Si: Decreased bowel tones; guaiac-positive stool

Crs: In acute ischemia, w/o surgery, nearly all die (Nejm 1969;281:309); some pts survive with surgery, especially those with incidents that are embolic in origin

Cmplc: r/o **mesenteric venous thrombosis** (Nejm 2001;345:1683) w abdominal pain and pos guaiac (50%), then bowel infarction; dx w abdominal CT (90% sens); rx w anticoagulation, and surgery if clinically forced

Lab: *Hem:* Elevated wbc
Paracentesis: Rbc's, wbc's; and bacteria late in course

Xray: Mesenteric arteriogram

Rx: of acute syndrome: Endarterectomy and limited bowel
resection

of abdominal angina: Frequent small feedings; surgery, preferably
in anginal stage before infarction

6.6   Large Bowel Diseases

Appendicitis

Nejm 2003;348:236; Jama 1996;276:1589

Cause: Obstructed appendix from fecolith, lymphoid hyperplasia from
viral illness

Epidem: 7% lifetime risk; incidence in ER pts w abdominal pain < age
60 yr = 25%, > age 60 yr = 4%

Pathophys:

Sx: Nausea, anorexia; pain, periumbilical at first, then migrates to
right lower quadrant; < 72 hr duration; sensation of constipation
and urge to defecate

Si: Fever 37.5-38.5°C; < 101°F. Right lower quadrant guarding and
rebound tenderness; tenderness may be only on pelvic/rectal
exam or w heel pounding; later rigidity and diminished bowel
sounds; mass; any or all may be absent especially in elderly pts.

Crs: 12-24 hr

Cmplc: Perforation (20-25%) w peritonitis; perforation increases
prevalence of infertility × 5 (Nejm 1986;315:1506)

r/o PID; intussusception in children < age 4 yr; mesenteric
adenitis, including *Yersinia* pseudoappendicular syndrome (p 563)
(Nejm 1989;321:16); diverticulitis; typhilitis, a cecal colitis seen
w aggressive chemoRx of leukemia

Lab: *Hem:* CBC not sens or specif, but usually wbc about
10,000-13,000 with some left shift

Urine: Urinalysis often shows hematuria, suggesting ureteral impingement

Xray (Ann IM 2004;141:537):

1st: Spiral CT after Gastrografin enema (Nejm 1998;338:141), or plain CT w rectal contrast; combined w US in children has 94% sens and specif (Jama 1999;282:1041); especially useful in women and whenever dx equivocal

2nd: Ultrasound, 25% false neg, 0% false pos? (Nejm 1987; 317:666)

KUB not helpful

Rx: Surgery; w cefoxitin prophylactically perioperatively if perforation likely? Neg pathology in 15-20% overall despite current diagnostics (Jama 2001;286:1748), and in 45% of young women

Pain meds ok to use while w/u in progress (Acad Emerg Med 1996;3:1086; BMJ 1992;305:554)

Ischemic Colitis

BMJ 2003;326:1372

Cause: Atherosclerotic disease w low-flow states; embolic

Epidem:

Pathophys: Partial or full inferior mesenteric artery occlusion

Sx: Crampy and often bloody diarrhea

Si: Guaiac-positive stool

Crs: After initial acute illness, gradual scarring with lumen narrowing, which gradually normalizes

Cmplc: Strictures sometimes, although most heal

Lab: *Noninv:* Endoscopy w bx quite specific

Xray: Barium enema rarely done but has classic "thumbprints" in colon wall from mucosal hemorrhages

Rx: Surgery usually not necessary; watch for stricture later

Ulcerative Colitis

GE Clin N Am 2004;33:235

Cause: Genetic component (Ann IM 1989;110:786)

Epidem: Age of onset = 20-40 yr, occasionally younger (Nejm 1971; 285:17). Lower incidence in smokers and other nicotine users! (Nejm 1983;308:361) and in pts s/p appendectomy before age 20 (Nejm 2001;344:808).

Pathophys: Autoimmune?

Sx: Bloody diarrhea; cramps, poorly relieved with bowel movement; arthritis (20%), especially of hip, knee, ankle, pip joints, and full ankylosing spondylitis syndrome; fever and weight loss

Si: Friable rectal mucosa (positive "wipe test," ie, when bowel wall is wiped, punctate bleeding sites are seen; w flexible sigmoidoscope, usually manifested simply as more than usual "scope trauma"); clubbing; erythema nodosum; uveitis, though less common than in regional enteritis

Crs: Depends on rx

Cmplc:
- Carcinoma (Nejm 1990;323:1228), especially if diffuse disease; may be more malignant than usual colon cancer since it has a 25% 5-yr mortality
- Strictures
- Perforation and peritonitis, and/or megacolon
- Sclerosing cholangitis (p 351) (Ann IM 1985;102:581)
- Stress and depression result, but do not cause (Ann IM 1991; 114:381)
- **Pyoderma Gangrenosum** in < 5% of toxic pts, may occur even when bowel quiescent; present also in RA, IBD, myeloproliferative d/o's, paraproteinemias; must biopsy to be sure not another type of ulcers since steroid rx bad for most other causes (Nejm 2002;347:1412)

r/o other causes of acute diarrhea (p 401): *C.difficile* colitis (p 574); **ulcerative proctitis**, similar disease isolated to rectum, can get above it on sigmoidoscoy, rx w steroid enemas and mesalamine (Rowasa) 500 mg pr bid (Gut 1998;42:195); post-colostomy diversion colitis in empty colorectal segments, rx with instillation of short-chain fatty acids (Nejm 1989;320:23)

Lab: *Serol:* Ameba titers to r/o before starting steroids if a local risk
Noninv: Colonoscopy

Xray: KUB to r/o megacolon (6-8 cm diameter)

Rx   (Nejm 1996;334:841): Screening and surveillance for cancer:
Colonoscopic (Gastrointest Endosc Clin N Am 1997;7:1:129);
    perhaps q 1-2 yr with q 10 cm biopsies for dysplasia after
    8-10 yr of pancolitis vs q 5-10 yr unless sx change
of disease
Salicylates:

* Sulfasalazine (Azulfidine) as 500 mg tabs, 2-4 gm po qd (Ann IM 1984;101:377) or more up to 12 gm qd, active metabolite is 5-aminosalicylic acid (5-ASA); prophylactically keeps disease in remission (25% recurrence/yr: Lancet 1992;339:1279); much cheaper than 5-ASA meds; adverse effects (increased when > 4 gm qd in slow acetylators: Nejm 1973;289:491): allergic worsening of sx (Nejm 1982;306:409), rash that can be desensitized with increasing doses (Ann IM 1984;100:512)

* 5-Aminosalicylic acid (5-ASA) as
  Coated mesalamine (Asacol) (Ann IM 1991;115:350)
      400 mg po t-qid, very effective and works moderately
      well at 400 mg po b-qid to prevent recurrence (Ann
      IM 1996;124:205); or as
  Retention enema 60 cc to help left-sided disease (Med Let
      1988;30:53); or as
  Pentasa 500 mg; or as

Olsalazine (Dipentum), the 5-ASA dimer, 500 mg po bid
up to 1 gm bid; adverse effects: diarrhea (Med Let
1990;32:103); cost $25/wk; or

Balsalazide (Colazal) (Med Let 2001;43:62), a precursor;
2.25 gm po tid

Steroid enemas or systemically, eg, prednisone 60-80 mg po
qd, or ACTH 120 U/24 hr iv for severe flare; chronically try to
get off entirely, at least < 10 mg po qd to avoid adverse effects
(p 1072)

Ciprofloxacin? (GE 1998;115:1072) 500-750 mg po bid ×6
mo for resistant flares

Human monoclonal anti-integrin antibody to prevent T cell
in-migration works modestly at least short term (Nejm 2005;
352:2499)

6MP if can't get off steroids; some small cancer risk as well as
reversible problems (Ann IM 1989;111:642); cyclosporine
4 mg/kg iv qd helps 80% within 1 wk of those who fail iv steroids
for 1 wk when flaring (Nejm 1994;330:1841)

Nicotine 14+ mg patch qd helps many (Ann IM
1997;126:364; Nejm 1994;330:811,856) during acute phase only,
does not prevent recurrences (Nejm 1995;332:988)

Surgical colectomy with ileostomy usually cures, although
when it should be done is debatable; for recurrent flares, must do
if both iv steroid and iv cyclosporine fail (Nejm 1994;330:1841)

Diverticulitis/Diverticulosis

Nejm 1998;338:1521

Cause: Diverticulosis, which may be congenital but is usually acquired

Epidem: Diverticulosis prevalence = 5-10% over age 45, 80% over
age 85. Right-sided disease more common in Asians.
Diverticulitis occurs in 20% of pts w divertiuclosis; 20% of pts w
diverticulitis are < 50 yr old.

Pathophys (Nejm 1975;293:83): Low-residue diet leads to increased intracolonic pressures causing outpocketings (diverticula); diverticultis caused by micro and macro perforations

Sx: Left lower quadrant pain usually, though may be anywhere; fever; diarrhea intially often, then constipation

Si: Tenderness, mass in left lower quadrant; fever

Crs: Variable; < age 50, 33% recur over 10 yr; higher recurrence in older pts

Cmplc: Perforation; partial obstruction; abscess; fistulas; bleeding from diverticulosis alone, dx by colonoscopy acutely (Nejm 2000;342:78)

r/o right-sided **angiodysplasia of the colon**, often seen in elderly pts and associated with aortic stenosis

Lab: *Hem:* Elevated wbc and L shift

Xray: CT scan; ultrasonography; tagged red cell scan or angiography (Nejm 1972;286:450) to localize diverticular bleeding

Rx: Prevent w high-fiber diet; avoid opiates
Antibiotics for acute disease, eg, ciprofloxacin + metronidazole × 7-10 d po, or iv ampicillin + gentamicin + metronidazole
CT-guided percutaneous drainage if abscess > 5 cm diameter
Surgically staged colonic resection with temporary colostomy for perforation/abscess

Irritable Bowel Syndrome

Nejm 2003;349:2136, 2001;344:1846; Ann IM 1995;123:688

Cause: Unknown, perhaps bowel motility deficits, perhaps psychiatric/stress

Epidem: 10-20% prevalence; females > males; associated w sexual abuse in women; and w other functional gi disorders (Ann IM 1995;123:688); adult onset, almost all before age 50

Pathophys: Probably a heterogeneous mix of disorders, psychiatric dx's seem to increase reporting of sx but not disease prevalence

Sx: Alternating constipation and diarrhea; and/or abdominal pain ×
12+ wk, w mucous stools but no blood; bloating and sense of
incomplete emptying; in women, irritable bowel or dyspeptic sx
are associated w h/o sexual abuse in > 50% (Ann IM
1991;114:828)

Si: Usually normal exam; no weight loss, fever or gi bleeding

Crs:

Cmplc: r/o *Giardia,* IBD, colon cancer, bowel ischemia, impaction,
laxative abuse, malabsorption

Lab: *Chem:* TSH, chemistry profile
Endo: Flexible sigmoidoscopy
Hem: CBC, ESR
Stool: Commercial screens to r/o laxative abuse; O + P; Sudan
stain for fat; leukocytes

Rx (Am J Gastroenterol 2002;97:S7-26): Bran or other bulking
agents, $Al(OH)_3$ antacids; psychiatric care (GE 1991;100:450)

if predominantly diarrhea present: Low-dose tricylic antidepressants; perhaps alosetron (Lotronex) 1 mg po bid (Med Let
2002;44:67, 2000;42:53), pulled from market in 2000 due to
ischemic colitis but back at lower doses for severe cases, 1 mg po
qd-bid w special monitoring; loperamide (Imodium) 2-4 mg po
qid or diphenoxylate (Lomotil). If sx still persist, get *Giardia* antigen on stool and consider bile salt binding.

if predominantly constipation: SSRIs, or tegaserod
(Zelnorm) (ACP J Club 2004;141:44; Med Let 2002;44:79) 6 mg
po bid; a cisapride-like drug; for short-term use, moderately helpful, NNT = 15-20

if pain: Antispasmodics like dicyclomine (Bentyl) 10-20 mg
po t-qid; Librax t-qid; Donnatol t-qid

Colon Polyps and Cancer

Nejm 2000;342:1960

Cause: Neoplasia; at least 20% are clearly genetic (Nejm
1985;312:1540), a small number are autosomal dominant

Epidem: After lung cancer, 2nd most common cancer in U.S.; 6% lifetime risk, 130,000 incidence/yr in U.S., 60,000/yr die in U.S. Most arise from adenomatous polyps over years and decades (Ann IM 1993;118:91) and occasionally from villous adenomas, not hyperplastic polyps? (Ann IM 1990;113:760 vs Nejm 2000; 343:162,169). Adenomatous polyps themselves are associated w high-animal-fat, low-fiber diets (Ann IM 1993;118:91); lower adenoma/cancer rates w increased dietary fiber (Nejm 1999;340: 169,223) but such a diet does not decrease recurrence after a 1st polyp is removed (Nejm 2000;342:1149,1156).

Associated with family h/o cancer or adenomatous polyps (Ann IM 1998;128:900; Nejm 1996;334:82) in a 1st-degree relative, 2-5 (5, under age 45) × baseline rate if one such relative. Autosomal dominant multiple gi polyposis syndromes (adenomatous or hamartomatous or nonpolyposis syndromes) (Nejm 2003;348:919): **Familial Colonic Polyposis** and **Turcot** (colonic polyps and CNS tumors: Nejm 1995;332:839) **Syndromes** (gene defects on chomosome 5: Nejm 1993;329:1982, 1990;322:904); **Gardner's Syndrome** with pigmented retinal lesions (Nejm 1987;316:661); and **Peutz-Jegher Syndrome** of hamartomas throughout the gi tract, pigmented spots on lips, with gi bleeding and gi as well as breast and gyn cancers developing in > 50% (Ann IM 1998;128:896; Nejm 1987;316:1511); **Lynch Syndrome** (Jama 2005;293:1979,1986,2008; Ann IM 2003; 138:560), hereditary nonpolyposis colon cancer 80% lifetime risk, and cancer of endometrium, ovary, stomach, small bowel, biliary tree (Jama 1997;277:915). Polyposis syndromes are generally associated with distal cancers, whereas nonpolyposis genetic types are associated with proximal cancers and other cancers (esp endometrial) in the same pt and 1st-degree relatives and have defects in DNA repair genes (Nejm 1998;338:1481).

Also associated with *Streptococcus bovis* septicemia, where cancer is present 85% of the time (Ann IM 1979;91:560); ulcerative colitis sx > 10 yr (p 386); elevated cholesterol in men (Ann IM 1993;118:481)

Not associated with inguinal hernia (Nejm 1971;284:369)

Sx: Change in bowel habits; blood in stool or on toilet paper (ask in ROS; positive response associated w 24% prevalence of significant pathology: Jama 1997;277:44); abdominal cramps and other obstructive sx early with left-sided tumor, late with right-sided tumor

Si: Acanthosis nigrans (see p 337 for differential dx); palpable rectal or abdominal mass; blood in stool, gross or by guaiac

Crs: Duke's stage A(I); $T_{1-2}N_0M_0$: confined to submucosal area, 90% 5-yr survival with surgery

Stage B(II)$_A$; $T_3N_0M_0$: through muscularis mucosa, 60-80% 5-yr survival

Stage B(II)$_B$; $T_4N_0M_0$: through serosa, 45-70% 5-yr survival

Stage C(III)$_A$; $T_{1-2}N_1M_0$: <5 pos nodes, 30-40% 5-yr survival

Stage C(III)$_B$; $T_{3-4}N_1M_0$: > 5 pos nodes, 25% 5-yr survival

Stage D(IV); $T_{any}N_{any}M_{1+}$: widely metastatic, 0% 5-yr survival

Cmplc: Metastases; *S. bovis* endocarditis (Ann IM 1979;91:560; Nejm 1977;297:800)

r/o anal canal cancer (Nem 2000;342:792) caused by HPV, rx'd w radiation and chemoRx

Lab:

Endo: Sigmoidoscopy or colonoscopy for primary prevention (p 918)

Colonoscopy q 3-5 yr in pts who have had an adenomatous polyp removed (Nejm 1993;328:901), whether large or small, since 30% will have proximal neoplasia (Nejm 1997;336:8). Screen if one or more 1st-degree relatives had colon cancer or adenomatous polyps (Ann IM 1998;128:900), start at age 40 (ACS; Nejm 1994;331:1669).

Path: Histologic staging as above, each worse if blood vessel invasion

Adenomatous and/or villous polyps deserve full bowel w/u (Jama 1999;281:1611)

Serol: CEA to monitor for recurrence, but does not change survival

Stool: Screening occult blood testing (p 918)

Xray: Air contrast barium enema for sx if colonoscopy unsuccessful

Rx: Prevent w:

- ASA 81-325 mg po qd or b-tiw (Nejm 2003;348:883,891) w greater benefit w higher doses, up to 650 mg po qd reduces risk by 50% (retrospective nurses cohort study: Ann IM 2004;140:157,224); or other NSAIDs like ibuprofen (GE 1998;114:441; Nejm 1995;333:609), sulindac (Clinoril) (Ann IM 1991;115:952 vs Nejm 2002;346:1054); all shown to decrease recurrent polyps but may not be worth the bleeding risks, probably work by inhibiting cyclooxygenase (COX-2) found in aggressive colon cancer (Nejm 2000;342:1960; Jama 1999;282:1254)
- Calcium qd in low-fat dairy products (Nejm 1999;340:101; Jama 1998;280:1074)
- Folate qd × yrs may reduce absolute risk ×30% after 15 yr (NNT-15 = 3) (Ann IM 1998;129:517); perhaps genetic screening for adenomatous polyposis coli gene if positive family hx (Nejm 1997;336:823). Vitamins E, C, and A (β-carotene) do not prevent (Nejm 1994;331:141).

Surgical excision by laparotomy or colonoscopy; prophylactic removal of adenomatous polyps, even those < 1 cm (Nejm 1993;329:1977), decreases cancer rate by 90%

Chemotherapy (Nejm 2005;352:476, 2004;350:2406; Med Let 2004;49:46) post-op for stage C(III) w adjuvant 5-FU and levamisole + radiation

Palliation of advanced disease prolongs median survival from 2 mo w 5-FU alone to > 21 mo but is it worth the $15,000/mo cost (Nejum 2004;351:317, 337)

Cytotoxic agents:

- 5-FU + leucovorin iv qd × 5 d q 4-5 wk; or
- Oral 5-FU (capecitabine); or
- Oxaliplatin (Eloxatin) (Nejm 2004;350:2343); or

Monoclonal antibodies vs endothelial growth factor like:

- Cetuximab (Erbitux) or evacizumab (Avastin) (Nejm 2004;350:2335), costs $1000/wk; or
- Irinotecan (Camptosar) (Nejm 2000;343:905) iv weekly ($1000/dose: Med Let 1997;38:8)

f/u after resection beyond pursuit of sx and q 3-5 yr colonscopy not justified (Nejm 2004;350:2375)

of liver mets: Resection then hepatitic artery chemoRx (Nejm 1999;341:2039)

in rectal cancer: Pre-op radiation (Jama 2000;284:1008; Nejm 1997;336:980) and chemoRx (Nejm 2004;351:1731) and AP resection, but latter has post-op sexual dysfunction in $^1/_3$ of pts; helped by adjuvant radiation and 5-FU more than colonic, but trade prolongation of life for toxicity (Nejm 1994;331:502, 1991;324:709)

Groin Hernias (Femoral, Indirect, and Direct Inguinal)

Jama 1997;277:663

Cause: Indirect is usually due to congenital failure to close processus vaginalis combined w increased intra-abdominal pressure, eg, from coughing or something else; direct from a defect in transversalis fascia

Epidem: Male/female = 25:1.

Pathophys: Direct inguinal protrudes anteriorly, often bilateral
Indirect goes down inguinal canal, can go to scrotum
Femoral (3%)

Sx: Fullness, bulge, pain

Si: Hernia present, at least w straining when standing

Crs:

Cmplc: Strangulation, most often in 1st 3 mo; most often w femoral type (> 50%)

Lab:

Xray:

Rx: Trusses for direct and indirect types help some
          Various surgical repairs; mesh repair has a 3-yr 23% recurrence rate, compared to 42% recurrence w suture repair? (Dutch: Nejm 2000;343:392); open repairs have a lower recurrence, but laparoscopic repairs allow faster recovery (Nejm 2004;350:1819, 1895)

6.7 Miscellaneous

Abdominal Pain, Nonsurgical

Causes: angioedema, hereditary and acquired; porphyria and lead poisoning; familial Mediterranean fever; thrombotic thrombocytopenic purpura; sickle cell crisis; paroxysmal hemoglobinuria (PNH); anaphylactoid purpura and other vasculitides; urticaria pigmentosa and all causes of urticaria; abdominal epilepsy?

Anal Fissure

Nejm 1998;338; 257

Epidem: Common, > 10% of rectal complaints

Pathophys: Once started, perpetuated by firm bowel movements. Associated w and perpetuated by spasm of internal (not external) anal sphincter (Nejm 1999;341:65)

Sx: Rectal pain

Si: Posterior (90%) fissure/ulcer between anal verge and dentate line; skin tag at anal verge; prominent proximal papilla

Cmplc: r/o inflammatory bowel disease, especially if not posterior

Rx (Nejm 1999;341:65):

- 1st: Nitroglycerine 0.2% ointment (nitropaste diluted ×10) bid × 6 wk; 60% cure; adverse effects: headache
- 2nd: Botulinum toxin injections (Nejm 1998;338:217) 20 U in each side of anal sphincter; 96% cure
- 3rd: Surgical lateral internal sphincterotomy; 90-95% cure; cmplc: permanent weakness of anal sphincter w gas, mucus, and rarely stool leakage

Colonic Distention, Acute Nonobstructive (Ogilivie's Syndrome), Pseudo-obstruction

Epidem: Hospitalized pts

Crs: 40% recur

Cmplc: 3% perforate and have 50% mortality

Xray: KUB shows colon diameter > 10 cm

Rx: Colonoscopic decompression helps 70%
Neostigmine 2 mg iv (Nejm 1999;341:137) helps 90%

Constipation

Nejm 2003;349:1360

Cause: Drugs, diet, colon lesions, hypothyroid, autonomic neuropathies, hypocalcemia

Sx: Abdominal cramps; < 3 stools/wk

Si: Abdominal mass from stool

Cmplc: Fecal impaction (Nejm 1989;321:658) with fever, dyspnea, encopresis (diarrhea around a fecal impaction) (Ped Rv 1998;19:22; Ped Clin N Am 1996;43:279; Clin Ped 1991;30:669) especially in children age 3-5

r/o hypothyroidism, Hirschsprung's in children (rarely have fecal incontinence)

Rx: Laxatives:
1st: Fiber 20-25 gm qd
2nd: Psyllium (Metamucil, etc)
3rd: Sorbitol (Cystosol) 70% soln, 30-60 cc po hs
- Lactulose (p 372) with fewer side effects and cheaper (Am J Med 1990;89:597)
- Polyethylene glycol (PEG) (Miralax, Colyte, GoLytely) tbsp/8 oz water qd
- Emollients like dioctyl Na succinate (Colace, Surfak)
- Lubricants like mineral oil
- Mg compounds like milk of magnesia
- Stimulant/irritants like cascara, senna, and castor oil
of **Encopresis:** Bisacodyl (Dulcolax) 5 mg ii tabs po qd with mineral oil; enemas if football-sized stool

Fecal Incontinence

Nejm 1992;326:1002

Cause: Diarrhea; overflow from impactions (encopresis—see above); rectal neoplasms; neurologic, eg, myelomeningocele, MS, dementia, CVA, neuropathy, cord lesions; abnormal pelvic floor, eg, congenital and trauma especially from obstetrics, aging, and pelvic floor denervation

Epidem: Especially common in elderly pts

Rx: 1st: High-fiber diet, loperamide (Imodium), diphenoxylate (Lomotil), enemas if impacted
2nd: Biofeedback
3rd: Surgery

Hiccoughs

Cause: Lower esophageal obstruction as in achalasia or stricture (Ann IM 1991;115:711)

Rx: 1 tsp dry sugar (Nejm 1971;285:1489)

Liver Bx Techniques

Nejm 2001;344:495, 1970;283:582 [Menghini]; place in w/u of elevated LFTs (Ann IM 1989;111:472)

Nausea and Vomiting

Also see rx for chemoRx induction p 440

- Vagal stimulation directly: Gagging or stomach distention > 20 mm Hg; uterine, bladder, renal distension; elevated CNS pressure

Rx: Diphenhydramine (Benadryl) 25-50 mg po q 6 hr, since both antihistamine and anticholinergic effects

- Labyrinthine stimulation causing cerebellar nausea, eg, motion sickness and all diseases affecting middle ear

Rx: Dimenhydrinate (Dramamine) best; scopolamine patch (Transderm V); or meclizine (Antivert) 25 mg po bid

- Medullary chemoreceptor trigger zone stimulation by morphine, digoxin, tetracycline, oncologic chemoRx, disulfiram (Antabuse), estrogens, uremia, radiation, cancer, toxins, anesthetics

Rx:

Phenothiazines like prochlorperazine (Compazine) 10 mg iv/im, better than promethazine (Phenergan) (Ann EM 2000; 36:89); chlorpromazine (Thorazine)

Metoclopramide (Reglan) iv helps during cisplatin chemoRx

Marijuana (Nejm 1975;293:795); tetrahydrocannabinol po or smoked (Ann IM 1979;91:819), better than Compazine? (Nejm 1980;302:135 vs Ann IM 1979;91:825)

Serotonin antagonists (Med Let 2004;46:27; Nejm 1990;322: 810,816) ondansetron, gransetron, palonosetron, or dolasetron, better than metoclopramide

Droperidol (Inapsine) (Med Let 2002;44:53) 0.625-1.25 mg iv, esp for post-op nausea and vomiting; adverse effects: QT prolongation and torsades

Nabilone 2 mg po q 6-8 hr (Nejm 1979;300:1295)

Peritonitis

Sx: Pain w cough (78% sens/specif-BMJ 1994;308:1336)

Si: Rebound, pain w pelvic shake, heel percussion pain

Diarrhea

See Nejm 2004;351:2421

Acute: Gastroenteritis causes and w/u: Am J Med 1999;106:670; Nejm 2004;350:38

Following list is grouped by fever and fecal leukocyte findings (see individual diseases on each cause as well). Work it up if fever, fecal blood, fecal leukocytes (73% sens, 84% specif for inflammatory disease) or immunoassay for neutrophil lactoferrin (92% sens, 79% specif), sx > 5 d, known exposures (Ann IM 1986;105:785), HIV-positive or otherwise impaired host, traveler on return home, severe volume depletion, or community outbreak.

if fever and/or fecal leukocytes present, consider empiric rx (Med Let 1998;40:47) on day 1 with ciprofloxacin 500 mg po × 1 dose (Lancet 1994;334: 1537) or bid × 3 d + loperamide (Imodium) ii 2 mg tabs, then i/stool up to 8 pills qd, lower doses for children (Ann IM 1991;114:731; safe in all adults: Ann IM 1993;118:377); unless it might be due to Salmonella, C. *difficile*, or O157:H E. *coli* where both antibiotic and antimotility rx worsen disease

if no fever, blood, or mucus, give loperamide as above w simethicone 250 mg/dose (Arch Fam Med 1999;8:243)

Rehydration and supportive care for all, like oral rehydration solution (p 1010); bismuth subsalicylate (Pepto-Bismol) 60 cc in adults or 1.14 cc/kg (100 mg/kg) in children helps speed recovery (Nejm 1993;328:1635, Peds 1991;87:18), as does zinc gluconate 20 mg po qd within 1st 3 d in 3rd World children (Nejm 1995; 333:839); perhaps racecadotril 1.5 mg/kg po q 8 hr in children (Nejm 2000;343:463)

Chronic (> 4 wk) (Nejm 1995;332:725)

Cause: In order of frequency: chronic infection, inflammatory and irritable bowel disease, steatorrhea, carbohydrate malabsorption, medications/food additives, previous surgery w bacterial overgrowth, endocrine (adrenal insufficiency, hyper/hypothyroidism, diabetes mellitus), laxative abuse, ischemic bowel, radiation enteritis, colon cancer, idiopathic/functional, microscopic colitis (Am J Med 2000;108:416) from either collagenous or lymphocytic colitis that presents as chronic watery diarrhea, have a normal-appearing mucosa on endoscopy but abnormal pathlogy on bx

Pathophys: Bacterial gut wall invasion; enterotoxin production; bacterial adherence to epithelial cell membrane cytotoxin production; unabsorbed solutes causing osmotic diarrhea; deconjugated bile salts and hydroxylated fatty acids; congenital/familial absorptive/ secretory abnormalities; Zollinger-Ellison syndrome, vasoactive intestinal peptide, calcitonin, carcinoid tumors; diabetic autonomic neuropathy; factitious from laxative use, or water dilution of stool (Nejm 1994;330:1418)

Crs: Of idiopathic diarrhea, if w/u neg, is benign and resolves in < 4 yr (Nejm 1992;327:1849)

Lab: *Chem:* Lytes, BUN/creat, TSH, T_4, gastrin, VIP if > 1 L/d
Hem: CBC, ESR
Endo: Sigmoid/colonoscopy w bx
Stool: For fecal leukocytes, O+P × 3 before barium studies, pH, 24-hr weight, 72-hr fat

Xray: KUB, UGIS and SBFT, BE

Rx: Somatostatin analog octreotide (Ann IM 1991;115:705); vera-pamil; loperamide (Imodium) 2 mg tabs up to 8 qd in adults; cholestyramine; antibiotics

6.8   Causes of Diarrhea

P = polys, B = bloody (see Nejm 2004;351:2421)

Amebic Diarrhea

P (p 633)

Epidem: Rare

Pathophys: Colonic wall invasion

Sx: Incubation period weeks to months

Si: Fever, fecal leukocytes often present; friable rectal mucosa; alter-nating constipation and diarrhea

Lab: Antibody titers best; O+P

Rx: Rehydration and supportive care; metronidazole (Flagyl), etc

Bacillus cereus Diarrhea

(p 529)

Epidem: Rare in U.S.; from refried rice

Pathophys: Heat-stable toxin produced on small bowel mucosa

Sx: Incubation period 1-6 hr for nausea and vomiting; 6-24 hr for diarrhea

Si: No fever, no fecal leukocytes present

Lab:

Rx: Rehydration and supportive care symptomatic

Campylobacter Diarrhea

PB (Ann IM 1983;98:360; Nejm 1981;305:1444) (p 546)

Epidem: 5% of all acute diarrheas; increased in gay males (Ann IM 1984;101:338)

Pathophys: Fecal-oral, via water; from domestic animals sometimes; present in ileum, jejunum, and colon

Sx: Incubation period 1-7 d

Si: Half have fever, fecal leukocytes present, can lead to chronic colitis, 20% last > 1 wk

Lab: Culture in 10% CO_2 for 48 hr on special medium

Rx: Rehydration and supportive care; cipro if lasts > 3 d, or erythromycin

Clostridium difficile

P (p 574)

Epidem: Common after antibiotic use, especially in elderly pts

Pathophys: Overgrowth usually after po antibiotics, especially clindamycin; produces toxin

Sx: Incubation period

Si: Fever, fecal leukocytes sometimes present

Lab: Stool toxin titer

Rx: Rehydration and supportive care; metronidazole; vancomycin if no response or severe illness

Clostridium perfringens Diarrhea

(p 575)

Epidem: 3rd most common cause of foodborne diarrhea after staph and salmonella

Pathophys: Toxin

Sx: Incubation period 12 hr

Si: No fever, no fecal leukocytes present, mild diarrhea only, no vomiting

Lab:

Rx: Rehydration and supportive care

Colitis, Ulcerative/Granulomatous

P (p 386)

Epidem: Incidence = 1-2/yr in primary care practice

Pathophys: Colon and/or small bowel IBD

Sx: Bloody diarrhea

Si: Fever sometimes, fecal leukocytes sometimes, friable rectal mucosa

Lab: Biopsy bowel

Rx: Rehydration and supportive care; steroids, salicylates

Colitis, Herpes II

P

Epidem: In gay males

Pathophys:

Sx: Incubation period days to weeks

Si: Often fever, fecal leukocytes present, severe pain, urinary hesitancy in 50% and/or sacral paresthesias in 25% (Nejm 1983;308:868)

Lab: Tzanck prep or culture

Rx: Rehydration and supportive care; acyclovir

Colitis, Ischemic

P (p 386)

Epidem: Rare, except in elderly pts

Pathophys: Inferior mesenteric occlusion

Sx: Incubation period minutes to hours

Si: Late fever, polys present, friable rectal mucosa

Rx: Rehaydration and other supportive care

Cryptosporidiosis *(Cryptosporidium parvum)*

Nejm 1995;332:855 (p 632)

Epidem: Animal- (especially young ones like calves) or human-contaminated public water supplies (Nejm 1996;334:19, 1989;320:1372), swimming pools (Jama 1994;272:1597) or animal-feces–contaminated food (Maine cider epidemic: Jama 1994;272:1592); more frequent in immunocompromised pts, eg, with AIDS, infants in day care, tropical developing countries; common, 25% of U.S. adults have antibodies

Pathophys: Oocytes are resistant to chlorine, takes only 30-150 to infect

Sx: Diarrhea, can be dehydrating in HIV pts

Si: Self-limited in immunocompetent pts (Nejm 1983;308:1252)

Cmplc: Chronic cholecystitis in AIDS pts, often fatal (Nejm 1996; 334:19)

Lab: *Bact:* Positive acid-fast stain of stool pos

Rx: Rehydration and supportive care; nitazoxanide or alternatives

E. coli (Invasive)

Especially 0157:H7; PB (p 548) (Am J Pub Hlth 1997;87:176; Ann IM 1995;123:698; Nejm 1995;333:364)

Epidem: Most common cause of infectious bloody diarrhea in U.S. From manure and manure dust (Jama 2003;290:2709) contamination of hamburger, drinking water, swimming beaches (Nejm 1994;331:579).

Pathophys: Colon wall invasion and toxin production

Sx: Incubation period 1-3 d

Si: Low-grade fever, fecal leukocytes often present, initial watery stool becomes bloody; hemolytic-uremic syndrome and TTP

Lab: Stool cultures on sorbitol-MacKonky agar; stool toxin titers

Rx: Rehydration and supportive care; cipro or Tm/S DS bid × 3 d (Ann IM 1987;106:216) if must but avoiding antibiotic rx may prevent HUS (Nejm 2000;342:1930)

E. coli (Toxigenic) Diarrhea

Epidem: Common

Pathophys: Toxin

Sx: Incubation period 12-24 hr

Si: No fever, no fecal leukocytes present

Lab:

Rx: Rehydration and supportive care; ciprofloxacin

Gonorrhea and Chlamydia Diarrhea

P

Epidem: In gay males (Nejm 1983;309:576)

Pathophys: Rectal wall invasion

Sx: Incubation period

Si: Fever, fecal leukocytes present, friable rectal mucosa; r/o syphilis

Lab: Gram stain and culture

Rx: Rehydration and supportive care antibiotics to patient and partners

Lymphogranuloma venereum Colitis

P

Epidem: High incidence in gay males

Pathophys: Rectal wall invasion

Sx: Incubation period

Si: Often fever, fecal leukocytes present

Lab: Titers, culture

Rx: Rehydration and supportive care; tetracycline, or erythromycin

Norwalk Virus Diarrhea

Ann IM 1982;96:756; Am J Pub Hlth 1982;72:1329

Epidem: Epidemic, $^1\!/_2$ of all nonbacterial epidemics; spread by fecal oral route, eg, contaminated oysters (Jama 1995;273:466); a calcivirus

Pathophys: Small bowel invasion

Sx: Incubation period 24-48 hr

Si: No fever, no fecal leukocytes present, vomiting > diarrhea in children, reverse in adults; r/o other viral gastroenteritis causes (Nejm 1991;325:252) including rotavirus, enteric adenovirus, and astrovirus especially in small children (Nejm 1991;324:1757)

Lab:

Rx: Rehydration and supportive care

Rotavirus Diarrhea

Epidem: Episodic in individuals, especially infants < 2 yr in 3rd World; 20 deaths and 50,000 hospitalizations annually in U.S.; nearly 1 million die annually worldwide in developing countries

Pathophys: Small bowel invasion; immunity develops w recurrent infections (Nejm 1996;335:1022)

Sx: Incubation period

Si: May have fever, no fecal leukocytes present

Lab: Stool ELISA antigen test

Rx: Tetravalent po vaccine; 60-80% effective in infants but causing intussceptions in 1/5000-10,000 (Nejm 2001;344:564) so
pulled from U.S. market in 1999
Rehydration and supportive care

Salmonella spp. Diarrhea

PB (p 567)

Epidem: 4% of all acute diarrheas, 2nd most frequent cause of food
poisoning after staph

Pathophys: Small bowel invasion

Sx: Incubation period 12-36 hr

Si: Fever, may have fecal leukocytes present

Lab: Culture

Rx: Rehydration and supportive care

Salmonella typhi Diarrhea

PB (p 566)

Epidem: Rare

Pathophys: Colonic wall invasion

Sx: Incubation period 12-36 hr

Si: Fever, may have fecal leukocytes present

Lab: Culture

Rx: Rehydration and supportive care; ciprofloxacin

Shigella Diarrhea

PB (Nejm 1971;285:831)

Epidem: 3% of all acute diarrheas, especially in children and
retarded pts

Pathophys: Wall invasion

Sx: Incubation period 1-2 d

Si: Fever, fecal leukocytes present

Lab: Cultures

Rx: Rehydration and supportive care; Tm/S

Staphylococcal Diarrhea

Epidem: Very common; most common form of food poisoning

Pathophys: Small bowel heat-stable toxin; only toxin that does not stick to bowel wall

Sx: Incubation period 2-8 hr

Si: No fever, no fecal leukocytes, nausea and vomiting often worse than diarrhea

Lab: None indicated

Rx: Rehydration and supportive care

Vibrio cholera and *parahemolyticus* Diarrhea

(p 571)

Epidem: Rare

Pathophys: Toxin inhibits Na pump

Sx: Incubation period 1-3 d

Si: No fever, no fecal leukocytes present

Lab:

Rx: Rehydration and supportive care; tetracyline?

Vibrio mimicus, etc, Diarrhea

Ann IM 1983;99:169

Epidem: Handlers of seawater, especially in oysters

Pathophys:

Sx: Incubation period 3-72 hr

Si: Half have fever, sometimes fecal leukocytes present, otitis media often

Lab: Culture

Rx: Rehydration and supportive care; tetracycline?

Yersinia Colitis

PB (p 563)

Epidem: Rare, except occasionally in epidemics

Pathophys: Cholera-like enterotoxin in small bowel

Sx: Incubation period long

Si: Fever, fecal leukocytes present, indolent despite rx; immune complex si and sx

Lab: Cultures best; antibody titers (30% false neg)

Rx: Rehydration and supportive care; tetracycline

Other Rare Causes of Diarrhea, Especially in Immunocompromised Hosts

Intestinal spore-forming protozoa:
- *Cyclospora cayetanensis* (p 633)
- *Enterocytozoon bienensis*, intracellular microsporidial protozoan; causes diarrhea and cholangitis (Nejm 1993; 328:95; Ann IM 1993;119:895); effectively rx'd w fumagillin (Nejm 2002;346:1963)
- *Isospora belli* (p 633)

Anaerobes:
- *Plesiomonas*, invasive anaerobe (Ann IM 1986;105:690)
- *Aeromonas*, toxin producer, facultative anaerobe (Ann IM 1986;105:683)

GASTROENTEROLOGY

Chapter 7

Geriatrics

D. K. Onion and K. Gershman

7.1 Osteoporosis

Ann IM 1995;123:452 (men); Nejm 1992;327:620; Bull Rheum Dis 1988;38(2):1

Cause: See Table 7.1 (D. Spratt 9/95)

Table 7.1   Causes of Osteoporosis

Acromegaly	Hyperthyroidism
Alcoholism	Idiopathic, at least some of which is
Anorexia (Ann IM 2000;133:790)	genetic in structure of bone matrix
Cushing's disease/syndrome (even 10 mg	protein (Nejm 1998;338:1016)
prednisone qd enough), including	Malabsorption
chronic steroid use even inhaled in	Myeloma
asthmatics (Nejm 2001;345:941) and	Puberty, late onset, at least in men
rheumatoid arthritis (Ann IM 1993;	(Nejm 1992;326:600)
119:963)	Renal calcium leak (rx'd w thiazides)
Diabetes, type I	Scurvy
Estrogen deficiency in postmenopausal	Vitamin A chronic excessive intake
women or amenorrheic athletes (Nejm	> 3000 μgm/d (Jama 2002;287:2815;
1984;311:277); hypogonadotrophic	Ann IM 1998;129:770)
hypogonadism in men	Vitamin D wintertime deficiency (Jama
Homocystinuria (Nejm 2004;305:2033,	1995;274:1683)
2042)	Vitamin D antagonist meds like
Hyperparathyroidism	phenytoin

Epidem: More in female smokers from changes in estrogen metabolism (Nejm 1994;330:387, 1985;313:973); less frequent in blacks and Polynesians because they start with higher adolescent bone densities (Nejm 1991;325:1597). Osteopenia/porosis present in 42%/7% of U.S. women > age 50 (Jama 2001;286:2815).

Pathophys (Nejm 1988;318:818): Perhaps from increased prolactin premenopausally (Nejm 1980;303:1571) and/or simple estrogen deficiency postmenopausally. In athletes and other younger women, the problem is either the estrogen deficiency and/or progesterone deficiency from short or absent luteal phase regardless of whether pt is athlete (Nejm 1990;323:1221).

Sx: Bone pain, especially vertebral; fractures

Si: Decreased height/kyphosis from vertebral compression fractures, measure w rib–pelvis distance ≤ 2 fingerbreadths (Jama 2004; 292:2890)

Crs: Chronic, slowly progressive

Cmplc: Rib and vertebral fractures (Nejm 1983;309:265)
r/o causes listed in Table 7.1 when premature, ie, in men < 70 and women < 60 yr

Lab: *Chem:* PTH, serum and urine calcium to r/o hyperparathyroid and renal calcium leak in asx postmenopausal type (D. Spratt 9/95)

Xray: Osteopenic bones and fractures
Screening debatable (NIH/CDC: Jama 2001;285:785), using:
- Densitometry (Nejm 1991;324:1105; 1987;316:212) w dual xray absorptiometry (Med Let 1996;38:103) of hip most important since vertebrae often falsely dense though if very low, should pursue secondary causes aggressively; T scores (standard deviation from mean density of 30-yr-old woman); fx risk varies by a factor of 2 for each SD above or below the T score mean; osteopenia = 1-2.5 SD's below that mean, osteoporosis

≥ 2.5 SD's below mean w a $5^+\times$ increased risk of fx; Z score is SD's from same age group; scores take $2+$ yr to change w rx (Jama 2000;283:1318) and are not useful to follow (Jama 2000; 283:1318); cost = $50

- Quantitative CT scan, but is not standardized or useful (UCLA 9/02)

Rx (Med Let 2000;42:97; Nejm 1998;338:736): All preventive or instituted to slow the progression (Med Let 1992;34:101) and work to prevent the steroid-induced type as well (Nejm 1993; 329:1406)

Weight-bearing exercise (Nejm 1996;124:187; Ann IM 1988;108:824)

Smoking cessation; helps exercise and allows protective effect of estrogens (Ann IM 1992;116:716)

Calcium replacement therapy (Med Let 2000;42:29), as $CaCO_3$, 1-1.5 gm of elemental Ca^{++}/d; milk has 300 mg Ca^{++}/cup; chewable Tums 200 or 500 mg/tab; Oscal 500 mg/tab (Med Let 1989;31:101); Ca citrate (Citracal) 315 mg/tab, but absorbed better especially in pts on PPI/achlorhydrics/elderly (Nejm 1985;313:70); all come w 200 IU vitamin D/500 mg of Ca^{++}; $5-7/mo. Substantial effect even without estrogen (Ann IM 1994; 120:97), eg, 50% less loss/yr (Nejm 1993;328:460).

Vitamin D as 225-400 IU qd (400 IU in multivitamins) or calcitriol (D_3) 0.25 µgm po bid markedly decreases fractures without producing stones by preventing increased PTH of winter at least (Nejm 1993;327:1637, 1992;326:357, 1989;321:1777; Ann IM 1991;115:505); one RCT finds no effect? (Ann IM 1996;124:400)

Bisphosphonates; long-term (10+ yr) side effects unknown; all around $55/mo

- Alendronate (Fosamax) (Med Let 2001;43:26; Nejm 1995; 333:1437) 10 mg po qd or 70 mg q 1 wk clearly helps prevent progression over 10 yr, NNT-3 = 10-30 (Nejm 2004;350:1189;

Lancet 1996;348:1535), or 5 mg po qd or 35 mg q 1 wk for prevention in osteopenic and/or high-risk women (eg, on steroids); adverse effects: various gi sx, rarely chemical esophagitis esp if not taken w lots of fluids and pill sits on esophageal mucosa (Nejm 1996;335:1016)

- Risedronate (Actonel) (Med Let 2002;44:87; Jama 1999; 282:1344) 2.5-5 mg po qd, or 35 mg/wk; decreases hip fx in elderly women, NNT-3 = 90 (Nejm 2001;344:333) vs NNT-1 = 12 (J Am Ger Soc 2004;52:1832)
- Etidronate (Didronel) (Nejm 1997;337:382)
- Pamidronate (Aredia), esp if on steroids or leuprolide (Nejm 2001;345:948) rx; 60 mg iv q 3-12 mo
- Zoledronate (Zometa) (Nejm 2002;346:653; Med Let 2001;43:110) 2-4 mg iv q 1-12 mo; like generic pamindronate but infuses over 15 min unlike 2 hr w pamindronate; cost $850/4 mg

Calcitonin (Cibacalcin) 100 IU sc/im or 200 IU nasally qd; also relieves acute fx pain possibly via opiate effect (J Fam Pract 1992;35:93), not as good as alendronate (J Clin Endocrinol Metab 2000;85:1783); nasal $60/mo, sc/im $225/mo

Statin drug rx of increased cholesterol also helps slow osteoporosis? (Jama 2000;283:3205,3211,3255; Lancet 2000;355:2185 vs Ann IM 2003;139:97; Jama 2001;285:1850)

Thiazides help bone density and fx rate (Ann IM 2003;139:476, 2000;133:516) w/o adverse lipid effects (J Am Ger Soc 2003;51:340) as do β-blockers (Jama 2004;292:1326)

Folic acid 5 mg po qd and B_{12} to lower homocysteine levels (Nejm 2004;350:2033,2042,2089) and fx rates (NNT = 14) (Jama 2005;293:1082,1121)

Estrogen replacement therapy (p 838) is a substantial benefit during rx (Jama 2004;291:2212) but not worth the cardiovascular and breast cancer risks (Jama 2003;290:1739); or selective estrogen receptor modulators (p 838) like raloxifene (Evista) (Med Let 1998;40:29) 60 mg po qd; or androgens in men if hypogonadal

Strontium ranelate 2 gm po qd (Nejm 2004;350:459,504) perhaps; still in trials in Europe

NaF in slow-release form 25 mg po bid (Med Let 1996;38:3) or 20 mg qd, 12 mo on, 2 mo off, appears to decrease fx rates in spine when given w 1000+ mg Ca (Ann IM 1998;129:1, 1995; 123:401,466), but is controversial

Parathyroid hormone sc daily either as 40 μgm of the 34 aa fragment, or 100 μgm of the full 84 aa PTH, NNT = 10 (Nejm 2001;344:1434; Arch IM 2002;162:2297); effects inhibited by concurrent bipohosphonate rx (Nejm 2003;349:1207,1216,1277)

Vertebroplasty w polymethylmethacrylate (J Neurosurg 2003;98:36; Clin Ger Med 2004;12:32)

7.2 Falls in the Elderly

Ann IM 1994;121:442; Nejm 1994;331:821

Cause (J Am Ger Soc 1988;36:266): Accidents especially in home (37%), weakness/balance/gait problems (12%), drop attacks (11%), unknown (8%), dizziness or vertigo (7%), orthostatic hypotension (5%), CNS events (1%), syncope (1%); and (combined = 18%) acute illnesses, confusional states, visual impairments (Nejm 1991;324:1326), and drugs (> 4 meds a risk factor) such as long-acting benzodiazepines (J Am Ger Soc 2000; 48:682), tricyclics, and phenothiazines (Nejm 1987;316:363) as well as other psychoactive drugs (J Am Ger Soc 1999;47:30) especially in nursing homes (Nejm 1992;327:168); trazodone and SSRIs only slightly less risky than TCAs (Nejm 1998;339:875); and paradoxically increased by restraints (J Am Ger Soc 1999;47: 1202; Ann IM 1992;116:369). Bifocal glasses increase rates by 40% (J Am Ger Soc 2002;50:1760).

Epidem: 30% of elderly > 65 yr, 50% of those > 80 yr living in the community fall each year (Nejm 1997;337:1279); 10% of those sustain serious injury, 6% fracture something. Over 50% of all nursing home pts fall during their stay (J Am Ger Soc 1995;43:

1257) because of greater frailty and better reliability of reporting (J Am Ger Soc 1988;36:266); in nursing homes, higher rates at shift change and w lower staffing ratios (Primary Care 1989; 16:377; J Am Ger Soc 1987;35:503).

Majority occur during mild–moderate activity, especially in bedroom or bathroom, walking, stepping up or down, or changing position; 70% at home; 10% on stairs, descending worse than ascending (Age Aging 1979;8:251); > 50% accidents are due to environmental hazards: cords, furniture, small objects, optical patterns on escalators, stairs, floors (Clin Ger Med 1985;1:555).

Females > males, whites > blacks

Active elderly at greater risk of injury than frail elderly? (J Am Ger Soc 1991;39:46)

Pathophys: Fx risk from falls increased in elderly because of decreased energy absorption capability of tissue and impaired protective responses like reaction time, muscle strength, level of alertness, cognition (J Gerontol 1991;46:M164)

Sx: H/o hypotensive sx posturally, postprandially, on micturation; may have h/o PAT, SSS, AS, hemiplegia, neuropathy, seizures, anemia, hypothyroidism, poor nutritional status, ETOH abuse, intercurrent illness (UTI, pneumonia, CHF); or medications (use of antihypertensives, antidepressants, sedatives, hypoglycemics, phenothiazines, or carbamazepine)

Si: Evaluate environment: stairs, floors (slippery from urine, highly polished linoleum, thick-pile rugs), low-lying furniture, pets, shower, lighting, stairway handrails, toilet grab bars, footwear/slippers

Inability to balance on 1 leg correlates w marked increase in risk of fall (J Am Ger Soc 1997;45:735)

Tinetti Gait/Balance Assessment

Balance:

- Upon immediate standing (if abnormal, r/o myopathy, arthritis, Parkinson's, postural hypotension, deconditioning, hip disease, hemiparesis)

- With eyes closed and feet together (if abnormal, r/o multisensory deficit or diminished proprioception)
- With sternal nudge (r/o Parkinson's, NPH, CNS disease, back problems), turning 360°
- Sitting down (if abnormal, r/o impaired vision, proximal myopathy, ataxia)
- Neck turning (r/o cervical arthritis or spondylosis, vertebrobasilar insufficiency)
- Back extension
- Reaching up, bending down, standing on one leg for higher-functioning individuals (J Am Ger Soc 1986; 34:119)

Gait:
- Step height

  Frontal lobe gait, seen in dementia: wide-based, slightly flexed, small shuffling steps, hesitant steps, can't initiate step, "glued to floor," most common gait abnormality (Nejm 1990;322:1441)

  Spastic gait, seen in stroke; circumduction, scrape foot along floor, hand–arm spasticity

  Parkinsonian gait, lacks arm swing, turn in many small steps, get stuck while walking especially in open spaces like doorways, 4th most common gait abnormality

  NPH, short steps, decreased velocity of stride length and associated shoulder movements, increased sway, poor balance, difficulty turning

- Path deviation: Observe from behind, one foot at a time in relation to midline; abnormal path deviation from midline in

  Vestibular gait, seen with sensory ataxia, 2nd most common gait abnormality; broad-based, foot stamping, pt looks at feet, pos Rhomberg

Peripheral neuropathy, 3rd most common gait abnormality, unsteady on one side and then the other

Muscle weakness, slow unsteady swagger, use furniture to grab onto when walk

- Postural sway; observe from behind for truncal side-to-side motion; w:

Cerebellar gait, 5th most common gait disturbance; wide-based, irregular, unsteady, veering, truncal titubation

Antalgic gait, seen with arthritis of hip when cane held incorrectly on same side throwing trunk out over affected hip and resulting in stress on hip and lower back (Ger Med Today 1985;4:47); or broad-based waddling gait seen with severe arthritis, myositis, PMR

- Hysterical gait; hemiparesis without circumduction, hemiparetic arm normal during walking, good strength lying down but ataxia when walking, staggering a long time to get to opposite wall, tightrope walking, pt drags person assisting down to the ground

Crs:

Cmplc: Hip fx (p 420)

Falls are the 6th leading cause of death in elderly (Ann Rv Pub Hlth 1992;13:489); clustering of falls associated with high 6-mo mortality (Age Aging 1977;6:201); 1% result in hip fx, 5% other fx, 5% serious soft tissue injury (Nejm 1988;319:1701)

Prolonged lies waiting for help (< 10% of falls), if > 1 hr may cause dehydration, pressure sores, rhabdomyolysis, pneumonia (J Gerontol 1991;146:M164)

25% of fallers subsequently avoid ADLs and IADLs for fear of falling again (J Gerontol 1994;49:M140; Nejm 1988;319:1701)

Nursing home admissions (Nejm 1997;337:1279; Am J Pub Hlth 1992;82:395); increased use of health care services (Med

Care 1992;30:587); ~50% pts hospitalized for falls are discharged to nursing homes (Emerg Med Clin N Am 1990;8:309)

Lab: Routine w/u: CBC w diff, UA, chem screen, stool guaiac, sTSH, B12 and ESR (to r/o PMR), EKG, CXR, and/or CT as history indicates

Noninv: No need for Holter monitoring; prevalence of ventricular arrhythmia is 82% in both fallers and nonfallers; no sx reported with these arrhythmias (J Am Ger Soc 1989;37:430)

Rx: Prevent; fall reduction programs reduce falls by $\geq \frac{1}{3}$ (J Am Ger Soc 2004;52:1487; Jama 1997;278:557; Nejm 1994;331:821); pt education handouts (Am Fam Phys 1997;56:1815)

- Minimizing number of medications with lowest posssible doses
- Exercise programs to increase muscle strength and flexibility (J Am Ger Soc 2003;51:1685, 1693); balance and gait training especially getting in and out of chairs, turning around; nursing home standard PT is of moderate benefit (J Am Ger Soc 1996; 44:513; Jama 1994;271:519)
- Assistive aids: Walker use s/p hip fx by advancing 20-30 cm, then moving weak leg first; front-wheeled walker for Parkinson's, which avoids retropulsion and tripping. Cane use s/p hip fx only if ipsilateral upper extremities and contralateral lower extremities are strong, < 25% of pt's weight should be placed on cane; when going up or down stairs keep good leg up higher, ie, "up with good, down with bad." Trochanteric pads decrease hip fx's (p 420).
- Proper shoes, sneakers ok (J Am Ger Soc 2004;52:1495)
- Chairs should have armrests
- Obstacle-free, glare-free, adequately lit environment
- Avoid physical and pharmacologic restraints (Ann IM 1992; 116:369; Jama 1991;265:468); alternatives: special areas for walking, lower beds, floor pads, alarm systems (Am Fam Phys 1992;45:763), surveillance by staff; hospital alternatives: use of family visitors, professional sitters, lower beds, "functional" ICUs

7.3 Hip Fracture

Am Fam Phys 2003;67:537; Nejm 1996;334:1519

Cause: Falls + osteoporosis

Epidem: Rates lower in blacks; rates increased by thinness (Nejm 1995;332:767), pos family hx, alcohol use, CVA hx (Nejm 1994;330:1555), smoking (Nejm 1987;316:404), hyperthyroidism, inactivity, caffeine use, visual impairment (J Am Ger Soc 2003;51;356; Nejm 1991;324:1326), and drugs such as long-acting benzodiazepines (J Am Ger Soc 2000;48:682), tricyclics, SSRIs (Lancet 1998;351:1303), and phenothiazines (Nejm 1987;316:363) as well as other psychoactive drugs especially in nursing homes (Nejm 1992;327:168); paradoxically may also be increased by restraints (Ann IM 1992;116:369). Associated w being on feet < 4% of the day, higher pulse rates (Nejm 1995;332:767).

Pathophys: 45% femoral neck (intracapsular), 45% intertrochanteric (good blood supply), 10% subtrochanteric

Falls and fractures occur in the elderly because

- Slow gait results in more falls on hips rather than other body parts,
- Diminished protective responses,
- Less fat/muscle protection, and
- Diminished strength (J Gerontol 1989;44:M107)

Sx: H/o fall; hip pain, but may be vague in the elderly

Si: External rotation of the leg w shortening; pain w motion

Crs: 25% of fall-induced hip fractures result in death within 6 mo, 25% in subsequent functional dependence; 50% are walking independently 1 yr postfracture (Am J Med 1997;103:205). Usually fatal unless repaired. Prefracture mental status and physical functional level are best predictor of eventual outcome (J Am Ger Soc 1992;40:861).

Cmplc: After fx, frequently develop in hospital (J Gen Intern Med 1987;2:78) confusion (49%), UTI (33%), arrhythmia (26%), pneumonia (19%), depression (15%), CHF (7%), DVT

r/o, if xrays neg, stress fx, pubic ramus fx, acetabular fx, greater trochanteric fx, and trochanteric bursitis or contusion

r/o apparent or occult dementia, 50% prevalence (J Am Ger Soc 2003;51:1227)

Lab:

Xray: Plain films, AP and lateral or AP w 15-20° internal rotation show fx, often subtle, especially if impacted; after 72 hr, bone scan or MRI if dx still in doubt

Rx: Prevent 1st episode or recurrence w rx of osteoporosis (p 411) (Nejm 1992;327:1637) w:

- Hip protectors in high-risk pts (BMJ 2003;326:76; Nejm 2000; 343:1506,1562; Lancet 1993;341:11); worn in special underpants, 30% refuse to use but when do, 60% reduction in hip fx's, NNT-5 = 8; vs Dartmouth study finding no significant help (Jama 2003;289:1957)
- By treating osteoporosis (p 411)
- Avoid use of slippery throw rugs in the home and restraints (Ann IM 1992;116:369)

Surgical reduction, pinning/fixation, or arthroplasty if badly displaced intracapsular; within 48 hr if possible w 48 hr perioperative antibiotics

Postsurgery consider heparin, LMW heparin 12 hr pre-op and 1 mo post-op (Nejm 1996;335:696), warfarin DVT prophylaxis (p 52), or perhaps hirudin 30 min pre-op (Nejm 1997;337: 1329); as well as compression stockings (Arch IM 1994;154:67); weight bearing in 1-2 d and early rehab in hospital, rehab unit, or NH (Jama 1998;279:847, 1997;277:396) w extended resistance training (Jama 2004;292:837)

7.4 Dementias

Alzheimer's Dementia (Dementia, Alzheimer's Type) (DAT)

Nejm 2004;351:56, 2003;349:1056 (best rv); Clin Ger 2004;92:450;
    J Am Ger Soc 2003;51:S281; Ann IM 2003;138:400,411

Cause: Unclear but several genes implicated, on chromosomes 1, 14
    (Nejm 1995;333:1283), and amyloid A_4 protein deposition
    (Lancet 1992;340:467; Ann Neurol 1992;32:157) gene on
    chromosome 21 (Nejm 1989;320:1446)

        Early onset (< 60 yr):

- Amyloid precursor protein (APP) gene on chromosome 21
- Presenilin single- or two-gene (PSEN1, PSEN2) type (40% of
early-onset cases)

        Late onset (> 60 yr):

- Apolipoprotein-E gene, E4 allele hetero- and homozygotes on
chromosome 19 (Nejm 2000;343:450)
- Chromosome 9q22, UBQLN1 gene (Nejm 2005;352:884)

Epidem: Prevalence = 5% at age 70 yr, 20% at 80 yr, 50% at 90 yr
    (Jama 1995;273:1354) vs 40% of population at age 85 yr (Nejm
    1999;341:1670) but varies depending on which criteria used
    (Nejm 1997;327:1667); 20-50% incidence in family members of
    late-onset Alzheimer's patients (Ger 2000;55:34; Ann IM 1991;
    115:601); males = females; 100% of Down's syndrome pts age
    > 35 yr (Science 1992;258:668) probably secondary to trisomy of
    chromosome 21 for amyloid protein

        Increased incidence in pts w elevated plasma homocysteine
    levels (Nejm 2002;346:476)

        Decreased incidence w 1-6 alcoholic drinks/wk (Jama 2003;
    289:1405)

        50+% of elderly dementia is Alzheimer's, 15+% is vascular
    multi-infarct type, 15% is Lewy-Body type, 25% is Parkinson's
    type, and many cases are mixtures of several causes

Pathophys (Nejm 1991;325:1849): Neuronal dropout; decreased acetylcholine synthesis (Nejm 1985;313:7), hence anticholinergics worsen (Nejm 1985;313:7)

E4 allele of apolipoprotein E (Nejm 1996;334:752,791; Jama 1995;273:1274) facilitates β amyloid protein deposition in injury-induced (eg, boxers) neurofibrillary tangles (Nejm 1995; 333:1242), concentrations of which correlate w cognitive decline (Jama 2000;283:1571)

Sx: Loss of social skills and memory usually unacknowledged by patient; repetitive questions and behaviors observed by family (97% sens-J Am Ger Soc 2003;51:32)

Si: Abnormal mental status (Psych Clin N Am 1991;14:309; 1-page test: Ann IM 1977;86:40) w memory loss > 6 mo + ≥ 1 other cognitive function impairments (DSM-IV; Am Psychiatr Assoc 1994;142; Neurol 1984;34:939) in language, calculations, orientation, and/or judgment (See Table 7.2 and 7.3)

- Memory deficits: Recent much worse than remote; including orientation to time (day, mo, yr) (day of week is 53% sens, 92% specif-Ann IM 1991;115:122); recall 3 items
- Construction deficits: Perceptive/spatial disorientation, eg, answers to "how do you get there from here?"; clock face drawing; copy interlocking pentagons; gets lost
- Language impairments: Anomias/paraphasias/aphasias, which often result in neologisms or circumlocutions
- Abstraction impairments: "What does it mean to give someone the cold shoulder?", categorization, calculations
- Praxis impairments: Inability to perform complex movements necessary for behaviors like writing, meal preparation, dressing
- Prosody defects: Trouble conveying and reading facial expressions of emotions, affect changes
- Executive function problems (Lancet 1999;354:1921): Frontal lobe difficulty creating and executing complicated goal-directed behaviors. Test w ability to draw (not copy) a clock

showing 2:10 (impaired person draws hands to 2 and 10 rather than 2 and 2), and other tests.

Hallucinations in up to 20%, esp, in 1st 2 yr; delusions in up to 50% (J Am Ger Soc 2003;51:953)

Pupillary dilatation > 20% within 30 min to 1/100 diluted tropicamide gtts, even 1 yr before measurable DAT, 95% sens/specif (Sci 1994;266:1051) vs not helpful and not being used clinically (Arch Neurol 1997;54:165)

Table 7.2   Mini Cognitive (Minicog) Exam

Test	Content	Points
1. Recall	3 unrelated items, being sure registered by repeating	0-3
2. Spatial/executive function	Clock draw with all 12 numbers plus hands at 8:20	0-2
Interpretation: 0-2 = dementia, 3-5 = maybe no dementia		

(Internat J Ger Psych 2001;16:216, 2000;15:1021)

Crs: Slowly progressive; mean survival from first sx = 10 yr; shorter, the more severe it is (Ann IM 1990;113:429). 33% 5-yr survival w MMSE ≤ 17, 55% 5-yr and 33% 10-yr survival w MMSE ≤ 25 (Ann IM 2004;140:501)

Stages (Am J Psych 1982;139:1136) 1 and 2: Forget familiar names and places

Stage 3: Coworkers aware

Stage 4: Difficulty w finances

Stage 5: Need assistance dressing

Stage 6: Incontinence, delusional

Stage 7: Grunting, nonambulatory

Cmplc: Depression in caregivers, prevalence = 50%
r/o: reversible causes (Adams: Nejm 1986;314:1111):

Table 7.3   Mini Mental Status Exam

Test	Content	Points
Time orientation	Year/month/day of week/season/date	5
Place orientation	State/county/town/building/floor	5
Registration	3 objects (table, hat, apple)	3 (for immediate repeat)
Attention	serial 7's, or spell "world" backward	5
Recall	Recall above 3 objects	3
Naming	Name 2 objects (watch, pen)	2
Repetition	Repeat "no ifs, ands, or buts"	1
Command	3-part command (left hand to right ear and stick out tongue)	3
Written command	Sign that says "close your eyes"	1
Composition	Write a sentence	1
Spatial orientation	Copy interlocking pentagons	1
Total		30

Normal: 23-26 for uneducated; 29+ for college educated; impaired < 23; in AD, scores decrease by 4 pts/yr

(J Psych Res 1975;12:189)

- Mild cognitive impairment (J Intern Med 2004;256:183; Neurol 2004;63:115)
  ADLs and IADLs intact
  Pt able to describe episodes in detail
  Pt more concerned than family
  Normal MMSE
  No trouble operating equipment
  Recent memory of events intact
  Some word-finding troubles
- Delirium (p 773), if < 1 mo, in which alertness may fluctuate from fear, lethargy to hypervigilance, delusions and distortions, easily distracted because attention span is most prominent deficit; test by serial 7's; serial digits up to 7, eg, phone numbers; spell "world" or do days of wk or mos of year backward

- Depression pseudodementia (p 432); more "I don't know" answers than the guesses of DAT; often both occur together; language preserved; psychomotor retardation. If MMSE score ≥ 21, pts are more responsive to antidepressants.
- Drugs, single or multiple (6/100)
- Myxedema (4/100)
- Toxins like occult solvent/paint exposure, lead, arsenic, mercury, manganese, thallium, carbon monixide
- Subdural hematoma (2/100)
- Frontal/temporal tumor
- Tertiary syphilis
- AIDS
- B_{12} deficiency
- Wernicke-Korsakoff w antegrade memory loss, alcohol hx; may recover partially over 1 yr (Nejm 1985;312:16)

Other dementias:

- Frontal/frontotemporal (subcortical) dementias (J Am Ger Soc 1998;46:98), which show preservation of spatial sense but loss of executive control function (socially inappropriate and disinhibition prominent early), forgetfulness, and motor findings 1st (Arch Neurol 1993;50:873), unlike amnesia and language deficits in DAT; eg, Parkinson's; Huntington's; Wilson's; **olivopontine degeneration**; normal-pressure hydrocephalus (may be partially reversible); **Lewy body dementia** (J Am Ger Soc 1998;46:1449; Neurol 1996;47:111) w attention deficits, hallucinations that worsen w antipsychotics, and Parkinsonism, rapid (months) onset. **Pick's disease**, similar to Alzheimer's but with less memory impairment and more behavioral change, is rare and anatomic changes are isolated to frontal and temporal lobes.
- Multi-infarct dementia when stepwise crs, emotional lability prominent, and h/o HT, CVA, or ASHD
- Creutzfeld-Jakob dementia (p 430)

- Primary progressive aphasia (Nejm 2003;349:1535) w crs like Alzheimer's but deficits in 1st 2 yr only in language/word finding

Lab: *Chem:* TSH, T$_4$, chemistry panel, lytes if acute, B$_{12}$ level w f/u MMA levels if borderline (p 447)

Hem: CBC

Noninv: Unnecessary but EEG occasionally helpful to distinguish DAT (slow waves) from depression (normal)

Path: Brain histology at postmortem shows neurofibrillary tangles, senile plaques with eosinophilic amyloid; experimental apo-E genotyping is 65% sens/specif (Nejm 1998;338:506)

Serol: Perhaps VDRL, HIV antibody if young

Xray: Head CT or MRI distinguishes from multi-infarct dementia (Neurol 1993;43:250) in all pts (Nejm 1986;314:964) but very low yield of reversible disease, eg, < 1/250 (Ann IM 1994;120:856)

Rx: Preventive:
- Regular exercise, eg, walking > 1 mi qd (Jama 2004;292:1447)
- Statin rx of increased cholesterol may prevent or slow onset (Arch Neurol 2000;57:1410,1439; Lancet 2000;356:1627)
- NSAIDs (not ASA or acetaminophen) may decrease risk (Jama 1998;279:688; Neurol 1997;48:626) if taken × 2+ yr (NNT-2 = 16) (Nejm 2001;345:1515,1567) but don't help once demented (Jama 2003;289:2819)
- "Use it or lose it" intellectual activity may delay/prevent vs predict (Nejm 2003;348:2489,2508)
- Screening/preventive rx of other diseases must be truncated to acount for overall prognosis and risk benefits (Jama 2000;283:3230)
- ERT no help, may worsen (Jama 2004;291:2947,2959,3005)
- Apolipoprotein-E screening not appropriate (Jama 1997;277: 832; 1995;274:1627)

Memory meds (Nejm 1999;341:1672):

- Acetylcholinesterase inhibitors (eg, physostigmine); all modestly helpful (J Am Ger Soc 2003;51:S289, 737 [DBCT]; Jama 2003;289:210) so try to use early and continuously (UCLA 9/02), also help w vascular dementias (ACP J Club 2004; 141:39); not useful in NH (J Am Ger Soc 2003;51:133); all cost $130/mo

  Donepezil (Aricept) (Arch IM 1998;158:1021; ACP J Club 1998;129(3):68; Med Let 1997;39:53) 5-10 mg po hs; no long-term effects on crs, no help w behavioral sx, but improved clinical state and quality of life, NNT-6 = 5 (Neurology 2001;57:613); cmplc: least NV+D, agitation/insomnia, myalgias unlike galantamine and rivastigmine (Clin Ger Med 2001;17:346); metabolism slowed by paroxetine (Paxil)

  Galantamine (Reminyl) (Med Let 2001;43:53) 4 mg po bid, increase to 8-12 mg bid; adverse effects like donepezil but more NV+D

  Rivastigmine (Exelon) (Med Let 2000;42:93) 1.5-6 mg po bid; minimal drug interactions w p450 drugs like phenytoin, carbamezepine, ketoconazole; adverse effects: most NV+D, weight loss

- Antiglutamatergics (eg, amantadine):

  Memantine (Namenda) (Jama 2004;291:317; Med Let 2003; 45:73; Nejm 2003;348:1333) 5 mg, increase to 20 mg over 8 wk po qd; slows progression in pts w MMSE $\approx$ 15 modestly like acetylcholinesterase drugs and has additive effect; adverse effects: dizziness, severe headache, constipation, confusion, expensive

- Vitamin E 2000 IU po qd (Nejm 1997;336:1216) but not helpful in preventing progression of MCI to Alzheimer's, an early enthusiasm may be misplaced (Nejm 2005;352:2379,2439)

Perhaps:

- Ginko biloba extract 40 mg po tid helps modestly over 1 yr by DBCT (Jama 1997;278:1327) but others (Med Let 1998;40:63) skeptical of study design and results and not helpful in healthy elderly (Jama 2002;288:835); adverse effects: coma when used w trazodone
- Selegeline 10 mg po qd (Nejm 1997;336:1216), can prolong independent living of agitated behavior:

  Respirodone (Respirdal) 1-3 mg po bid; or olanzapine (Zyprexa); or quetiapine (Seroquel)

  Carbamazepine (Tegretol) 25 mg po bid up to 200 tid to a level of 6-7 mg % following CBC and LFTs (J Clin Psych Neurol 1990;51:115)

  SSRIs

Other options depending on predominant sx in decreasing order of desirability:

- Gabapentin (Neurontin)
- Clozapine, avoids extrapyramidal sx but causes agranulocytosis, hypotension, and seizures (J Ger Psych Neurol 1994;7:129)
- Phenothiazines (p 940) in order of increasing extrapyramidal and decreasing sedation/anticholinergic/hypotensive effects. Haloperidol (Haldol) 1-3 mg/d is effective for psychosis and disruptive behavior (Am J Psych 1998;155:1512) but tardive dyskinesia 3-5× higher in elderly compared to younger pts.
- Trazodone 50 mg po b-qid (J Clin Psych 1986;47:4)
- Benzodiazepines such as oxazepam (Serax) 10 mg po tid, or lorazepam (Ativan), but diminished effect after several months
- Propranolol 60-600 mg po qd (Can J Psych 1992;37:651; Psych Ann 1990;20:446)
- Estrogen perhaps for sexual aggression in men? (J Am Ger Soc 1991;39:1110)

  In NH, wandering can also be managed by "wandering areas," sign posts, pictures of residents on resident room doors, tape barriers, half-doors, coded locks

of inanition: Tube feedings no help and risky (Nejm 2000; 342:206; Jama 1999;282:1365)

Creutzfeldt-Jakob Disease

Nejm 1998;339:1994, 1997;337:1821

Cause: A transmissable spongiform encephalopathy caused by a small slow virus, similar to measles's progressive multifocal leukoencephalopathy, kuru (Nejm 1986;314:547, 1972;287:429), and scrapie; or prions (proteinaceous infectious particles); or a virino consisting of a nucleic acid/host protein combination. Human growth hormone extracts caused it before recombinant types were available. Fibrillary structures in brain (Nejm 1985;312:73); rare cases are thought genetic, autosomal dominant (Nejm 1991; 324:1091) plus additional genetic impact on incubation period and infectivity.

Epidem: Growth hormone rx from brain extracts caused an epidemic in U.S. (Nejm 1985;313:728), 10,000 young people have now received potentially contaminated HGH in U.S. Not entirely inactivated by heat, formalin, or cold.

From eating beef infected w **Mad Cow Disease** (bovine spongiform encephalitis); 20+ cases in U.K., esp in young adults (Jama 1997;278:1008), but not in the U.S. (Jama 1999; 281:2330); this new variant is much more rapidly progressive

Natural incidence = 1-2/1 million population; 100× as frequent in Libyan Jews

Pathophys: Corticostriatospinal atrophy

Sx: Onset usually age > 35 yr, all > 20 yr except in new-variant C-J disease; dementia; myoclonus; psychiatric sx; ataxia

Si: Dementia and myoclonus plus occasionally long tract si's and/or parkinsonism and/or anterior horn cell degeneration

Crs: Rapid progression over a few weeks time; most die in 6 mo, all by 3 yr

Cmplc: r/o anoxic damage, syphilis (by CSF exam), inclusion encephalitis (in children and adolescents), Alzheimer's (slower course), lipid storage disease (by positive family hx), AIDS

Lab: *CSF:* LP may be normal, but distinctive CSF proteins (14-3-3 protein) can distinguish from all other dementias, 96% sens/specif in demented pts (Lancet 1997;348:846; Nejm 1996; 335:924, 1986;315:279)

Noninv: EEG shows diagnostic slow waves in bursts; may be focal

Path: Brain bx shows slow virus marker proteins by Western blot, 0% false pos, occasionally false neg occur (Nejm 1986; 314:547); or prion protein by Western blot in vivo bx of cribiform plate/olefactory bulb (Nejm 2003;348:711)

Rx: None available (Nejm 1985;312:1035)

Normal-Pressure Hydrocephalus

Cause: Idiopathic, or postsurgical, trauma, or infection

Epidem:

Pathophys: A "communicating hydrocephalus" (in contrast to foraminal or aqueductalstenosis) and obstruction is therefore at cisterna. Hence, 4th ventricle may dilate, causing cerebellar si's.

Sx: First, trouble walking (ataxia) and may remain as only sx; or may then develop progressive dementia and incontinence

Si: Horizontal nystagmus, normal discs, spasticity, frontal lobe si's

Crs: Progressive dementia

Cmplc:

Lab: *CSF:* Transient improvement with removal of 50 cc (Acta Neurol Scand 1987;75:566) 1-3× in 1 wk; neurosurgeons not doing shunt unless see improvement with this first

Xray: CT scan shows big ventricles (100%); cisternogram shows delayed or no movement of dye out over hemispheres, but there are false neg

Rx: Surgical shunt, 80% success (Jama 1996;44:445; Nejm 1985;312:1255); cmplc: infections in 3-5%

Depression in the Elderly

Jama 2002;287:1568

Cause: Often situational; hypothalamic/pituitary/adrenal axis and circadian rhythm disruption; drugs (Med Let 2002;44:59) including alcohol, amantadine, antipsychotics, cimetidine, clonidine, cytotoxic agents, digoxin, alphamethyldopa, propranolol, sedatives, steroids, reserpine

Epidem: Prevalence is 10-15% in the geriatric population

Pathophys: MAO activity is increased in brains of elderly (Am J Psych 1984;141:1276)

Sx: Major depression has at least 5 of the following sx × 2 wk unless recent major loss:
- Impaired sleep, often w early morning awakening
- Diminished interest (anhedonia)
- Diminished energy
- Impaired concentration and/or appetite
- Feelings of guilt
- Agitation
- Psychomotor retardation
- Diminished self-esteem (J Am Ger Soc 1986;34:215)
  Masked depression may present as somatization syndrome

Si: Depression scales (Clin Ger Med 1986;5:165); weight loss

Crs:

Cmplc: Suicide, 20% fatal

r/o grief reaction, dysthymia, schizophrenia, drug reactions

Lab: *Chem:* TSH, B_{12} level

Hem: CBC

Rx: Medications: tricyclics (p 942), generally use $^1/_3$ usual adult doses (demethylation is decreased in the elderly); beware drug interactions

1st: • SSRIs like sertraline (Zoloft) 25-50+ mg po qd; paroxetine (Paxil) 10-20+ mg po qd (DBRCT: Jama 2000;284:1519); citalopram (Celexa) not helpful (DBCT Am J Psych 2004;161:2050)

• Trazodone (Desyrel) up to 150 mg po qd; soporific

• Desipramine (Norpramin) 25-150 mg po qd; useful if sleeping too much

• Imipramine (Tofranil) up to 150 mg po qd; especially if also has urge incontinence

2nd: • Nortriptyline (Pamelor, Avantyl) 10-35+ mg po qd

• Amoxapine (Asendin), especially good to get eating, cf Ritalin

• Mirtazapine (Remeron) 15-45 mg q hs; sedates, increased appetite

• Buproprion (Welbutrin) 50 mg po bid

• Enhancers: L-thyroxine 0.025 mg po qd, methylphenidate (Ritalin) 5-10 mg po q am and noon (Clin Therap 2000;22:A25; Am J Psych 1995;152:929), or lithium up to 300 mg po tid following 12 hr postdose levels

Electroshock therapy (ECT) is very effective in the elderly (Nejm 1984;311:163)

7.5 Miscellaneous

Abuse of Elderly

Detection and rx (J Am Ger Soc 1996;49:65; Nejm 1995; 332:437)

Activities of Daily Living (ADLs)

Katz functional assessment (Gerontol 1970;10:20) records loss of independence in 6 skills (bathing, dressing, toileting, transferring, continence, feeding) in the order in which they are usually lost, and regained in reverse order; assess actual capacity, not reported performance (J Gerontol 1983;38:385). Speed and pain in performing ADLs in arthritis pts (J Chronic Dis 1978;31:557); rehab for ADLs (Arch Phys Med Rehab 1988;69:337).

Instrumental Activities of Daily Living (IADLs)

More complex activities like shopping, seeking transportation, preparing food, climbing stairs, and managing finances, housework, telephone, medications, and job (Fillenbaum IADLs: J Am Ger Soc 1985;33:698). Other IADL scales: home assessment (Clin Ger Med 1991;7:677); nutrition (Am Fam Phys 1993;48:1395); driving (Clin Ger Med 1993;9:349).

ASHD

Rx in the elderly: HT rx of pressures > 140/90, even though prevalence > 50%, helps prevent MIs and CVAs, NNT-5 = 18 (Jama 1994;272:1932); lifestyle changes, then thiazides, then β-blockers? (Jama 1994;272:842; HT 1994;23:275)

Albumin Levels

< 3.5 gm % predict > 50% 5-yr mortality vs 10-20% if > 4 gm % (Jama 1994;272:1037)

Asx Bactiuria

Rx: No evidence that rx improves female outcomes in elderly and/or diabetics (Nejm 2002;347:1576)

Congestive Heart Failure in the Elderly

Pathophys: $^2/_3$ due to diastolic dysfunction, ie, EF > 50% (Ann IM 2002;137:631; Jama 2002;288:2144), although 5-yr survival better than w systolic dysfunction (nl = 90%, diastolic dysfunction = 62%, systolic dysfunction = 45%)

Code status: Durable power-of-attorney applications; mail to pts > 65 yr old after hospitalization (Nejm 1994;271:209). CPR in elderly > 70 yr success so low not worth it? (Ann IM 1989;111:193,199 vs Jama 1990;264:2109). Prior competent choice vs best-interest standard is moving focus to pts' subjective experience at time of therapy (J Am Ger Soc 1998;46:922).

Driving by Elderly

J Am Ger Soc 2004;52:143, 2003;51:1499

Accident risk increased from 6-50% as go from 0/3 to 3/3 pos answers to following: (1) ability to copy interlocking pentagons, (2) walk > 1 block qd, and (3) 2+ structural abnormalities of feet (Ann IM 1995;122:842). Visual tracking techniques can also help stratify cognitively impaired pts (J Am Ger Soc 1998;46:556, 1997;45:949). Not at night, not in traffic, informally test regularly (Jama 1997;45:949, 1995;273:1360).

Incontinence

Jama 2004;191:986, 996; Nejm 2004;350:786

Innervations: bladder, parasympathetic (cholinergic); internal sphincter, α-sympathetic; external sphincter, voluntary S_{2-3} roots

Urge incontinence (detrussor instability, irritable bladder)

Cause: Decreased CNS inhibition, eg, dementia, Parkinson's, CVA; or parasympathomimetic drugs such as bethanechol (Urecholine); or irritation from cytitis, prostatitis, BPH, bladder tumor

Pathophys: Detrusor instability w or w/o impaired contractility

Lab: Cystometrics show spastic contractions

Rx: Antibiotics for any infection only if recent change in incontinence pattern or other evidence of symptomatic UTI (Ann IM 1995;122:749)

Anticholinergics (parasympathetic inhibition):
  Antimuscarinics (all cause dry mouth sx):
  • Imipramine 25-50 mg po hs
  • Oxybutynin (Ditropan) 2.5-5 mg po tid; long-acting (Med Let 2001;43:28) and transdermal (Ocytrol) (Med Let 2003;45:38) forms not as effective; $22/mo generic, $90/mo trade

  Muscarinic receptor antagonists (much less dry mouth):
  • Darifenacin (Enablex) 7.5-15 mg po qd; no better than cheaper ones; $100/mo
  • Flavoxate (Urispas)
  • Solifenacin (VESIcare) 5 mg po qd; no better than cheaper ones; $100/mo
  • Tropsium chloride (Sanctura) (Med Let 2004;46:63) 20 mg po bid; poor gi absorption; $90/mo
  • Tolterodine (Detrol) (Med Let 1998;40:101) 1-2 mg po bid; long-acting forms not as effective (Med Let 2001;43:28); $100/mo

  Biofeedback (Ann IM 1985;103:507) or behavioral training (Kegel anal sphincter contraction w abdominal muscle relaxation) (Jama 2002;288:2293); better than medications (Jama 2004;191:986,996; J Am Ger Soc 2000;48:370) vs no clear benefit (Cochrane Library meta-analysis: ACP J Club 1999;130:67)

  Estrogens vaginally no help by DBCT (Jama 2005;293:935)

Overflow incontinence

Cause: Bladder outlet obstruction, eg, BPH, uterine prolapse, constipation, α-stimulant drugs, neuropathy (impaired sensory input to sacral micturation center); or diminished detrusor strength (flaccid due to lower motor neuron disease or meds such as anticholinergics, calcium-channel blockers, smooth-muscle relaxants)

Sx: Obstructive w diminished urinary stream, frequency; if neuropathic, will have no sensation of bladder fullness

Lab: Postvoid residuum > 100 cc; cystometrics show no contractions w 400+ cc when due to diminished sensation

Rx: Self-catheterization (J Am Ger Soc 1990;38:364)
Stool softeners for constipation
Rx prolapse or BPH
Increase detrusor strength w parasympathomimetics, bethanechol (Urecholine) 10+ mg po tid, or phenoxybenzamine (Dibenzyline) 10 mg po qd
Block sphincter constriction (α blockade) w doxazosin (Cardura) 2-8 mg po qd, prazosin (Minipres) 1-2 mg po tid, tamsulosin (Flowmax) 0.4-0.8 mg po qd, or terazosin (Hytrin) 1 mg increasing to 5-10 mg po qd-bid; all $30-50/d

Stress incontinence (Urol Clin N Am 1998;25:625; Am Fam Phys 1998;57:2675)

Cause: Estrogen deficiency effect on urethral mucosa; or pelvic relaxation after childbirth or urologic surgery; neuropathies; α-blocking meds

Pathophys: Sphincter insufficiency

Sx: Loss of urine w cough, sneeze, laugh

Si: Cystocele on physical exam if due to pelvic relaxation

Rx: Estrogen vaginally no help by DBCT (Jama 2005;293:935); Kegel exercises qid (J Am Ger Soc 1983;31:476); pessaries (Am

Fam Phys 2000;61:2723); surgery (suburethral sling or open retropubic culposuspension)

of neuropathic types: Imipramine 25+ mg hs (α stimulation, parasympathetic inhibition); or biofeedback (Ann IM 1985;103:507)/behavioral therapy (Jama 2003;290:345)

Functional incontinence

Cause: Can't get to toilet

Si: All normal

Rx: Schedules plus reinforcement, if oriented ×1 and can identify 1 of 2 objects, prompting can decrease incontinence from 25% to 6-9% (Jama 1995;273:1366)

Knee Replacement Rehab

Rx: Weekly testoterone 100 mg im × 4 wk much improves rapid recovery and rehab (J Am Ger Soc 2002;50:1698)

Smell Impairment

Epidem: 25% prevalence > age 55, 63% > age 80 (Jama 2002;288:2307)

Chapter 8

Hematology/Oncology

D. K. *Onion*

8.1 Chemotherapy

MANAGING CANCER AND CHEMOTHERAPY

Cachexia/Wasting Syndromes

Nejm 1999;340:1740

Assess diet; r/o other disease; if testosterone deficient, replace w testosterone enanthate 300 mg im q 3 wk (Ann IM 1998;129:18), not scrotal patch (Am J Med 1999;107:130)

Other possible aids:

- Megestrol (Megace; a progestin) 40 mg po qid or liquid 40 mg/cc up to 800 mg qd, stimulates appetite and weight gain (Ann IM 1994;121:393,400)
- Androgens: Nandrolone (Jama 1999;281:1275) 100 mg im q 1 wk, in renal failure; oxandrolone (Jama 1999;281:1282) 20 mg qd po in AIDS
- Growth hormones possibly in AIDS (Ann IM 1996;125: 865,873,932), but cost $1000/wk
- Marijuana, marinol, tetrahydrocannabinol (THS); no apparent detrimental effect in AIDS (Ann IM 2003;139:258)
- Thalidomide? (Am J Med 2000;108:487)
- TPN during chemoRx of questionable (Ann IM 1984;101:303) or no (Ann IM 1989;110:734) benefit

Fetal Damage

None in oncology nurses (Nejm 1985;313:1173); no increase in cancer (Nejm 1998;338:1339) or anomalies (Nejm 1991;325:141) in offspring conceived by pts later in life after chemoRx, except maybe anomalies after dactinomycin

Fevers

Require stat w/u and rx (p 491)

Mucositis and Keratinized Tongue

Occurs w chemoRx for hematologic cancers and is diminished by palifermin iv prophylaxis (Nejm 2004;351:2590)

Nausea and Vomiting

Prophylaxis (eg, some emetogenic drugs like cisplatinum) and rx (Med Let 2004;46:27), usually use several together:

- Dexamethasone, 1st, 8-20 mg iv 30 min before, then 4 mg po bid (Nejm 2000;342:1554), or 10 mg qid × 24 hr; or 10 mg iv before chemoRx with metaclopramide 10 mg po qid afterward is better than ondansetron (Nejm 1993;328:1076)
- 5-HT (serotonin) antagonists:

  Ondansetron (Zofran) (Med Let 2003;45:62) 0.15 mg/kg iv over 15 min once ($200) or 8 mg iv ($50), then 8 mg po bid (Nejm 2000;342:1554), or 4 mg po tid (Ann IM 1993;118:407); start $\frac{1}{2}$ hr before chemoRx; better w dexamethasone w 1st dose; or 8 mg po b-tid (Nejm 1993;328:1081), with metopimazine (a phenothiazine) 30 mg po qid (Nejm 1993;328:1076); twice as good as metaclopramide (Ann IM 1991;114:834); adverse effects: headaches, constipation, elevated LFTs all limit use (ACP J Club 1997;127:65)

  Dolasetron (Anzemet) (Med Let 1998;40:53) 100 mg iv ($206) or po ($72) ×1

Granetron (Kytril) (Nejm 1995;332:1) 3 mg iv ($120) or
2 mg po ($90) ×1
Palonosetron (Aloxi) (Med Let 2004;46:27) 0.25 mg iv ×1
($305)
- Aprepitant (Emend) (Med Let 2003;45:62) 125 mg po day 1,
80 mg qd days 2+3 1 hr before chemoRx; a substance P/NK
inhibitor; adverse effects: esthenia, hiccups; $300/crs

Also reported to help:
- Hypnotic desensitization (Nejm 1982;307:1476)
- Marijuana or other cannabinoids (BMJ 2001;323:16) like
dronabinol (Marinol = tetrahydrocannabinol) 10-20 mg po q
4-6 hr (Ann IM 1997;126:791)
- Prochlorperazine 5-20 mg po, pr, im, or occasionally iv
- Accupuncture w or w/o electrostimulation qd reduces emesis
by $^2/_3$ in DBCT (Jama 2000;284:2755)

Pain

Nejm 1996;335:1124

WHO analgesic ladder (dosing, p 1067–1072):
1st: NSAID
2nd: Add opiate (codeine, oxycodone)
3rd: Add stronger opiate (morphine, oxycodone, fentanyl) +
tricyclic or anticonvulsant

Chemotherapeutic Drugs

Listed by tumor type and toxicities: Med Let 2000;42:83
Generally administered under the direction of an oncologist and
used in combination with one another in complex regimens, not as
single agents; doses adjusted for each cycle depending on the other
agents being used and patient response

Alkylating Agents

Several increase leukemia risk by 6-20× up to 8 yr after treatment ends; risk is increased by splenectomy and minimally affected by

radiation rx; but overall fewer than 2% get leukemia after chemoRx (Nejm 1990;322:1,7)

- Busulfan (Myleran); adverse effects: marrow suppression, pulmonary fibrosis, some alopecia
- Chlorambucil (Leukeran) po; adverse effects: marrow suppression, pulmonary fibrosis
- Cyclophosphamide (Cytoxan); or analog ifosfamide (Ifex); adverse effects: marrow suppression; alopecia; pulmonary fibrosis; hemorrhagic cystitis, and bladder cancer risk = 5% at 10 yr, 10% at 12 yr, 16% at 15 yr after rx (Ann IM 1996;124:477), give with mesna to detoxify urine so bladder spared (Med Let 1989;31:98)
- Melphalan (Alkeran); adverse effects: marrow suppression, especially of platelets; leukemia risk 10 times more than for cyclophosphamide (Nejm 1992;326:1745)
- N-mustard; adverse effects: marrow suppression, some alopecia
- Thiotepa; adverse effects: marrow suppression

Antimetabolites

- Azathioprine (Imuran) and 6-MP (mercaptopurine) po, but absorption erratic (Nejm 1983;308:1005); adverse effects: marrow suppression, gi ulcerations, cholestasis, increased effect with allopurinol, excessive toxicity in the 1/300 homozygous for catabolic enzyme deficiency (Ann IM 1997;126:608)
- Cytosine arabinoside Cytarabine); adverse effects: marrow suppression
- 5-Fluorouracil (5-FU) iv, or as capecitabine (Xeloda) (Nejm 2005;352:2696) po; adverse effects: marrow suppression, gi ulcerations
- Gemcitabine (Gemzar) (Med Let 1996;38:102) iv weekly; for pancreatic Ca where it improves pain and functional status and marginally prolongs life, also in breast, bladder, and pulmonary small cell Ca; cmplc: marrow suppression, NV+D; cost $600/wk

- Methotrexate (Nejm 1983;309:1094) po or intrathecal; adverse effects: marrow suppression; gi ulcerations, aspirin increases effect (protein binding is decreased); in rheumatoid arthritis EBV lymphomas, which regress w withdrawal of mtx (Ann IM 1993;328:1317); reversible pneumonitis
- Thioquanine; adverse effects: marrow suppression, excessive toxicity in the 1/300 homozygous for catabolic enzyme deficiency (Ann IM 1997;126:608)

Anthracyclines

- Daunorubicin (Daunomycin); adverse effects: marrow suppression; red urine; alopecia; cardiotoxicity (Nejm 1998;339:900) especially at doses > 40 mg/kg, age-related, decreased by 2-4 d infusions (Ann IM 1982;96:133); in children, long-term adverse cardiac effects (Ann IM 1996;125:47; Nejm 1991; 324:808)
- Doxorubicin (Adriamycin) iv; adverse effects: marrow suppression; cardiotoxicity at all doses (Ann IM 1996;125:47) especially > 350 mg/m^2 total, preventable w dexrazoxane (Med Let 1991;33:85)
- Epirubicin (Ellence) (Med Let 2000;42:12); analog of doxorubincin used for breast Ca; less cardiotoxic, more expensive
- Idarubicin (Idamycin); similar to daunorubicin for AML (Med Let 1991;33:84)

Arabines (Purine Analogs)

- Cladribine (Leustatin) (Ann IM 1994;120:784); for hairy cell leukemia, CLL, and T-cell lymphomas
- Fludarabine (Fludura) iv for CLL (Med Let 1991;33:84)
- Vidarabine

Epipodophyllotoxins

Nejm 1991;325:1682

- Etoposide (a podophyllin) (Med Let 1983;25:48); for testicular cancer, small cell, ALL, etc; adverse effects: marrow suppression; AML in 4-12%, especially if given weekly
- Teniposide; for ALL; adverse effects: AML in 4-12%, especially if given weekly

Other

- Asparaginase (Med Let 1978;20:103) iv; adverse effects: hemorrhagic pancreatitis, hepatitis, anaphylaxis, transient decrease in thyroid-binding globulin (Nejm 1979;301:251)
- BCG (Nejm 1974;290:1413); mainly for superficial bladder cancer
- Bleomycin (Ann IM 1979;90:945); adverse effects: pneumonitis, fibrosis
- Bortezomid (Velcade) (Med Let 2003;45:57); a proteasome inhibitor used for refractory myeloma
- Carboplatin (Med Let 1989;31:83); for ovarian cancer after cisplatinum fails or as 1st drug
- Carmustine (BCNU) iv; adverse effects: pulmonary fibrosis, most manifest within the first 3 yr after rx but may not appear for up to 15 yr (Nejm 1990;323:378); delayed suppression of polys and platelets
- Cisplatin (Ann IM 1984;100:704) iv or intraperitoneal; for testicular Ca cures and in combination rx of oat cell, head and neck, ovarian, and cervical Ca; adverse effects: renal damage (Ann IM 1988;108:21); neuropathy, prevent with ACTH analog (Nejm 1990;322:89); pulmonary fibrosis; low Mg^{++} (Ann IM 1981;95:628); MIs and CVAs (Ann IM 1986;105:48); rarely leukemia (Nejm 1999;340:351)
- Cyclosporine (Nejm 1989;321:1725); for immunosuppression in organ transplants; use w diltiazem or ketoconazole to reduce cyclosporine dose costs (Nejm 1995;333:628); adverse effects: lymphomas develop in 13% (Nejm 1984;310:477); nephropathy, severe and progressive when dose ≥ 5 mg/kg/d, or is con-

tinued in face of increasing creatinine, or age > 30 yr (Nejm 1992;326:1654; Ann IM 1992;117:578); increased uric acid and gout (Nejm 1989;321:287); hypertension (Nejm 1990; 323:693); levels increased by grapefruit consumption

- Dacarbazine (DTIC); adverse effects: marrow suppression
- Dactinomycin (Actinomycin D); adverse effects: marrow suppression, mucous membrane ulcerations
- Docetaxel used for hormone-resistant mets from prostate Ca (Nejm 2004;351:1502)
- Estramustin, like docetaxel
- Hydroxyurea; adverse effects: marrow suppression, leg ulcers (Ann IM 1998;128:29)
- Imatinib (Gleevec) (Nejm 2002;346:645,683; Med Let 2001; 43:49) po; tyrosine kinase inhibitor against Rous sarcoma virus-like oncogenes (Nejm 2002;347:462,472,481); used in CML and gi sarcomas
- Mithramycin (Plicamycin) iv; for testicular Ca, hypercalcemia; with hydroxyurea for CML blast crisis (Nejm 1986;315:1433); adverse effects: marrow suppression, especially of platelets, causing bleeding
- Mitomycin; adverse effects: marrow suppression
- Mitoxantrone; used for hormone-resistant metastatic prostate Ca (Nejm 2004;351:1502); adverse effects: marrow suppression, cardiotoxic, blue urine and nails
- Mycophenolate mofetil (CellCept) (Med Let 1995;37:84); used w cyclosporine instead of azathioprine for organ transplant
- Oxaliplatin (Eloxatin) (Nejm 2004;350:2343; Med Let 2003;45:7) w 5-FU and leukovorin for metastatic colon Ca
- Paclitaxel (Taxol) (Nejm 1995;332:1004) and similar docetaxel (Taxotere) (Med Let 1996;38:87) iv q 3 wk; used vs breast and ovarian cancers as adjuvant rx and for palliation; adverse effects: neutropenia, hypersensitivity reactions, peripheral neuropathies; cost: $1200-2000/dose

- Pegascargase (Oncaspar); a polyethylene glycol–conjugated asparagenase, which makes it less sensitizing (Med Let 1995; 37:23)
- Procarbazine (Matulane) (Ann IM 1974;81:796); adverse effects: marrow suppression, crosses blood–brain barrier, MAO inhibitor
- Semustine (Lomustine, methyl-CCNU); adverse effects: delayed suppression of polys and platelets
- Sirolimus (Rapamune) (Med Let 2000;42:13); immunosuppressant like cyclosporine; used in transplant pts w steroids and cyclosporine
- Tacrolimus iv/po; immunosuppressant like cyclosporine; used w steroids, eg, for liver transplant (Nejm 1994;331:1110), and topically for atopic dermatitis (p 179) (Med Let 2002;44:48)
- Topotecan (Hycamtin); used in late ovarian Ca (Med Let 1996;38:96)
- Vinblastine (Velban) weekly iv; adverse effects: marrow suppression
- Vincristine (Oncovin) (Ann IM 1974;80:733) weekly iv; adverse effects: peripheral neuropathy (rx to loss of reflexes), constipation

Biologic Response Modifiers: Cytokines

- Interferons; for multiple, rapidly expanding tumors, eg, α-interferon for Kaposi's sarcoma in AIDS (Ann IM 1990;112: 812) and macrophage activation (Nejm 1991;324:509); adverse effects: various autoimmune diseases (Ann IM 1991; 115:178), depression helped by preventive SSRI rx (Nejm 2001;344:961)
- Interleukin-2 with or without lymphocyte-activated killer cells for metastatic melanoma and renal cell cancer; adverse effects: sepsis due to impaired granulocytic chemotaxis (Nejm 1990; 322:959)

- Tumor necrosis factor
- Granulocyte colony-stimulating factors: Filgrastim (Neupogen) and sargramostin (Leukin); use after chemotherapy to increase polys and decrease infections (Ann IM 1994;121:492; Med Let 1991;33:61)
- Monoclonal antibodies:
  - Bevacizumab (Avastin) (Med Let 2004;49:46; Nejm 2004;350:2335,2407); a monoclonal antibody vs vascular endothelial growth factor, used for colon Ca w 5-FU regimens; $1000/wk
  - Cetuximab (Erbitux) (Med Let 2004;49:46); used in colon Ca; $2000/mo
  - Gemtuzumab (Mylotarg) (Med Let 2000;42:67); for AML, currently approved for pts > 60 yr in 1st relapse; a recombinant human monoclonal antibody directed type
  - Rituximab (Rituxan)
  - Trastuzumab (Harceptin)
  - Erlotinib (Tarceva) and gifitinib (Iressa) (Med Let 2005; 47:25); for non-small cell lung cancer
- Protease inhibitor
  - Bortezomid (Nejm 2005:352;2487,2534,2546) for myeloma

Radio-immunoconjugates

- Tositamomab Iodine-131 (Bexxar) (Med Let 2003;45:86); for follicular, non-Hodgkin's lymphomas
- Tinxetan (Zevalin) (Med Let 2002;44:101); to get micro/local rad rx ($30,000/rx)

8.2   Vitamin Deficiency Anemias

B_{12} Deficiency Anemia

Nejm 1997;337:1441, 1966;275:978

Cause:

- s/p gastric resection, even yrs later may develop, probably the most common cause now (Ann IM 1996;124:469), or post–gastric bypass or even plication
- Pernicious anemia (PA) with no intrinsic factor (IF): Congenital juvenile type (Nejm 1972;287:425) and adult autosomal dominant, atrophic gastritis type; both genetic but unrelated (Ann IM 1974;81:372)
- *Diphylobothrium latum* competition for gut B_{12}
- Dietary deficiency, very rare, perhaps only in strict non-ovolacto-vegetarians (Nejm 1978;299:317)
- Distal small bowel absorptive defect, limited to as little as 10-20 cm in some patients
- Blind loop bacterial consumption (Ann IM 1977;87:546)
- Drugs: PAS, neomycin, colchicine (Nejm 1968;279:845)
- "Pancreatic intrinsic factor" deficiency of enzyme to break down salivary protein-B_{12} complex so can bind IF in stomach (Nejm 1971;284:627)
- Malabsorption of food/protein-bound B_{12} very common (15% prevalence) in elderly (Am J Clin Nutr 1994;60:2)

Epidem: PA increased in Scandinavians and blood group A people; prevalence in all races in U.S. ~ 0.1% (Nejm 1978;298:647; Ann IM 1971;74:448), 1.9% over age 60

Pathophys: B_{12} is a crucial coenzyme for ribonucleotide reductase (RNA to DNA) and propionic catabolism, lack of which may cause CNS demyelination first in posterior, then in lateral columns. In PA, antigastric parietal cells (where IF is made), as well as H^+/K^+-ATPase antibodies

Sx: of anemia, sore mouth; mean age of onset of PA = 60 yr; 20% of PA pts have pos family hx; diarrhea and other malabsorption sx

Si: Anemia, glossitis, stomatitis, fair complexion, vitiligo

Crs: Sx onset after 2 yr of total deficiency

Cmplc: CHF due to profound anemia; thrombocytopenic purpura; stomach Ca with adult PA; subacute combined degeneration (case: Nejm 2003;348:2204) of cortex and posterior and lateral (corticospinal) columns of spinal cord w sx of distal paresthesias and numbness, paraplegia, vibratory sense and position sense loss, pos Rhomberg, psychiatric sx and dementia, and peripheral neuropathy, seen even without macrocytosis (Nejm 1988;318: 1720,1752); carcinoid-secreting tumor due to chronic gastrin stimulation (Nejm 1997;336:866)

r/o (Nejm 1973;288:764) other macrocytic anemias: Folate deficiency, orotic aciduria (Nejm 1990;322:1641,1652), di Guglielmo's syndrome, anti-DNA drugs

Lab: *Chem:* Gastrin levels sky high (no acid inhibition since acid-secreting cells hit harder than gastrin secretors: Nejm 1970;282: 358). HgbF and A$_2$ increased; B$_{12}$ by RIA < 100 pg/cc, but levels < 300 pg/cc may be significant if elevated MMA levels; increased LDH, Fe, bilirubin, serum methyl malonic acid (MMA; > 271 nM/L), and homocyteine levels elevated before overt B$_{12}$ deficiency (Ann IM 1996;124:469)

Gastric: Aspirate shows no acid, no false negatives?

Hem: Macrocytic anemia, neutropenia, and hypersegmented polys, normal or sometimes low platelets (ineffective production) unlike Fe deficiency; r/o myelodysplastic syndromes

Path: Marrow is megaloblastic with red cell precursor nuclei still open, ie, not pyknotic in late normoblastic stage, Howell-Jolly bodies, giant "C" metamyelocytes. In PA, stomach shows lymphatic infiltration early; CNS shows multifocal myelin degeneration with microcavities and glial scar.

Serol: Elevated intrinsic factor antibodies in PA

Schilling test: Rarely done anymore; first load with im B$_{12}$, then 3 hr later give hot B$_{12}$ po and measure excretion in 24-48 hr urine sample, normal > 15%; then repeat with intrinsic factor to see if corrects

Rx   (J Am Ger Soc 2002;50:1789): Preventive: Avoid unnecessary folate replacement, which helps anemia but masks subacute
combined degneration (Nejm 2003;348:2204)

B_{12} 1000-2000 μgm qd loading dose × 7 d im or weeks po,
or q 3 d ×4, or nasal spray (Nascobal) 500 μgm q 1 wk (8
doses/bottle); po as good as im even if no intrinsic factor (Acta
Med Scand 1968;184:247; Nejm 1959;260:361); then ≤ 500-
1000 μgm/mo po/im/nasal maintenance

Consider gastroscopy at least at diagnosis, maybe regularly to
pick up cancer in situ, which has 85% 5-yr survival

Folic Acid Deficiency

V. Herbert, Trans Assoc Am Phys 1962;75:307

Cause:

- Dietary: Poor, pregnant (18% of Boston City Hospital pregnant females: Nejm 1967;276:776), and/or alcoholic
- Inadequate absorption: Small bowel disease, throughout
  length, eg, sprue, blind loop
- Antifolate drugs, most of which inhibit deconjugase in gut mucosa since only monoglutamic folate is readily absorbed (Nejm
  1969;280:985): Alcohol, Dilantin, mysoline, birth control pills
  (Nejm 1970;282:858), triamterine (Ann IM 1970;73:414),
  pyramethamine, chemoRx especially with methotrexate

Epidem:

Pathophys: Minimum daily requirement is 50 μgm/d in adults and
children; 400 μgm/d in pregnancy. Reserves last 3-6 mo.
Polyglutamic folic acid is present in meat, eggs, cow's (not goat's)
milk products, vegetables (prolonged steaming will leach out);
necessary for thymidylate synthesis (the important one), histi-
dine catabolism (FIGLU is an intermediate), methionine synthesis, and two steps in purine metabolism.

Sx: of anemia; sore tongue and mouth, diarrhea

Si: Glossitis, stomatitis, hemolytic jaundice

Crs: Anemia in 20 wk after intake becomes zero; megaloblasts and some anemia after 40-60 d (R. Hillman, Nejm 1971;284:933)

Cmplc: Bleeding in pregnancy (Nejm 1967;276:776); increased MI and other ASCVD risk even w/o anemia, probably via increased homocysteine (Jama 1996;275;1893)

r/o other megaloblastic anemias (Nejm 1973;288:764): B_{12} deficiency, orotic aciduria (Nejm 1990;322:1641,1652), di Guglielmo's syndrome, anti-DNA drugs

Lab: *Chem:* Serum folate level by radioimmunoassay (Nejm 1972;286:764)

Hem: Anemia, macrocytic with macro-ovalocytes; neutropenia and hypersegmented polys; platelets normal or low, unlike Fe deficiency

Path: Marrow is megaloblastic with giant "C" metamyelocytes (bands); macrocytic cells elsewhere too, eg, gut mucosa (Nejm 1970;282:859)

Rx: Being added to cereal products to decrease congenital spinal abnormalities and for possible beneficial effects on heterozygous homocysteinemia

Monoglutamic folic acid 1 mg po qd is twice the adequate replacement dose; **beware:** doses of 15 mg qd will reverse B_{12} anemia but not the neurologic deficits (Arch IM 1960;105:372)

Iron Deficiency Anemia

Nejm 1999;341:1986; in infancy and childhood: Nejm 1993;329:190

Cause: Insufficient Fe for heme and related coenzyme synthesis because of gi blood loss from cancers, benign diseases like ulcers, eg, chronic *H. pylori* gastritis (Jama 1997;277:1135); or in runners (Ann IM 1984;100:843); or from cow's milk–induced gi bleeding in infants < 1 yr old; or because of absorptive defects in mucosa, as in sprue

Epidem: U.S. prevalence (Jama 1997;277:973): Children age 1-2 = 3%, adolescent girls = 2%, childbearing women = 5%

Increased prevalence in:

- Areas of low dietary Fe (Maritime Provinces)
- Children in 1st year of life with Fe-deficient mother and/or diet
- Adult women with heavy menses, pregnancy, nursing, or dieting
- Adult men with occult gi bleed, especially cancers
- Pica eaters, since starch, clay, etc, absorb Fe
- Post-gastric surgery, 50% at 10 yr due to rapid transit and absent H+, which is necessary for Fe absorption
- Any patient with colon, esophageal, or other gi cancer

Pathophys: Fe absorption is a balance between the reticuloendothelial system storage and gi mucosal cells' shedding of ferritin, a storage form (Nejm 1971;284:1413)

Sx: of anemia; sore mouth or tongue; pica, eating of starch, clay, etc (cause or effect? Ann IM 1968;69:435)

Si: Angular stomatitis, glossitis, nail spooning (r/o hyperthyroidism)

Crs: With rx, reticulocytes increase in 5 d, hgb increases 0.2 gm/d

Cmplc: Plummer-Vinson syndrome, seen in women, with esophageal webbing between cricoid and arch of aorta causing dysphagia. In children, Fe % saturations < 10% w anemia, even if corrected, correlate w poor later school performance (Nejm 1991;325:687).

r/o **Colon Cancer Always,** w colonoscopy or air contrast BE unless UGI sx, in which case w EGD 1st; hypoproliferative normochromic normocytic **Anemia of Chronic Disease** (Nejm 2005; 352:1011) caused by depressed erythropoietin (< 100) (Nejm 1990;322:1689) and treatable w po Fe and erythropoietin 150 U sc biw (Nejm 1996;334:619); also other microcytic anemias: thalassemia, lead intoxication, inherited hemoglobin E, paroxysmal nocturnal hemoglobinuria

Lab: *Chem:* Serum iron < 120 mg %, TIBC > 340 mg %, % saturation < 8% (between 8% and 20% may be hypoproliferative
low reticuloendothelial system Fe release). Ferritin decrease
(reflects marrow Fe but can be falsely elevated with inflammation). Erythropoietin levels elevated.

Hem: Anemia w hgb < 11%, hct < 32%; diagnostic trial of iron
should lead to normal crit in < 2 mo

Platelets increased (Nejm 1970;282:492) due to throm-
bopoietin effect of erythropoietin

Polys decreased in severe disease

Rbc's show microcytes, hypochromia, targets, pencil
forms; indices show MCHC < 30 mg %, decreased MCH
and MCV; r/o β-thalassemia, hemoglobin C or D disease,
spherocytosis, lead poisoning, and chronic aluminum toxicity (Nejm 1997;336:1556)

Path: Marrow shows no intracellular iron

Rx: $FeSO_4$ or ferrous gluconate 300 mg tid po, or qd if no rush;
use elixir if rapid transit causes poor absorption; with vitamin C
to increase absorption in elderly pts or unusual—especially
achlorhydric—conditions; avoid taking w tea, which decreases
absorption by 75%

Fe dextran iv only (not im), rarely need

Pyridoxine-Deficient/Responsive Anemias

Br J Hem 1956;2:86

Cause: Pyridoxine-deficient type is genetic. Responsive/not deficient
type is genetic, X-linked; drugs like INH induce it by complexing
with pyridoxine.

Epidem:

Pathophys: Pyridoxine is necessary for tryptophan, 5-HIAA, alanine,
nicotinic acid, and ALA synthetase synthesis, as well as mitochondrial Fe use. In deficient type, unknown reason for increased

requirements, but the problem fully corrects on low-dose replacement. In responsive/not deficient type, the problem never fully corrects; perhaps the defect is distal to pyridoxine and a large load partially overdrives the reaction.

Sx: Deficient type: Peripheral neuropathy

Si: Deficient type: Anemia
Responsive/not deficient type: Hepatosplenomegaly, anemia

Crs: Deficient type: Corrects with low dose (5 mg/d); reverts in 2-3 mo if rx stopped
Responsive/not deficient type: Partially corrects with high dose (300 mg/d)

Cmplc: Responsive/not deficient type: Iron overload states

Lab: *Chem:* Fe and TIBC levels elevated
Hem: Normal rbc survival, hypochromic anemia in both types. Reticulocytes normal or increased in deficient type; low in responsive/not deficient type.
Path: Marrow shows ring sideroblasts (normoblasts with Fe free in mitochondria), r/o idiopathic, myelodysplastic (Nejm 1999;340:1649), or alcohol-induced anemias (Nejm 1976;295:881)
Urine: Xanthurenic acid with tryptophan load is normal in deficient type but increased in responsive/not deficient type. Porphyrins increased in deficient type; decreased in responsive/not deficient type.

Rx: Pyridoxine 300 mg po qd

8.3 Hemoglobinopathies

Hemoglobin C Disease

Cause: Genetic, autosomal recessive (trait may manifest if coincident with sickle trait)

Epidem: In black Africans, perhaps up to 15% with disease in some areas; 3% of U.S. black population

Pathophys: Single amino acid alteration in β chain of HgbA

Sx:

Si: Splenomegaly; compensated hemolytic anemia

Crs:

Cmplc: Increased thrombotic disease; proliferative peripheral retinopathy
r/o hemoglobin D disease, similar but rarer

Lab: *Hem:* Hemolytic anemia with elevated reticulocytes and bilirubin, and erythroid hyperplasia in marrow; peripheral smear shows targets, microcytes; hgb electrophoresis shows characteristic HgbC

Rx: Transfusions for crisis; folic acid

G_6PD Hemolytic Anemia

Nejm 1991;324:169

Cause: Hereditary, nonspherocytic anemia:
Type I: Genetic; sex-linked recessive (women show only some decreased reducing power)
Type II: Genetic plus drug precipitants like antimalarials, eg, primaquine, sulfonamides, nitrofurans, ASA and aminopyrines, sulfones, dimercaprol, naphthalene, phenylhydrazine, probenecid, vitamin K, chloramphenicol, fava beans (only in whites), α-MeDopa (Nejm 1967;276:658), etc. In 11% of U.S. blacks; much higher prevalence in several Near Eastern groups, eg, Kurds (62%). This type exists because of balanced polymorphism from a selective advantage in females against falciparum malaria.

Epidem: Racial prevalence: Blacks, 15%; Sardinians, 14%; Sephardic Jews (Nejm 1967;277:1124), up to 20%; Ashkenazi (Polish-Russian) Jews, <1%; Greeks; Egyptians

Pathophys: In Caucasians, G6PD is decreased in all rbc's, leading to profound anemia through vulnerability to oxidative damage because G_6PD reduces NADP and thus provides the cell-reducing power to maintain sulfhydryl (SH) groups and help detoxify free radicals and peroxides. A deficiency also exists in other body cells (Nejm 1969;281:60). In contrast, G_6PD is decreased in only older (> 60-day-old) rbc's in blacks.

  Drugs are all redox catalysts taking TPNH → TPN, hgb → met-hgb. Cell membranes injured by oxidizing thiols (SH→ SS). Injured cells then phagocytized by liver and spleen.

Sx: Acute jaundice and anemia with infection or drug use in type II. Newborn jaundice can cause kernicterus.

Si: Anemia, color blindness

Crs: Sickle trait protects, and vice versa (Nejm 1972;287:115)

Cmplc:

Lab: *Hem:* Hemolytic anemia with increased reticulocytes, bilirubin, and marrow red cell series; low haptoglobin. Peripheral smear shows Heinz bodies (precipitated hemoglobin: Nejm 1969;280:203), helmets. G_6PD enzyme assay.

Rx: Stop drug; avoid infection and other sources of aplastic crisis; vitamin E no help (Nejm 1983;308:1014). Exchange transfusion in neonates with icterus.

Sickle Cell Anemia

Nejm 1999;340:1021; 1997;337:762

Cause: Genetic, autosomal

Epidem: In U.S. blacks, 7% have trait, 0.5% are homozygous. Genetic distribution in world correlates with history, geography, and malaria (Ann IM 1973;79:258).

Pathophys: Val substituted for Glut in β chain leading to hemoglobin (hgb) S, unstable at low O_2, which causes polymer precipitation, which in turn sickles cells. These sickled cells stick to vessel walls, causing clots and infarctions. Splenic infarcts produce diminished antibody formation, which leads to increased infections. HgbF ($\alpha_2\gamma_2$) may persist as a survival mechanism into adult life. Heterozygous cells sickle only in severe hypoxia or if HgbC or HgbD present. Renal damage to medulla causes decreased concentrating ability, K^+ loss, papillary necrosis, etc. α-Thalassemia trait protects, and vice versa (Nejm 1982;307:1441).

Sx: Painful crises in 60%; frequency correlates w worse prognosis (Nejm 1991;325:11)

Si: Retarded growth and sexual maturation (Nejm 1984;311:7); frontal bossing; skin ulcers, especially lower legs; angioid streaking of fundi indicates neovascularization (r/o Paget's, pseudoxanthoma elasticum)

Crs: 50% live to age 45 yr, longer if fetal hgb > 8.6% (Nejm 1994;330:1639); heterozygotes have no clinical disease

Cmplc:
- Acute chest pain syndrome (Nejm 2000;342:1854); most common cause of death; includes hypoxia, ARDS, and pneumonia
- Aplastic crises associated w parvovirus B19 infection in children, and with severe pain
- Pneumococcal and salmonella sepsis/infections, especially osteomyelitis (Nejm 1973;289:803)
- CVAs, which may be predictable by intracranial Doppler studies, then perhaps prevent with transfusions (Nejm 1992;326:605)

- Renal failure, 25% have proteinuria that may progress to renal failure (Nejm 1992;326:910)
- Bony infarcts, necrosis
- Gout (increased uric acid production)
- Gallstones
- Pulmonary hypertension chronically (Nejm 2004;350:886)
- Sudden death rate with heavy exertion increased to 32/10,000 in heterozygotes in contrast to 1/100,000 in whites (Nejm 1987;317:781)
  - Myonecrosis and myofibrosis (Ann IM 1991;115:99)

Lab: *Hem:* ESR low, sickled cells in peripheral smear; hemoglobin electrophoresis shows HgbS + increased HgbF (Nejm 1978;299:1428)

Urine: UA w hematuria, low specific gravity due to inability to concentrate even in heterozygotes

Xray: Long-bone infarcts/necrosis, "hair on end" skull, step fractures of vertebrae

Rx: Preventive maneuvers:
- Amniocentesis and abortion of affected fetuses (Nejm 1983;309:831)
- Penicillin (or Tm/S, or macrolide) prophylactically until age 5 (Jama 2003;290:1057)
- Pneumococcal vaccine (Nejm 1977;297:897); or phenoxymethyl penicillin 125 mg bid works age 4 mo-3 yr? (Nejm 1986;314:1593)
- Pre-op exchange transfusion helps (Nejm 1990;322:1666), but prophylactic transfusion in pregnancy does not work (Nejm 1988;319:1447)
- Hydroxyurea (Jama 2001;286:2099, 1995;273:611; Nejm 1995;332:1317) 10-25 mg/kg/d gradually increased to just start suppressing polys; stimulates fetal hemoglobin production (Nejm 1990;322:1037); improves survival over 8 yr (Jama 2002;289:1645)

Butyrate (short-chain FA) is ineffective (Nejm 1995;332:1606)
of surgical crisis: Transfuse to normal hematocrit (Nejm 1995;
333:206)

of anemia:

- Transfusions, but rx limited by sensitization, less with
  black blood donors (Nejm 1990;322:1617)
- Marrow transplant perhaps worth the risk because it
  works if patient survives (Nejm 1996;335:369, 426);
  90% w compatible donor survive

of nephropathy: ACE inhibitors to prevent progression (Nejm
1992;326:910)

of sepsis: Ceftriaxone im in children as outpts (Nejm 1993;
329:472)

of crisis: iv fluids, NSAIDs, narcotics; possibly steroids (Nejm
1994;330:733); possibly poloxamer 188 (Jama
2001;286;2099), possibly inhaled nitric oxide/O_2, 80%/20%
× 4 hr (Jama 2003;289:1136)

of stroke: Transcranial Doppler ulstrasound and transfusions
(plain or exchange) (Nejm 1998;339:5)

Hereditary Spherocytosis

Cause: Genetic, autosomal dominant in 75%; recessive in 25% (Nejm
1982;306:1170)

Epidem: In Europeans mainly; 5/100,000

Pathophys: Rbc membrane protein ("ankyrin": Nejm 1988;318:230)
deficiency causes Na permeability increase, which increases
intracellular Na so that cellular swelling results (Nejm
1986;315:1579); similar defect in nonspherocytic anemia (Nejm
1968;278:573). The swollen spherocyte is quickly phagocytized
by spleen.

Sx: Anemia, aplastic crisis

Si: Jaundice, splenomegaly, occasionally leg ulcers

Crs:

Cmplc: Aplastic crisis; r/o very similar **Elliptocytosis**, secondary hemolytic anemias

Lab: *Hem:* Microcytic smear has spherocytes. Osmotic fragility increased, glucose corrects. Coombs test neg.

Rx: Transfuse
Surgical splenectomy helps anemia though cellular defect remains

α-Thalassemia

Nejm 1976;295:710

Cause: Genetic

Epidem: Increased prevalence in Asians, Shiite Arabs (Nejm 1980;303:1383), and all populations exposed to malaria because of heterozygous individuals have some resistance

Pathophys: Impaired α-hgb chain synthesis, absolute or qualitative, and often associated with mental retardation (gene linkage) or fetal hydrops (Nejm 1981;305:607, 638). Thus homozygote unable to make HgbA ($\alpha_2\beta_2$), HgbA$_2$ ($\alpha_2\delta_2$), or HgbF ($\alpha_2\gamma_2$).

Sx: Homozygotes: Severe disease at birth with hydrops fetalis, ie, anasarca due to anemia
Heterozygotes: None or mild anemia

Si: Homozygotes: Splenomegaly, increased marrow proliferation and space

Crs: Homozygotes: Perinatal death

Cmplc: Heterozygotes: Severe disease when combined with another hemoglobin abnormality; hemosiderosis/iron overload

Lab: *Hem:* In both homo- and heterozygotes, peripheral smear shows rbc stippling (RNA and mitochondria), siderocytes, targets, "ghosts," and bizarre forms

In heterozygotes, MCV < 73 m^3, HgbA$_2$ < 3.5%; Fe levels normal (Nejm 1973;288:351); normal hgb proportions, or HgbH (β_4) increased (r/o acquired HgbH, rarely in erythroleukemics: Nejm 1971;285:1271)

In homozygotes, hgb electrophoresis shows no HgbA, HgbA$_2$, or HgbF; hgb Barts (γ_4) (Nejm 1990;323:179) and/or HgbH may be present; both of the latter are incompetent O$_2$ carriers

Rx: Transfusions, beware of iron overload

β-Thalassemia

Nejm 1999;341:99; Ann IM 1979;91:883

Cause: Genetic, autosomal. Homozygote = thalassemia major, Cooley's anemia. Heterozygote = thalassemia minor or thalassemia trait.

Epidem: Caucasians, especially Mediterraneans, eg, Greeks and Italians: up to 60% gene prevalence in some villages. Blacks: 1% of U.S. black population carries. Southeast Asians: 2-10% gene prevalence (Found Blood Res 10/86). Sustained by partial malaria resistance in heterozygotes.

Pathophys: β-Hemoglobin chain synthesis blocked in homozygotes so they are unable to make HgbA ($\alpha_2\beta_2$) but can make HgbA$_2$ and HgbF. Heterozygote has some decreased β-chain synthesis.

α/β-Thalassemia interaction: In β-thalassemia, $\beta/\alpha = 0.5$, but can be $> 0.5 \rightarrow 1$ if concomitant α-thalassemia gene as well, since this decreases inclusion production and thus intramedullary ineffective rbc production, leaving only a hypochromic, microcytic pattern (Nejm 1972;286:586)

Sx: Thal major: Onset age 3-6 mo when HgbA replaces HgbF
Thal minor: Asx unless α precipitants (Nejm 1974;290:939)

Si: Thal major: Skull bossing (marrow proliferation)
Thal minor: Splenomegaly

Crs:

Cmplc:

Thal major: Hemochromatosis/siderosis w transfusions leading to diabetes, insulin resistance (Nejm 1988;318:809), and hypopituitarism with impaired puberty and 2° amenorrhea; prevented with Fe-binding rx begun before age 10 (Nejm 1990;323:713); r/o thal trait plus HgbE, which looks like thal homozygote, **Hemoglobin E** is present in 40% of Southeast Asians (Found Blood Res 10/86); B_{12}; folate deficiency

Thal minor: Sickle/thal disease ($\frac{1}{4}$ as common as SS disease). Fe deficiency decreases α chain production, which in turn worsens the disease (Nejm 1985;313:1402). B_{12}, folate deficiency. Most commonly presents as a mild microcytic anemia so r/o other causes (p 453).

Lab: *Amniotic fluid:* To detect affected fetus, DNA probes works 85% of time, no false pos or neg (Nejm 1983;309:384, 1983; 308:1054)

Chem: In thal major, iron and % saturation both increased; bilirubin, urine, and stool urobilinogen all increased

Path: Liver bx to monitor iron load (Nejm 2000;343:327)

Hem: In both, MCV < 79 m^3, rbc stippling (RNA and mitochondria); siderocytes (hemosiderin-laden) in peripheral blood; targets; rbc "ghosts"; teardrops if spleen still in, vacuoles if not (Nejm 1972;286:589)

Hgb electrophoresis: In thal minor, HgbA$_2$ ($\alpha_2\delta_2$) persists at $\geq 2\times$ normal %; > 3.5% is diagnostic (Nejm 1973;288:351). In thal major, no significant HgbA; HgbF may persist.

Xray: Skull films show "hair-on-end" evidence of marrow space increase

Rx: Prevention (Nejm 2002;347:1162): In high-risk populations, w PCR analysis of chorionic villus sampling, abortion, and genetic counselling

of thal major: splenectomy and transfusions to keep hgb > 10 and thus diminish bone fragility (Nejm 1972;286:586); marrow transplant, 25% mortality (Nejm 1990;322:417), but only ~6% if transplanted early in course before liver damage (Nejm 1993;329:840); 5-azacytidine iv over 4 d q 1 mo increases HgbF (Nejm 1993;329:845) as does hydroxyurea and butyrate iv qd (Nejm 1993;328:81)

of Fe overload: *Avoid Fe rx*; tetracycline po to decrease gi absorption (Nejm 1979;300:5); deferoxamine sc with pump hs decreases diabetes, late liver and heart disease (Nejm 1994;331:567,574), but can cause dose-dependent deafness and blindness (Nejm 1985;313:869); or possibly deferiprone po (Nejm 1998;339:417, 1995;332:918), but not effective and adverse effects: agranulocytosis, hepatic fibrosis

8.4 Porphyrias

Hepatic Porphyrias (Acute Intermittent Porphyria, Variegate Porphyria, Porphyria Cutanea Tarda)

Ann IM 2005;142:439; Nejm 1991;324:1432

Cause: All 3 are genetic, autosomal dominant (VP: Nejm 1978;298:358)

Epidem: Acute intermittent porphyria (AIP): More women than men
Variegate porphyria (VP): Increased in South African Caucasians and in alcoholics (Nejm 1978;298:358)
Porphyria cutanea tarda (PCT): Increased in cirrhotics and hepatoma pts

Pathophys: Generally excess porphyrins cause skin sensitization; and excess ALA and porphobilinogen (PBG) cause neurologic damage. Impaired mitochondrial enzyme systems: succinyl CoA +

glycine (with ALA synthetase, the rate-limiting enzyme) →
ALA → PBG → UroPG I-III → CoproPG III → ProtoPG III →
ProtoPorph → heme (pathways: Nejm 1970;283:955). In AIP,
drug/diet induces ALA synthetase increase, and deficiency of
UroPG synthetase (PBG deaminase), causing increased ALA and
PBG, in turn causing demyelination and perhaps pain. In VP,
decreased conversion PPG → PP (Nejm 1980;302:765). In PCT,
decreased conversion UPG → CPG in rbc (Nejm 1978;
299:1095) and liver (Nejm 1982;306:766); skin damage from UV
and/or traumatic activation of complement (Nejm
1981;304:213).

Sx: Precipitated by barbiturates, sulfas, griseofulvin, alcohol (even in
mouthwashes: Nejm 1975;292:1115), estrogens and preg-
nancy, infections, weight reduction (Nejm 1967;277:350)

AIP: Onset age 20-40, abdominal colic, vomiting, constipation,
urine becomes brown on standing after voiding; no skin
involvement

VP: Onset age 11-30, abdominal colic, rash like PCT

PCT: Dermal sensitivity w bullae and scars, hyperpigmentation,
red urine, photosensitivity (differential dx: p 209)

Si: AIP alone: HT, tachycardia, low-grade fevers

AIP and VP: Peripheral motor and sensory neuropathy,
psychoses, and neuroses

PCT: Rashes, hirsutism, scarring, vitiligo, milia especially on
hands

Crs: AIP: 25% 5-yr mortality after first attack; worse in younger
patients

Cmplc: AIP: Respiratory paralysis, infections

VP and PCT: r/o scleroderma; congenital erythropoietic porphyria (Nejm 1986;314:1029); protoporphyria (Nejm
1991;324:1432); naprosyn, tetracycline, or nalidixic acid
photosensitization or similar skin changes seen with
hemodialysis and in all of which urine tests will be neg

Lab: *Hem:* in PCT: hgb, Fe, and TIBC increased often

Urine: in AIP and VP: red-brown on standing (pyrroles condense to porphyrins); single-void rapid semiquantitative PBG level elevated and, if positive, get other tests for precursors (ALA porphyrin and PBG), plus plasma porphyrins, fecal porphyrins, and rbc PBG deaminase levels. 24-hr urine PBG level > 2× normal during acute attack; urine porphyrins between attacks less helpful.

in PCT: PBG tests negative; chromatography shows increased UPG and CPG in urine

Rx: Prevent attacks of AIP and VP by avoiding multiple precipitating drugs, weight loss, infections, and drugs; test relatives; warn about pregnancy and oral contraceptives. In VP and PCT, avoid skin changes with protective clothing.

for PCT: phlebotomize 500 cc q 2 wk; unknown mechanism perhaps via hepatic Fe metabolism (Nejm 1968;279:1301). Chloroquine 250-500 mg qd × 5-8 d, exacerbates, then long remissions (Jama 1980;223:515).

of AIP/VP attacks: iv 10% glucose. Hemin (Panhematin) iv inhibits ALA synthetase.

8.5 Hemolytic Anemias

Aplastic Anemia

Ann IM 2002;136:534; Nejm 1997;336:1365

Cause: A stem cell disease. Autoimmune via drugs, infectious agent, or chronic immune disease, eg, quinidine (Nejm 1979;301:621), phenylbutazone, chloramphenicol, gold salts; viral hepatitis, EB virus (Ann IM 1988;109:695), parvovirus 19 (Ann IM 1990; 113:926; Nejm 1989;321:484,519,536); thymomas, rheumatoid arthritis (Ann IM 1984;100:202), SLE, myasthenia gravis, myxedema, viral hepatitis (Nejm 1997;336:1059).

Epidem: Pregnancy may induce relapse, but still possible

Pathophys: Sudden insult to stem cell from lymphocytic immune response; rarely folate-responsive in adult type (Nejm 1978; 298:469); perhaps antibody to erythropoietin in some cases

Sx: Recent PNH (15%); petechiae, infection, anemia

Si:

Crs:

Cmplc: Hematologic and solid tumors after marrow transplant or immunization (Nejm 1993;329:1152); PNH (p 468) (Ann IM 1999;131:401,467) in 25% of immunologically mediated aplastic anemias

Lab: *Hem:* Pancytopenia, ncnc anemia, retics < 2%, nucleated rbc's, normal Fe and TIBC

Path: Marrow shows marked decrease in rbc precursors, E/M ratio << 1:3

Serol: B_{19} parvovirus IgM and IgG titers (p 686); or by DNA hybridization studies of serum if immunosuppressed (Ann IM 1990;113:926)

Rx (Nejm 1991;324:1297):

- Marrow transplant if young and compatible donor, 69% 15-yr survival (Ann IM 1997;126:107)
- High-dose cyclophosphamide 50 mg/kg iv qd × 4 d; 65% complete remission (Ann IM 2001;135:477)
- Antilymphocyte globulin + prednisone + cyclosporine (Jama 2003;289:1130; Nejm 1991;324:1297), 68% response, 55% 7-yr and 38% 15-yr survival (Ann IM 1997;126:107); same response in older pts although mortality higher (Ann IM 1999; 130:193)
- Transfusions; use irradiated blood to prevent graft-vs-host disease from transfused lymphocytes
- Androgens, probably help only when hypoplasia not aplasia, eg, stanozolol 2 mg qd; try others if one doesn't work

Immune Hemolytic Anemia

Cause: Autoimmune in one of several different ways (see below) via drugs, cold agglutinins, idiopathic immune globulins

Epidem:

Pathophys:

- Autoimmune: Perhaps spontaneously, eg, in SLE, perhaps induced by unknown agents
- Drug induced: Methyldopa (antibodies are vs Rh antigens, 20% have positive Coombs after 5 mo rx, dose related but much lesser % of hemolysis because of coincident RES impairment: Nejm 1985;313:596), procainamide (20%: Nejm 1984; 311:809)
- Hapten type: Drug or virus (Nejm 1971;284:1250) attaches to rbc and antibody is directed vs this combination; eg, penicillin, especially high-dose iv (Nejm 1972;287:1322)
- "Innocent bystander": Agent/drug loosely attaches to rbc, antibody + C' attaches to rbc antigen–agent combination, agent/drug falls off, leaving antibody + C'-coated rbc, which is then picked up and lysed by RES rather than intravascularly; occasionally similar coincident platelet injury; eg, penicillin (ibid), tetracycline (ibid), cephalothins (Ann IM 1977;86:64), quinine, quinidine, sulfas (Nejm 1970;283:900)
- Cold agglutinin disease: Usually IgM, unlike above, which are usually IgG (Ann IM 1987;106:238)

Sx: of anemia

Si: Splenomegaly, jaundice

Crs: Drug types resolve with drug withdrawal; others respond to rx of primary disease, splenectomy, and steroids

Cmplc: Pulmonary emboli are most common cause of death; infections

Lab: *Chem:* Bilirubin increased

Hem: Smear shows spherocytes, "too many to be congenital spherocytosis"; retics increased; Coombs often positive, although
can be negative if antibody pulled off rbc by test serum;
anti-C′3 Coombs positive; in innocent bystander type,
increased osmotic fragility; IgG coating of rbc, 35-200 mole-
cules/rbc too few to give positive Coombs but can be detected (Nejm 1971;285:254), debate about what number is
significant and what false-pos/neg rate at each level, may be
useful to follow autoimmune and drug-induced types

Rx: Steroids (often relapse on moderate doses); cyclophosphamide (Nejm 1976;295:1522); androgens like danazol 600-800 mg
qd until better, then 200-400 mg qd maintenance (Ann IM
1985;102:298)

Splenectomy, 50% permanent remission, although Coombs
may remain positive; takes 3 wk to help, unlike rbc-defective hemolytic anemias, probably because needs time for antibody levels
to diminish

Paroxysmal Nocturnal Hemoglobinuria

Nejm 1991;325:991

Cause: A somatic mutation of PIG-A gene on the X chromosome in a
hematopoietic stem cell (Nejm 1994;330:249)

Epidem: Rare; onset usually age 20-40 yr

Pathophys (Ann IM 1999;131:467; Nejm 1990;323:1184): Somatic
mutation clonal deficiency in rbc membranes as well as
megakaryocyte and myeloid series; 2 cell populations, lysed cells
are young, survivors are normal. Rbc's of normal pts transfused
into PNH patients survive; PNH cells transfused to normal pts
lyse. Lysis due to C′3 inhibitor absence (DAF or decay accelera-
tion factor) from cell surface because the absent protein normally
glues C′ inhibitor and other proteins to cell surface membrane
(Nejm 1994;330:249).

Periodic massive hemolysis causes hemoglobinuria; correlates with sleep and with local acidosis (increased C'3 activity with slight decreases in pH)

Thrombosis, multiple microscopic and gross, perhaps due to lipid from rbc broken down membrane (thromboplastin) or platelets lysed and/or activated by C'3 system (Nejm 1972;286:180)

Sx: Weakness; pain (microthrombi) in lumbar back, chest, abdomen

Dark urine in the morning from hemoglobinuria; present initially in 50% of adults, 15% of pts < age 20; eventually 65% < age 20 develop it. Aspirin can precipitate attack.

Si: Unexplained hemolytic anemia or Fe deficiency; occasionally splenomegaly; occasionally icterus

Crs (Nejm 1995;333:1253): Chronic, median survival = 10 yr, 15% spontaneously remit; death from venous thrombosis, bleeding, or renal failure

Cmplc:

- Marrow failure present on presentation in 25% of adults and 60% of pts < age 20. Eventually most manifest marrow aplasia, which is not caused by PNH; rather, immune aplasia allows PNH clones to proliferate (Ann IM 1999;131:401,467). May present as an aplastic crisis or as infection (agranulocytosis). Fe and folate deficiencies also develop from losses in urine.
- Venous thrombi (50% at postmortem) in bowel, extremities, and liver causing liver failure and varices
- diGuglielmo's syndrome (Nejm 1970;283:1329) or CML
  r/o cold hemoglobinuria (IgG antibody fixes to rbc in cold and lyses when warmed, causing gangrene of digits and extremities; common in tertiary syphilis)

Lab: *Chem:* LDH elevated, from rbc's; AST (SGOT) increased, from liver damage

Hem: Plasma brown with methemalbumin; pancytopenia with low alk phos in polys; macrocytosis (decreased folate); hypochromia (Fe loss in urine); retics increased to 10-16%

Ham test: A diagnostic test; patient's rbc's broken down by normal serum acidified to pH 5.5-6.0. Thrombin worsens, Mg worsens (Nejm 1973;288:705).

Sugar water test: A screening test; PNH cells lyse in isosmolar sugar water with no lytes, normals don't (C′3 activated more easily in absence of lytes)

Flow cytometry and PIG-A gene product assays much more sens now than Ham and sugar water tests (Ann IM 1999;131:401,467)

Path: Renal biopsy shows Fe deposits

Urine: Intermittent hemoglobinuria, persistent hemosiderinuria from tubular cells; positive for Fe by nitroprusside blue; UUB > 1/64

Rx: • Avoid heparin since increased C′3 activation; warfarin can be used. Acutely can transfuse with washed rbc's (avoid wbc antigens, which when combined with antibody can activate C′3). Replace folate and Fe; but not too much, since iron can worsen because it increases retics, which themselves are more sensitive to hemolysis.

• Eculizumab, a recombinant human monoclonal antibody that inhibits C′ activation; iv q 1-2 wk; perhaps? (Nejm 2004;350:552)

• Androgens may help

• Marrow transplants work (Ann IM 1984;101:193) but risks compared to natural crs may not be worth it (Nejm 1995;333:1253)

• Streptokinase for acute venous thrombosis, eg, Budd-Chiari and inferior vena cava, can be used safely (Ann IM 1985;103:539)

8.6 Clotting Disorders

Screening Tests of Clotting Function

Activation Sequences:

Stage 1 (intrinsic system): XII → XI → IX* $\overset{VIII}{\to}$ X* activation (VIII acts as an enzymatic enhancer of IX → X)

Stage 1 (extrinsic system): VII* + tissue thromboplastin → X* activation

Stage 2: X* $\overset{V}{\to}$ II* (prothrombin) activation (V acts as an enzymatic enhancer of X → II)

Stage 3: II* → I (fibrinogen) + XIII activation

- Tourniquet test: BP cuff at 100 mm Hg × 5 min, normal is no petechiae; tests vessels and platelets (Nejm 1970;283:186)
- Bleeding time (BT), Ivy (Nejm 1972;287:155; rv of all platelet function tests: Nejm 1990;324:27): normal ∼ 4 min; tests vessels and platelets; a linear function of platelet numbers between 10,000 and 100,000; NSAIDs and aspirin (by far the worst) prolong via platelet effect that lasts platelet lifetime (3-d half-life: Nejm 1969;280:453). ASA tolerance test: Normal result is BT still < 15 min; greater elevation probably reflects underlying clotting disorder.
- Clotting time: Normal < 10 min; tests primarily stage 1 but stage 2 changes will also increase it
- Prothrombin time (PT): Normal = 11-14 sec, tests extrinsic system and stages 2 and 3
- Fibrinogen level: Normal > 200 mg %
- Activated partial thromboplastin time (aPTT): Normal = 30-40 sec; tests stages 1-3 without VII or platelets; stage 1 if PT ok
- Fibrin split products

* = Vitamin K–dependent factors.

Classic Hemophilia (Hemophilia A)

Nejm 1994;330:38

Cause: Genetic, sex-linked recessive causing factor VIII deficiency

Epidem: 80% of all patients with lifelong bleeding diathesis (Ann IM 1966;65:782); 1/7000-10,000 male births, only ⅓ have complete factor VIII deficiency

Pathophys: Intrinsic system defect (p 471) caused by deficiency of functioning factor VIII, although present in plasma immunologically (defective protein). Factor VIII is synthesized in blood vessel endothelial cells; circulates complexed to von Willebrand protein, which enhances VIII synthesis; protects it from proteolysis; and concentrates it at sites of active hemostasis.

Sx: Male; positive family hx in ⅔ (⅓ are due to new mutations). Wide spectrum from postsurgical bleeding to chronic bruising, joint bleeds, and crippling arthritis; gu bleeding (usually insignificant); no bleeding after minor cuts.

Si: Bleeding after trauma. Spontaneous hemarthroses only in severe disease.

Crs: Lifelong, 1995 prognosis nearly comparable to normal population if don't get HIV or Hep B (Ann IM 1995;123:823)

Cmplc: Psychiatric conditions related to chronic illness; hepatitis B (Ann IM 1977;86:703) and C; AIDS; flexion contractures of joints; intracranial bleeding, the cause of death in 25%

Lab: *Hem:* Prolonged PTT but normal PT and platelet count; r/o factor VIII autoantibody inhibitor, factor XI deficiency, antiphospholipid antibodies, lupus anticoagulants, or factor XII deficiency

Factor VIII levels: None detectable = severe disease; 1-4% of normal = moderate disease; 5-25% of normal = mild disease

Rx: Preventively avoid ASA and other NSAIDs; prenatal dx and abortion (Nejm 1979;300:937), in 1st trimester with DNA probe (Nejm 1985;312:682); detect female carriers by recombinant DNA techniques

Comprehensive outpt programs save money and lives; try to keep VIII > 15% w recombinant DNA VIII, no viral contamination risks (Nejm 1993;328:453; Med Let 1993;35:51), cost $20,000-$100,000/yr

Desmopressin (DDAVP) (Nejm 2004;351:683, 1998;339:245) 0.3 μgm/kg over 30 min iv or sc, or 150 μgm in children, 300 μgm in adults via nasal spray (Ann IM 1991;114:563) increases VIII transiently within 1 hr, eg, perisurgically or after trauma (Ann IM 1985;103:228); adequate alone in 80% (Ann IM 1985;103:6); adverse effects: water intoxication, MI/angina

Recombinant activated factor VII (rFVIIa; NovoSeven) (Med Let 2004;46:33) 90 μgm/kg; also being used off-label for traumatic bleeding; cost = $1500/mg so $10,000 to rx a 70-kg patient

of VIII antibody formation (IgG) (Nejm 2002;346:662, 702), in 10% and up to 50% of those w severe disease; rx with activated prothrombin concentrates (Konyne); or big doses of VIII; can also use plasmapheresis, steroids, and cyclophosphamide; not yet clear if will be an issue with recombinant VIII (Nejm 1993; 328:453)

Von Willebrand's Disease (Pseudohemophilia)

Cause: Genetic, autosomal dominant; or acquired, eg, with lymphoma (Nejm 1978;298:988)

Epidem: Prevalence = 1/25,000. Associated with mitral valve prolapse and Marfan's, both inherited connective tissue defects (Nejm 1981;305:131).

Pathophys: von Willebrand protein normally complexes and circulates with factor VIII, which enhances synthesis of VIII, protects it from proteolysis, and concentrates it at sites of active home-ostasis (Nejm 1994;330:38)

Platelets have decreased adhesiveness, probably due to a coenzyme deficiency, normally provided by factor VIII. No factor VIII inhibitors develop.

Types (Nejm 1983;309:816): I = decrease in VIII protein; II A and II C = decreased ability to form large VIII multimers; II B = increased removal rate of large multimers

Sx: Bleeding, some menstrual and/or birth-related bleeding despite normal increase in VIII during pregnancy

Si: Severe bleeding from abrasions, mucous membranes, postsurgery; rarely into joints like true hemophiliacs

Crs: Much less morbidity than hemophiliacs with similar VIII levels

Cmplc: Blood loss, spontaneous CNS or abdominal bleeding

Lab: *Hem:* VIII deficiency by levels and clot workup (p 471); antigen/function ratio ≤ 1, unlike hemophilia (Ann IM 1978;88:403)

Clotting studies: Normal PT and platelets; prolonged PTT; bleeding time may be normal, but not after ASA when BT > 15 min reliably, normals don't (D. Deykin, 1978); ristocetin test shows abnormal platelet function

Immunol: Deficient von Willebrand's factor by immunoassay, also called "factor VIII antigen"

Rx (Nejm 2004;351:683): Avoid ASA, indomethacin, phenyl-butazone, and other NSAIDs

Keep trough factor VIII levels > 30% for minor surgery and spontaneous bleeds; keep > 50% for major surgery, obstetrical delivery and dental extractions

Desmopressin (DDAVP; vasopressin analog) (for dosing, see rx for hemophilia), for type I and IIA only, worsens other types through platelet aggregation (Ann IM 1985;103:228; Med Let 1984;26:82)

Factor VIII w vW factor content, eg, Humate-P

Factor XI Deficiency and Factor IX Deficiency (Hemophilia B)

Factor XI: Nejm 1991;325:153

Cause:

XI: Genetic, autosomal recessive, incomplete penetrance

IX: Genetic, sex-linked recessive, several types of mutants (Nejm 1970;283:61); or acquired in nephrotics (Ann IM 1970;73:373) and pts w amyloid (binds factor IX) and big spleen, rx w splenectomy (Nejm 1979;301:1050)

Epidem:

XI: Common in Ashkenazi Jews, 1/190 people have in Israel; rare in others, < 1/1 million

IX: Prevalence = 1/10,000; 16% of all lifelong bleeding diathesis pts

Pathophys: Intrinsic system defect (p 471)

Sx: XI: Rarely spontaneous bleeding; usually only postsurgery

IX: Severe w trauma, surgery; hemarthroses, hematuria

Si:

Crs:

Cmplc: r/o circulating antibody inhibitors due to SLE, or multiple myeloma

Lab: *Hem:* Clotting w/u (p 471)

Xray:

Rx: Avoid ASA, indomethacin, phenylbutazone, and other NSAIDs

Refrigerated blood or plasma since both more stable than factor VIII

of IX deficiency: Alphanine; danazol 600 mg qd increases endogenous production (Nejm 1983;308:1393); keep levels 5-15% all the time, > 40% for surgery

Other Factor Deficiencies: I (Fibrinogen), II (Prothrombin), V, VII, X, XIII

Nejm 1970;282:57, 1969;280:405

Cause: All genetic, except occasionally due to amyloid (Nejm 1979; 301:1050, 1979;304:827); all autosomal recessive

Epidem: All very rare, < 1/1 million

Pathophys: (p 471)

Sx: I and VII: No or little bleeding
II: Mild bleeding, especially postsurgery
V and X: Mild bleeding but hemarthroses
XIII: Severe bleeding, hemarthroses, poor wound healing

Si:

Crs:

Cmplc: With II deficiency; r/o SLE anti-II antibodies

Lab: *Hem:* Clotting w/u (p 471)

Rx: For II, deficiency Konyne (p 473)

8.7 Purpura and Platelet Disorders

Disseminated Intravascular Coagulation (DIC)

Nejm 1999;341:586

Cause: 2 requirements: (1) reticuloendothelial system blockade by pregnancy, endotoxin, radiation, steroids, colloid; and (2) clotting system activated by:
- Thromboplastin releaser, eg, frozen tissue, placenta, tumors, trypsin, snake venom (Nejm 1975;292:505), open brain trauma (Nejm 1974;290:1043), renal transplant rejection (Nejm 1970; 283:383); or

- Defibrination agent, eg, amniotic fluid; or
- Platelet factor 3 (phospholipid) release, eg, platelet clot, hemolysis, fat embolism, immune reaction; or
- Activation of factor XII, eg, by exo- or endotoxin from sepsis

Epidem: More common than TTP. Increased incidence in OB especially with septic abortions, abruptio, eclampsia, mole, amniotic fluid embolus, missed abortion, retained dead fetus, fatty liver of pregnancy (Ann IM 1983;98:330); leukemias, cancers, and all cases of severe tissue damage; freshwater drownings; gram-negative sepsis

Pathophys: Fibrinogen is low due to consumption and rapid lysis; tissue damage especially in CNS, lung, and kidneys from thrombotic ischemia

Sx: Bleeding, coma; fever only if there is a secondary cause of fever, unlike TTP

Si: Palpable purpuric rash (r/o allergic vasculitis); shock, hypotension; oozing/bleeding at all sites

Crs: Acute, hours to days

Cmplc: Renal cortical necrosis, ATN, Sheehan's syndrome, acute cor pulmonale, adrenal insufficiency (rarely fatal)
r/o other microangiopathic anemias: TTP, HELP, HUS, malignant HT, and chemoRx-induced types

Lab: *Hem:* Smear shows microangiopathic anemia with helmets and other fragments. Platelets < 100,000. ESR = 0 (afibrinogenemia). PT very sensitive (R. Hillman 3/86), and PTT prolonged. Fibrinogen < 40 mg %; low levels of II (hence PT long), VIII, V (< 50% is diagnostic). Fibrin split products (D-dimers) markedly elevated; prolonged thrombin time. Elevated antithrombin III (Hillman 3/86).
Urine: Hematuria, isosmolar anuria late when ATN develops

Rx: Treat primary problem; replace factors, eg, fresh-frozen plasma and platelets; perhaps heparinize at low doses like 300-400 U/hr or w

LMW heparin, possibly antithrombin III, to break the consumption cycle; never do so in face of liver disease, and only as a last resort if chronic cause and uncontrollable bleeding

Thrombotic Thrombocytopenic Purpura (TTP)

Nejm 2002;347:589

Cause: von Willebrand factor cleaving protease (ADAMTS-13) IgG inhibitor (acquired type) or deficiency (familial type) (Nejm 1998;339:1578,1585,1629)

Epidem: Incidence is 4/1 million; 1/1000 autopsies, male/female = 2:3. Associated with IgG platelet antibodies in Graves' and Hashimoto's diseases (Ann IM 1981;94:27); with *E. coli* 0157:H7 infections (Ann IM 1995;123:698); occasionally w drugs, eg, ticlopidine rx (Jama 1999;281:806; Ann IM 2000;132:794), or rarely clopidogrel (Plavix) (Nejm 2000;342:1766)

Pathophys: von Willebrand factor multimers build up due to lack of cleaving protease, cause platelet aggregation/consumption and fibrin arteriolar plugging (Nejm 1998;339:1578,1585,1629, 1982;307:1432)

Sx: Fever, abdominal pain, bleeding especially in urine and gi tract, syncope (95%), headaches (34%), visual changes (8%) from retinal hemorrhages, seizures (8%)

Si: Fever usually (80%) < 102°F; purpura; retinal hemorrhages; neurologic si's in 90% (Curr Concepts Cerebro Dis 1977;12:17); coma (31%), mental changes (26%), paresis (20%), aphasia (11%), dysarthria (7%)

Crs: < 90 d in 80%, 90-365 d in 13%, > 1 yr in 7%. Mortality ~ 90% without rx, 10% with rx (Nejm 1991;325:398); nearly 20% of cases are recurrent, 36% recurrence over 10 yr (Ann IM 1995; 122:569)

Cmplc: Renal failure; occasionally Stokes-Adams attacks due to bundle of His degeneration

Lab: *Chem:* Bilirubin (85%) and BUN (90%) elevated; LDH markedly increased

Hem: Smear shows microangiopathic anemia with red cell fragments, burr cells, helmets, and nucleated rbc's. Hgb < 10.4 gm. Retics increased a lot, eg, ~20%. Platelets < 120,000 (97%). Wbc ~ 4000-5000 or less. Clot studies normal except mildly increased fibrin breakdown products. von Willebrand factor cleaving protease deficiency or inhibitor present (unlike HUS).

Noninv: EKG and EEG, both may be nonspecifically abnormal

Path: Gingival biopsy may show fibrin plugs; 60% false neg, 0% false pos (Ann IM 1978;89:500). Marrow shows increased megakaryocyte numbers.

Urine: Active nephritic sediment with protein, rbc's, wbc's, casts

Rx (Nejm 1991;325:398): Plasma (which has von Willebrand factor cleaving protease) as FFP, cryosupernatant, solvent-treated plasma, or plasma exchange (Am J Med 1999;107;573)

Immunosuppression to inhibit IgG antibody to von Willebrand factor clearing protease, w:

- Steroids iv, eg, 200 mg prednisone qd
- Cyclophosphamide + ritaximab (Ann IM 2003;138:105) possibly
- Splenectomy perhaps for recurrence (Ann IM 1996;125:294)

Hemolytic-Uremic Syndrome

Nejm 2002;347:589, 2002;346:23, 1990;323:1161

Cause:

- Postinfectious or postpartum (Nejm 1985;312:1556) via endotoxin; vero (shiga) toxin produced by 0157:H7 *E. coli* (Ann IM 1995;123:698; Nejm 1995;333:364, 1987;317:1496) infection from petting cows (Nejm 2002;347:555); hamburger and milk results in HUS in 6-30% of those children infected, and

also causes TTP; also caused by other *E. coli* (Nejm 1996; 335:635), shigella, pneumococcus, salmonella
- Relapsing
- Drug-induced TTP/HUS syndrome, esp w quinine (Ann IM 2001;135:1047, 1993;119:215)

Epidem: Increasing incidence; most under age 5 where now incidence = 6/100,000; day care clusters occurring. 65% of all types are postinfectious.

Pathophys (Nejm 2002;346:23): Relapsing type very similar to TTP and associated w circulating very large von Willebrand factor multimers, but predominant renal involvement (Nejm 1991;325:426). Diarrhea-associated types show a shiga toxin-induced thrombogenesis and vasculitis, with 4 systems involved: kidney, skin, joints, bowel.

Tissue plasminogen activator is elevated (Nejm 1993;327:755) because is complexed and inactivated

Drug-induced types probably due to drug-induced antibodies

Sx: Diarrhea (86%), vomiting (75%), bloody diarrhea (59%), abdominal cramps (50%), fever (49%), seizures (17%)

Postinfectious type may have h/o viral or bacterial infection 1-2 wk before

Si: As above; oligo/anuria

Crs: 2 wk average; < 5% mortality if supported; ie, is self-limited

Cmplc: Renal failure, 47% require dialysis temporarily and 25+% have long-term renal impairment (Jama 2003;290:1360); shock, cardiac arrest, blindness, CVAs

Lab: *Chem:* Elevated BUN and creatinine
Hem: Crit < 30%; microangiopathic picture with red cell fragments, platelets < 150,000; if wbc's > 15,000, prognosis worse. von Willebrand factor cleaving protease function nor-

mal (unlike TTP) (Nejm 1998;379:1578). Elevated D-dimer.

Urine: Hematuria, proteinuria

Rx (Nejm 1991;325:398): Prevent by avoiding antibiotic rx of O157 *E. coli* diarrhea (Nejm 2000;342:1930 vs Jama 2002; 288:996) and antimotility drugs

Supportive; dialysis; steroids may help by decreasing edema; plasma exchange transfusions help (Am J Med 1999;107:573)

No help: Antihistamines, anti-shiga toxin (Jama 2003; 290:1337)

Henoch-Schönlein or Anaphylactoid Purpura

Nejm 1997;337:1512; Semin Arth Rheum 1991;21:103; Arthritis Rheum 1990;33:1114

Cause: Perhaps an IgA immune complex disease precipitated by URI, strep throat, medications, or food allergies; but none of these is clearly associated

Epidem: Mostly in children, but up to 30% in adult? (Med Clin N Am 1986;70:355)

Pathophys: A small-vessel IgA immune complex vasculitis, with 4 systems involved: renal focal proliferative GN, skin purpura, joint arthritis, bowel edema and bleeding

Sx: H/o viral or bacterial infection 1-2 wk before (65%). Diffuse extensive purpura; abdominal pain, with nausea and vomiting often as 1st si; gi bleeding; hematuria; joint pain and swelling; fever

Si: Purpuric rash, palpable in 85%, especially over legs, arms, and buttocks; in adults, the rash blisters and ulcerates more, and more often involves the trunk; joint swelling

Crs: Usually benign and self-limited; < 10% recurrence. In adults, morbidity and mortality may be higher, all from renal disease (Clin Nephrol 1989;311:60); others find outcomes similar in adults and children (Semin Arth Rheum 1991;21:103).

Cmplc: Bowel obstruction due to intussusception, may look like appendicitis; glomerular nephitis, nephrotic syndrome, and end-stage renal disease (5%)

r/o other small-vessel vasculitis (p 1142)

Lab: *Chem:* BUN and creatinine increased in 10-20%

Hem: Platelets normal

Path: Polys around, but usually not in small arteriole walls; this finding helps distinguish it from **Leukocytoclastic Vasculitis**, which is seen in most systemic small-vessel vasculitis (p 1142)

Stool: Guaiac-positive

Urine: Hematuria and proteinuria in 50%

Rx: Steroids w azathioprine may help; antihistamines no help. Plasma exchange transfusions may help when rapidly progressive GN.

Immune (Idiopathic) Thrombocytopenic Purpura (ITP)

www.hematology.org/practice/idiopathic.cfm; Nejm 2002;346:995; Ann IM 1997;126:319

Cause:

- Autoimmune direct antiplatelet antibodies; part of hemolytic anemia spectrum (Nejm 1977;297:517), SLE, lymphoma, CLL, cancer, HIV; a type II direct cytotoxic antibody (p 518)
- Hapten type and innocent bystander immune reactions (type III, IgG immune complexes: Nejm 1985;313:1375, 1984;311:635) involving transfusions (Nejm 1972;287:291); drugs like gold, heparin (Nejm 1976;295:237), quinidine, thiazides, sulfas; perhaps transient viral infections

Epidem: Chronic form, 70% women, 70% < age 40 yr; childhood type onset around age 5, usually abrupt onset, remits in 70% within 6 mo; males = females

Pathophys: Antiplatelet IgG coats platelets, decreases half-life from 3-5 d to < half-day because macrophages gobble up; delayed (type IV) hypersensitivity reaction may also play some role

Sx: Easy or spontaneous bruising

Si: Petechiae, purpura

Crs: Remission spontaneously in 85% children, 10% adults

Cmplc: Spontaneous bleeding only when platelet counts < 10,000-20,000 (Nejm 1997;337:1870); in pregnant pts, follow antibody levels and platelet counts (Nejm 1990;323:229, 264)
     r/o other causes of thrombocytopenia:

- Impairments of production: Hypoproliferative production, eg, pernicious anemia, PNH; or ineffective production, eg, alcoholics
- Impairments of distribution, eg, splenic pooling
- Consumption, eg, immune destruction (ITP); vascular destruction (DIC); or delayed-onset heparin-induced thrombocytopenia associated w high thrombotic risk (Ann IM 2002;136:210)

Lab: *Chem:* Plasma glycocalicin increased (50-250% of normal range), a fragment of platelet membranes, increased in all consumptive thrombocytopenias (Nejm 1987;317:1037)

Hem: Platelets decreased in number, increased in size (immature). Bleeding time unnecessary but will be normal because, although numbers are decreased, stickiness is increased. Coomb's test may often be positive since low-grade hemolytic anemia may be present as well (Nejm 1977;297:517); as Evan's syndrome, seen in SLE, pregnancy.

Serol: HIV, maybe ANA

Path: Marrow shows increased megakaryocyte numbers but usually not indicated except over age 60

Rx: Consider when platelet counts consistently < 30,000/cc (Ann IM 1997;126:307; Nejm 1993;328:1226)

1st: Prednisone, ~100 mg po qd × 1-2 wk or to response then taper; or, in resistant cases, dexamethasone 40 mg po daily × 4 d helped 85%, and 50% long-term remission (Nejm 2003;

349:831); if platelet count at 10 d < 90,000, then q 28 d
repeats may help (Nejm 1994;330:1560)

2nd: Splenectomy works in 75% (60% complete and 15% partial
remissions) (but only 14% of SLE: Ann IM 1985;102:325);
response is predicted by response to high-dose iv IgG
(1 gm/kg iv qd ×2) (Nejm 1997;336:1494); must balance
against later fear and risk of sepsis (death in 1-2% lifelong
before pneumovax, unknown what it is now)

Transient: Immunoglobulin rx w plasmapheresis transient help;
or high-dose iv IgG, will overwhelm RES and produce transient remission, eg, for surgery, very expensive (Nejm
1982;306:1254): $3000-4000/dose; or iv anti-Rh(D) IG,
which costs ½ as much and, in Rh-positive pts, saturates
spleen w coated rbc's so can't consume platelets (Med Let
1996;38:6); Fc receptor monoclonal IgG (Nejm
1986;314:1236)

Maybe: ChemoRx with cytoxan, azathioprine, colchicine, vincristine, vinblastine; or MOPP or CMOPP regimen—all
doubtful help (Ann IM 2004;140:112)

in pregnancy: Steroids iv, immune globulin, and cesarean section
all potentially useful but only justified if sx in mother (Nejm
1990;323:229,264)

in children: Usually just observaton; rarely iv immune globulin or
steroids at 4 mg/kg/d × 4 d

8.8   Myeloproliferative Disorders

Thrombocythemia

Nejm 2004;350:1211

Cause: A clonal myeloproliferative disease, most due to a "gain of
function" mutation of JAK2 gene on short arm of chromosome 9
which may manifest as P. vera, thrombocythemia, or myelofibrosis (Nejm 2005;352:1779)

Epidem: Incidence = 4/10,000/5 yr while that of benign thrombocy-topenia = 8/10,000/5 yr (Ann IM 2003;139:470).

Pathophys: Excess clonal production of defective platelets

Sx: Bruises, melena, hematemesis, etc

Si: Purpura, bleeding; splenomegally (40%)

Crs: Benign in young

Cmplc: CVA and seizures (Ann IM 1984;100:513); **Erythro-melalgia =** attacks of redness and burning of extremities relieved for days by one aspirin, a platelet microvascular disorder (Ann IM 1985;102:466)

r/o vast majority of elevations, are transient or benign thrombocythemias (Ann IM 2003;139:470); reactive causes of elevated platelets, all w no effect on clotting: stress, acute blood loss, acute infection, exercise, malignancy, Fe deficiency, s/p splenectomy, hemolytic anemia, chronic infection, drugs like vincristine

Lab: *Chem:* Pseudohyperkalemia, acid phosphatase, and LDH ele-vated; plasma levels normal but increased in test tube due to platelet contraction

Hem: Platelets, some giant, increased usually > 1 million but function may be diminished, eg, by thromboplastin genera-tion test or response to epinephrine (Ann IM 1975;82:506); levels between 400,000 and 1 million are usually reactive in etiology

Basophils increased > 40/mm³. Marrow shows increased megakaryocyte size, inappropriately large for platelet count, unlike CML and reactive causes of elevated platelets.

Rx: ASA 100 mg po qd

of sx like recurrent thrombosis or abnormal clotting studies and planned surgery:

• Hydroxyurea even though leukemia risk present (Nejm 1995;332:1132)

- Anagrelide 1-1.5 mg po q 6 hr × 5-12 d until platelets decrease to normal, then 1.5-4 mg po qd (Nejm 1988;318:1292)
- Alkylating agents (busulfan, melphalan) rarely, but leukemia risk
- Interferon-α rarely

Polycythemia Vera

Cause: A clonal myeloproliferative disease; most due to a "gain of function" mutation of JAK2 gene on short arm of chromosome 9 which may manifest as P. vera, thrombocythemia, or myelofibrosis (Nejm 2005;352:1779)

Epidem: Male > female. Incidence = 3/10,000/5 yr, while that of benign idiopathic polycythemia = 51/10,000/5 yr (Ann IM 2003;139:470).

Pathophys: Caused by loss of Bcl-X_L apoptosis regulator genes dependence on erythropoietin of (Nejm 1998;338:564,572,613). Excessive production of rbc's causes elevated crit, sludging at crits > 60% only (Nejm 1970;283:183); increased cellular breakdown causing gout; venous distention and headache; increased atherosclerosis, why?

Sx: Headache, dizziness, warm bath–induced pruritus (Nejm 1972; 286:845)

Si: Splenomegaly (75%), hepatomegaly, red sclerae (r/o conjunctivitis), plethora

Crs: 3% annual mortality, 3.5%/yr incidence of thrombotic events (Ann IM 1995;123:656)

Cmplc: Gout; thromboembolic diseases; erythromelalgia (p 485); Budd-Chiari due to hepatic venous occlusion even in occult myeloproliferative disease, ie, may be first sx especially in young female (Ann IM 1985;103:329)

r/o other etiologies of high crit:
- Hypovolemia: Pheochromocytoma, Addison's, stress

- Increased erythropoietin causes (can rx all by adenosine receptor inhibition of erythropoietin effect by theophylline: Nejm 1990;323:86)
- Hgb abnormalities with increased O_2 affinity, eg, hgb Rainier, Chesapeake, Kempsey, Yakima, M
- Hypoxia due to lung disease, etc = 95% of polycythemics; esp in smokers (Nejm 1978;298:6)
- Tumor producing erythropoietin, eg, of posterior fossa of brain, hepatoma, renal, uterine fibroid
- Renal transplant

Lab: *Hem:*
- White count increased to 30,000 with increased or normal leukocyte alkaline phosphatase (LAP) activity
- B_{12} high due to increased binding protein in all myeloproliferative diseases and some leukemoid reactions (Ann IM 1971;765:809)
- Platelets elevated (80%)
- Basophils, elevated > $40/mm^3$ is diagnostic of myeloproliferative disease although some false negs (Clem Finch, 1972)
- Erythropoietin levels, low to normal = 3-5 U/d in 24-hr urine; elevated to 30 U/d in anemia or secondary polycythemia; useful in 2nd-stage w/u of polycythemia (Nejm 1986;315:283)
- Plasma volume increased in 60% of P. vera (decreased in stress polycythemia)
- Rbc volume increased in P. vera and secondary causes, normal in stress polycythemia
- Hgb electrophoresis or blood gases at 37°C (graph: Ann IM 1976;84:518) to r/o abnormal hgb
- Carboxy hgb level to r/o smoking cause (Nejm 1978;298:6)
- Marrow shows larger megakaryocytes, unlike CML and secondary causes of elevated platelets (Finch); erythroid hyperplasia; no fat; no Fe

Rx: Maintain crit < 45% with phlebotomies; ASA 81-325 mg po qd halves thromboembolic cmplc rates (Nejm 2003;350:113)

Possibly interferon-α2b sc tiw (Ann IM 1993;119:1091)

ChemoRx worsens prognosis by increasing neoplasms (Ann IM 1995;123:656) but over age 60-70 yr hydroxyurea stroke prevention may be worth the AML risk

Myelofibrosis with Myeloid Metaplasia

Nejm 2000;342:1255

Cause: A clonal myeloproliferative disease, most due to a "gain of function" mutation of JAK2 gene on short arm of chromosome 9 which may manifest as P. vera, thrombocythemia, or myelofibrosis (Nejm 2005;352:1779)

Epidem: Older people (age > 50 yr); most common cause of splenomegaly in this age group. May interconvert with P. vera, debatable (p 486).

Pathophys: A clonal stem cell disorder causes ineffective erythropoesis, dysplastic megakaryocytes, immature granulocytes, and reactive myelofibrosis. Hematopoiesis moves to liver and spleen as marrow fibroses.

Sx: Bleeding, bruising; abdominal masses; failure to thrive

Si: Hepatosplenomegaly, anemia, purpura/ecchymoses, hypermetabolic cachexia in later stages

Crs: Slow, median survival 3-6 yr

Cmplc: Gout, renal stones, and failure

Lab: *Hem:* Anemia; smear shows bizarre rbc's, droplet forms diagnostic (r/o other infiltrative macrocytic disease of marrow, eg, metastatic cancer), immature granulocytes, nucleated rbc's

Wbc increased to < 50,000, except terminally can be ≥ 100,000

Leukocyte alkaline phosphatase (LAP) normal to elevated

Platelets often increased with giant forms and megakaryocytes on peripheral smear

Rx: of pain or hypersplenism: Perhaps splenectomy, or irradiation, and hope that liver and marrow can take over, but danger of thrombocytosis post splenectomy

of anemia: Transfusions, androgens

of leukocytosis: Hydroxyurea, interferon-α

Chronic Myelogenous Leukemia (CML)

Nejm 1999;340:1330, 1999;341:164; Ann IM 1999;131:207

Cause:

Epidem: Median age of onset = 53 yr, but wide range down to childhood; incidence = 1-2/100,000/yr; 15% of adult leukemia. 95% are due to a Philadelphia (Ph) chromosome (22 from 9 crossover, opening up oncogene: Nejm 1985;313:1429); also increased incidence in Down's syndrome trisomy 21, and with atom bomb or P^{32} exposure.

Pathophys: Unregulated signal transduction by a tyrosine kinase formed as a result of a chromosome 22 and 9 translocation. Marrow invasion, leads to decreased rbc's, platelets, and wbc's. Single-cell origin suggested by G_6PD type A or B enzyme exclusively in Ph-positive cells (Nejm 1973;289:307).

Sx: Fatigue, anorexia/weight loss, purpura, hives, and pruritus (histamine release); but 40% are asx when found on CBC

Si: Splenomegaly (50%), anemia, purpura, swollen gums (cellular infiltrate); no lymphadenopathy; "chloroma," red-brown skin papule becomes green when blood squeezed out of it (Nejm 1998;338:969)

Crs: Median survival ~40 mo; then acute blastic crisis develops; w rx, 50% 5-yr survival, 30% 10-yr survival

Cmplc: Pulmonary and endocardial fibrosis with eosinophilic variety. Lymphoid blast crisis (B or T cells).

Lab: *Chem:* Serum B_{12} markedly increased, often > 1000 pg/cc, r/o
cancer if > 20,000 pg/cc (Nejm 1974;290:282). Uric acid
increased.

Hem:

- Smear not diagnostic, may have elevated wbc's; wbc =
  50,000-250,000, mostly myelocytes; blastic phase =
  30+% blasts; ^{2}/$_3$ AML type, ^{1}/$_3$ ALL type which determines
  rx choices and prognosis
- Basophils elevated > 40/mm^3 plus marrow mast cells also
  increased (Ann IM 1978;88:753)
- Platelets increased in number although function impaired
- LAP decreased even when in relapse, r/o infectious mono,
  PNH, and slight decrease in sickle cell disease (Nejm
  1975;293:918)
- Marrow has positive Ph chromosome prep in all; all erythroid and myeloid elements increased; even erythroblasts
  have Ph chromosome

Rx (www.nccn.org):

- Marrow transplant (Ann IM 1997;127:1080, Nejm
  1998;338:962), potentially curative in young pts so 1st choice
  there; 50-75% 5-yr survival
- Interferon-α (Nejm 1997;337:223, 1994;330:820; Ann IM
  1996;125:541) im qd × 28 d then tiw (Ann IM 1994;
  121:736); or w cytarabine
- Imatinib (Gleevec) (Nejm 2002;346:645,683; Med Let 2001;
  43:49); currently best option short of transplant
- Antimetabolites like cytosine arabinose

DiGuglielmo's Syndrome (Myelodysplastic Syndrome, Erythroleukemia, Sideroblastic Anemia, Siderochrestic Anemia, Refractory Normoblastic Anemia)

Nejm 1999;340:1649

Cause: Neoplastic; may be a member of the myeloproliferative disorders; PNH patients may evolve to diGug's (Nejm 1970;283:1329)

Epidem:

Pathophys: Erythromyelosis (is still erythropoietin-dependent), erythroleukemia, and myeloblastic leukemia develop progressively

Sx:

Si: Progressive anemia

Crs: Years

Cmplc: Myeloblastic leukemia (50%)
r/o aplastic anemia

Lab: *Chem:* Fe and TIBC increased; IgG increased in ¹/₃
Hem: Smear shows erythroblasts, NCNC anemia, may be moderately macrocytic

Marrow is megaloblastic with vacuoles in normoblasts; erythroblastic hyperplasia; increased myeloblasts; ring sideroblasts, normoblasts with free iron in mitochondria, ie, not incorporated into hgb (r/o acute alcohol toxicity, pyridoxine-responsive anemia, pernicious anemia, INH, chloramphenicol toxicity, lead toxicity)

Platelets decreased, often due to ineffective production
Leukocyte alkaline phosphatase low; neutropenia

Rx: Oxymethalone or other androgens; recurrent transfusions; antithymocte globulin iv qd × 4 d perhaps (Ann IM 2002; 137:156)

Lenalidomide (a thalidomide) improves anemia, thrombocytopenia, and neutropenia in pts w myelodysplastic syndrome resistant to erythropoietin (Nejm 2005;352:549)

8.9   Lymphomas/Leukemias

Agranulocytosis and Neutropenia

Cause:
- Allergic directly as with chloramphenicol or via lupus, eg, from procainamide (Ann IM 1984;100:197)

- Autoimmune antibodies and occasionally, perhaps, killer T cells (Ann IM 1985;103:357); idiopathic usually; ibuprofen induced, reversible (Nejm 1986;314:624)
- Direct drug toxic effect from chemotherapy, chloramphenicol

Epidem: Autoimmune type associated with rheumatoid Felty's syndrome

Pathophys:

Allergic type: Delayed-hypersensitivity T cells kill in marrow; drugs can act as hapten to induce

Autoimmune type: Antibodies especially to HLA surface antigens

Sx: Malaise, sore throat

Si: Pharyngitis, recurrent infections

Crs: Idiopathic autoimmune type very benign

Cmplc: Sepsis
r/o genetic cyclic neutropenia (Nejm 1989;320:1306)

Lab: *Hem:* Polys < 500/mm^3

Rx: To prevent sepsis:
- Protective isolation, probably no benefit, but at least eliminate salads (Nejm 1981;304:433)
- Antibiotic prophylaxis: Trimethoprim/sulfa (Ann IM 1980;93:358); or fluoroquinolone + penicillin (Jama 1994;272:183); or ofloxacin + rifampin (Ann IM 1996; 125:183);
- Granulocyte colony-stimulating factor (Nejm 1992;327:99), eg, filgrastim (Neupogen), long-acting form Neulasta ($3000/shot) or sargramostim (Leukin) (Med Let 2002;44:44); often used w some multiple-drug regimens
- Lithium po increases production of polys; level 0.7-1.4 decreases infections and increases survival (Nejm 1980; 302:257)

- Transfusions of polys no help even with documented infection (Ann IM 1982;97:509)

  of allergic type: Steroids, cyclophosphamide

  of autoimmune type: Splenectomy helps, 70% by decreasing IgG (Nejm 1981;304:580; Ann IM 1981;94:623)

  of direct toxic type: Stop offending medication

  of fever/sepsis (Ann IM 2002;137:77,123): Ceftazidime (Ann IM 1994;120:834) or imipenem alone; or with aminoglycoside but less often used now (ACP J Club 2003;138:45); or piperacillin/tazobactam (Zosyn); or ciprofloxacin; or aztreonam/vancomycin. Oral Augmentin w or w/o ciprofloxacin as good or better than iv regimens (ACP J Club 2005;142:32; Nejm 1999;341:305,312,362) at least when is short-lived during cancer chemoRx. If not better in 4+ days, add antifungal rx like amphotericin (Nejm 1993;328:1323), or less toxic fluconazole (Am J Med 2000;108:282) or itraconazole (Ann IM 2001;135:412) or voriconazole (Nejm 2002;346:225), or caspofungin (Nejm 2004;351:1391).

Acute Nonlymphocytic Leukemia (Including Myeloblastic [AML] and Monoblastic)

AML: Nejm 1999;341:1051

Cause:

Epidem: Increased incidence in patients treated for Hodgkin's, multiple myeloma, Waldenström's, and ovarian cancers treated with radiation, MOPP (4% at 10 yr get it: Ann IM 1970;72:693), and alkylating agents like melphalan, chlorambucil, thiotepa, and cyclophosphamide (Nejm 1990;322:1,7); may be preceded by a myelodysplastic syndrome associated w somatic chromosomal deletions. 2.4 cases/100,000/yr in U.S.; 12.6/100,000/yr over age 65.

Pathophys: Perhaps a defect in a maturation stimulator so cells don't die as normally would

Sx: Weakness, bleeding, fever, infections

Si: Anemia; petechiae and ecchymoses (83%); sternal tenderness, lymphadenopathy, hepatosplenomegaly; testicular, skin, meningeal, gum and perianal infiltration especially with monocytic types

Crs: Grim, although still 10% 5-yr survival; grimmer if alkylating agent-induced (Ann IM 1980;93:133), if preceded by myelodysplasia, or if monomyelocytic

Cmplc: CNS involved (7%); sepsis always; significant bleeding

Lab: *Chem:* Elevated B_{12}, uric acid, phosphate; low calcium with rx due to PO_4 released by dead cells

Hem: Anemia; decreased platelets; smear shows blasts, if > 200,000 needs leukophoresis. Marrow shows blasts > 30%; Auer rods sometimes and nucleoli in myeloblasts.

Immunol: Circulating immune complexes correlate with worse prognosis (Nejm 1982;307:1174)

Rx (www.nccn.org):

Induction w cytarabine + daunorubicin: If decide to do, takes 1 mo in hospital, make aplastic and septic usually, 65% chance of inducing 6-14 mo remission. In a small subset (10%) of pts (promyelocytic), tretinoin (all-*trans*-retinoic acid) matures the leukemic clone (Nejm 1997;337:1021, 1993;329:177).

Maintenance: Marrow transplant (Ann IM 1985;102:285) with autologous marrow, or HLA-matched sibling, or unrelated donor, as good as (44% have > 4-yr survival) continued intensive chemotherapy? (Nejm 1998;339:1649 vs 1995;332:217)

Acute Lymphocytic (Lymphoblastic) Leukemia (ALL)

Nejm 2004;350:1535, 1998;339:605

Cause: 2 types: child and adult

Epidem: Adult type represents 15% of adult leukemias. Incidence of childhood type is 32/1 million/yr (Nejm 1991;325:1330); no increased incidence near power lines (Nejm 1997;337:1).

Pathophys: CNS involvement more common (40%) than in AML (7%)

   78% are B-cell types; 17% are T-cell types; 5% have no markers using monoclonal antibodies (Nejm 1991;324:800); some also have myeloid antigens, which correlate with worse prognosis

   Associated with chromosome 9 deletion that has interferon-α and -β genes (Nejm 1990;322:77)

Sx: Malaise, fever ($^1/_3$ due to sepsis, $^2/_3$ due to tumor)

Si: Pallor; hepatosplenomegaly

Crs: In children, now much higher cure rates, 70+% 5-yr survival (Nejm 1993;329:1289; 1991;325:1330) unless Philadelphia chromosome positive (Nejm 2000;342:998). In adults, prognosis is much worse than in children; T-cell types have worst prognosis, rest susceptible to rx; 30-40% cure currently.

Cmplc: Varicella zoster disease with 7% mortality (Nejm 1980;303:355); *Pneumocystis carinii;* CMV, progressive multifocal leukoencephalopathy; AML after chemoRx in 4% (Nejm 1989; 321:136), 2nd primary in 0.5% of children (Nejm 1991;325:1330); sterility (Nejm 1989;321:143)

Lab: *Hem:* CBC shows anemia, low platelets, increased wbc's

   Marrow shows invasion; tissue cultures of treated pts predict relapse if grow blasts with original tumor surface markers (Nejm 1986;315:538)

   Lymphocyte terminal deoxynucleotidyltransferase, a primitive lymph enzyme normally present in thymus, is present in childhood and T-cell ALL and occasionally in blast crisis of CML

   Flow cytometry to tell B cells from T cells and the subtypes

Rx (www.nccn.org):

    Induction: Prednisone, vincristine, asparaginase (or its less sensitizing conjugate, pegaspargase [Oncaspar]: Med Let 1995;37:23), daunorubicin (hard on children's hearts: Nejm 1991;324:808) + methotrexate (mtx) > 80% remission

    CNS (asx) rx: Irradiate + intrathecal mtx after in remission

    Maintenance: Mtx, teniposide, and cytarabine (Nejm 1998; 338:499); can stop after in remission × 3 yr

    Marrow transplant (allogenic or autologous) in 2nd remission if recurs, 50% work (Nejm 1994;331:1253)

Chronic Lymphocytic Leukemia (CLL)

Nejm 2005;352:804

Cause: Genetic mutations

Epidem: Adults, males > females, 90% age 50+ yr, median age at onset = 65 yr ; very rare in Asians

Pathophys: B-cell leukemia. Platelets decreased due both to autoimmune and splenomegaly mechanisms

Sx: Onset insidious, asx for years; rash and/or ulcer; no fever from tumor unless infected (M. Turck 1/69)

Si: Stage 0: Lymphocytosis > 15,000
      Stage I: Above + adenopathy
      Stage II: Above + hepato- and/or splenomegaly
      Stage III: Above + anemia
      Stage IV: Above + depressed platelets (purpura)

Table 8.1　RAI Staging

Stage	0	I	II	III	IV
At presentation (%)	31	35	26	6	2
Median survival (yr)	10+	9	5	6	2

(Nejm 1998;338:1506)

Crs: Correlates with abnormal karyotypes (Nejm 2000;343:1910)

Cmplc: 2nd malignancy; sepsis especially with encapsulated organisms like H. flu and pneumococcus; ichthyosis; cardiac involvement (25%) rarely diagnosed premortem

r/o rare T-cell types, often associated with retrovirus infections (Nejm 1995;332:1744,1749) or **Sézary syndrome** from chromosome 14 inversion (Nejm 1986;314:865), the only type that involves the skin (Ann IM 1974;80:685)

Lab: *Chem:* Elevated uric acid

Hem: Ncnc anemia in ²/₃; Coomb's-positive, steroid-responsive anemia in ¹/₃ (C. Finch, 1969); thrombocytopenia; wbc's > 15,000, by definition, usually > 100,000 with 75-90% lymphs, prolymphocytic variant may have up to 54% prolymphocytes, if more than that is prolymphocytic CLL and has a bad prognosis; marrow shows monotonous lymphocytic infiltration. Flow cytometry to identify monoclonal surface markers. CD5 markers on cells identify B-cell CLL and r/o reactive lymphocytosis.

Rx: Only if sx or progression beyond stage I or II; in future will base rx on cell markers/mutations

Prophylactic pneumovax; rapid antibiotic rx of infections

Chemotherapy (www.nccn.org) for stage II+–III+ only, no help for stages 0, I, and II unless progressive (Nejm 2000; 343:1799, 1998;338:1506); usually with fludarabine (Nejm 2000;343:1750) or chlorambucil + prednisone, which gives a 60-80% response; but < 10% are complete and overall survival is not improved. Then busulfan, cyclophosphamide, vincristine; interferon-α often w AZT especially for T-cell types (Nejm 1995;332:1744, 1749); 70% response rate

Radiation, total body; 50% response but less toxic than above

Non-Hodgkin's Lymphoma [Including Diffuse Histiocytic, Hairy Cell, Lymphosarcoma (gastric type p 337)]

Cause: Hepatitis C virus induces B-cell type (Ann IM 1997;127:423); reversible w rx of Hep C (Nejm 2002;347:89)

Epidem: 35,000/yr in U.S. Occurs in older (less tolerant of rx) pts than Hodgkin's, although does represent 7% of all childhood/ adolescent tumors (500/yr in U.S.)

    Increased incidence in pts with diminished immune responses: AIDS, Sjögren's syndrome (Ann IM 1978;89:888), sarcoid, malaria, celiac disease, radiation + chemotherapy–treated Hodgkin's pts (Nejm 1979;300:452)

Pathophys: 80% are B-cell types and include all those associated with Sjögren's (Nejm 1978;299:1215)

Sx: Adenopathy

Si: Splenomegaly, adenopathy

Crs: 5-yr survival = 32-83% depending on age, stage (like Hodgkin's staging), LDH, functional status, and cell type. Indolent lymphomas have long survival but no cure; aggressive lymphomas, the opposite.

Cmplc: Leukemia
    r/o **bovine babesiosis** in splenectomized patients (Ann IM 1981;94:326); cutaneous T-cell lymphomas (p 402)

Lab: Stage like Hodgkin's
    Chem: Marked increase in LDH, unlike myeloma (Ann IM 1989; 110:521)
    Hem: Ncnc anemia
    Path: Low grade:
- Small lymphocyte (CLL)
- Follicular small cleaved cell
- Follicular mixed cell

Intermediate grade:
- Follicular large cell
- Diffuse small cleaved cell
- Diffuse mixed cell
- Diffuse large cell

High grade:
- Immunoblastic
- Lymphoblastic (ALL)
- Small noncleaved (Burkitt's, etc)

Serol: M spike, or κ or λ chains in a small % (Nejm 1978;298:481)

Rx (www.nccn.org):
- Observation alone is an option for low-grade asx types until or unless sx or progress
- ChemoRx, depending on the aggressiveness of the lymphoma grade:

  CHOP (cyclophosphamide, doxorubicin [hydroxydaunorubicin], vincristine [Oncovin], prednisone) (Nejm 1993; 328:1002, 1992;327:1342) × 3 cycles followed by field irradiation; in pts > 60 yr as well (Ann IM 2002;136:144)

  ACVBP (doxorubincin [Adriamycin], cyclophosphamide, vindesine, bleomycin, prednisone) (Nejm 2005; 352:1199) may be better than CHOP

  Interferon-α w COPA (same as CHOP) + fludarabine (Fludara) for low and intermediate grades (Nejm 1993; 329:1608, 1992;327:1330) like Sézary's syndrome and mycosis fungoides

- Immunotherapy with anti-idiotype antibodies for B-cell lymphomas (Nejm 1989;321:851), eg, rituximab (Rituxan) (Med Let 1998;40:65) iv q 1 wk × 4; $11 000; ie, after remission induced, immunize w im injections of the portion of the IgG specific to that tumor class (Nejm 1992;327:1209). Or radioimmunoconjugates (p 447).

- Marrow transplantation (Nejm 1987;316:1493,1499) w chemoRx for recurrence improves 5-yr event-free survival from 12% to 50% (Nejm 1995;335:1540)
- Autologous stem cell transplantation combine w above chemoRx for aggressive types (Nejm 2004;350:1287)
- Irradiation, total body or involved field, combined w CHOP (Nejm 1998;339:21)

of hairy cell type leukemia: 2-Chlorodeoxyadenosine (2-eda); or interferon-α

Burkitt's Lymphoma

Cause: Epstein-Barr virus in B lymphocytes (Nejm 1976;295:685)

Epidem: Endemic in Africa and New Guinea; less frequent in U.S. and U.K.

Pathophys: A subtype of non-Hodgkin's lymphoma; malignant lymphoma of undifferentiated B lymphocytes; solid extranodal growth, no leukemia; a phytohemagglutinin type of transformation of lymphocytes

Sx: Jaw mass (50% of African cases); abdominal tumors (most common presentation in U.S., 2nd after jaw in Africa)

Si: Stage I: Single tumor mass
Stage II: 2 or more masses
Stage III: Intrathoracic, abdominal, or osseous (excluding facial bones) involvement
Stage IV: CNS and/or marrow invasion

Crs: Rapid onset and progression without rx
Stages I and II remit with rx in 80%
Stages III and IV remit with rx in 50%
Cure possible, perhaps 50% overall

Cmplc: Marrow invasion (50% in U.S., 10% in Africa); leukemia (< 1% in Africa, 10% in U.S.)

r/o developing-country **Immunoproliferative Small Bowel Disease** and subsequent "Mediterranean" lymphoma (Nejm 1983;308:1401)

Lab: *Bact:* EBV isolatable

Path: "Starry sky" pattern = macrophages interspersed among undifferentiated tumor cells

Serol: Diminished primary antibody responses, increased IgG, decreased IgM. Normal delayed hypersensitivity. Increased antibody titers to EBV.

Rx (www.nccn.org): "World's fastest-growing tumor"; start rx within 48 hr

Surgical debulking very important

ChemoRx with cyclophosphamide, methotrexate including intrathecally, or cytosine arabinoside intrathecally

Hodgkin's Disease

Cause: Neoplasia w genetic predisposition precipitated by unknown viral infection (Nejm 1995;332:413); EBV associated, and probable cause in 50±% in young adults (Nejm 2003;349:1329)

Epidem: Pattern like polio virus; increased in wealthy, small families, etc. Perhaps patient-to-patient contacts, or shared contacts; extensively examined in NY school studies (Nejm 1973;289:499,532) but questioned (Nejm 1979;300:1006). Male/female = 2:1; 3200 deaths/yr in U.S.; bimodal age incidence, peaks at age 15-30 yr and ~50 yr

Pathophys: Possibly a retroviral infection or other perturbation of T and/or B cells, which become a Reed-Sternberg line arising in lymph nodes and spreading in contiguous groups of nodes

Sx: Fever (classic Pel-Epstein fever = 2 wk on, 2 wk off, occurs in 15%), night sweats or weight loss (any of these 3 make it stage B), nodes, pruritus

Si: Lymphadenopathy (painless, firm and rubbery), fever, 25% are stage I or II when present

Stage I: Limited to 1 anatomic area

Stage II: 2 contiguous anatomical areas, 1 side of diaphragm

Stage III: 2 or more contiguous areas on 2 sides of diaphragm but involving only nodes and spleen

Stage IV: Extranodal sites, diffuse infiltrations, eg, of liver

Crs: Overall 1992 cure rate = 75% with current w/u and rx

Cmplc:

- Leukemia or non-Hodgkin's lymphoma after rx, 1%/yr but plateaus after 15 yr, although solid tumor rate remains steady (Nejm 1988;318:76) and may even increase for breast Ca especially if rx'd as a child (Nejm 1996;334:745,792)

- Sepsis, especially if had staging splenectomy (10% get: Nejm 1977;297:245), and stages III and IV are unresponsive to pneumovax (Nejm 1978;299:442)

- Late, post-radiation (Jama 2003;290:2831):

  Thyroid disease, especially myxedema after radiation rx (Nejm 1991;325:599)

  Cardiac valvular insufficiency/stenosis late

  Carotid and/or subclavian stenosis

  Breast Ca risk when women < 30 yr w intact ovaries treated (Jama 2003;290:465)

  r/o toxoplasmosis, phenytoin (Dilantin) syndrome, other lymphomas, immunoblastic lymphadenopathy, AIDS

Lab: *Hem:* ESR > 30 mm/hr before and especially after rx predicts (50%) relapse within 18 mo (Ann IM 1991;114:361). Bone marrow to look for infiltration.

Path: Node bx shows Reed-Sternberg cells, aberrant macrophages (Nejm 1978;299:1208), multilobed dark nuclei with inclusions

Xray: CT of abdomen and thorax, PET scan

Rx (www.nccn.org): Preventively immunize with 23 valent pneumococcal vacine, *H. influenza* vaccine, and tetravalent meningococcal vacine 10 d before rx if can, otherwise after rx completed (Ann IM 1995;123:828)

ChemoRx (Nejm 1993;328:560) with 6+ cycles of ABVD (Adriamycin, bleomycin, vinblastine, dacarbazine) (Nejm 1993; 327:1478), or the former gold standard, MOPP (mustard, Oncovin [vincristine], procarbazine, prednisone). Other regimens being tried alternating with MOPP to further increase survival and cures include ABVD (Adriamycin, bleomycin, vinblastine, dacarbazine) or BCVPP (Ann IM 1984;101:447). Adverse effects: sterility and decreased testosterone in males (Nejm 1978; 299:12); female productivity affected less (Nejm 1981;304:1377); leukemia risk w MOPP.

Radiation, 3000-4000 rads over 4 wk, for stage Ia and some IIs. Cardiac function impaired 10 yr later (Nejm 1983;308:569); radiation pneumonitis.

8.10 Immunologic Diseases

Jama 1997;278:22

Multiple Myeloma

Nejm 2004;351:1860; 1997;336:1657

Cause: Neoplastic B cells

Epidem: 10,000 deaths/yr in U.S.; incidence in blacks twice that in whites. Older pts, peak incidence in 50-60-yr age group; benzene workers (Nejm 1987;316:1044).

Pathophys:

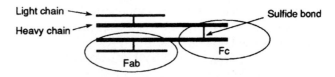

Figure 8.1 Immunoglobulin structure.

Natural evolution of MM: From normal plasma cells to "monoclonal gammopathy of unknown significance (MGUS)" by chromosomal translocation or deletion; then, after years, to MM as osteoblastic and angiogenesis capacities of cells increase

of all M-protein disease: 50% IgG (60% with Bence-Jones protein), 24% IgA (70% with BJ), Bence-Jones protein only (21%), IgD (3%), no M protein (1.5%), IgM + Waldenstrom's (0.5%)

IgG and IgA have specific heavy chains and common light (λ and κ) chains. M protein is a homogeneous protein electrophoresis spike. Myelomas in which one can identify a specific antigen to which the M component is directed (eg, ASLO, RA, cold agglutinin anti-I) raise interesting questions of pathogenesis (Nejm 1971;284:831).

Sx: Recurrent infections; skeletal pain and pathologic fractures; Raynaud's if M component is an IgG cryoprotein; arthritis, first sx in 5% (R. Ritchie 1975)

Si: Bone pain (infiltration), hepatosplenomegaly

POEMS syndrome seen with myeloma and plasmacytomas: **P**olyneuropathy; **O**rganomegaly especially adenopathy, splenomegaly, and hepatomegaly; **E**ndocrinopathy including hypogonadism and hypothyroidism; **M**onoclonal gammopathy; **S**kin changes including hyperpigmentation and thickening

Crs: Die < 2 yr of diagnosis; probably takes 5-10 yr for isolated lesion to spread and kill. With rx, 30 mo mean survival, 2% 10-yr survival (Nejm 1983;308:314).

Cmplc: r/o benign monoclonal gammopathy (Nejm 2002;346:564) w < 3 gm % monoclonal protein, < 10% marrow plasma cells; present in 2% of the population > 50 yr; 1%/yr progress to myeloma or related diseases

- Sepsis especially with H. flu and pneumococcus, at least with IgG type
- Anemia
- Pancytopenia
- Renal failure: ATN often precipitated by IVP, RTA, Fanconi's syndrome, urate deposition, amyloid
- Hypercalcemia
- Amyloidosis (10%)
- Neuropathy due to myelin antibodies (Nejm 1980;303:618)
- Leukemia in 15% at 4 yr after rx (Nejm 1979;301:743)
- Hyperviscosity (9% of IgG) correlates with Sia water test (Ann IM 1972;77:853)
- Angioneurotic edema due to autoantibody against M component, consumes C'1 inhibitor (p 234)

Lab: *Chem:* Anion gap low, cationic proteins increased (Nejm 1977;296:858)

Hem: Anemia with decreased rbc half-life due to IgG coating; peripheral smear shows plasma cells (5%). Marrow shows > 10% atypical plasma cells in 90%, usually immature. ESR increased in most, although may be temperature dependent if cryoprecipitate and hence low at room temperature.

Serol: SPEP shows > 3 gm monoclonal protein; false pos in 0.1% at age 40 yr, 5% at age 80 yr; spurious spikes from aggregated IgG after standing, fibrinogen or bacterial or hgb contamination in β area, hyperlipidemia in α_2 area.

Urine protein electrophoresis: Monoclonal light-chain (κ or λ), Bence-Jones protein; either this or SPEP is positive in 99% (r/o amyloid, malignant lymphomas, occasionally benign)

Xray: Skull, spine show osteolytic (punched-out) lesions and/or diffuse osteoporosis

Rx: < age 65, high-dose chemoRx followed by autologous stem cell transplant (Nejm 2003;348:1875,2495,2551)

over age 65-70 only if anemia, elevated creatinine or calcium, w melphalan + steroids, VAD (vincristine, doxorubicin, dexamethasone), or perhaps w bortezomib proteasome inhibitor (Nejm 2005;352:2487) or thalidomide (Nejm 1999;341:1565) for refractory cases or relapses

IgG iv prophylactically may prevent infection (Lancet 1994; 343:1059) but costs $25,000/yr (Ann IM 1994;121;suppl 2:32)

of anemia: Erythropoietin tiw helps (Nejm 1990;322:1693)

of bone pain and hypercalcemia, and perhaps w initiation of chemoRx: Pamidronate iv (Nejm 1996;335:1836) or other biphosphonate (Ann IM 2000;132:734)

of pathologic fx's: Coincident monthly pamidronate infusion w chemoRx (Nejm 1996;334:488).

Waldenström's Macroglobulinemia

Cause: Lymphomas

Epidem: Onset at age 40-60 yr; rare

Pathophys: Plasma cell clone production of IgM; $\frac{1}{3}$ are cryoglobulins, coating of rbc's causes rouleaux formation, IgM + coagulation factors clump; all 3 lead to peripheral sludging. If in glomerular capillaries (unlike in tubules with multiple myeloma), can cause renal failure.

Sx: Masses, fatigue, Raynaud's, bleeding, urticaria (cryoglobulins)

Si: Lymphadenopathy, hepatosplenomegaly, anemia, purpura, abnormal fundi with patchy venous bulges, microaneurysms, and hemorrhages

Crs: Remissions up to 5 yr

Cmplc (cf diabetes): CNS circulatory impairments (sludging), CHF, peripheral neuropathy and myopathy, infection, visual loss, gi bleeding, renal failure, amyloid

r/o **Heavy-chain Disease (Franklin's Disease)** (Nejm 1993;329:1389), a B-cell lymphoma that produces IgA or IgG heavy chains; the latter causes developing-country gi lymphadenopathy or **Immunoproliferative Small Intestinal Disease;** uvular edema a prominent sx

Lab: *Hem:* Anemia, Coomb's positive; decreased rbc survival; elevated ESR; elevated white counts, frequently reaching leukemic levels with atypical cells ("lymphocytoid" plasma cells)

Serol: IgM spike on SPEP and IEP; cold agglutinins ($^1/_3$). Sia water test pos in 50%; forms "parachute" unlike IgG "cloud" when add 1 drop serum into distilled water (C. Janeway, Nejm 1966;275:652).

Urine: Proteinuria with BJ protein (10%)

Xray: No osteoporosis

Rx: Plasmapheresis stat to decrease viscosity until rx takes effect (Nejm 1984;310:762)

1st: Chlorambucil + prednisone po; 50% response in previously untreated pts, 50% 5-yr survival

2nd: Fludarabine or rituxan, 40% response after above fails; or 2-chlorodeoxyadenosine (Ann IM 1993;118:195) qd × 7 d, twice, yields a 60% response even in previously treated, but adverse effects: neutropenia

Agammaglobulinemias

Ann IM 1993;118:720 (acquired)

Cause: Common variable immunodeficiency (acquired) (Nejm 1995; 333:434): Primary, or secondary to protein loss via malnutrition nephrotic syndrome, exfoliative dermatitis, or enteropathy
Congenital (Nejm 1995;333:431): Genetic, X-linked mutation in Bruton tyrosine kinase gene; occasionally autosomal recessive from MU heavy-chain gene mutation on chromosome 14 (Nejm 1996;335:1486)

Epidem: Acquired: Males > females, family h/o SLE, ITP, IgA deficiency
Congenital: Sx at age 5-6 mo

Pathophys:
Acquired: Absent B lymphs
Congenital: Defect in B-cell development (Nejm 1987;316:427) from a cytoplasmic signal-induced molecule mutation

Sx:
Acquired: Onset at age 8+ yr; recurrent purulent infections, especially sinus and lung, and ECHO virus of CNS (Nejm 1977;296:1485); sprue syndrome and giardia
Congenital: Onset at age 6-12 mo, rarely as late as 4 yr; RA-like sx often 1st; recurrent purulent sepsis, leads to bronchiectasis; sprue syndrome and giardia

Si:
Acquired: Lymphadenopathy, hepatosplenomegaly, eczema
Congenital: Lymphadenopathy in older pts, hepatosplenomegaly, *Pneumocystis carinii*, hypoplastic tonsils

Crs:

Cmplc:
Acquired: Pernicious anemia (33%), ITP, hemolytic anemia, neutropenia, noncaseating granulomas (Ann IM

1997;127:613), gi tumors, gastric cancer, mycoplasma RA syndromes, bronchiectasis, pneumocystis infections (Nejm 1992;326:999)

Congenital: Bronchiectasis, increased neoplasias, polio from live viruses

r/o **severe combined immunodeficiency** (Nejm 1995;333:435) rx'd w marrow transplant (Nejm 2000;342:1325) or gene therapy (Nejm 2002;346:1185), **X-linked Wiskott-Aldrich syndrome** (Nejm 1998;338:291), **DiGeorge syndrome** rx'd w thymus transplant (Nejm 1999; 341:1180), and **hereditary thymic aplasia and dysplasia** (Nejm 1984;311:235,300)

Lab: *Path:* No plasma cells in marrow or RES

Serol: Diminished or absent IgG (< 100 mg %), and absent IgA and IgM

Xray: Congenital: Lateral neck shows diminished lymphoid tissue

Rx: Prevention: Carrier detection by recombinant DNA probes of B cells can work (Nejm 1987;316:427).

IgG 300-600 mg/kg in adults, 400-800 mg/kg in children iv q 4 wk (Ann IM 2001;135:165) can result in nearly normal life; beware of IgE antibodies to IgA, which can cause anaphylaxis (Nejm 1986;314:560)

in acquired: Cimetidine helps some by suppressing suppressor T cells (Nejm 1985;312:198); interleukin-2 weekly sc (Nejm 1994;331:918)

Dysgammaglobulinemias

Cause: Type I: Genetic, X-linked recessive (Bruton type) or autosomal; or acquired

Epidem: Type II: Subclass deficiencies becoming more frequently recognized; 1% of pediatric allergy clinic populations

Pathophys: In both, the absence of IgA leads to giardia infections and villous changes

>   Type I: Diminished or absent IgA and IgG; elevated IgM; in genetic type, defect in switch cells, whose job is to change B cells' IgM production to IgA and IgG production (Nejm 1986;314:409)

>   Type II: Diminished or absent IgA and IgM; IgG normal, but $\frac{1}{4}$ may lack subsets of IgG and others may lack only these IgG subsets, leading to pulmonary infections and disease (Nejm 1985;313:720,1247)

Sx: Type I: Recurrent pyogenic and opportunistic (especially *P. carinii*) infections

>   Type II: Diarrhea, intermittent

Si:

Crs:

Cmplc:

>   Type I: Thrombocytopenia, hemolytic and aplastic anemia, neutropenia (responds to granulocyte colony-stimulating factor) IgM plasma cell tissue invasions; r/o hereditary ataxia telangiectasia (p 735) for type III)

>   Type II: Sprue-like syndrome w gi lymphoid hyperplasia, *Giardia lamblia* infections, PA and stomach cancer (Nejm 1988;318:1563)

Lab: *Immunol:* Immuno and protein electrophoresis:

>   Type I: No IgA or IgG; IgM = 150-1000 mg % but is diffuse w/o a spike; IgE and IgD increased in many

>   Type II: No IgA or IgM, IgG normal or decreased

>   *Path:* Type I: Plasmacytoid lymphocytes

>   Type II: Decreased plasma cells in hyperplastic lymph nodes

Xray:

Rx: Symptomatic of giardia; no IgA replacement since can lead to anaphylaxis to the IgA; can occur even w blood transfusions

Type I: Steroids may help acquired type if due to increased suppressor T cells, marrow transplant (Nejm 1995;333:426)

Chronic Granulomatous Disease

Nejm 2000;343:1708, 1991;324:509

Cause: Genetic, ^{2}/$_3$ are sex-linked recessive; ^{1}/$_3$ are autosomal recessive (Nejm 1970;283:217)

Epidem:

Pathophys: Defect in leukocyte NADH oxidase or other similar enzymes leads to impaired killing, although phagocytosis ok, and thus purulent infections especially with staph, klebsiella-enterobacter, *E. coli,* and serratia (Nejm 1983;308:245; 1971; 285:789)

Sx: Frequent and severe pyogenic infections from early childhood on

Si:

Crs: Usually fatal

Cmplc: Malabsorption and B_{12} deficiency (Nejm 1973;288:382)
r/o **Chédiak-Higashi Syndrome**, a similar failure of poly-degranulation with secondary neutropenia and pyogenic infections, rx with ascorbate (Nejm 2000;343:1710)

Lab: *Hem:* NBT test: nitroblue tetrazolium is not reduced to blue formazon in vitro by affected granulocyte fraction; female carriers of sex-linked type have intermediate NBT tests although asx; carriers of autosomal recessive type are NBT normal and asx

Immunol: DHS skin tests normal, as are immunoglobulin levels by serum protein electrophoresis

Path: Liver bx shows chronic granulomas, often calcified; small bowel bx shows lamina propria histiocytes and granulomas; r/o Whipple's (Nejm 1973;288:382)

Rx: Prevent w 2nd-trimester detection and abortion (Nejm 1979; 300:48)

HEMATOLOGY/ONCOLOGY

Rx with interferon-γ, which activates macrophages, sc tiw; or marrow transplant (Nejm 2001;344:881)

8.11 Miscellaneous

HEMATOLOGY

Anemia W/u in Primary Care

1st: CBC, w indices, peripheral smear exam, and retic count
2nd: Folate and B_{12} and/or iron and TIBC if indicated by 1st
3rd: Bone marrow aspiration and bx

Eosinophilia

Nejm 1998;338:1592

Cause: Allergic, helminth parasitic infections, malignancy, vasculitis, idiopathic, drug allergy usually reversible except for tryptophan-induced eosinophilia/myalgia syndrome (Ann IM 1990;112:85) (p 1093); interleukin-5–producing T-cell clones (Nejm 1999;341:1112)

Pathophys: Nejm 1991;324:1110

Lab: *Hem:* $> 350/mm^3$ is abnormal, $> 1500/mm^3$ needs w/u and rx

Rx: of idiopathic type with counts $> 1500/mm_3$ to prevent heart disease (Ann IM 1982;97:78) w steroids, hydroxyurea, vincristine, or interferon-α (Ann IM 1994;121:648), interleukin-5 antibodies like mepolizumab (Nejm 2003;349:2334)

Erythrocyte Sedimentation Rate

Methods and rare utility (Ann IM 1986;104:515); acute-phase reactants probably better measured by C-reactive protein elevations (> 10 mg/L) (Nejm 1999;340:448)

Erythropoietin (Epogen, Procrit)

Med Let 2001;43:40

50-150 U/kg iv/sc tiw, or darbepoetin (Aranesp) (Med Let 2001; 43:109) 0.45-4.5 μgm/kg/wk sc/iv; helps in renal failure, cancer chemoRx, HIV disease, presurgical, or all ICU pts w hgb < 8.5? (Jama 2002;288:2827,2884); adverse reactions: development of erythropoietin antibodies can lead to total shutdown of erythropoiesis (Nejm 2002;346:469); cost: $100/wk

Methemoglobinemia, Acquired

Nejm 2000;343:337

Epidem: Rare, induced by oxidizing drugs like benzocaine, dapsone, sulfonamides, and nitrates even in foods (Nejm 2004;351:2429) especially in pts predisposed to hemolysis like G_6PD-deficiency pts

Sx: SOB

Si: Ashen pallor

Lab: O_2 sat decreased; brown serum

Rx: Methylene blue 2 mg/kg iv or po

Normal Marrow Ratios

Marrow/fat = 1:1, erythroid/myeloid (granulocytic) series = 1:3

Platelet Transfusions

Leukocyte reduction and UVB irradiation decrease antibody formation and increase survival (Nem 1997;337:1861); as does cross-match before, can do with HLA typing or simply serum and platelet cross-match in aggregometer (Nejm 1975;292:130); freeze and keep, eg, draw when well, transfuse when on chemoRx (Nejm 1978;299:7); cmplc: bacterial sepsis from contamination (Nejm 2002;347:1075)

Red Blood Cell Indices

Calculations: MCV = hct/rbc, MCH = hgb/rbc, MCHC = hgb/hct

Transfusions of Red Blood Cells

At what hgb level? RCT shows keeping > 7 gm % better than higher levels in critically ill pts (Nejm 1999;340:409, 467)

of autologous red cells: draw 1 U q 1 wk, can harvest 4-6 U in 3 wk for elective surgery using supplemental recombinant erythropoietin rx if initial hct < 39% (Nejm 1997;336:933), especially helpful in women and children (Nejm 1989;321:1162) but risks may not warrant unless odds of needing tfx high (Nejm 1999;340:525); or 4 wk prior to surgery, weekly erythropoietin + iron polysaccharide complex 150 mg po tid, w/o banking units also helpful (Ann IM 2000;133:845)

Viral infection risk (www.bloodsafety.org) < 1/200, 000+ U w screened blood, 95% of risk is for Hep B, and rest is Hep C and HIV risk (1/2 million for each); 23 cases of West Nile virus transmission via packed red cells and FFP now prompts possible screening of donor blood (Nejm 2003;349:1236)

2,3-DPG

Increases with increased pH and decreased pO_2, and causes easier O_2 dissociation, hence compensates for anemia (Nejm 1970;283:165); HgbF binds 2,3-DPG poorly relative to HgbA, which explains increased O_2 binding by fetal blood (Nejm 1971;285:589)

ONCOLOGY

Cancer Induction

- Oncogenes (clear reviews: Nejm 1994;330:328; Ann IM 1984;101:223), viral (v-onc) and cellular (c-onc); tumor suppressor gene mutations correlate especially w sarcomas (Nejm 1992;326:1301,1309); retinoblastoma gene is on chromosome 13 (Nejm 1991;324:212)
- Dioxin, perhaps in low levels (Nejm 1991;324:212)

Marrow Transplant

Nejm 1994;330:827

HLA matched (Nejm 1990;322:485; Ann IM 1989;110:51). Useful for various conditions: Wiskott-Aldrich syndrome, aplastic anemia, combined immunodeficiency (even non-HLA matched works: Nejm 1999;340:528), Fanconi's anemia, Hurler's disease, possibly thalassemia major (40-50% survival), possibly sickle cell disease, hematologic cancers, some solid tumors like breast, ovarian, melanoma, and glioma. Costs $150,000-$500,000 and for some diseases may be no better than standard rx.

Placental/cord blood source more available and often better w less GVH disease (Nejm 2001;344:1818, 2000;342:1846), 75% success (Nejm 1998;339:1565; Med Let 1996;38:71), especially if can't match (Nejm 2004;351:2265,2276,2328)

Peripheral blood stem cells from a donor after filgrastim (granulocyte colony-stimulating factor) are better source for transplant (Nejm 2001;344:175; Ann IM 1997;126:600)

Cmplc:

- Rejection: Use methotrexate + prednisone + antithymocyte globulin (Nejm 1982;306:392); avoid transfusion of blood or platelets beforehand, which diminishes success from 75% to 25% (Ann IM 1986;104:461)
- Graft vs host disease (rv: Nejm 1991;324:667) including bronchitis (Nejm 1978;299:1030), skin, gi tract, and liver (venooclusive disease: Ann IM 1979;90:158), latter prevented w ursodiol prophylaxis (Ann IM 1998;128:975)
- B-cell lymphoproliferative syndromes from "mono" to lymphoma (Nejm 1991;324:1451)
- Solid tumors (melanoma, squamous cell, thyroid, bony, CNS) all increased × 2.5-4, 5-10 yr out (Ann IM 1999;131:738; Nejm 1997;336:897)

Rx: Prophylactic pneumovax against increased pneumococcal disease (Ann IM 1979;91:835); acyclovir against herpes simplex

(Nejm 1981;305:63); CMV immune plasma against CMV (Ann IM 1982;97:11).

Filgrastim, a granulocyte-stimulating factor, can reinduce transplanted marrow growth (Nejm 1993;329:757)

Vitamin Prevention of Cancer

No diminished cancer rate with:
- Vitamin A or β-carotene (Nejm 1996;334:1145, 1150), although possibly low dietary vitamin A intake may increase breast Ca rate and po A may help in that small way (Nejm 1993;329:257); with vitamin E (Nejm 1994;330:1029)
- with vitamin C rx by Pauling (Nejm 1985;312:137)

IMMUNOLOGY

Allergy testing

Rv: Ann IM 1989;110:304
- Skin prick testing for wheal/flare mediated by IgE; easiest and best 1st test to up to 30 allergens; if patient intolerant, use RAST tests
- Intradermal tests if above neg; problem is false pos
- Total IgE levels somewhat helpful if extreme, eg, if < 50 μgm/L then atopic disease excluded, if >900 μ gm/L then likely
- Provocation tests, eg, bronchial or oral occasionally helpful
- Skin patch testing for DHS contact dermatitis helpful if substance is not irritating
- IgG levels useful only to measure antivenom blocking antibody

Cryoglobulinemia

Ann IM 2002;137:571; Nejm 1997;337:1512

Cause: 98% have hepatitis C (p 356) as the cause (Ann IM 1992; 117:573) if no clear other cause like SBE, HIV in 23% (Ann IM

1999;130:226), or leprosy. Both types II and III are associated w hepatitis B and C, Sjögren's, and Waldenström's (Nejm 1992; 327:1490).

Pathophys: Small-vessel vasculitis due to circulating immune complexes of IgG (the antigen) and IgM (the rheumatoid factor autoantibody), hence "mixed cryoglobulinemia." Type II IgM is polyclonal; type III is monoclonal and 10% of the time can evolve to B-cell lymphoma. Chronic viral infection may stimulate or select a genetic translocation that precipitates the lymphoma.

Sx: Arthralgias

Si: Purpura, neuropathic weakness (Ann IM 1977;87:287)

Cmplc: Membranoproliferative glomerulonephritis, and porphyria cutanea tarda (Ann IM 1995;123:615,625, 1992;117:573; Nejm 1993;328:465); debatably Sjögren's/sicca syndrome, polyarteritis; B-cell lymphomas

Lab: Type I: Monoclonal IgG, usually associated w malignancy
Type II: Mixed, polyclonal IgG and IgM rheumatoid factor
Type III: Mixed polyclonal IgG and monoclonal IgM rheumatoid factor
Complement: C_4 very low but normal C_3

Rx: NSAIDs, steroids, cyclophosphamide; if systemic disease, possibly interferon-α2a helps esp in hepatitis C types (Nejm 1994; 330:751)

Plasmapheresis

Expensive and not clearly beneficial in many situations for which promoted (Nejm 1984;310:762); may help chronic but not acute (Guillain-Barré) inflammatory demyelination polyradiculoneuropathy (Nejm 1986;314:461)

Protective Isolation

No benefit for granulocytopenias (Nejm 1981;304:448) (p 491)

Types of Hypersensitivity Reactions

I: Anaphylactic, IgE on mast cells, eg, anaphylaxis from bee sting

II: Cytotoxic, antigen contained in or on cell surface; eg, Rh hemolysis

III: Immune complex, eg, serum sickness

IV: Delayed hypersensitivity (DHS), eg, IPPD tubercular skin test

Chapter 9

Infectious Disease

D. K. Onion and S. Sears

BACTERIOLOGY

9.1 Antibiotics

Drug prices are average wholesale prices quoted in Medical Letter are for generic type if available; current retail prices may vary widely.

Penicillins

Amoxicillin 250-500 mg po bid adequate; less diarrhea than ampicillin; cheap

Amoxicillin + clavulanic acid (Augmentin) po 250 mg/125 mg or 500/125 tid; spectrum includes β-lactamase organisms, ie, is resistant to penicillinase, thus used against H. flu, staph, *B. fragilis, E. coli*; for OM, UTI, sinusitis, and for animal and human bites. Ok in pregnancy; not effective vs pseudomonas, enterobacter, serratia; adverse effects: diarrhea; $130/10 d for 500 mg tid.

Ampicillin 250 mg qid po/1-2 gm q 2-6 hr iv; penicillinase sensitive; very cheap

Ampicillin + sulbactam (Unasyn) 2 gm/1 gm iv q 6 hr; $47/d

Penicillin G po/iv/im; if parenteral form in short supply, can substitute ampicillin

Phenoxymethyl penicillin (Pen V) po; gastric acid resistant; $2-5/10d

Penicillinase-Resistant, Antistaph Penicillins

Nafcillin iv; resistant to penicillinase; adverse effects: ASA-like
platelet impairment (Nejm 1974;291:265); dose-dependent
neutropenia; glucose and alkali increase its degradation, so give
it in saline (Nejm 1970;283:118); adverse effects: hard on veins

Oxacillin po or iv/cloxacillin 500 mg qid po; resistant to penicillinase; adverse effects: hepatitis, reversible, anicteric, occurs at
> 1 gm qd (Ann IM 1978;89:497); hard on veins; $23/10 d po

Dicloxacillin 250 mg po qid; $8/10 d

Anti-Pseudomonal/Extended-Spectrum Penicillins

Piperacillin (Med Let 1982;24:48) 2-5 gm q 4 hr, iv/im; $430/7 d
Piperacillin + tazobactam (Zosyn) (Med Let 1994;36:7)
3 gm/375 mg iv q 6 hr; spectrum and cost like Timentin
Ticarcillin + clavulinic acid (Timentin); spectrum includes
staph, gram-neg organisms, and anaerobes; $60/d

First-Generation Cephalosporins

Some resistance but generally all are good vs *E. coli*, klebsiella,
Proteus mirabilis, gram-positive cocci except methicillin-resistant
staph and enterococcus; MIC vs staph < 0.5 μgm/cc

Cefadroxil (Duricef) 1-2 gm/d po divided bid; $30-70/10 d
Cefazolin (Ancef) 1-8 gm/d iv divided q 8 hr
Cephalexin (Keflex) 1-4 gm/d po divided qid; trade = $80/10 d,
generic = $5
Cephalothin (Keflin) 2-12 gm/d iv divided q 6 hr, im is painful;
$400/10 d iv
Cefradine (Velosef) 1-4 gm/d po divided; $12/10 d generic

Second-Generation Cephalosporins

MIC vs staph = 1-2 μgm/cc
Cefaclor (Ceclor) 1-4 gm/d po; vs H. flu; not as effective as other
2nd-generation ones and higher incidence of hypersensitivity reactions; $42/10 d for 500 mg tid

Cefotetan (Cefotan) (Med Let 1986;28:70) iv q 12 hr; vs anaerobes, *neisseria*, gram-positives and -negatives, but not listeria
or enterococcus; adverse effects: rare vitamin K–reversible
increase in protime; $41/d

Cefoxitin (Mefoxin) (Ann IM 1985;103:70) 3-12 gm/d iv; spectrum includes gc, anaerobes (80%); $500/10 d iv

Cefprozil (Cefzil) (Med Let 1992;34:63) 250 mg po q 12 hr; 2nd
or 3rd choice for otitis media or bronchitis; $122/10 d for
500 mg bid

Cefuroxime (Zinacef) 0.75-3 gm q 8 hr iv, or 125 mg po bid (as
Ceftin); spectrum includes penicillin-resistant gc, H. flu, and
moraxella *(Moraxella catarrhalis)*; $350/10 d iv; $136/10 d
500 mg bid

Loracarbef (Lorabid) (Med Let 1992;34:87) 200 mg po q 12 hr;
no better than others; $60/10 d

Third-Generation Cephalosporins

All good vs gc, *Moraxella catarrhalis*, H. flu; ok vs klebsiella,
E. coli; miss anaerobes, listeria, pseudomonas, enterococci, atypicals
(legionella, mycoplasma, chlamydia). MIC vs staph = ~5+ µgm/cc
for all except for ceftriaxone, which is lower. All $50-$70/d.

Cefdinir (Omnicef) (Med Let 1998;40:85) 300 mg or 7 mg/kg po
bid; similar spectrum to cefpodixime; $82/10d

Cefditoren (Spectracef) (Med Let 2002;44:5) 400 mg po bid;
similar profile to others; $65/d10 d

Cefepime (Maxipime) (Med Let 1996;38:84); no advantages over
others

Cefixime (Suprax) (Med Let 1989;31:73) 400 mg po ×1; ok vs
gc (Nejm 1991;325:1337), but no good vs pseudomonas,
staph, or anaerobes; $85/10 d

Cefoperazone (Cefobid); biliary excretion—hence for biliary
infections; q 8-12 hr

Cefotaxime (Claforan) 2-12 gm iv/im qd divided

Cefpodoxime (Vantin) (Med Let 1992;34:107) 100-400 mg po bid; good vs methicillin sens staph and intermediately penicillin sens pneumococcus, for gc (single dose), 2nd choice for OM/sinusitis (R. Holmberg 9/93); $91/10 d 200 mg bid

Ceftazidime (Fortaz); good vs pseudomonas but high MIC for staph so not reliable for it

Ceftibuten (Cedax) (Med Let 1996;38:23) 400 mg po qid; poor vs staph and pneumococcus (Med Let 1998;40:85), no advantages over others; $78/10 d

Ceftizoxime (Cefizox) iv q 8-12 hr

Ceftriaxone (Rocephin) iv/im qd-bid; good CSF penetration—hence best for blind rx of childhood meningitis (Nejm 1990; 322:141), can be used for penicillin-sensitive strep SBE, useful outpt drug (Jama 1992;267:264); adverse effects: pseudocholecystitis and true gallstones (Ann IM 1991;115:712), very rare severe acute hemolysis (Med Let 2002;44:100)

Aminoglycosides

Work well vs gram-negative bacilli; some activity against staph, penicillin-resistant diphtheroids, enterococci with a penicillin. All renal and vestibular toxic. Once-daily dosing reasonable and perhaps less toxic (BMJ 1996;312:338; Ann IM 1996;124:717, 1992;117:693).

Amikacin 24 mg/kg/24 hr; useful for resistant gram-neg

Gentamicin 3-5 mg/kg iv q 24 hr iv or q 2 half-lives (half-life = 4× creatinine in mg %); get peak, half hr after dose, 6-9 μgm/cc; and get trough, half hr before dose, < 2 μgm/cc. Vestibular toxicity is worse than auditory nerve toxicity.

Tobramycin; same dosing as gentamicin; $60/gm, 10× gentamicin cost; less renal toxicity, monitor levels with goal = 5-10 μgm/cc

Carbapenems

Imipenem + cilastatin (Primaxin) 0.5-1 gm iv q 6 hr; resistant to penicillinase; broader spectrum than 3rd-generation cephalosporins, good vs strep, staph, anaerobes, resistant gc, and H. flu, most gram-negs, gets into CSF; pseudomonas resistance develops, inadequate vs penicillin-resistant pneumococcus, methicillin-resistant staph, enterococcus, mycoplasma, chlamydia; adverse effects: seizures; $123/d

Meropenem (Merrem) (Med Let 1996;38:88) 1 gm iv q 8 hr; similar to imipenem/cilastin but a little better vs gm negs and a little less good vs gm pos organisms, ok vs *Listeria*; renal excretion; cost $155/d

Ertapenem (Invanz) (Med Let 2002;44:25) 1 gm iv qd; can be used for community-acquired pneumonias like ceftriaxone qd in elderly (J Am Ger Soc 2003;51:1526); similar spectrum to other carbapenems BUT misses *Pseudomonas* and *Acinetobacter spp.* so not useful for nosocomial infections; $50/d

Fluoroquinolones

Nejm 1991;324:384

Avoid all in pregnant women and children under 18 (cartilage damage)

1st Generation:

Norfloxacin (Ann IM 1988;108:238); 200-400 mg bid po; for UTI and gc; $60/10d

2nd Generation:

Ciprofloxacin 250-750 mg po bid, or 400 mg iv q 12 hr (Med Let 1991;33:75); no good vs anaerobes, enterococcus, chlamydia, staph (resistance develops quickly: Ann IM 1991; 114:424), or strep, but gets all else including gonorrhea and other gram-negatives including *Pseudomonas aeruginosa* in UTI, sputa of cystic fibrosis pts, and chronic external otitis; as prophylaxis in leukemias (Ann IM 1987;106:1,7); adverse effects: causes increases in theophylline levels; $61/10 d po

Ofloxacin (Floxin) (Med Let 1992;34:58, 1991;33:71) 400 mg po × 1 for gc, or 400 mg po bid × 1+ wk; good vs gc, all H. flu, gi pathogens except *C. difficile*, mycoplasma, and chlamydia;

no good vs anaerobes or pseudomonas, less helpful vs staph
and strep; $3/400 mg pill

3rd Generation (mainly for resistant pneumococcus):

Gatifloxacin (Tequin) (Med Let 2000;42:15); 400 mg po or iv qd;
like levofloxacin, covers atypicals, resistant pneumococcus,
H. flu, and moraxella, but not as good as cipro vs gm negs;
may prolong QT; can cause hypoglycemia, as can other
quinolones in pts on oral hypoglycemics, and rarer hyper-
glycemia in normal pts; $70/crs po, $115/3 d crs iv

Gemifloxacin (Factive) (Med Let 2004;46:78) 320 mg po qd ×
7-10 d; as effective as levo-, gati-, and moxifloxacin vs resistant pneumococcus; adverse reactions: rash in > 3% esp
young women, more than than others in class; similar LFT
elevations in 2%, QT prongations, gi sx; $132/wk

Levofloxacin (Levaquin) (Med Let 1997;39:41) 500 mg po/iv qd;
like others, is active isomer component of ofloxacin, better
than cipro vs gram-pos cocci, covers atypicals, resistant
pneumococcus, H. flu, and moraxella, but not as good as
cipro vs gm negs; $100/10 d po

Moxifloxacin (Avelox) (Med Let 2000;42:15) 400 mg po qd, like
levofloxacin, covers atypicals, resistant pneumococcus,
H. flu, and moraxella, but not as good as cipro vs gm negs;
can prolong QT interval; $75/wk

Trovofloxacin (Trovan) (Med Let 1998;40:30) 100-200 mg po qd
or 300 mg iv qd, or 100 mg po × 1 for UTI; effective vs gram
positives including resistant pneumococcus, as well as vs
anaerobes (only quinolone w such coverage); adverse effects:
fatal allergic hepatitis and pancreatitis, esp if > 21 d use,
which has caused FDA to severely restrict use

Immunologic Agents

Immune globulin (Nejm 1991;325:110,123); 100+ mg/kg/mo im
to keep trough IgG > 400 mg %; used for IgG deficiencies,
in AIDS children (Nejm 1991;325:73), Kawasaki's disease,

ITP, immune neutropenia, and sometimes in CLL (Nejm 1991;325:81) but may not be worth it; $100-1000 per dose

Interferon-α2a; for hepatitis B and C disease; adverse effects: marrow suppression, flu-like illness, depression, sometimes irreversible autoimmune disorders like thyroiditis (1-2%)

Interferon-γ; adjunct in atypical tbc, leprosy, toxoplasmosis, leishmaniasis (Nejm 1994;330:1348), and other persistent intracellular infections as well as chronic granulomatous disease (Ann IM 1995;123:216)

Activated protein C recombinant (Xigris) (p 611)

Macrolides

Med Let 1992;34:45

Beware cardiotoxic effects (long QT, p 107) when given w terfenadine and other nonsedating antihistamines (Jama 1996;275:1339), or alone esp in women (Jama 1998;280:1774)

Azithromycin (Zithromax) po or iv, 500 mg or 10 mg/kg × 1, then 250 mg or 5 mg/kg po qd × 4 d; or 1-2 gm po × 1 for chlamydial cervicitis and urethritis (Nejm 1992;327:921), *Mycobacterium avium*, legionella, gonorrhea; also available iv; less gi sx than erythromycin; less good than erythromycin for staph and strep; $40/crs

Clarithromycin (Biaxin) 250-500 mg po bid, also available as qd XL though levels lower; spectrum like erythromycin; fewer gi sx; $65/10 d for 250 mg bid

Dirithromycin (Dynabac) (Med Let 1995;37:109) 500 mg po qd; adverse effects: gi intolerance, probable interactions w nonsedating antihistamines like other macrolides; $27/7 d

Erythromycin 250-500 mg po/iv qid; adverse effects: increased digoxin, theophylline, warfarin, and carbamazepine levels (Med Let 1985;27:1); $7.50/10 d

Telithromycin (Ketek) (Med Let 2004;46:66) 800 mg po qd × 5 d for sinusitis or bronchitis, 10 d for community-acquired pneumonia; really a ketolide, works for penicillin-resistant pneumococcus; adverse effects: gi, blurred vision, prolongs statin and benzodiazapam half-lives; $115/10d

Monobactams

Aztreonam (Med Let 1987;29:45) used vs aerobic gram negs; $50/d

Oxazolidinones

Linezolid (Zyvox) (Ann IM 2003;138:135; Med Let 2000;42:45) 600 mg po or iv bid; vs MRSA and other vancomycin-resistant organisms; adverse effects: NV+D, a MAO inhibitor so avoid w tyramine foods and several antidepressants; $100-150/d

Sulfas

Sulfisoxazole (Gantrisin) 8 gm in 24-hr load, then 4 gm qd maintenance po divided; vs UTIs; adverse effects: allergies, migrating pulmonary infiltrates

Trimethoprim/sulfa (Septra, Bactrim) po, iv; adverse effects: resistance develops in gi tract organisms with prophylactic use, decreased polys with azathioprine (Imuran) due to folate metabolism interference (Ann IM 1980;93:560); hyperkalemia at high doses (Ann IM 1993;119:291, 296) or even standard doses (20% have K > 5.5 mEq/L) especially if renal failure (Ann IM 1996;124:316); cheap

Miscellaneous

Chloramphenicol 3 gm qd iv/im (im as good as iv: Nejm 1985; 313:410) or 100 mg/kg/24 hr divided, eg 150 mg qid; vs anaerobes, *E. coli*, salmonella, rickettsia; liver excretion; adverse effects: sideroblastic marrow aplasia, dose related or allergic; so rarely used in developed world; $21/d

Clindamycin; vs anaerobes, especially with gentamicin, as well as soft tissue and bone infections w staph and strep; adverse effects: *C. difficile* colitis

Dapsone; a sulfone used for dermatitis herpetiformis, leprosy, or w Tm/S for pneumocystis

Doxycycline 100 mg po bid; adverse effects: similar to tetracycline

Fosfomycin (Monurol) (Med Let 1997;39:66) 3 gm po in water × 1; no better than Tm/S or cipro for UTI

Metronidazole (Flagyl) (Nejm 1980;303:1213); 500 mg po as good as iv (Nejm 1981;305:1569) or topically as gel 5 gm bid × 5 d; tinidazole (p 631) similar; vs trichomonas, giardia, amoebic abscess, most anaerobes especially B. *fragilis*; adverse effects: Antabuse effect, decreased warfarin metabolism

Minocycline (Ann IM 1993;119:16) 100 mg po qd; adverse effects: similar to tetracycline, gi intolerance, rare allergic pneumonitis (Ann IM 1992;117:476), vestibular sx

Mupirocin (Bactroban) topically tid for impetigo; as good as po antibiotics; $10/15 gm tube (Med Let 1988;30:55)

Quinupristin/dalfopristin (Synercid) (Med Let 2000;42:45, 1999;41;109) iv, active vs MRSA and vancomycin-resistant enterococci; lots of drug interactions; cost $3000/10 d

Rifabutin (Med Let 1993;35:36) 300 mg po qd; used to prophylact AIDS pts vs M. *avium*

Rifampin 600 mg qd/bid; vs tbc, meningococcal carrier; adverse effects: elevated liver function tests, depressed white count, hearing loss, tbc resistance, increased warfarin metabolism

Spectinomycin; vs gc in penicillin-allergic patients

Tetracycline 250-500 mg po qid; adverse effects: photosensitivity, discolors children's teeth, fatty liver in pregnancy (Ann IM 1987;106:703), adsorbed by milk, antacids, and po iron; gi intolerance; cheap

Vancomycin (Med Let 1986;28:121) 1 gm iv q 12 hr or 125-500 mg po qid; vs clostridium enterocolitis, S. *viridans* SBE if penicillin allergic, methicillin-resistant staph, ok alone vs enterococcus; $800/10 d iv, $20/d po

9.2 Gram-Positive Organisms

Anthrax

Ann IM 2003;139:337; Nejm 2001;345:1607,1621

Cause: *Bacillus anthracis*

Epidem: Soil organism w long-lived endospores; biologic weapon

Pathophys: Infected by skin contact, inhalation of spores, or contact w infected animals or their meat. Endospores germinate and multiply in macrophages, leading to septicemia w exotoxin production including "edema toxin."

Sx: No sore throat and no rhinorrhea. Painless skin papule at contact site, then black eschar and edema.

(r/o brown recluse spider bite, erythema gangrenosum in neutropenic pts w *Pseudomonas aeruginosa* bacteremia, furuncle, ecthyma; nausea and vomiting; dyspnea; neurologic sx

Si: gi ulcerations and edema; fulminant pneumonits and mediastinitis (Jama 2001;286:2549,2554) after 5-10 d incubation

Crs: Skin, 80-90% benign resolution w antibiotics; gi disease resolves in 10-14 d; pulmonary, fatal

Cmplc: Meningitis; skin scarring; gi perforation

Lab: *Bacti:* Gram-pos rods in long chains ("bamboo"); grows like *Bacillus cereus;* lab may call it a contaminant unless warned
Skin tests: 82% pos 1-3 d after sx; 99% by 4 wk

Rx (Nejm 2002;287:2236; Med Let 2001;43:87,91): Vaccine 0.5 cc sc at 0, 2 and 4 wk; then 6, 12, and 18 mo; then q 1 yr
Prophylaxis after exposure w doxycycline 100 mg po bid, or ciprofloxacin 500 mg po bid, × 4 wk if vaccinated at the same time, or 60 d otherwise; in pregnant women, give cipro or tcn × 2 wk then amoxicillin 500 mg tid
of disease: Penicillin and doxycycline; if allergic to penicillin, chloramphenicol, erythromycin, + cipro

Bacillus Cereus Food Poisoning

Jama 1994;271:1074; Nejm 1978;298:143

Cause: *Bacillus cereus*

Epidem: Commonly reported in Europe, rare in U.S.

Pathophys: Heat-stable toxin produced in unrefrigerated rice: stays when fried and causes nausea and vomiting; perhaps an entero-toxin causing the diarrhea

Sx: Nausea and vomiting: h/o eating fried rice; 1-6 hr incubation
Diarrhea: 6-24 hr incubation

Si: No fever; NV+D

Crs: 24-36 hr duration

Cmplc: Fulminant liver failure and rhabdomyolysis (Nejm 1997;336:1142).
If diarrhea, r/o clostridial or staph toxin colitis, which also lack fever.

Lab: *Bact:* Gram-pos rods

Rx: Symptomatic

Diphtheria (Membranous Croup)

Ann IM 1989;111:71; Nejm 1988;318:12,41

Cause: *Corynebacterium diphtheria,* gravis and midas strains lysogenic for a specific phage (other species are opportunistics in debili-tated patients) (Ann IM 1969;70:919)

Epidem: Epidemically present in U.S., and resurging in Russia; immu-nization of > 50% of population begins to decrease incidence; peak incidence at age 15-39 yr; female/male = 2:1. Seattle epi-demic (> 1100 cases) in alcoholics (Ann IM 1989;111:71). Human carriers are reservoirs; acutely ill patients are communica-ble only ~2 wk. Skin lesions can also be both portal of entry and source of carrier state (Nejm 1969;280:135).

Pathophys: Exotoxin produced by phage hits conducting cells, eg, heart and nerves. Resulting anatomic changes in heart increase incidence of arrhythmias and failure years later. Gravis strain causes more lymphadenopathy, especially in pharynx, and hits heart more often.

Sx: Weakness, slight sore throat (90%), low-grade fever (85%), dysphagia and nausea (25%), headache (18%)

Si: • Fever.
  • Membrane: Exudate flows over tonsils, where it thickens in 2-3 d to classic fibrin pharyngeal waxy material, blue-white bleeds when peal, but has minimal inflammation
  • Edema of neck (18%)
  • Conjunctivitis
  • Infected skin lesions

Crs: 2-5 d incubation period

Cmplc:
  • Airway obstruction, especially with midas strain
  • Cardiac arrhythmias and myocarditis, especially with gravis strain; EKG abnormal in 65%; 10% fatality rate from cardiac arrest
  • Neuropathies: Peripheral (15%); rarely palatal motor impairment in first days of illness; cranial nerves III, VI, VII, IX, and X motor in 2-3 wk; Guillain-Barré rarely months later
    r/o mononucleosis, which can mimic membrane
  (L. Weinstein 3/85)

Lab: *Bact:* Smear shows club-shaped, nonmotile gram-pos bacilli, close to actinomycetes; culture on Loeffler's slant can detect within 12 hr if holding rx; if already treated with penicillin, may grow in 1 wk on tellurite slant, sharply selective

Rx: Prevent w active immunization of infants with toxoid in DPT 4-shot series, booster at school age, or over age 7 with 3-shot dT series; 80% of U.S. population now immunized; no deaths in patients with at least 1 immunization; q 10 yr thereafter with tetanus as dT (rv CDC: Ann IM 1985;103:896)

for carrier state: Penicillin as Bicillin × 1, or erythromycin (resistance developed in Seattle) 250 mg qid × 7 d (89% effective), or clindamycin 150 mg qid × 7 d

for active disease: Penicillin or erythromycin (resistance developed in Seattle), of questionable help (L. Weinstein 3/85); antitoxin ineffective if given > 48 hr after onset (Weinstein) and probably not worth complication risk anyway but can be done w 50,000 U antitoxin for acute gravis in first 24 hr and repeated in 24 hr × 1

Enterococcal Infections

Cause: *Enterococcus faecalis* and *faecium*, a group D strep

Epidem: Fecal organism; increasing resistance

Pathophys: In mixed infections, often "selected out" by cephalosporins

Sx: Abscesses, cellulitis, septic arthritis, UTIs

Si:

Cmplc: SBE

Lab: *Bact:* Gram-positive cocci

Rx: Aminoglycoside plus a penicillin essential for synergy; many β-lactamase producing, gentamicin-resistant strains are appearing now, treatable w vancomycin or ampicillin/sulbactam (Unasyn) (Ann IM 1992;116:285), although vancomycin resistance is now common (Nejm 2000;342:710), for which can use quinupristin/dalfopristin (Synercid) or linezolid (Zyvox)

Listerial Infections

Nejm 1996;334:770

Cause: *Listeria spp.*

Epidem: Present in most soils, animal gi tracts, and raw milk from infected cows, although it can occur even if pasteurized (Nejm 1997;336:100, 1985;312:404), or cheese (Mexican cheese epidemic in Calif: Nejm 1988;319:823)

Increased in pregnant women, elderly, neonates (Nejm 1971;285:599), and immunocompromised pts (Ann IM 1992;117:466)

Pathophys: Intracellular pathogenesis, usually picked up by gut macrophages and spread from there

Sx: Of sepsis, meningitis (p 560)

Si: Sepsis, meningitis esp in children < age 6 mo (p 560)

Crs:

Cmplc: Meningitis, sepsis, spontaneous abortion

Lab: *CSF:* Gram-pos rods, tumbling motility; often < 80% polys

Rx: Ampicillin is 1st choice; Tm/S is 2nd choice or used w ampicillin

Staph Food Poisoning

Nejm 1984;310:1368,1437

Cause: *Staphylococcus aureus*

Epidem: Most common type of food poisoning

Pathophys: Heat-stable enterotoxin produced by staph in food after preparation, eg, potato salad. Lack of fever indicates a toxin disease.

Sx: 8-hr incubation period. Nausea, vomiting, and some diarrhea without fever. Excess nausea and vomiting relative to diarrhea suggest staph rather than others.

Si:

Crs:

Cmplc: r/o clostridial and *Bacillus cereus* food poisonings, both of which also lack fever

Lab: None unless need to work up for public health reasons, then Gram stain and culture the food

Rx: Symptomatic

Staph Tissue Infections

Nejm 1998;338:520

Cause: *Staphylococcus aureus*

Epidem: Normal inhabitant of skin and upper respiratory track; 90% resistant to penicillin; cluster of MRSA infections in St. Louis Ram football team (Nejm 2005;352:468)

Pathophys: Multiple exotoxins increase its pathogenicity, including β-lactamase, coagulase, hyaluronidase, other proteases, leukocidin, lipases, staphylokinase. Hair follicles infected because fibrin restrains spread but retards healing.

Sx: Pain, swelling, may have fever

Si: Abscesses, carbuncle, furuncle, pneumonia, and empyema; acute endocarditis involving healthy valves; osteomyelitis, usually metaphyseal; septicemia

Crs: Bacteremia mortality = 11-43%

Cmplc: DIC, endocarditis including R-sided especially in drug users, metastatic infections, necrotizing fasciitis (Nejm 2005;352:1445)

Lab: *Bact:* Gram-positive cocci clusters, coagulase positive; methicillin resistance present in > 50% in some ICUs (Nejm 1998;339:520)

Rx:

Prevention: Mupirocin (Bactroban) topical rx to anterior nares of carriers (30% of population) pre-op reduces nosocomial post-op infection rates (Nejm 2002;346:1871,1905; Ann IM 1991;14:101,107 vs Ann IM 2004;140:419)

Surgical drainage

β-Lactamase–resistant drug like nafcillin/oxacillin iv, later go to po cloxacillin or diclox. Cephalosporin, clindamycin, Tm/S, erythromycin.

of methicillin-resistant staph (MRSA): (1) community-acquired type (Nejm 2005;352:1436,1455,1485), which often causes skin, soft tissue, and post-influenza pneumonia infections and is sensitive to quinolones, Tm/S, and clindamycin (beware clindamycin "sensitive" but really resistant if erythromycin resistant = "D test"); and (2) hospital-acquired type, where must use vancomycin w or w/o rifampin, but resistance appearing (Nejm 1999;340:493,517)

of vancomycin-resistant MRSA (Nejm 2003;348:1342): Linezolid (Zyvox) or Synercid

of recurrent abscesses: Prevent w rifampin 600 mg bid × 5 d (Nejm 1986;315:91) + vancomycin or Tm/S (Ann IM 1982;97:317)

of infected orthopedic appliances: Pencillinase-resistant penicillin + rifampin × 2 wk then quinolone + rifampin f/u rx × 3-6 mo (Jama 1998;279:1537)

Toxic Shock Syndrome

Nejm 1998;339:527; Ann IM 1982;96(2), 1982;97:608

Cause: *S. aureus;* occasionally strep-induced (Nejm 1987;317:146) by group A *S. pyogenes*, which produces scarlet fever toxin A (Nejm 1991;325:783, 1989;321:1)

Epidem: Initially 97% cases were associated with tampon use during menses, now none is w change in tampon manufacture, but some cases still associated w menstruation. Associated w influenza (Jama 1987;257:1053).

Pathophys: Enterotoxins produced at any body site

Sx: Diarrhea (98%), vomiting (92%), headache and sore throat (77%), myalgias

Si: Fever (87%), hypotension, scarletiniform rash that later desquamates

Crs: 10-15% mortality

Cmplc: Hepatitis and renal failure. Recurrent (25%). Chronic headache/memory changes (Ann IM 1982;96:865).

r/o Kawasaki's disease (p 887)

Lab: *Bact:* S. *aureus* in cultures of infected site, blood cultures usually negative

Rx: Fluids, staph antibiotics like clindamycin, which shut down toxin production; perhaps steroids, perhaps gamma globulin

Staphylococcus Epidermidis Infections

Ann IM 1989;110:9

Cause: *Staphylococcus epidermidis* (coagulase-negative staph)

Epidem: Normal skin inhabitant. Most common cause of hospital-acquired bacteremia; often catheter, prosthesis, or vascular graft associated.

Pathophys: Enmeshes in glycocalyx coating of catheters and prosthetics

Sx:

Si: Infections of implanted prosthetics

Crs:

Cmplc: 30% mortality with bacteremia

Lab: *Bact:* Culture, coagulase-negative staph. r/o S. *saprophyticus*, also a pathogen at least in urinary tract

Rx: > 60% are methicillin resistant; 1st vancomycin (Ann IM 1982;97:503), but some resistance (Nejm 1987;316:927); rifampin; gentamicin

Group B Strep Infections

Nejm 2000;343:175,209, 1990;322:1857

Cause: *Streptococcus agalactiae*, a group B strep

Epidem: 0.6/1000 births; 2000/yr in U.S.; 15-40% of pregnant women are colonized. Increasing incidence of serious (21% mortality)

infections in nonpregnant adults as well as pregnant women; a minority of group B strep infections in the U.S. now are in infants. Affects elderly and/or sick adults (Nejm 1993;328:1807,1843), especially diabetics.

Pathophys: Vaginal colonization leads to newborn and maternal infections

Sx: Floppy baby

Si: Newborn sepsis, and maternal chorioamnionitis, endometritis, and post-C/S wound infections

Crs:

Cmplc: r/o *E. coli, Listeria, S. epidermidis*

Lab: *Bact:* Gram-positive cocci in chains; usually β-hemolytic; PCR assay 45 min test now possible at presentation in labor (Nejm 2000;343:175,209)

Rx: Perhaps prevent someday by immunization with group B polysaccharide vaccine (Nejm 1988;319:1180), but pneumovax to mothers doesn't help (Nejm 1980;303:173)

Ampicillin iv (Nejm 2002;347:233,240,280, 2000;342:15, 1986;314:1665) intrapartum and to baby, in women with 35-37 wk prenatal positive vaginal/rectal cultures, and fever, and/or premature labor (< 37 wk), and/or prolonged (> 12 hr) ruptured membranes or various other risk-based or rx-all-carriers strategies, all of which tend to decrease group B strep newborn sepsis but increase incidence of resistant *E. coli* sepsis

Rat Bite Fever

Am J Med 1988;85:711; Lancet 1987;2:1361

Cause: *Streptobacillus moniliformis*, occasionally *Spirillum minor* (a spirochete)

Epidem: Rat bite or contaminated dairy products (Haverhill fever). In low-socioeconomic groups and in medical researchers working with rats.

Pathophys:

Sx: Bitten 2-3 d before, heals in 10-12 d; very inflamed bite in case of *Spirillum;* chills; arthralgias in large joints

Si: Fever, macular rash on palms and soles

Crs:

Cmplc: Endocarditis and other cardiac infections
r/o rickettsia, coxsackie B

Lab: *Bact:* Blood culture positive; spirillum can be seen on peripheral smear

Rx: Use gloves preventively
Penicillin for both types (Ann IM 1985;102:229)

Pneumococcal Infections

Cause: *Streptococcus pneumoniae,* especially types 3 and 6 (most virulent)

Epidem: Population carriers disseminate to pts w diminished resistance; 50% of population carries in upper respiratory tract at some time

Increased incidence in blood group A types because pneumococcus has A-like antigens, and in pts after splenectomy because residual RES requires increased antibody coating before phagocytosis can occur (Nejm 1981;304:245)

Pathophys (Nejm 1995;332:1280): Invasive w pyogenic response; little toxin production; pathogenic via numbers alone; polysaccharide capsule in virulent strains makes phagocytosis hard

Sx: Meningitis: Fever, confusion
Otitis media: Ear pain
Pneumonia: Fever, chills, sudden onset of pleurisy

Si: Meningitis: Fever, confusion
Otitis media: Hot ear
Pneumonia: Bloody sputum unlike viral or mycoplasma

Crs: Pneumonia: Xray clears in 6 wk (Nejm 1970;283:798)

Meningitis: 50% mortality

Cmplc: Triad w endocarditis, meningitis, and pneumonia often fatal (Am J Med 1963;33:262); empyema

r/o multiple myeloma if crit low

Lab: *Bact:* Gram-pos diplococci; culture shows optochin-sensitive/bile salt-soluble colonies

Rx: Prevent w vaccine, which is inducing a decline in the rate of invasive disease in all age groups, including HIV-pos children (Nejm 2003;348:1737,1747, 2003;349:1341)

- Adult pneumococcal 23 valent vaccine (Prevnar) (Med Let 1999;41:84), 65% overall effective (Nejm 1991;325:1453; Ann IM 1988;108:653, 1986;104:1-118) at least for elderly (> 65 yr) and people at increased risk, eg, splenectomy, COPD, alcoholics, diabetes, chronic renal pts on dialysis, CHF (Ann IM 1984;101:325,348); in all pts? (Ann IM 1986;104:106 vs Jama 1996;275:194); ineffective in many sick pts who need it the most, eg VA COPD pts (Nejm 1986;315:1318). Revaccinate if vaccination in doubt or once 5 yr later at least for high-risk pts and those who got 1st dose before age 65 (Mmwr 1997;46:1); local reactions in ~10% of those revaccinated (Jama 1999;281:243).
- Pediatric conjugated 7 valent vaccine (Jama 2000;283:1460) @ 2, 4, 6, and 12 mo, or single dose thereafter; even single dose dramatically decreases pneumococcal infection rates under age 5 (Jama 2004;291:2197) including otitis media by 20+% (NNT-2 = 5)(Nejm 2001;344:403)

of disease: Since penicillin resistance now is so widespread albeit regionally variable, 25% nationally (Nejm 2000;343:1917), until know sensitivities, rx w ceftriaxone + vancomycin for life-threatening infections like meningitis; or vancomycin iv w po levofloxacin 500 mg po qd × 7-14 d, or 3rd-generation fluoro-quinolone. Then, if sensitive, switch to penicillin or another β-lactam antibiotic, although quinolone resistance is appearing and can even develop during the crs of rx (Nejm 2002;346:747).

Scarlet Fever

Nejm 1970;282:23, 1977;297:365

Cause: *Streptococcus pyogenes* (rarely *S. aureus*, which causes no sore throat)

Epidem: Respiratory droplets and wound infections. Occurs in children only, since adults usually are already immune.

Pathophys: Erythrogenic toxin produced by bacteria lysogenized by a specific phage, which causes bacterial capsular dilatation, rupture, and toxin release

Sx: Sore throat, fever, rash

Si: Rash, trunkal, especially in creases (Pastia's lines), palpable, viral-like. Spots on soft palate. "Strawberry" tongue. Circumoral pallor.

Crs:

Cmplc:
- Acute glomerular nephritis
- Rheumatic fever, in old days 3% in epidemic and ½% in endemic type if no rx; now < 1/10,000 w/o rx, and < 1/100,000 w rx in adults
- Peritonsillar abscess (Quincy abscess), and tonsillar vein phlebitis leading to pulmonary emboli, rx with tonsillectomy (L. Weinstein 3/85)
- Toxic shock syndrome (p 534), which may just be the extreme variant (Nejm 1991;325:783)

    r/o other childhood exanthems: roseola, rubeola, rubella, erythema infectiosum (5th disease)

Lab: Sore throat w/u protocol (Ann IM 1980;93:244)
Bact: Throat culture, single swab positive in 75%, 2 swabs in 85% β-hemolysis on culture plates. Positive culture may still be

just a carrier. Rapid office tests take 10 min–1 hr, cost $2-3 plus lots of time (Med Let 1985;27:49) but may still have to culture if negative (J Peds 1987;111:80).

Hem: Eosinophils increased often

Rx: Penicillin, erythromycin. If sick, treatment speeds healing (Jama 1975;227:1278); but no mild cases (Am J Med 1951;10:300).

Streptococcal Pharyngitis

Nejm 2001;344:205, 1991;325:783; Ann IM 1989;110:612

Cause: *Streptococcus pyogenes,* group A, β-hemolytic, rarely group C or D

Epidem: Respiratory droplets; occasionally foodborne (Nejm 1969;280:917); 15% of the population carry in pharynx

Pathophys:

Sx: Sore throat, fever[1] > 100°F, no cough[2]

Si (Jama 2004;291:1587, 2000;284:2912): Pharyngeal and/or tonsillar exudate[3] (50% sens, 80% specif), anterior cervical tender and/or enlarged nodes[4] (50% sens, 70% specif), T° > 101°F (38°C) often (50% sens and specif). Findings 1-4 = Centor score and are crucial (Ann IM 2001;134:506,509).

Crs: 10 d without rx

Cmplc:
- Acute glomerular nephritis
- Rheumatic fever, in old days 3% in epidemic and 1/2% in endemic type if no rx; now < 1/10,000 w/o rx and < 1/100,000 w rx in adults
- Peritonsillar abscess (Quincy abscess) and Lemierre syndrome (Nejm 2004;350:1037) w fusobacterium anaerobic bacteremia, including septic pulmonary emboli from jugular phlebitis 5-7 d after acute sore throat

  r/o (A. Komaroff, 1985) chlamydia (21%) especially TWAR, viral (17%) (rhinovirus, coronavirus, adenovirus, parainfluenza virus, respiratory syncytial virus, echo, coxsackie, acute primary HIV infection), mycoplasma (11%), mononucleosis (EBV) (10%), non-group A strep (9%), legionella (3%), gonorrhea (1-2%), diphtheria; or *Arcanobacterium haemolyticum* (a diphtheroid) pharyingitis and scalatiniform rash, esp common in adults, rx w erythromycin

Lab: Sore throat w/u protocol and rx strategies (Jama 2004;291:1587; Ann IM 2001;134:506,509); rapid strep test for all children and adults w Centor scores of 3+, rx positives; but if rapid test neg, get full throat culture in children

Bact: Rapid office throat swab strep tests take 10 min, cost $2-3; are 90+% specific but in practice only 60-70% sensitive (30-50% sens, 95% spec-Jama 1992;267:695) so may need to culture negatives especially in children (Med Let 1991;33:40; J Peds 1987;111:80). New optical immunoassay test 80% sens, 95% specif compared to culture, which is 70+% sens and 99% specif (Jama 1997;277:899).

Full throat culture, single swab positive in 75%, 2 swabs in 85%. β-Hemolysis on culture plates. Positive culture may still be just a carrier.

Rx: Penicillin V or erythromycin 250 mg po t-qid, × 10 d at least if want rheumatic fever prophylaxis, even bid may be enough (Peds 2000;105:E19), although 20-40% resistance to erythromycin is now being reported (Nejm 2002;346:1200, 1992;326:292); or azithromycin. Rx immediately (Ann IM 2001;134:506,509) if h/o fever, adenopathy, no cough, and exudate; or, if 2-3 of these 4 criteria met, get rapid strep and rx only if pos.

Tonsillectomy and adenoidectomy does decrease recurrence of strep throats in children with 3 or more documented strep throats/yr over several yr (Nejm 1984;310:674, 717)

of hyperendemic outbreak, eg, Marine boot camp (Nejm 1991;325:92): Benzathine penicillin 1 million U q 1 mo or po erythromycin to all group members

Streptococcal Erysipelas, Cellulitis/Wound Infections, Necrotizing Fasciitis, and Impetigo

Nejm 2004;350:904 [cellulitis],1996;334:240

Cause: *Streptococcus pyogenes*, group A, β-hemolytic

Epidem: Erysipelas and cellulitis are common; necrotizing fasciitis (NF) is rare, 1/yr in big hospital. Invasive strep infections in 1.5/100,000/yr in general population, 3/1000 of household contacts (Nejm 1996;335:547); but invasive cases are just the tip of the iceberg since same strain will be found causing much more pharyngitis in the community (Jama 1997;277:38).

Pathophys: Erysipelas: Mainly in lymphatics
Cellulitis: In subcutaneous tissues
NF: Infections dissect along fascial planes, so skin is last to go, and look deceptively benign; $^1/_3$ of the time NF is associated with anaerobic bacteria as well
Impetigo: A superficial skin infection, starts in a break in the skin

Sx: Pain, fever, and rapid spreading in erysipelas, cellulitis, and NF; in impetigo, sx are of a weeping rash usually in a child

Si: Erysipelas: Has sharp limits, symmetric swelling, usually across bridge of nose
Cellulitis: Has little edema and indistinct limits; may be perianal in children
NF: Has edema, fever, redness, gas crepitation (in 50%), anesthesia (nerve infarction), ecchymosis (thrombosis)
Impetigo: Rash has bullae with honey yellow exudate

Crs: In NF, 75% die without surgical debridement within 1-2 d

Cmplc: Toxic shock syndrome (p 534) and acute glomerular nephritis can occur with all
Erysipelas: r/o **Erysipeloid** (hands, exposure to raw meat and animals, slower spread; gram-positive rod, culture skin biopsy; rx with penicillin, etc)

Cellulitis: Erythema nodosum and endocarditis; r/o acute axillary lymphadenitis (Nejm 1990;323:655), vibrio saltwater infections, pasturella from animal bites, pseudomonas in diabetic feet, mouth anaerobes from human bites, **aeromonas cellulitis** from leeches or freshwater abrasions rx'd w cipro or imipenenem/cilastin

NF: r/o gas gangrene

Lab: *Bact:* In all, culture, and gram-positive cocci in chains on Gram stain

Path: For NF, frozen section biopsy

Serol: ASO titers elevated

Rx: Prevention w bacitracin dressing no better than vaseline (Jama 1996;276:972)

for all, antibiotics like penicillin, erythromycin although 20-40% resistance now in Finland (Nejm 1992;326:292)

of impetigo: Mupirocin (Bactroban) ointment (not cream) topically tid as good as po antibiotics; $10/15 gm tube (Med Let 1988;30:55); debated if need to cover for resistant staph, especially nonbullous type (Lancet 1991;338:803)

of NF: Extensive surgical debridement first; clindamycin helps decrease toxin production

9.3   Gram-Negative Organisms

Whooping Cough

Nejm 2005;352:1215

Cause: *Bordetella pertussis* (similar to hemophilus); occasionally sporadically by adenovirus (Nejm 1970;283:390). From respiratory tract of infected persons, especially during catarrhal stage; 90% attack rate.

Epidem: Worldwide, worst in developing countries. Highest incidence in children < 5 yr. Female morbidity > male. In U.S., increased to $> 11,000$ cases/yr in 2003, $5\times$ that in 1980, w many infections in adults.

Pathophys: Rapid bacterial multiplication causes decreased tracheal and bronchial ciliary action, which in turn causes infection by strep, staph, etc. Endotoxin produced and released when bacteria die, causing cell irritation and occasional death; perhaps neurotoxic effects on CNS.

Coughing causes anoxia, which somehow causes hemorrhages

Sx: Catarrhal stage (mild cough) $\times$ 2 wk; then paroxysmal coughing lasting weeks to months.

In adults (Ann IM 1998;128:64), nonproductive intermittent chronic cough (> 2 wk), 12-21% of those w that sx? (Jama 1996;275:1672, 1995;273:1044); diaphoresis (50%)

Si: Spasmodic coughing—long, drawn-out with rapid sharp inhalations (whoops); small petechial hemorrhages throughout body. No fever.

Crs: Paroxysmal stage lasts > 2 wk, 27% still have cough at 90 d ("cough of 100 days")

Cmplc: Seizures; secondary pulmonary infection and atelectasis; meningitis; in infants, apnea and death 75% are < 1 yr, 40% are < 3 mo (Ann IM 1972;76:289)

r/o croup (p 886)

Lab: *Bact:* Culture, if sx ≤ 4 wk, of sputum or nasal/pharyngeal swab during catarrhal stage, and/or PCR tests of same

Hem: Wbc's increased with high % (usually $> 50\%$) lymphocytes, looks like CLL in a child

Serol: ELISA IgG antibody titers increased after 3 wk although cutoffs for dx on a single titer controversial

Rx: Preventively (CDC rv: Ann IM 1985;103:896):
- Immunize with antigens 1, 2, and 3 in children between age 6 wk and < 6 yr; use acellular pertussis as DTaP for immuniza-

tions beginning at 2 mo, 70-90% effective compared to placebo, while whole-cell vaccine is only 40-60% effective and has encephalitic/neurologic cmplc's (Nejm 1996;334:341,349, 391, 1995;333:1045; Jama 1996;275:37). No cross-placental transfer.

- Tdap boosters in adolescents and adults to control in the wider population (Jama 2005;293:3003)
- Hyperimmune globulin
- Antibiotics prophylactically or to sick pts to decrease infectivity, do shorten course: erythromycin 40 mg/kg in children, 1 gm/d in adults; or azithromycin; or Tm/S × 10 d, 8 mg/ 40 mg/kg in children, 320/1600 in adults

Campylobacter Diarrhea

Ann IM 1983;98:360, 1983;99:38; Nejm 1981;305:1444

Cause: *Campylobacter jejuni*

Epidem: Contaminated water, surface water, and municipal water supplies (Ann IM 1982;96:293); similar epidemiology to giardia. Also may be sporadic, foodborne, often by eggs. Cattle, goats, horses, and perhaps wild animals excrete in feces. 3× more frequent than giardia; more common than salmonella and shigella (Harvard Medical School CME lecture 3/85).

Pathophys:

Sx: 1-7 d incubation period
Diarrhea (100%), cramps (95%), fever (80%), bloody diarrhea (29%)

Si:

Crs: 20% last over 1 wk

Cmplc: Chronic colitis; Guillain-Barré syndrome (Nejm 1995;333:1374; Ann IM 1993;118:847); **immunoproliferative small bowel disease** (alpha-chain disease), a mucosa-associated lymphoid tissue (MALT) lymphoma w plasma cell infiltration of bowel wall and monoclonal α-heavy chain, prevalent around Mediterranean, causes a chronic wasting diarrhea, can cause diffuse B-cell lymphomas and is rx'd w combinations of antibiotics like amoxicilin + clarithromycin + metronidazole

r/o ulcerative colitis relapses

Lab: *Bact:* Culture in 10% CO_2 × 48 hr, special media

Rx: Erythromycin if sx > 3 d; ciprofloxacin (Arch IM 1990;150:541), or other quinolone although drug resistance appearing because of their use in poultry industry (Nejm 1999;340:1525)

Granuloma Inguinale

Ann IM 1985;102:705

Cause: *Calymmatobacterium granulomatis*

Epidem: Venereally spread, ie, an STD; highest rates in low-income areas

Pathophys:

Sx: Painless ulcer

Si: Genital papule, inguinal nodes. Skin breaks down into granulation tissue.

Crs: Long term even with rx

Cmplc:

Lab: *Path:* Biopsy shows diagnostic intracellular organisms, called Donovan bodies

Rx (Med Let 1994;36:1):

1st tetracycline; 2nd streptomycin

Traveler's Diarrhea

Nejm 2000;342:1716, 1993;328:1821

Cause (Jama 1999;281:811): *E. coli* enterotoxigenic type (50+%), rarely invasive type; (p 549) *Salmonella sp.*, campylobacter, rotavirus, et al

Epidem: In salads, sewer-contaminated water (Crater Lake epidemics: Ann IM 1977;86:714). 30% of all travelers to Mexico get one type or the other, usually within 2 wk of arrival (Nejm 1976; 294:1299). Most of acute childhood diarrhea in Brazil (Nejm 1975;293:567).

Pathophys: A toxin is produced while the organisms are attached to gut wall much like *C. perfringens*; heat-labile toxin type is delayed in onset like cholera; heat-stable types cause immediate onset (Nejm 1975;292:933). In the unusual invasive types, colonic wall invasion causes bloody mucus, like shigella.

Sx: Toxin-producing types: clear, watery diarrhea may become bloody later; fever (50%)
Invasive types: Bloody mucus, fever in most, pain

Si: Toxin-producing types: Sometimes low-grade fever
Invasive types: Fever

Crs:

Cmplc: r/o other gi infections (p 401–409)

Lab: *Bact:* Stool smear shows polys in invasive types, none in noninvasive types; if polys present, culture for pathogens on sorbitol–MacConkey agar, O157 antiserum test of cultured *E. coli* (Nejm 1995;333:364)

Rx (Med Let 1994;36:41):
Prevent in travelers w:

- Avoidance of high-risk foods, eg, ice, salads, milk, street foods, hot sauces (Ann IM 2002;136:884); of questionable benefit (Jama 1999;281:811)
- Antibiotic prophylaxis if willing to risk rx cmplc:
  Ciprofloxacin, 1st choice, 500 mg po × 1 dose (Lancet 1994; 334:1537) or qd; or ofloxacin (Floxin) 300 mg po qd; or norfloxacin 400 mg po qd

INFECTIOUS DISEASE

Doxycycline 100 mg qd × 5 wk (90% effective: Nejm 1978; 298:758) but resistance common in 1993; gi excretion means can use in face of renal or hepatic disease

Bismuth subsalicylate (Peptobismol) 60 cc or ii tabs qid (75% effective), has 2 ASA equivalents/60 cc (Med Let 1980;22:63); salicylate probably inhibits prostaglandins, hence effect or antibiotic effect of bismuth

Rifaximin 200 mg po qd-bid (Ann IM 2005;142:805); not absorbed, prevents 75%

Tm/S single strength po qd in children, risks allergic reaction of diarrheal sx when traveling, may be the better approach, w:

- Loperamide HCl (Imodium) 4 mg po then 2 mg after each stool up to 16 mg po qd used with any antibiotic below doesn't hurt, may help (Ann IM 1993;118:377, 1991;114:731); diphenoxylate + atropine (Lomotil) may worsen some types, eg, shigella (Jama 1973;226:1575) and

- Ciprofloxacin, 1st choice, 500 mg po bid × 3 d (Ann IM 1991;114:731), also gets campylobacter, salmonella, and shigella as well as the pathogenic *E. coli*; or norfloxacin 400 mg po bid × 3 d; or levofloxacin 500 mg po qd × 3 d, or ofloxacin (Floxin) 300 mg po bid × 3 d; all about $33/crs, or

- Azithromycin 1000 mg po ×1, or 500 mg po qd × 3 d; $32/crs generic

- Tm/S (Septra) DS bid × 3-5 d (Ann IM 1987;106:216; Nejm 1982;307:84); resistance more common than with cipro

- Rifaximin (Xifaxan) (Med Let 2004;46:74) 200 mg po tid × 3 d; nonabsorbed refampin-like antibiotic as good as cipro for nonbloody diarrhea w/o fever, but not adequate if fever or blood; $33/crs

E. Coli Invasive Diarrhea

Cause: Toxin-producing types like O157:H7 (Nejm 1995;333:364)

Epidem: O157:H7 type (Ann IM 1995;123:698), in manure dust (Jama 2003;290:2709), hamburger (Jama 1984;272:1349), cattle coats (petting zoo outbreak: Nejm 2002;347:555), sprouts (Ann

IM 2001;135:239), drinking water, and swimming lakes (Nejm 1994;331:579). Most common cause of infectious bloody diarrhea in U.S.

Pathophys: Colonic wall invasion and toxin production causes bloody mucus, like shigella

Sx: Incubation period 1-3 d. Bloody mucus, fever in most, pain.

Si: Low-grade fever, fecal leukocytes present, initial watery stool becomes bloody

Crs:

Cmplc: Hemolytic-uremic syndrome (in 10% vs 15%: Jama 1994; 272:1349 vs Nejm 2002;347:555) or TTP
r/o other gi infections (p 401–409)

Lab: *Bact:* Stool smear shows polys; if polys, culture for pathogens on sorbitol–MacConkey agar and do O157 antiserum test of cultured *E. coli* (Nejm 1995;333:364); stool toxin titers

Rx: Rehydration and supportive care; at least in children, antibiotic rx increases risk of hemoytic-uremic syndrome (Nejm 2000;342: 1930), can use ciprofloxacin or Tm/S DS bid × 3 d (Ann IM 1987;106:216)

Chancroid

Ann IM 1985;102:705, 1983;98:973

Cause: *Haemophilus ducreyi* (Ann IM 1981;95:315)

Epidem: Venereally spread, ie, an STD, associated with syphilis in 15%

Pathophys:

Sx: Painful ulcer after 2-15 d incubation

Si: Adenopathy; tender, "dirty," necrotic ulcer(s); tender bubos (40%)

Crs: Self-limited

Lab: *Bact:* Culture positive in 80%

Rx (CDC: Ann IM 2002;137:255; Med Let 1999;41:89):
for patient and contacts: Ceftriaxone 250 mg im once; or azithromycin 1 gm po once; or ciprofloxacin 500 mg po bid × 3 d; or erythromycin 500 mg qid × 7 d
in AIDS: Azithromycin, cipro, or erythro as above

Nonspecific Vaginitis (Vaginal Bacteriosis, Bacterial Vaginosis)

Nejm 1997;337:1896

Cause (Med Let 1999;41:86): *Gardnerella vaginalis, Mobiluncus,* mycoplasmas, ureaplasmas, and other anaerobes that themselves may be primary cause. These are all endogenous flora, not necessarily venereal, since occur in 15% of virginal women.

Epidem: 3rd most common cause of vaginitis after trichomonas and monilia

Pathophys: Diminished presence of lactobacilli, corresponding increase in pH leading to *G. vaginalis, Mycoplasma hominis* (Nejm 1995;333:1732,1737), and anaerobe (esp. *Bacteroides*) overgrowth

Sx: Vaginitis with watery discharge, no dyspareunia

Si: Watery discharge evenly coats walls; vinegar-like smell

Crs:

Cmplc: Increased incidence of premature labor (< 37 wk) and low birth weight
r/o trichomonal (p 643), monilial (p 191), and other (p 848) vaginitis causes

Lab: *Bact:* Vaginal discharge smear shows clue cells (100%: Lancet 1983;2:1379); pH > 4.5-5.0; positive amine ("whiff") test, ie, discharge smells of ammonia (70-80%); few polys. Culture positive in 40% (Obgyn 1984;64:271).

Rx (Med Let 1994;41:86):

Preventive: Unclear if screening as rx for asx pregnant women decreases prematurity and LBW babies (Am J Prev Med 2001;20:62); rx at least women at high risk for preterm labor since rx decreases incidence from 50% to 30% (Nejm 1995; 333:1732 vs 2000;342:534,581)

of disease (Ann IM 2002;137:255):

- Metronidazole (Flagyl) 2 gm qd × 1 → 75% cure; or 500 mg bid × 7 d → 95% cure (Lancet 1983;2:1379), costs $5; 30% recur in 1 mo, at least if partner not rx'd, although partner rx not clearly helpful (Ann IM 1989;111:551). Or as metronidazole vaginal gel 5 gm qd × 5 d, costs $20; or
- Clindamycin 300 mg po bid × 7 d; or as 2% vaginal cream 5 gm q hs × 7 d; costs $27

in pregnancy: Metronidazole 250 po tid × 7d, or clindamycin po as above

Haemophilus Respiratory Infections

Nejm 1990;323:1415; Ann IM 1973;78:259

Cause: *Haemophilus influenzae*, unencapsulated or encapsulated (type B) (Mmwr 1985;34:201)

Epidem: Airborne from respiratory tract of infected person. Worldwide distribution. Infections with unencapsulated type occur in all age groups and are common in people with COPD. Infections with more invasive and malignant encapsulated type now becoming rare with advent of vaccine in children; most now in adults (Ann IM 1992;116:806). Before Hib vaccine, incidence was 100/100,000 and meningitis in 60/100,000 under age 5.

Pathophys:

Sx:

Si: Otitis media, bronchitis, sinusitis. Encapsulated type can also cause acute epiglottitis (p 235), sore throat with dysphagia, meningitis,

pneumonia, but only rarely otitis media (10% of all H. flu otit
is media).

Crs: Meningitis has 5% mortality and 30% incidence of neurologic
sequelae

Cmplc: Encapsulated type causes:
- Sudden death with epiglotitis, especially if sedated or kept
  supine, or throat stick gags throat, due to cardiac arrest
  (L. Weinstein 3/85) and airway obstruction
- Retropharyngeal abscess resulting in "quacking" voice, breathe
  better supine (Weinstein 3/85)

Lab: *Bact:* Gram-negative coccobacilli; capsule may be visible in
encapsulated type

Xray: Lateral neck soft tissue view to look for epiglottis involvement

Rx: Passive prophylaxis for encapsulated-type disease possible w
rifampin (Nejm 1987;316:1226) or hyperimmune globulin (Nejm
1987;317:923)

Active immunization: Hib vaccine conjugated with diphtheria
protein to give better immune response in infants (Nejm
1987;317:717); give MSD Pedvax Hib at 2 and 4 mo with
DPT and boost at 12 mo (Med Let 1991;33:5), perhaps a
shot at 6 mo if using one of the other vaccines; all appear
interchangeable (Jama 1995;273:849). Vaccinating mother
in 3rd trimester may help where risk is high (Jama 1996;
275:1182).

of active disease: Ampicillin, but 8-20% of all U.S. isolates now
resistant; in life-threatening illness, ceftriaxone or rarely
used chloramphenicol. Tm/S if mild infection and may be or
is resistant to ampicillin.

of cmplc's: Steroids and tracheotomy for acute airway obstruction; steroids for meningitis, like dexamethasone 0.15 mg/kg
iv 20 min before antibiotic, then q 6 hr × 4; decreases
cmplc, especially deafness (Nejm 1990;319:968)

Klebsiella Pneumonia

Cause: *Klebsiella pneumoniae* (enterobacteriaceae)

Epidem: Fecal contamination usually; a normal inhabitant of large bowel and often in upper respiratory tract

> 1% of all pneumonias; increased incidence in males > 40 yr

Pathophys:

Sx: Brown-red, thick ("currant jelly") sputum; fever, chills; pleurisy

Si: Fever; consolidation si's, often much less impressive than xray

Crs: Rapidly progressive; 25-50% mortality

Cmplc: Empyema; multiple-drug resistance acquisition in hospital (Ann IM 1971;74:657)

Lab: *Bact:* Gram stain shows gram-neg rods w capsule
> *Hem:* Wbc may be low

Xray: Chest consolidations may be convex, "swollen lobar consolidation"

Rx: Gentamicin + cephalosporin, fluoroquinolone, or 3rd-generation cephalosporin until know sensitivities

Legionnaires' Disease (Legionellosis)

Nejm 1997;337:682; J Infect Dis 1992;165:736

Cause: *Legionella pneumophilia,* etc

Epidem: Airborne or drinking water-borne (Nejm 1992;326:151)
> Epidemic and endemic. Male > female; summer/fall peaks; many unrecognized cases, 5% of all community-acquired pneumonias; spread by air-conditioner systems (Nejm 1980;302:365). Increased incidence in patients on dialysis, with DM, COPD, over age 50, on chemotherapy.

Pathophys:

Sx: 2-10 d incubation. Diarrhea* ($^2/_3$); cough without sputum, pleurisy, headache, recurrent rigors; r/o mycoplasma and psittacosis

*Most important findings for dx

Si: Pneumonitis,* fever,* slow pulse, confusion, wound infections (UVM: Ann IM 1982;96:173)

Crs: High fatality rate if immunocompromised

Cmplc: r/o other atypical pneumonia agents, eg, Pittsburgh agent (Ann IM 1980;92:559) and very similar **Pontiac Fever** (Ann IM 1984;100:333)

Lab:

> *Bact:* Sputum Gram stain shows polys without bugs; gram-neg rod when pick culture, won't stain in tissue. Fluorescent antibody stains of transtracheal aspirate or sputum, pos in 26% (Ann IM 1979;90:1). Culture requires special media, very fastidious.
>
> *Chem:* LFTs increased ($\frac{1}{2}$); Na < 130 ($\frac{2}{3}$)
>
> *Hem:* ESR increased ($\frac{1}{3}$); polys increased ($\frac{2}{3}$) with left shift
>
> *Serol:* Titer > 1/250 IgG and IgM
>
> *Urine:* 3+ protein (20%), rbc's. Urine antigen by RIA or ELISA, 70% sens, 100% specif; is the clinically most useful test.

Xray: Chest shows bilateral pneumonia, $\frac{1}{3}$ w pleural effusion

Rx (Nejm 1998;129:328):

> Azithromycin, clarithromycin, or erythromycin × 10-14 d; ciprofloxacin 400 mg iv q 8 hr or 750 mg po bid, or newer fluoroquinolone; doxycycline, but less effective. Add rifampin in severe disease.

Moraxella Infections

Cause: *Moraxella (Branhamella, Neisseria) catarrhalis*

Epidem: High carrier rates in the population

Pathophys: Major pathogen in COPD/chronic bronchitis; 3rd most common bacterial pathogen in otitis media after pneumococcus and H. flu

Sx: Increased sputum production, cough

*Most important findings for dx

Si: Fever fairly uncommon

Crs:

Cmplc:

Lab: *Bact:* Gram-neg diplococci
Hem: Wbc usually < 10,000

Xray:

Rx: Ciprofloxacin, 2nd-generation cephalosporins, macrolides, Tm/S, tetracyclines

Gonorrhea

Cause: *Neisseria gonorrhea*

Epidem: Venereal; common; bacteremia associated with deficient complement factors, eg, C'_5, C'_6, C'_7, C'_8 (Ann IM 1983;99:35); prevalence = $\frac{1}{2}$% in U.S. (Jama 2004;291:2229) but higher in blacks. Coincident *Chlamydia* infection in 15-20% male heterosexuals, 25-40% females (Ann IM 2003;139:178; Nejm 1984; 310:545).

Pathophys: Infects mucous membranes of gu tract (Nejm 1985; 312:1683). IgA protease on surface distinguishes infectious *Neisseria* from commensals (Nejm 1978;299:973), as do pili. Septicemia more commonly with strains with fewer gu sx, leading to rash, polyarthralgias with negative joint taps (an immune complex disease: Ann IM 1978;89:28); later one joint may evolve to a single hot infected joint (Nejm 1968;279:234).

Sx: Male: Urethral discharge, but ⅔ asx (Nejm 1974;290:117); anal infections, more often asx (Ann IM 1977;86:340); pharyngitis (Nejm 1973;288:181)
Female: Bartholin cyst (80% of acute Bartholin's gland cyst infections are due to gc); vaginal discharge, dysuria, pelvic inflammatory disease, pain typically occurring with menses or pregnancy, abnormal menstrual bleeding due to endometritis

Si: Urethral, anal, or pharyngeal discharge; in female, abdominal distention, "chandelier sign" (severe pain w cervical motion), pus in cervix

Crs: 2-7+ d latent period

Cmplc:

- Bacteremia with purpuric or vesicular pustule on broad erythematous base or later, hemorrhagic bullae
- Endocarditis, 80% have arthritis too; with monoarticular arthritis, 3% will have endocarditis
- **Fitzhugh-Curtis Syndrome**, hepatic capsule inflammation (Nejm 1970;282:1082)
- Polyarthritis and tenosynovitis (rv of all septic arthritis: Nejm 1985;312:764)

    r/o trichomonas, candida, chlamydia (Nejm 1974;291:1175), syphilis, Reiter's, appendicitis in female

Lab: *Bact:* Gram stain, in male 1st, culture only if unclear on Gram stain; in female, smear of cleanly wiped cervix to look for > 3 polys/hpf with intracellular gram-neg cocci, has 67% sensitivity, 98% specificity

Culture: In women; in male only if unclear on smear. Reculture all after rx and recheck VDRL if negative 1st time. Penicillinase-producing strains now in U.S.

Serol: Screen for associated complement deficiencies with CH_{50} level (Nejm 1983;308:1138)

Rx: Preventive tetracycline, in neonates, 1% ointment once, or erythromycin; are better than $AgNO_3$ (Nejm 1988;318:657) of disease (Ann IM 2002;137:255), general rules: regimens now must be good vs penicillinase-producing organisms; 1st-generation cephalosporins and phenoxymethyl penicillin are ineffective; tetracycline inadequate for gc but treat all with azithromlycin 1 gm po × 1, or doxycycline 100 mg bid × 7 d to get chlamydia; or in pregnancy erythromycin 500 mg po qid × 7 d or amoxicillin 500 mg po tid × 7 d

1st line:

- Ceftriaxone 125-250 mg im × 1 ($10); gets syphilis, and both pharyngeal and resistant gc; or
- Cefixime (Suprax) 400 mg po × 1 ($5); or
- Levofloxacin 250 mg po × 1
- Ciprofloxacin 300-600 mg po × 1; no good vs syphilis; resistance appearing (Ann IM 1996;125:465)
- Ofloxacin 400 mg po × 1

2nd line: Spectinomycin 2 gm im × 1; if penicillin allergy and pregnant; no good vs syphilis or vs gc pharyngitis, resistance develops quickly (Nejm 1987;317:272)

of cmplc's (Mmwr 1993;42:STD supplement:1): Arthritis and/or septicemia, hospitalize and tap joint, irrigate it if worsens. 10 million U aqueous penicillin until afebrile × 3 d then 7 d cefoxitin 1 gm qid iv, or spectinomycin 2 gm bid im.

Adult Meningitis (Meningococcal et al)

Nejm 2004;351:1849, 2001;344:1378

Cause (Nejm 1997;337:970):

Age 20-60: 1st pneumococcus, 2nd *Neisseria meningitidis* (Serogroup Y > C > B > A), 3rd *Listeria;* rarely *Haemophilus influenzae*

Age 60+: 1st pneumococcus, 2nd *Listeria,* 3rd others

Epidem: Meningococcal: Serogroup A in epidemics in developing countries; rare in U.S., 1/100,000/yr or < 3000 cases/yr; groups B (ET-5 strain: Jama 1999;281:1493) Y, and C are sporadic and in epidemics in U.S. (Jama 1995;273:383,390)

From respiratory tract of carriers (< 3% of general population) or pts with meningococcal pneumonitis (Ann IM 1979;91:7). Increased after influenza infection (Nejm 1972;287:5). Bacteremia recurs in pts with complement deficiencies of C'_6, C'_7, or C'_8 (40% of all adult meningitis is nosocomial, often gram negative, although meningococcal never is).

Increased by exposure to tobacco smoke

Pathophys: Meningococcal: IgA protease on surface distinguishes infectious from commensal meningococcus (Nejm 1992;327:864). Impaired protein C activation in sepsis (Nejm 2001;345:408).
URI leads to bacteremia 1st, then:

- Metastatic infections of meninges, eye, pericardium, joints, and/or cardiac valves
- Immune complex arthritis w/o permanent damage

Sx: Fever, changed affect/mental status (85%), stiff neck, headache (95% have at least 2/4 sx)

Si: T° > 100°F (95%), stiff neck (88%), petechial rash with central focal necrosis (66%) (purpura fulminans—pictures: Nejm 1996;334:1709), focal neurologic deficits (28%), seizures (23%)

Crs: Without rx, death in hrs; w rx, 25% meningococcal mortality; pneumococcal mortality higher and morbidity > 50%

Cmplc:

- CNS thrombophlebitis with focal seizures and deficits, cranial nerve neuropathies (Nejm 1972;286:882), communicating hydrocephalus
- Meningococcal myocarditis in 75% at postmortem, 20% have aseptic pericardial effusions (Ann IM 1971;74:212)
- Adrenal hemorrhage and insufficiency (Waterhouse-Friderichsen syndrome w meningococcal)
- Chronic meningococcal bacteremia without CNS involvement, fever, or rash
    In compromised host, r/o listeria, cryptococcus, toxoplasmosis, and other treatable causes of meningitis

Lab: *Bact:* CSF has > 10 white cells/mm^3, usually (87%) > 200, mostly polys; glucose < 40 mg % (50%); protein > 45 mg % (96%), usually > 100 mg %; Gram stain, CSF culture (for meningococcal, best in 10% CO_2), blood cultures

Xray: CT scan if focal si's before LP (Nejm 2001;345:1727), but *start antibiotics 1st*

Rx:

Prevent meningococcal in epidemic or in endemic areas by:

- Decreasing intimate contact
- Immunizing w quadrivalent conjugated vaccine (Menactra) (Med Let 2005;47:29) or unconjugated (Menomune) (Med Let 2000;42:69) if conjugated unavailable, 0.5 cc sc × 1; vs serogroups A, C, Y, and W-135; 85% effective in epidemic but under age 3 immunogenicity is less (Jama 2001;285:177, 1998;279:435); used in epidemics, routinely in army, and in dorm-living college students especially dorm-living freshmen (Jama 2001;286:688); $82/dose
- Administering prophylactic antibiotics (Nejm 1982;307:1266) to family, day care companions, and close friends, not school or hospital personnel unless 2 cases occur in a school (Jama 1997;277:389): 1st, ciprofloxacin 500 mg po × 1; 2nd, rifampin 600 mg po qid × 2 d; or ceftriaxone

of acute unknown adult meningitis (Med Let 1999;41:96):

- Cefotaxime or ceftriaxone pending cultures, w vancomycin up to 4 gm qd to cover resistant pneumococcus. With sensitivities, can truncate to penicillin 24 million U iv qd in q 2 hr bolus × 1 d then q 4 hr for meningococcal type and covers 64% of pneumococcus as well (Nejm 1997;337:970) or can add vancomycin to cover resistant pneumo until cultures back; doesn't eliminate carrier state; same choices in head trauma since most likely organism is pneumococcus; rarely chloramphenicol if penicillin allergic, but alarming appearance of chloramphenicol-resistant meningococcus appearing (Nejm 1998;339:868) in developing countries
- Dexamethasone 10 mg q 6 hr × 4 d improves outcomes (Nejm 2002;347:1549) in all types of bacterial meningitis (ACP J Club 2003;138:60)

of other gram-neg types (Ann IM 1990;112:610):

Cefotaxime, ceftizoxime, or ceftriaxone for non-pseudomonas types but not listeria (requires 3 wk penicillin). Ceftazidime and gentamicin for pseudomonas. Ampicillin + chloramphenicol or ceftriaxone or cefotaxime for H. flu, and drop the 2nd drug if organism turns out to be ampicillin sensitive.

Pediatric Meningitis

Ann IM 1990;112:610

Cause (Nejm 1997;337:970):

Age < 1 mo: 1st group B strep; 2nd Listeria; 3rd pneumococcus; 4th vaginal flora, listeria, and S. *epidermidis*

Age 2-24 mo: 1st pneumococcus, 2nd meningococcus, 3rd group B strep, 4th H. flu

Age 2-18: 1st meningococcus, 2nd pneumococcus, 3rd H. flu

Epidem: Overall incidence much reduced now since H. flu vaccines (Nejm 1997;337:970)

Increased incidence in premies

Pathophys: Age 6-24 mo: Cranial bruits due to increased intracranial pressure

Sx: Age < 6 mo: Poor appetite, seizures (30%)

Age 6-24 mo: Seizures (30%), petechial rash especially with H. flu and N. *meningitidis*

Si: Age < 6 mo: No stiff neck, no fontanelle bulge

Age 6-24 mo: Bulging fontanelle, stiff neck, cranial bruits (20% false neg and pos: Nejm 1968;278:1420)

Crs (Nejm 1997;337:970): Age < 6 mo has worse mortality than age 6-24 mo

Cmplc (Nejm 1997;337:970): Age < 6 mo has significantly worse morbidity than age 6-24 mo

In both, morbidities include cranial nerve palsies especially of VI, VII, and VIII; sensorineural hearing loss 6% w H. *flu*, 32% w pneumococcus, 10% w N. *meningitidis* (Nejm 1984;311:869); detect w evoked potentials (Peds 1984;73:579); subdural empyemas and effusions, hydrocephalus, retardation, seizures. *H. flu* morbidity > 6 yr later = 20% (Peds 1984;74:198).

Lab: CSF protein increased, glucose decreased, wbc > 10/mm³; Gram stain

Rx: Preventive: Age 6 mo-6 yr: Rifampin to intimate contacts of *H. flu* pt as well as meningococcal cases and to pt on hosp discharge to clear nose (Mmwr 12/24/84)

   Therapeutic (Med Let 1999;41:96): See individual organism pages

Age < 6 mo (Med Let 1999;41:96): Ampicillin and ceftriaxone, or cefotaxime plus gentamicin

Age 6 mo-6 yr (Med Let 1999;41:96): Ceftriaxone 100 mg/kg iv qd, or cefotaxime w vancomycin to cover resistant pneumococcus pending cultures

In both: Dexamethasone 0.15 mg/kg iv 20 min before antibiotic, then q 6 hr × 4; decreases cmplc especially deafness in *H. flu* types (Nejm 1990;319:968)—and perhaps other bacterial types as well (Lancet 1993;342:457; Nejm 1991;324:1525) esp pneumococcal (Jama 1997;278:925)

Bite Wound Infections

Nejm 2004;350:904, 1999;340:85,138

Cause: Anaerobes, *Pasteurella multocida* and *canis*, *viridans* strep, staph, *Moraxella*, and *Neisseria*

Epidem: *P. multocida* is the organism in > 50% animal bite wound infections, especially from cats; can also induce infections in scratches

Pathophys:

Sx:

Si: Cellulitis

Crs: 70% develop within 1 d, 90% in 2 d, 100% in 3 d

Cmplc:

Lab:

Rx: dT shot if indicated
        Prophylactic antibiotics reasonable if deep punctures (esp
    from cats), hand wounds, or surgical repair needed, w:
        1st: Augmentin (amoxicillin and clavulinic acid) po, or Unasyn
        (amp + sulbactam) iv; or
        2nd: For human bites: Penicillin + cephalosporine
        For animal bites: Moxifloxacin + clindamycin

Tularemia (Rabbit Fever)

Nejm 2001;345:1637, 1993;329:940; Vt. epidemic:
    Nejm 1969;280:1253

Cause: *Francisella (Pasteurella) tularensis*

Epidem: From infected rodents and lagomorphs, by eating or handling,
    or by being bitten by arthropod (tick) vector (50% of transmis-
    sions occur in this way). Worldwide wherever large rabbit/rodent
    populations, eg, muskrats in Vermont; endemic in Martha's
    Vineyard, Mass., rabbits (Nejm 2001;345:1601, 1979;301:827).

Pathophys: Endotoxin production and rapid multiplication, transient
    bacteremias lead to all parenchymous organ involvement

Sx: 5 d incubation
        Fever (97%), malaise (60%), headache (23%), nausea and
    vomiting (8%), pleuritic chest pain (5%)

Si: Ulcerated papule (94%) at site of entry, very infective; re-
    gional lymphadenopathy (70%); fever and septicemia

Crs: 2 wk duration on average; 15% relapse later

Cmplc: Tularemic pneumonia, probably need to inhale to get

Lab: *Bact:* Gram-negative bacilli; culture of blood, sputum, or local
    ulcer on special medium
    Serol: Available from health departments, agglutinin titers

Rx: 1st choice, streptomycin 15 mg/kg im bid × 14 d, or gentamicin; 2nd choice, tetracycline or chloramphenicol

Bubonic Plague (Black Death)

Cause: *Yersinia (Pasteurella) pestis*

Epidem:
- Rats, which eventually die of it, via flea vector; or
- Skin-to-skin contact; or
- Inhalation of respiratory droplets from infected person; or
- Ingestion of respiratory tract excretions
     Endemic in western U.S. rodents; found in farm animals too

Pathophys: Endotoxin production (Ann IM 1973;79:642), causes DPN inhibition so cell respiration blocked

Sx: 5-7 d incubation

Si: Bubo (large node); fever and septicemia; heart block and other conduction abnormalities

Crs: 90% die over 6 d

Cmplc: Pneumonia due to infected thromboemboli or direct infection from others (die in 3 d)

Lab: *Bact:* Gram stain shows gram-neg cocci; culture difficult from blood, nodes; phage diagnosis is specific
Serol: Fluorescent antibody

Rx (Med Let 1999;41:15):
Preventive: Vaccinate (not available to civilians)
of acute disease: 1st choice, streptomycin im bid or gentamicin im tid, × 10 d; also tetracycline, chloramphenicol; multidrug resistance reported in Madagascar (Nejm 1997; 337:677)

Yersinia Gastroenteritis

Nejm 1989;321:16

Cause: *Yersinia* (a pasteurella) *enterocolitica*

Epidem: Fecal/oral; associated with poor sanitation; can live and reproduce at 4°C, hence can occur in winter. Animal reservoirs, especially pigs (Nejm 1990;322:984). Contaminated chocolate milk in NY school epidemic (Nejm 1978;298:76); meat and milk products, fecally contaminated water. Person-to-person transmission rare, but can occur especially w blood transfusions.

Pathophys: Bowel wall invasion

Sx: Headache, sore throat, fever (FUO occasionally), abdominal pain, chronic and recurrent diarrhea

Si: Exudative pharyngitis especially in adults (Ann IM 1983;99:40), fever, erythema nodosum, polyarthritis (Bull Rheum Dis 1979;29:100)

Crs: 2+ wk, even with antibiotic rx

Cmplc: Misdiagnosed as appendicitis and as regional enteritis (Nejm 1990;323:113). Massive gi bleed or perforation; thyrotoxicosis (Ann IM 1976;85:735); bacteremia, especially if iron overloaded, which fuels growth—50% fatal; postinfectious arthropathy (HLA B27–associated)
    r/o other, more common forms of gastroenteritis (NV+D) like viral, esp from "small round-structured viruses" (Jama 1997;278:563)

Lab: *Bact:* Gram-neg rod, an enterobacteriaceae; grows best at 25°C in 24-48 hr; facultative anaerobe
    Serol: Passive hemagglutinin titer > 1/512 diagnostic but 30% false negatives

Rx: Questionable that rx helps uncomplicated cases
    In patients with focal, extraintestinal infections or bacteremia: 1st gentamicin + doxycycline pending sensitivities; maybe fluoroquinolones, maybe chloramphenicol or tetracyclines alone

Pseudomonas Infections

Ann IM 1975;82:819

Cause: *Pseudomonas aeruginosa* (rv of rare species: Ann IM 1972;77:211)

Epidem: From respiratory or gi tract droplets; normal skin flora
   Very old, very young, and immunocompromised pts most frequently infected. Occasional hospital epidemics from anesthesia bags, hot and cold nebulizers (Nejm 1970;282:531). Hot-tub folliculitis epidemics (Arch IM 1985;135:1621).

Pathophys: Exotoxin A production causing some of pathogenesis; antibody to it offers some protection (Nejm 1980;302:1360)

Sx: Pneumonias, septicemia, skin and wound infections

Si: Cutaneous ecthyma gangrenosum (in a very small %) w black necrotic center, indurated, in groin or axilla; r/o mucor and aspergillosis

Crs:

Cmplc: r/o "pseudobacteremia" with *Burkholderia (Pseudomonas) cepacia,* which grows in povidone/iodine prep solution (Nejm 1981;305:621) or in albuterol neb bottles (Ann IM 1995;122:762)
   r/o **Meliodosis,** tropical *Burkholderia (Pseudomonas) mallei* causes subcutaneous "farcy" infections; recrudesces up to 10 yr later, and as "glanders" it cavitates in liver, spleen, and lung hence looks like tbc; skin abscesses. In lab personnel too (Nejm 2001;345:256, 1981;305:1133).

Lab: *Bact:* Gram-neg rod

Rx: Preventive: Avoid hot/cold nebulizers; there is no effective decontamination
   of acute disease: Tobramycin (or gentamicin) + piperacillin (or mezlocillin, ticarcillin, or azlocillin); or ceftazidime + ciprofloxacin if penicillin allergic

of *P. pseudomallei:* Tetracycline or chloramphenicol × 1-6 mo at
  high doses

Typhoid (Enteric) Fever

Nejm 2002;347:1770

Cause: *Salmonella typhae*

Epidem: Fecal/oral, from carriers (2-3% of recovered population),
  probably resides in gallbladder

  Increased incidence in U.S. foreign travelers, cirrhotics, pts
  with tumors especially of CNS, hemolytic anemias especially
  sickle cell anemia, aortic aneurysms especially thoracic

Pathophys: Endotoxin production; intracellular organisms; ingestion
  results in gi lymph nodes picking up and the nodes' subsequent
  necrosis over 2 wk leading to septicemia and further node
  involvement plus ulceration

Sx: 7-14 (3-60 min/max) d incubation period

  T° > 38.5°C (100°F); constipation, more rarely diarrhea;
  malaise, headache

Si: Fever (100%), bradycardia P < 100 (80%), spleen (75%),
  hepatomegaly (30%), macular rash (rose spots) over lower
  chest (5%)

Crs: Fever gradually up, then gradually down over 7+ days even
  with rx

Cmplc: Mortality even with rx especially if septicemia; relapse (10%);
  metastatic infections to lung, brain, joints, aorta (10%); gi hemorrhage (7%); perforation (3%); pneumonia and/or multiple pulmonary emboli

Lab: *Bact:* Blood culture (15 cc), 50-80% positive in 1st 2 wk; marrow
  (26%) positive even when blood negative. Stool culture
  goes positive in 80% after 1 wk. Gram stain shows gram-neg
  rods. Stool mucus methylene blue stain shows wbc's, mostly

mononuclear unlike polys of salmonellosis, shigellosis, and ulcerative colitis (Ann IM 1972;76:697).

Serol: Widal's test positive after 2 wk, an antibody vs O, H, and Vi antigens

Rx:

Preventive:

Keep carriers away from food, water; chlorinate water; cholecystectomy, or ampicillin 6 gm qd with 2 gm probenecid (Med Let 1968;10:51), or ciprofloxacin (Nejm 1991;324:392) for carriers

Immunize (Med Let 1994;36:41) w:

- Live attenuated Ty21a vaccine (Vivotif) po qod × 4 beginning at least 2 wk before departure, good for 5 yr; or
- Capsular polysaccharide conjugated vaccine (Vi-rEPA) im × 2, 6 wk apart, ~95% effective even in children age 2-5 (Nejm 2001;344:1263, 1322)

of active disease:

- Ciprofloxacin, no resistance yet (Jama 2000;283:2668); or
- 3rd-generation cephalosporins like ceftriaxone, no resistance yet (Jama 2000;283:2668); or
- Chloramphenicol 4 gm qd × 4 wk; 15 gm/d when acute; or 15 gm qd × 14 d (Nejm 1968;278:171), some resistance (Nejm 1973;289:463)
- Ampicillin as good as chloramphenicol although some resistance (Nejm 1969;280:147)
- Tm/S (Nejm 1980;303:426)

of delirium leading to coma and/or shock, dexamethasone 3 mg/kg × 1, then 1 mg/kg q 6 hr × 48 hr, decreases mortality from 55% to 10% (Nejm 1984;310:82)

Salmonellosis, Paratyphoid

Cause: *Salmonella paratyphi* and other nontyphoid species

Epidem: Fecal/oral from carriers, $^1/_3$ carry for 1 yr after infection, some forever; pet reptiles, 90% carry (ME Epigram 3/99); birds, especially poultry from gi tracts and including chicken eggs, eg, ice cream epidemic when pre-mix was transported in tank truck that had just carried eggs (Nejm 1996;334:1281); cider (Mmwr 1997;46:4); orange juice (Jama 1998;280:1504); beef/hamburger, (Nejm 1987;316:565), especially in pts on antibiotics; carmine dye (ground-up insects) in food; marijuana (Nejm 1982;306: 1249); sprouts (Ann IM 2001;135:239)

Increased incidence in cancer patients (Nejm 1967;276: 1045), 1/400 leukemics, lymphomas, and colon cancer patients; 1/2000 patients with other cancers; 1/9000 patients without cancer

2nd most common food poisoning after staph and before clostridial

Pathophys: Endotoxin production by intracellular organisms in small and large bowels

Sx: Nausea, vomiting, diarrhea

Si: Diarrhea, may be as watery as in cholera

Crs: 12-72 hr incubation, unlike staph; several days duration; recover spontaneously after 1 wk

Cmplc: Septic arteritis and aneurysms (Nejm 1969;281:310)
r/o staph (less diarrhea) and clostridial food poisoning

Lab: *Bact:* Gram-neg rods on stool culture. Stool smear with methylene blue shows polys unlike typhoid fever but like other colitis, eg, ulcerative, shigella, *E. coli*, etc (Ann IM 1972;76:697).

Hem: White counts in normal range, no correlation with severity

Rx: Antibiotics contraindicated (ACP J Club 1999;130:15) because if rx, then carry in stool longer (27% vs 11% at 31 d), and in vivo resistance develops in 10% (Nejm 1969;281:636); but ciprofloxacin or Tm/S is used if fecal leukocytes, fever, and other

measures of severity are bad (Arch IM 1990;150:546); ciprofloxacin does help, but prolongs convalescent excretion (Ann IM
1991;114:195), and quinolone resistance now appearing, probably
due to use in animal feeds (Nejm 2002;346:413, 1999;341:1420)

Opiates could theoretically worsen due to decreased motility

Serratia Infections

Nejm 1979;300:887

Cause: *Serratia marcescens* (family enterobacteriaceae, tribe klebsiella)

Epidem: Frequent skin inhabitant; opportunistic infections, eg, iv
catheters (Nejm 1968;279:386) and ultrasonic nebulizers (Ann
IM 1970;73:15) in pts with compromised immune systems
including drug users (Ann IM 1976;84:29)

Pathophys:

Sx:

Si: Guaiac-negative red sputum; septicemia, meningitis, UTI, pneumonia, endocarditis (Ann IM 1976;84:29)

Crs: With septicemia, 36% mortality

Cmplc:

Lab: *Bact:* Gram-neg rods; culture and test for local sensitivities

Rx: Prevent w nebulizer wash with acetic acid, perhaps effective
(Nejm 1970;282:528,531)

of acute disease: Gentamicin best, or ceftazidime or
imipenem; in serious infections use in combinations; resistant to
tetracycline (100%), cephalothin (100%), ampicillin (91%),
streptomycin (86%), chloramphenicol (42%); but multidrug
resistance developing

Shigellosis

Cause: *Shigella spp.* (*dysenteriae, flexneri, boydii, sonnei*)

Epidem: Fecal/oral especially via water supplies, die fast with drying;
or person to person. Increased incidence in Asia (*dysenteriae*),

also most malignant; *sonnei* most benign. Infective dose low (~100 organisms) when compared w other bacterial diarrheas.

Pathophys: Shiga endotoxins, noninvasive so no bacteremias; superficial mucosal ulcerations, can produce DIC, hemolytic anemia, renal microangiopathy (Nejm 1978;298:926)

Sx: Nausea, vomiting, and severe diarrhea with cramps (75%); fever (75%); 50% of cases have both

Si: Bloody stool, watery like cholera

Crs: Incubation period = 8+ hr, average 2-4 d; duration ~1 wk

Cmplc: Incapacitating with low mortality, except *dysenteriae* often fatal

Reiter's syndrome precipitation; perhaps causes ulcerative colitis?

Lab: *Bact:* Gram-neg rods; stool culture. Stool smear shows polys (Ann IM 1972;76:697).

Rx: Symptomatic: Oral or iv lyte/fluid replacement, opiates to slow diarrhea, although theoretically could worsen by decreasing motility

Antibiotics: Ciprofloxacin (Ann IM 1992;117:727) 500 mg po bid × 5 d for *S. dysenteriae*, 1 gm po × 1 ok for other species; or azithromycin 500 mg po on day 1, 250 mg qd on days 2-5 (Ann IM 1997;126:697); or Tm/S (Nejm 1980;303:426); ampicillin 500 mg qid, questionably effective

Cholera

Nejm 1985;312:343; Ann IM 1981;94:656

Cause: *Vibrio cholerae* or new non O-1 strains

Epidem: Sewage in drinking water. Carriers (in gallbladder) = 3-5% of world population (Ann IM 1970;72:357); primarily in Asia, S. America, and N. Africa; increasing number of cases/yr in U.S. (Jama 2000;284:1541). Many asx cases.

Pathophys: Na pump inhibition by entero/exotoxin; glucose important to that pump (Nejm 1985;312:28)

Sx: Diarrhea; sometimes fever

Si: "Rice water" diarrhea up to 15 L/d; "dishwater hands" from volume depletion

Crs: Benign if replace H_2O and salt iv or via NG tube

Cmplc: Mortality significant in symptomatic disease without rx; increased anion gap acidosis (Nejm 1986;315:1591)

Lab: *Bact:* Gram-neg rods, flagellated; culture carriers post-Mg^{++} purge (30% false neg: Ann IM 1970;72:357)
Chem: Stool cyclic AMP increased

Rx (Mmwr 1991;40:562; Med Let 1991;33:107):
  Vaccination w live attenuated oral vaccine (vBS-WC), 78% effective (Nejm 2005;352:757; Lancet 1990;335:958)
of acute disease:

* Oral rehydration solutions (p 1010); catch up, then stool output + 100 cc q 1 hr (Ann IM 1975;82:101) or iv Ringer's lactate
* Antibiotics: Doxycycline 300 mg po × 1 or 100 mg po bid × 3 d; or in children, Tm/S 5 mg/25 mg/kg po bid × 3 d; or ciprofloxacin

Vibrio Diarrhea and Wound Infections

Ann IM 1988;109:261,318, 1983;99:464; Nejm 1985;312:343

Cause: *Vibrio vulnificus* and *parahaemolyticus*

Epidem: Southern seawater exposure. Various species live in sea— hence gi disease from raw oyster ingestion (Mmwr 1996;45:621), shell cut wound infections, swimming (Ann IM 1983;99:169).

Pathophys:

Sx: Nausea, vomiting, diarrhea with cramps within 4 d of consumption; bloody diarrhea in < 50%; fever, headache; ear pain; wound pain

Si: Otitis media, cellulitis, gangrene

Crs: 2-4 d (Nejm 1985;312:343)

Cmplc: Septicemia, often fatal, especially in compromised host (Nejm 1979;300:1) like alcoholics in whom can cross gut barriers

Lab: *Bact:* Culture with special medium (TCBS) broth

Rx: Preventive: Avoid raw oyster eating by the immunocompromised

Tetracyclines (Med Let 1991;33:107)

9.4   Anaerobes

Actinomycetes Infections

Cause: *Actinomyces spp.*

Epidem:

Pathophys: "Lumpy jaw disease" in cattle

Sx: Submaxillary gland swelling; occasionally IUD-associated PID (Jama 1982;247:1149); gastroenteritis

Si:

Crs:

Cmplc: Abscesses

Lab: *Bact:* Anaerobe; gram-positive branching forms
Path: "Sulfur" granules in affected tissues (Nejm 1970;282:593)

Rx: Penicillin po, or tetracycline, or streptomycin, or clindamycin (Ann IM 1973;79:853)

Botulism

Ann IM 1998;129:221

Cause: *Clostridium botulinum* (types A, B, E are the most common human pathogens)

Epidem: Heat-resistant spores contaminate:
- Canned foods or opened cans kept for days unrefrigerated (Ann IM 1996;125:558), leading to bacterial proliferation of exotoxin, which then is ingested without further heating—eg, homemade salsa, relish, canned vegetables or meats, garlic in oil
- Wounds characterized by bacterial proliferation and exotoxin production (80% type A, 20% type B)

  Spores common in dirt and dust

Pathophys: Exotoxin is heat-labile, extremely toxic (< 1 lb could kill the world); inhibits transmitter release at all cholinergic endings

In infants and occasionally in adults (Nejm 1986;315:239) with impaired gastric acid, can generate toxin in human gi tract

Sx: Incubation period of 12 hr to several days; mild gi sx; descending paralysis of motor and autonomic nerves starting w cranial nerves: double vision, dysphagia, dysarthria; upper respiratory tract paralysis with trouble breathing and swallowing

Si: "Myasthenia gravis that doesn't respond to edrophonium (Tensilon)," although some pts may respond a little (Ann IM 1981;95:443); flaccid paralysis

Crs: Pts can survive and recover with respirator and other supportive care for weeks to months

Cmplc: r/o myasthenia, Guillain-Barré, diphtheria, CVA, Eaton-Lambert syndrome; intoxication w organophosphates, CO, paralytic shellfish toxins

Lab: *Bact:* Smear of food shows gram-pos bacilli; food and/or stool culture grows obligate anaerobe; extract kills mice

CSF: Normal

Noninv: EMG shows low-amplitude response to nerve stimulation increased by 50/sec repetitive stimulation (Nejm 1970; 282:193); 15-40% false neg

Rx: Preventively heat all canned food prior to serving; immunization impractical on widespread scale of disease: Passive immunization with polyvalent horse anti-toxin helps before severe sx set in, available from CDC; type-specific if possible. Debride wounds. Gastric lavage if food recently ingested. Supportive care, eg, respirator, etc for weeks to months usually successful; guanidine not helpful (Nejm 1971; 285:773).

Pseudomembranous Colitis

Nejm 2002;346:334, 1994;330:257

Cause: *Clostridium difficile*

Epidem: Associated with antibiotic rx, usually broad-spectrum types and especially clindamycin (Nejm 1999;341:1645), and/or cancer chemoRx. Also the cause of 20% of all antibiotic-associated diarrhea without pseudomembranous colitis.

Pathophys: Proliferates when there is suppression of normal bowel flora by various broad-spectrum antibiotics; cytotoxic toxin production. IgG antibody to the toxin develops variably and is protective (Nejm 2000;342:390).

Sx: H/o antibiotic use, esp cephalosporin or clindamycin > 6 d before loose but not watery diarrhea onset; occasionally fever, abdominal pain

Si: Raised plaques (pseudopolyps) on sigmoidoscopy or colonoscopy, "swollen rice grains," bleed when scraped; rectum may be spared often

Crs:

Cmplc: 15-20% relapse rate w rx

Lab: *Bact:* Fecal leukocytes by methylene blue stain or Gram stain of stool

Chem: Toxin assayable in stool by various methods; by tissue culture assay, 94-100% sens, 99% specif; by latex agglutination assay (poorest test but most often used), 50% sens, 99% specif; by enzyme-linked methods, 75% sens, 99% specif; order if positive fecal leukocytes stain

Hem: Increased polys

Rx (Med Let 1989;31:94):

Prevent by restricting clindamycin use (Ann IM 1994; 120:272)

of colitis: Stop antibiotics and give metronidazole (Flagyl) 250 mg po qid × 10-14 d, perhaps iv if ileus. More expensive: vancomycin 125 mg po qid × 10-14 d, increase to 500 mg qid in resistant cases but do not give iv since is not secreted into bowel where the organism is. New quinolone resistant strains recur frequently and require rifampin 300 mg po bid as well.

Gas Gangrene

Nejm 1973;289:1129

Cause: *Clostridium perfringens* (*C. welchii*), or *C. novyi*; via wound contamination with dirt

Epidem (Nejm 1972;286:1026): In most soils; 8% of people carry in stool. Frequent agent in septic abortions.

Pathophys: Exotoxin produced in tissues leading to cell necrosis via lecithinase, which splits cell walls, collagenase, and other enzymatic activity. CO_2 produced in wounds. Obligate anaerobes; need to live in dead tissue.

Sx: Severe pain

Si: Fever, severe toxemia, necrotic skin; sweet smell

Crs: Rapid spread leading to death in hours or days

Cmplc: Shock, rapid hemolysis

r/o more benign anaerobic crepitant cellulitis (Ann IM 1975;83:375) in diabetics when *E. coli* or *Klebsiella* anaerobically metabolizes glucose; other anaerobes (p 578)

Lab: *Bact:* Smear shows large gram-pos sporulating bacilli, which in culture produce lecithinase and CO_2
Chem: Elevated bilirubin (hemolysis)

Xray: Gangrene: Tissue gas throughout muscle after 18 hr; unlikely to be gas gangrene if occurs earlier and/or without edema and inflammation (Nejm 1968;278:758)

Rx: Gangrene: Hyperbaric O_2 inactivates the toxin; antitoxin 75,000 U iv q 6 hr may stop the hemolysis? Antibiotics: high-dose penicillin + gentamicin. Urgent surgery to excise dead tissue.

Clostridial Food Poisoning

Nejm 1973;289:1129

Cause: *Clostridium perfringens,* via food (food poisoning) contamination with dirt

Epidem (Nejm 1972;286:1026): In most soils; 8% of people carry in stool. 3rd most common type of food poisoning after staph and salmonella.

Pathophys: Exotoxin produced in food before or rarely after ingestion, causing watery diarrhea via Na pump effects. Obligate anaerobes; need to live in dead tissue.

Sx: 12 hr incubation period, then diarrhea without vomiting; no fever

Si:

Crs: Mild, only 1% call doctor; lasts 12 hr

Cmplc: r/o other diarrheal illnesses (p 401–409)

Lab: *Bact:* Smear shows large gram-pos sporulating bacilli, which in culture produce lecithinase and CO_2

Xray:

Rx: Fluid replacement oral or iv

Tetanus, Lockjaw

Nejm 1973;289:1293, 1969;280:569

Cause: *Clostridium tetani,* via wound contamination with dirt

Epidem: Present in most soils; 535 cases in 1965 in U.S.; ~4 cases/100 million, mainly in southern states; Texas had 56% of cases; highest incidence in very young and very old (inadequate immunization); < 3% of pts have hx of ever having had tetanus toxoid;

increased incidence in "skin-popping" drug addicts. Females >
males.

Pathophys: Exotoxin production that is transported both via circulation to CNS (probably most significant in humans) and along motor nerves to CNS (but can't correlate wound distance from CNS with morbidity and mortality in humans)

Sx: Puncture wound or laceration (58%), or postpartum, post-surgery, skin ulcers

1-54 d incubation period, median = 8 d, 88% within 14 d; short incubation period in pts < age 50 is poor prognostic sign

Si: Spastic paralysis; tonic convulsive contractions precipitated by intrinsic or extrinsic muscle movement; no or rarely fever

Crs: 60% mortality

Cmplc: r/o **"Stiff Man Syndrome,"** autoimmune antibodies against GABA neurons (Ann IM 1999;131:522; Nejm 1990;322:1555) that induce muscle spasms over years, seen with hypopituitarism, IDDM, Graves disease, and other endocrinopathies (Nejm 1988; 318:1012,1060, 1984;310:1511), occasionally is an autoimmune paraneoplastic syndrome in breast cancer (Nejm 1993;328:546); rx w iv immunoglobulin (Nejm 2001;345:1870) and diazepam

r/o malignant neuroleptic syndrome (p 17)

Lab: *Bact:* Smears show gram-pos bacilli; culture shows fastidious anaerobe, pos in 32% of proven cases

Rx: Prevent w toxoid vaccine (CDC rv: Ann IM 1985;103:896) im, primary series of 3 over 1 yr, then q 10 yr, more frequently increases risk of reaction without increasing protection (Nejm 1969;280:575); some argue that routine dT booster is unnecessary in adults (Lancet 5/11/85, p1089); booster of dT is enough even for dirty wounds if last dT was less than 5 yr ago (Nejm 1983; 309:636)

Tetanus human immune globulin 250 U im, for dirty wounds with vaccine if not sure has had primary series; give coincident with vaccine in different im area

of disease: Metronidazole 500 mg iv q 6 hr (Nejm 1995;332:812); human immune globulin; respirator (Ann IM 1978;88:66)

Anaerobic Infections (Except Clostridial)

Cause: *Bacteroides fragilis* and other species; anaerobic streptococcus; microaerophilic streptococcus

Epidem:

Pathophys: Abscess formation very often; almost always 2 or more organisms; perivascular localization causes thrombophlebitis

Sx: Brain abscess; extrasubdural empyema; peridontal abscess; lung abscess; appendiceal/diverticular abscesses; hepatic abscess (Lancet 1/16/82, p134); PID/septic abortion; sinus abscess

Si: Putrid pus (fatty acids); palpable gas in tissues, but r/o gas gangrene, or *E. coli* gas formers in diabetic

Crs: Indolent, may be relatively asymptomatic for months

Cmplc: Thrombophlebitis often
r/o clostridial gas gangrene, which has incubation < 3 d, marked toxemia, severe pain, lots of swelling, necrotic blistered skin, minimal gas, sweet smell, gas extension and infection into muscle, which is all in contrast to anaerobic infections

Lab: *Bact:* Culture anaerobically

Rx: Anticoagulate with low threshold because of DVT predisposition
Antibiotics (Med Let 1999;41:95):

- Clindamycin; with gentamicin if may have aerobes; ampicillin alone ok in PID if not too toxic; better than penicillin in pulmonary abscess (Ann IM 1983;98:466; maybe not: Ann IM 1983;98:546); often used with penicillin for brain abscess

- Metronidazole (Flagyl) po or iv (Med Let 1981;23:13); cidal vs all anaerobes except microaerophilic gram-positives; diffuses well into abscess spaces
- Amoxicillin + clavulanci acid (Augmentin)/ampicillin + sulbactam (Unasyn)/piperacillin + tazobactam (Zosyn)
- Penicillin G, or ampicillin, ~10 million U qd; for brain abscess, perhaps with chloramphenicol
- Chloramphenicol; can be used alone for brain abscesses or w penicillin
- Cefoxitin or cefotetan; are 90% effective vs bacteroides
- Imipenem + cilastatin (Primaxin)

9.5   Acid-Fast Organisms

Tuberculosis

Am Rv Respir Crit Care Med 2000;161:S221, 1994;149:1359; Ann IM 1993;119:400

Cause: *Mycobacterium tuberculosis* and *bovis*

Epidem: Inhalation of respiratory droplets, of infected persons; but once on drugs probably little infectivity despite positive smears (Nejm 1974;290:459). Reinfection may be as important as reactivation, at least in homeless. Epidemic description at Bath Iron Works (Ann IM 1996;125:114).

   Incidence = 25,000 new U.S. cases/yr; these rates are increased in the 1990s from HIV patients, prisons, homeless populations (Nejm 1992;326:703) and the foreign born (Jama 1997;278:304). ³/₄ cases involve pts with previous positive PPD. 25 million positive PPDs in U.S., only 5-10% ever result in active disease whereas HIV pos pts who contract tbc become active cases at a rate of 5-10%/yr. In elderly and foreign born, 90% of cases are reactivation, whereas only 60% are in younger pts and the homeless (Jama 1996;275:305), and ¹/₃ are recent infections

(Nejm 1994;330:1692,1703,1750); 3/4 are now due to exogenous reinfection (Nejm 1999;341:1174).

Incidence is higher (Mmwr 5/18/90) in diabetics, institutionalized, household contacts, HIV-infected (Nejm 1992;326:231, 1991;324:289,1644), alcoholics, gastrectomy, silicosis, immunosuppressed including pts on TNF agents (Nejm 2001;345:1098), postpartum (Ann IM 1971;74:764) pts, blacks (Nejm 1990;322:422), and w highly virulent strains (Nejm 1998; 338:633)

M. *bovis* now very rare due to pasteurization of milk

Worldwide: 33% prevalence and tbc causes 6% of all deaths (Jama 1995;273:220; Mmwr 1993;42:961)

Pathophys (Nejm 1967;277:1008): Primary infection by inhalation into lower lungs, leading to local node involvement and asx bacteremia, causing gradual hypersensitization via lymphocytic response and eventual calcification and scar = sterile Ghon complex

Secondary disease is a reactivation and hypersensitivity reaction to bacteria spread by asx bacteremia to lung apices and upper kidneys, where high O_2 concentrations prevent Ghon complex-type sterilization

Sx: Fever, weight loss, night sweats, cough, sputum production, hemoptysis

Si: Same as sx

Crs: Mortality = 6%/yr, 12% at 2 yr, but 50% at 2 yr for HIV-positive pts and 80% for AIDS pts (Jama 1996;276:1223)

Cmplc: Apical lung abscess; peritonitis (Nejm 1969;281:1091); meningitis; epididymitis; PID; endometritis; splenic and hepatic abscesses; nontender, scarring skin sores/abscesses; arthritis (especially M. *bovis*); pericarditis (Nejm 1964;270:327); osteomyelitis, especially of spine **(Pott's Disease)**; pleuritis (Am Rv Tbc 1955;71:616); laryngitis, very infectious (Ann IM 1974;80:708);

hypercalcemia (25%) from vitamin D sensitivity (Ann IM 1979; 90:324)

Antibiotic resistance, geographically variable, 25% of cases resistant to INH and/or rifampin (Nejm 1993;328:521, 527); multiple-drug resistance epidemics in AIDS patients (Nejm 1992;326:1514), esp in New York City (Jama 1996;276:1229)

Lab: *Bact:* Sputum or urine AFB smears; cultures of sputum, gastric aspirate, urine, peritoneal fluid (1 L spun down: Nejm 1969;281:1091). RIAs now possible in 3 wk.

Path: Liver bx is pos in high % of miliary, or peritoneum bx if ascites protein > 2.5 gm %

Serol: Interferon-$\gamma \geq$ 0.35 IU/CC (Jama 2005;293:2746,2756; 2001;286:1740) is more specif and sens than skin test even in BCG immunized

Skin tests: Intermediate strength (IPPD, 5 U), positive if $\geq$ 5 mm in HIV pts (Ann IM 1997;126:123) or pts w pulmonary scars or recent contacts, > 10 mm in others or perhaps even > 15 mm in pts w very low risk; repeat in 2-3 wk to get booster effect, $^1/_3$ more become positive in elderly (Nejm 1985;312: 1483) but of questionable significance in the young (Ann IM 1994;120:190). Ignore old BCG immunization in interpreting, esp if > 5-10 yr ago. False negs with overwhelming infection, sarcoid, or other anergy. Delayed reactivity (IPPD neg at 48 hr, pos at 6 d) in 25% of SE Asians (Ann IM 1996; 124:779).

Urine: Acid, sterile, wbc's and rbc's, protein

Xray: Chest shows apical scarring and/or Ghon complex
IVP characteristically shows beaded ureters

Rx (Am Rv Respir Crit Care Med 2000;161:S221):
Prevent w:

- Hospital preventive policies (Nejm 1995;332:92), respiratory isolation in negative-pressure rooms (debatably: Ann IM 2000; 133:779) until 3 negative smears of HIV pts w abnormal chest xray, plus regular skin testing programs (Nejm 1995; 332:92; Ann IM 1995;122:658)

- BCG vaccination X1 to entire at-risk population, 50% effective over 60 yr (Jama 2004;291:2086, 1994;271:698)
- INH 300 mg po qd × 9 mo for PPD reactors (10-20% lifetime risk: Nejm 2004;350:2060) and household contacts; hepatitis risk is small: < 1/1000 at < age 35, 2/1000 for age 35-65, 3/1000 at > age 65: (Jama 1999;281:1014), <1/50,000 die (Ann IM 1997;127:1058); supplement w pyridoxine only if alcoholic and/or malnourished, not for asthmatics on steroids (Ann IM 1976;84:261); in pts on immusuppressives (infliximab et al) or HIV-pos pts w pos PPD or anergy, 300 mg po qd w B_6 (pyridoxine) 50 mg po qd forever (Lancet 1993;342:268) decreases incidence by $^2/_3$ at 2 yr (Nejm 1997;337:801)
- Rifampin 600 mg alone × 4 mo; or + pyrazinamide 20 mg/kg po qd × 2 mo for pos PPD in HIV pts as effective as 12 mo of INH (Jama 2000;283:1445) but hepatitis risk much higher (26% vs 15%: Ann IM 2002;137:640)
- Other options for latent tbc: Rifampin 600 mg qd × 4 mo; rifabutin alone if on some protease inhibitors; pyrizinamide + ethambutol

of active disease (Jama 2005;293:2776; Nejm 2001;345:189): Contact local health dept, use 4 drugs initially in all and continuing in AIDS (Nejm 1999;340:367); use tiw directly observed rx for all cases to prevent further drug resistance (Jama 1995;274: 945; Nejm 1994;330:1179) or biw rx after 2 wk of qd rx; prevalence of drug resistance increases from 10% to 36% if take meds for < 1 mo (Nejm 1998;338:1641)

1st line:
- INH 300 mg qd × 6 mo or b-tiw × 9 mo, with pyridoxine only if > 300 mg qd to prevent neuropathy; adverse effect: hepatitis
- Rifampin 600 mg qd or b-tiw × 9 mo, less toxic than streptomycin or INH or longer-acting form, rifapentine (Priftin) (Med Let 1999;41:21) biw × 2 mo then q wk thereafter;

adverse reactions: drug interactions, red body fluids, increased urate; $90/mo

- Pyrazinamide 0.5-40 mg/kg/d or b-tiw × 2 mo, with above allows 6-mo cure courses (Am Rv Respir Dis 1991;143:700,707). Rifamate (INH + rifampin) or "Rifater," a combination pill of all 3 (preferable: Ann IM 1995;122:951). Cure rates ∼ 98% (Am Rv Respir Dis 1982;126:460).
- Ethambutol 15 mg/kg pos qd, use as 4th drug until know sensitivities (Med Let 1995;37-67); adverse effects: retrobulbar neuritis, check visual acuity regularly, rarely reversible
- Streptomycin 250-1000 mg im qd or 20 mg/kg biw

2nd line:

- Capreomycin
- Ciprofloxacin
- Clofazimine
- Cycloserine
- Ethionamide
- Kanamycin/amikacin
- Levofloxacin
- Ofloxacin
- Aminosalicylic acid
- Rifabutin
- Rifapentine

of antibiotic-resistant tbc: 3 drugs to which organism tests as susceptible × 12-24 mo; frequent now in AIDS pts (Nejm 1993;328:1137, 1992;326:1514; Ann IM 1992;117:177,191), must use 4 drugs (Ann IM 1987;106:25)

of meningitis: dexamethasone 0.15-0.3 mg/kg × 8 wk (Nejm 2004;351:1741) for adults and children, HIV positive or negative

Atypical Tuberculosis

Cause: Atypical *Mycobacterium spp.* (MOTT: mycobacterium other than tuberculosis)

Epidem:

M. *scrofulaceum* and *kansasii* (MSK) (Ann IM 1998;129:698): Endemic in soil *(kansasii)*; little person-to-person spread. In Midwest especially.

M. *avium* and *intracellulare* (MAI): Major problem in AIDS, where it is 3rd most common opportunistic infection after pneumocystis and Kaposi's (Nejm 1996;335:428)

M. fortuitum and other fast growers (FG) (Ann IM 1970;73:971): Normal throat inhabitant?

Pathophys:

Sx: MSK: Pulmonary, scrofula, skin ulcers. Seen in AIDS pts (Ann IM 1991;114:861).

MAI: Pulmonary, especially in COPD, AIDS, and previously damaged lung but not always (Nejm 1989;321:863)

FG: Pulmonary; subcutaneous abscess; corneal infection

Si: Pulmonary

Crs: MAI: Quite virulent in HIV pts

FG: Spontaneous resolution w/o rx or w debridement

Cmplc: MSK: Full gamut like regular tbc; drug resistance common

FG: r/o M. *marinum*, which causes **Swimming Pool Granuloma** (Nejm 1997;336:1065)

Lab: *Bact:* All are nicotinic acid nonproducers in contrast to M. *bovis* and *tuberculosis*. All are acid fast; grow at 25°C; are avirulent to guinea pigs; chromogen characteristics: MSK shows photochromogen

MAI: No chromogen. FG: No chromogen and fast growth (2-7 d); r/o scotochromogen types, which are rarely clinically significant.

Skin tests: MSK and MAI are specific and cause 2nd-strength PPD to be positive

Rx:

for MSK: Rifampin, etc (Ann IM 1971;74:758)

for MAI (big problem in AIDS pts): Prophylaxis (Nejm 1996;335:428), routinely in all AIDS pts w CD_4 counts $<$ 100-200/cc (Nejm 1993;329:828) or perhaps only if $<$ 100, if no disseminated M. *avium* complex disease yet; can d/c prophylaxis when $CD_4 > 100$ again after HIV rx (Nejm 2000;342:1085)

• Rifabutin, similar to rifampin, retards dissemination in AIDS pts (Med Let 1993;35:36) 300 mg po qd prophylaxis; prevents 55% of expected cases, no resistance develops but can induce rifampin resistance (Nejm 1996;334:1573)

- Clarithromycin 500 mg po bid (Nejm 1996;335:384) prevents 69%, resistance develops in 45%
- Azithromycin 1200 mg po q wk (Nejm 1996;335:392) prevents 59% of expected cases; or used w rifabutin prevents 85%; resistance develops in 11%

of disease: Surgery, if possible, + 3-4 drugs (Nejm 1996;335:377, 1993;329:898; Ann IM 1994;121:905) like clarithromycin or azithromycin + ethambutol + clofazimine or rifabutin or rifampin or cipro or amikacin; interferon-γ may also help (Nejm 1994;330:1348)

Leprosy

Cause: *Mycobacterium leprae*

Epidem: Unknown mode of transmission, seems to require prolonged (> 1 mo) exposure, probably skin and nasal discharge. 3-5 yr incubation. Tuberculoid type is not infectious (Ann IM 1978;88:538).

15 million in world; especially children and young adults

Pathophys:
- Lepromatous type like sarcoid and Hodgkin's, involves impaired delayed hypersensitivity. Granuloma formation leads to nerve compression? IgG and IgA increased, while IgM normal (Ann IM 1969;70:295; Nejm 1968;278:298). T lymphs in lesions are all suppressor cells.
- Tuberculoid type, in patients with strong response; all T cells in lesions are helper cells (Nejm 1982;307:1593).

Both types infect colder tissues—hence hands, feet, ears, nose, peripheral nerves.

Sx: Years incubation period; eczematous rash; numbness (85%)

Si: Lepromatous to tuberculoid spectrum: Nodular accumulations in skin, mucous membranes, and other organs, especially on face; organisms are in these "globi"; to thickened peripheral nerves; to decreased sensation in extremities leading to mutilation and loss, pain and temperature sensation diminished

Absent wheal and flare response; vitiligo

Crs:

Cmplc: Arthritis, septic with bacteria in joint histiocytes (Nejm 1973;289:1410); secondary amyloid; **Erythema Nodosum Leprosum** w painful skin nodules, fever, wasting, rx'd w thalidomide (Med Let 1996;38:15)

Lab: *Bact:* AFB-positive smears of globi as well as blood and buffy coat since bacteria both free and in wbc's in lepromatous type, decrease in numbers correlates with rx over months, average rx duration = 105 mo (Nejm 1972;287:159); and of marrow histiocytes (Nejm 1979;300:834)

Path: Skin bx of globi and/or nerve bx show epithelioid cell collections without distinct tubercles; nerves surrounded by microscopic tubercles

Serol: VDRL, cryoglobulin, rheumatoid factor often pos in lepromatous, not tuberculoid types

Rx: Prevent w BCG immunization?, questionable results (Ann IM 1978;88:538); isolation unnecessary; DDS (Dapsone = diaminodiphenylsulfone) effective prophylaxis for household contacts (Ann IM 1978;88:539)

of disease: Triple rx w clofazimine (Med Let 1987;29:77) 50-100 mg po qd, + sulfones, eg, Dapsone + rifampin; or combinations of minocycline, clarithromycin, ciprofloxacin, and Augmentin. Cmplc of rx: Erythema nodosum leprosum, rx w thalidomide (Med Let 1998; 40:104)

May become noninfectious in weeks (Ann IM 1976;85:82) to 3 mo; 2+ yr course, longer with lepromatous type

9.6 Spirochetes

Lyme Disease

Ann IM 2002;136:421 (Rob Smith); Nejm 2001;345:115,
  1993;329:936, 1989;320:133

Cause: *Borrelia burgdorferi* spread by *Ixodes dammini* tick bite (same
  tick also spreads babesiosis and patients may get both: Ann IM
  1985;103:374)

Epidem: Deer tick, also infests white-footed deer mice. Northeastern
  and northwestern U.S. HLA DR$_4$ and DR$_w$2 B-cell allotypes associated with increased CNS, cardiac, and arthritic involvement
  (Nejm 1990;323:219). Most common tickborne spirochetal disease in U.S.; attack rates up to 66% of people living in a highly
  endemic area over 7 yr (Nejm 1989;320:133); annual incidence
  = 20-80/100,000/yr; also common in N. Europe (Nejm 1995;
  333:1319).

Pathophys: Sometimes an immune complex disease, but organisms
  now identified in joints most of the time (Nejm 1994;330:229).
  Clinical syndromes very much like primary, secondary, and tertiary syphilis; but much overlap between stage 1 and 2 sx
  complexes.

Sx   (Nejm 1991;325:159): Tick bite (should remove w tweezers)
  hx in 80% (Nejm 1995;333:1319); disease rare if tick on < 24 hr,
  usually takes 72 hr and most ticks associated w disease have
  stayed on 1 week (Nejm 1992;327:543)
  Stage 1: Arthralgias (98%), malaise (80%), headache (64%),
      fever (60%), stiff neck (aseptic meningitis); ringworm-like
      rash erythema chronicum marginatum (ECM) in 77%
      (Nejm 1995;333:1319)
  Stage 2: Neurologic and cardiac
  Stage 3: Arthritis; chronic neurologic changes

INFECTIOUS DISEASE

Si: Stage 1: Fever, lymphadenopathy; and erythema chronicum migrans, a warm "ringworm" around bite (ECM), median diam = 15 cm (pictures: Ann IM 1991;114:490, 1983; 99:76), present in 60-80%

Stage 2: Neurologic: lymphocytic meningitis (15%) and meningoencephalitis, peripheral motor or sensory neuropathies, facial nerve palsies including Bell's palsy. And/or cardiac: myocarditis (8%), like rheumatic fever with heart block but valve disease rare or never; sometimes heart block is only sx, no fever or even malaise; usually transient, ~6 wk after primary infection.

Stage 3: Recurrent polyarthritis at 1st, then 1-2 large joints; onset up to 4-6 mo after skin rash with decreasing recurrences over years (Ann IM 1987;107:725). Late keratitis (Nejm 1991; 325:159).

Crs: Stage 1 lasts 3-4 wk. Sx and si of stages 2 and 3 may be chronic and recurrent over months–years. Even after rx, especially if given > 3 mo after sx, residual arthralgias, fatigue, memory problems may persist (Ann IM 1994;121:560). Very benign crs in children (Nejm 1996;335;1270).

Cmplc: Chronic myocardiopathy (Nejm 1990;322:249). Neurologic (Nejm 1990;323:1438): chronic encephalopathy in 90% of those who have stage 2 neurologic sx; also chronic polyneuropathy and leukoencephalitis.

r/o ehrlichiosis (p 602), babesiosis (p 631) as separate or concomitant infection (Nejm 1997;337:27; Jama 1996;275:1657)

Lab: *Hem:* ESR > 20 mm/hr (53%), crit > 37% (88%), wbc < 10,000 (92%)

Path: Pos silver stain or culture of rash edge for organisms in 86% (Jama 1992;268:1311)

Serol (Jama 1999;282:62; Ann IM 1997;127:1109): Need reliable lab; IgM and IgG ELISA titer increased (Nejm 1983;308: 733) and pos Western blot; rare false pos, most in low-prevalence populations, in syphilis, and SBE (Ann IM 1993; 119: 1079); ≤ 5% false neg especially in late stages (Ann IM 1987;107:730), seen if early po antibiotic rx or early in crs, or w some labs that run 10-50% false neg and up to 25% false pos (Jama 1992;268:891). Immune complex measurement (Jama 1999;282:1942).

Synovial fluid: Organisms usually present by PCR (Nejm 1994; 330:229)

Rx (Med Let 2005;47:41; Jama 1995;274:66; Ann IM 1991; 111:472): Prevent w (Nejm 2003;348:2424):

- Permethrin (Nix) rx of clothing and DEET at 75+% concentration (Med Let 1989;31:46)
- Remove ticks within 24 hr

  Prophylactic rx after tick bite perhaps, doxycycline 200 mg po × 1, if engorged and/or on > 36 hr and in high-prevalence area (Nejm 2001;345:79 vs 133)

  of stage 1 (Med Let 1989;31:57): To decrease post-rash arthritis and illness (Ann IM 1983;99:22):

1st: Tetracycline 250 mg qid or doxycycline 100 mg bid × 21 d; × 10 d (DBCT: Ann IM 2003;138:697) if erythema migrans alone; or, for children and pregnant women, amoxicillin 250-500 mg po tid × 21 d, but misses concomitant Ehrlichia infections

2nd: Erythromycin 250 mg po qid × 10 d, or penicillin 20 million U qd iv × 10 d, or cefuroxime 500 mg po bid × 21 d (Ann IM 1992;117:273); also misses ehrlichia

  of stages 2 and 3: Doxycycline 200 mg po bid or amoxicillin as above but for 4-6 wk (Nejm 1994;330:229) or ceftriaxone 2 gm iv/im × 14-21 d especially if bad arthritis or cardiac/neurologic findings, only 1/13 failures (Nejm 1988;319:1661); or penicillin G 20 million U qd iv × 10-21 d for cardiac or neurologic abnormalities and/or meningitis (Ann IM 1983;99:767), cures 55% of arthritis. Avoid intraarticular steroids (Nejm 1985;312:869).

of acute non-meningitis disseminated disease: Doxycycline 100 mg po bid × 21 d, equally effective as ceftriaxone 2 gm im qd × 14 d (Nejm 1997;337:289)

of heart block: Antibiotics and temporary pacer (Ann IM 1989;110:339) since usually transient

of chronic encephalopathy: 60-85% improve with ceftriaxone rx given even after several years

if pos titers or hx and chronic fatigue/fasciitis syndrome, antibiotic rx not helpful (DBCT: Nejm 2001;343:85; Ann IM 1993; 119:503,518)

Relapsing Fever

Nejm 1993;329:939

Cause: *Borrelia recurrentis*

Epidem: Epidemic form via louse vector carrying person to person; endemic form via tick vector carrying between animal reservoirs to humans; worldwide

Pathophys: Organism changes antigen structure q 1-2 wk and causes bacteremia, which causes antibody production leading to antigen–antibody rosettes, which cause vasculitis and then sx subside again

Sx: Headache, fever, chills, myalgias, arthralgias, abdominal pain

Si: Each attack is 3-5 d of fever, then 4-10 d afebrile. Rash may be macular, papular, or purpuric looking like meningococcal bacteremia.

Crs: 3-10 recurrent attacks unless rx'd

Cmplc: Epidemic type has > 50% mortality; endemic form has < 2% mortality

Lab: *Bact:* Buffy coat smear shows spirochetes, loosely coiled by dark field, or Giemsa or Wright stain. Rat inoculation shows positive buffy coat changes as above in 4 d.
Hem: Elevated wbc and ESR; low platelets

Rx: 1st: tetracycline; 2nd: streptomycin; 3rd: penicillin, which commonly causes Herxheimer's reaction (J Infect Dis 1978;137:573), like syphilis (p 593)

Brucellosis (Undulant Fever)

Nejm 2005;352:2325

Cause: *Brucella melitensis* (goats), *abortus* (cattle), *suis* (pigs)

Epidem: Via ingestion or contact with infected milk or meat. In rural areas; affects 4% of all U.S. cattle. Endemic in Mexico

Pathophys: Intracellular organism causes endotoxin production; granuloma formation; diffuse systemic infestations can cause osteomyelitis

Sx: Acute: Deep bone pain; fever
Chronic: Weakness, aches, anxiety. A great mimicker of all diseases.

Si: Acute: Fever, undulating to peaks in pm; deep bone pain; lymphadenopathy (7%); splenomegaly (16%); hepatomegaly (17%)
Chronic: Low-grade fever, focal arthritis, epididymitis

Crs:

Cmplc: Endocarditis

Lab: *Bact:* Blood culture (16% pos) and reticuloendothelial tissue grow gram-neg bacilli on culture
Hem: ESR low, r/o trichinosis, psittacosis, leptospirosis, CHF; cbc shows lymphocytosis
Serol: Hemagglutination antibody titer increased; DCR tests best
Chem: Elevated ALT+AST

Xray: Osteomyelitis

Rx (Ann IM 1992;117:25):
Doxycycline 100 mg po bid + rifampin 15 mg/kg/d po × 6 wk, or streptomycin 1 gm qd × 15 d w doxycycline kept up for 6 wk; or Tm/s w one or more of those; or cipro, or ofloxacin w rifampin

Leptospirosis (Weil's Disease)

Nejm 1984;310:524; Ann IM 1973;79:167,786

Cause: *Leptospira spp.* (many)

Epidem: Usually in young adults in warm seasons, from contact with or ingestion of water contaminated with animal urine or directly with the animals themselves: dogs, rats (causing urban epidemic foci: Ann IM 1996;125:794), cattle, pigs, frogs, squirrels, other wild animals, etc; worldwide

Pathophys: Biphasic illness; Weil's disease is the 2nd, immune phase with rash, hepatitis, renal failure, myocarditis, uveitis

Sx: 2-26 d (average = 10 d) incubation period; abrupt onset of "flu syndrome"; malaise; headache often severe; fever; nausea, vomiting, diarrhea (50%); dry cough; jaundice although not always clinical

Si: Icterus, fever, purpura and other rashes, tender organomegaly, conjunctivitis, severe muscle tenderness; r/o dengue, adenovirus, toxic shock, rubella, rubeola, Kawasaki's

Crs: 2-5% mortality without rx, rest eventually resolve

Cmplc: Weil's disease or syndrome: Elevated bilirubin and BUN, anemia, uveitis, hemorrhages, aseptic meningitis with mental status changes
  Myocarditis, renal failure, hepatic failure, meningitis

Lab: *Bact:* Culture of urine up to 6-8 wk after onset, or acute CSF or blood on special media from CDC at 30°C × 6 wk; or guinea pig (not rodent) injection causes icterus in 3-12 d
  Chem: CPK, bilirubin, BUN (25%), LFTs all increased
  CSF: Aseptic meningitis pattern
  Hem: ESR low, r/o brucellosis, trichinosis, psittacosis (Petersdorf 1971), CHF
  Serol: Agglutinin titer > 1/25 (Nejm 1967;276:838)
  Urine: Rbc's

Rx: Prevent w doxycycline 100 mg po bid × 1 wk (Ann IM
1984; 100:696; Nejm 1984;310:497) if likely exposed
of disease (Lancet 1988;1:433): 1st, tetracycline 2-4 gm qd,
or doxycycline as above; 2nd, penicillin

Syphilis (Lues)

K. Holmes rv: Jama 2003;290:1510; Nejm 1992;326:1060

Cause: *Treponema pallidum*

Epidem: Incidence = 20+/100,000 in U.S., increasing since 1985;
spread via direct contact (venereal) with primary (1°) or secondary (2°) lesion

Pathophys: In 2°, marked bacteremia is present. Tertiary (3°) types
probably represent hypersensitivity reactions since few organisms
are present. Gummas, from endarteritis obliterans that causes
necrosis, eg, in aortic media. Three types of neurosyphilis:
- **Tabes Dorsalis**
- Meningovascular
- **General Paresis of the Insane** (GPI), primary parenchymal
involvement
    All 3° complications are increased in AIDS (Nejm
1987;316:1600)

Sx: 1°: Painless chancre
2°: Rash, round with pigmented center; fever; headache; alopecia; eye pain from iritis

Si: 1°: Chancre with edema (looks like squamous cell cancer) and
nonsuppurative lymphadenitis
2°: Macular/papular/pustular rash with pustules, annular-
appearing as ages, on palms and soles; split papules at mouth
corners and other moist body areas (condyloma lata); diffuse
lymphadenopathy; meningitis
3°: • Neurosyphilis: Argyle-Robertson pupils (small, unequal, reactive to accommodation not light); general paresis dementia; meningovascular, strokes, meningitis, and cranial nerve

palsies (Nejm 1994;331:1469,1516) most commonly seen within 3-4 yr of primary infection especially in AIDS pts, tabes dorsalis with motor long tract and sensory losses usually in lower extremities

- Vascular including aortitis with AI and aneurysms in 10%
- Gummas in 15%; 75% are cutaneous

Congenital: Onset at age 14+ wk even if seronegative at birth; si: rash, fever, hepatosplenomegaly, rhinitis, lymphadenopathy, elevated LFTs, CSF cells, and protein (Nejm 1990;323:1299); notched permanent (Hutchinson's) teeth, in 25%; interstitial keratitis in 50%; saddle nose

Crs: 1°: 9-90 d, 20-30% develop secondary syphilis

2°: Months if no rx

Cmplc:

1°: r/o herpes and chancroid (both tender)

2°: Obstructive pattern hepatitis (Nejm 1971;284:1422); nephrosis from immune complex disease (Nejm 1975;292:449)

3°: Cirrhosis (Med Clin N Am 1964;48:613)

r/o **bejel/pinta** from *Treponema carateum*, spread by skin-to-skin contact with lesions, as well as by flies in pinta. Bejel in Arabia, pinta in Central and South America. Primary disease consists of a nonulcerating papule; secondary, pigmented skin lesions later becoming depigmented and hyperkeratotic; tertiary disease, cardiovascular and nervous system involvement. Rx w penicillin.

r/o **Yaws** from *T. pertenue*, spread by skin-to-skin contact in many tropical areas, especially affecting children. An ulcerating papule w "strawberry" scar formation. Rx w penicillin.

Lab: *Bact:* Dark field shows bacteria with 8-14 spirals, ~7 m long; false positives in mouth from normal treponema flora there

CSF: Do LP 1 yr post rx of 1° or 2° types if VDRL or FTA still positive; in meningovascular syphilis, elevated protein and cells are present; VDRL is positive in 50% but can be negative even if bacteria present—hence getting FTA is better.

Probably best to just rx for 3-4 wk without LP if asx (Ann IM 1986;104:86).

Serol (rv: Ann IM 1986;104:368):

- VDRL or RPR is positive in 76% of 1° cases (if negative, dark field still positive), 100% of 2° ses; and 75% of 3° cases; false pos ($>$ 1/16) in mononucleosis, alaria, collagen vascular diseases, sarcoid, leprosy, yaws, pint
- TPI is positive in 50% of 1°, 98% 2°, and 90% of 3° cases
- FTA (Nejm 1969;280:1086) is posi e in 90% of 1°, 99% of 2°, 98% of 3°; false positives in only % of VDRL false-positive pts, some with yaws, pinta, o 10% lupus but is atypical (beaded: Nejm 1970;282:1287); re ins positive all life

Xray: Congenital type has lytic areas (bites) in g bones, subperiosteal

Rx (Ann IM 2002;137:255; Med Let 1999;4 9): Same even if HIV positive (Nejm 1997;337:307)

Prevent by partner notification, usefulness ited (Ann IM 1990;112:539)

of early disease (1°, 2°, or latent $<$ 1 yr): 1st, zathine penicillin (Bicillin) 2.4 million U im $\times$ 1, or azithr ycin 1 gm po $\times$ 1 (Ann IM 1999;131:434); 2nd, doxycycline 1 mg po bid $\times$ 14 d; 3rd, erythromycin 500 mg po qid $\times$ 14 d

of late, short of neurosyphilis: 1st, benzathine pen lin 2.4 million U im weekly $\times$ 3 wk; 2nd, doxycycline 100 mg po bid $\times$ 4 wk

of neurosyphilis: Penicillin G 2-4 million U iv q 4 hr $\times$ 10-14 d; 2nd, procaine penicillin 2.4 million U im qd + probenecid (Benemid) 500 mg po qid $\times$ 10-14 d

of congenital: Penicillin G 50,000 U/kg im/iv q 8-12 hr $\times$ 10-14 d, or procaine penicillin 50,000 U/kg im qd $\times$ 10-14 d

If penicillin allergy: Ceftriaxone im qd $\times$ 10 d, or tetracycline 2 gm qd or doxycycline 100 mg po bid $\times$ 15 d (12% failure rate) or macrolide like erythromycin 2 gm qd $\times$ 10 d (30 d for

3°) (12% failure rate) or azithromycin but drug resistance clearly had developed to it (Nejm 2004;351:154). Rx for 28 d if late latent disease.

Rx crs: < 1% relapse; follow VDRL, goes negative in 3-6 mo; with CNS lues, follow CSF cells; Herxheimer reaction (endotoxin sx with fever) within hours after penicillin (Nejm 1976;295:21). Longer rx in AIDS where early neurosyphilis develops (Nejm 1994;331:1469,1488,1516; Ann IM 1991;114:872, 1988;109:855) and penicillin rx only transiently effective since long-term cure normally depends on immunity.

9.7 Mycoplasma/Chlamydia

Chlamydial Atypical Pneumonias and URIs

Jama 1997;277:1214; Clin Infect Dis 1992;15:757; Ann IM 1987;106:507; Nejm 1986;315:189

Cause: *Chlamydia pneumoniae* (TWAR agent), which was previously thought to be *psittaci* (Nejm 1986;315:161)

Epidem: 100,000 cases/yr in U.S.; nearly half of all adults have a titer

Pathophys: Pneumonia and bronchitis

Sx: 7-14 d incubation period
Sore throat and hoarseness often 1st sx; fever only early in crs; dry cough often late in crs

Si: Minimal findings on chest exam; worse in elderly

Crs: Long (weeks) even w rx

Cmplc: Chronic infections may increase MIs? (Ann IM 1996;125:979, 1992;116:273)
r/o mycoplasma (cold agglutinins)

Xray: Chest, may show atypical pneumonic infiltrate

Lab: *Serol:* Paired sera allow dx of nonspecific chlamydial infection retrospectively

Rx: Tetracycline or erythromycin 500 mg qid × 10-14 d

Psittacosis

Nejm 1986;315:189

Cause: *Chlamydia psittaci*

Epidem: Birds like parakeets, parrots, chickens, pigeons; fecal spread. 100-200 cases from birds/yr in U.S.

Pathophys:

Sx: 7-14 d incubation period
Prominent headache; fever; sore throat, dry cough

Si: Confusion, headache, and muscle spasms mimic meningitis. Pneumonitis. Bradycardia relative to temperature; r/o gm-neg shock, typhoid, yellow fever, Q fever.

Crs: 10-21 d, 20% fatal without rx

Cmplc: r/o mycoplasma (cold agglutinins), Q fever (antibody titers), strep, and staph

Lab: *Bact:* Culture blood, sputum
Hem: ESR low frequently, r/o trichinosis, leptospirosis, brucellosis (R. Petersdorf 1971), CHF
Serol: Complement-fixing antibody on paired sera; r/o lymphogranuloma venereum

Rx: Tetracycline or erythromycin 500 mg qid × 2-3 wk

Chlamydial Nonspecific Urethritis (NSU), Proctitis, Mucopurulent Cervicitis, Pelvic Inflammatory Disease

Nejm 2003;349:2424

Cause: *Chlamydia trachomatis*; in NSU in men, also *Ureaplasma* and *Mycoplasma spp.*

Epidem: Venereal; over 50% of nonspecific urethritis episodes in males; 11% of proctitis in gay males (Nejm 1981;305:195); 12% prevalence in Maine women (Maine Epigram 5/87); 7-15% in army women recruits (Nejm 1998;339:739); 4% overall in U.S. (Jama 2004;291:2229) and highest in Southwest and blacks. Rates of transmission from males to females, and vice versa, nearly equal, as are the asx infection rates (Jama 1996;276:1737).

Pathophys:

Sx: 80-90% are asx; dysuria and urethral discharge in men, vaginal discharge in women

Si: Urethral discharge in male; proctitis, mild in gays
          Cervix shows yellow mucopurulent discharge (14% false pos: Nejm 1984;311:1; Ann IM 1982;97:216) and hypertrophic cervical ectopy (ectropion)
          Pharyngitis, from fellatio (Ann IM 1985;102:757)

Crs:

Cmplc: Epididymitis (the etiology in ½ of cases of epididymitis); endometritis, PID, perihepatitis like Fitzhugh-Curtis syndrome of gonorrhea; male sterility (Nejm 1983;308:502,505; Am J Pub Hlth 1993;83:996) and female sterility (worse than gc). r/o gc and mycoplasma PID.

Acute conjuctivitis in newborn (ophthalmia neonatorum) (r/o *Herpes simplex* w ulcerations) from gc or chlamydia, latter more common, 5% of all U Wash deliveries; a smaller % have pneumonitis, from 1 to 60 d postpartum, average 15 d, rx w erythromycin × 14 d (Med Let 1995;35:117)

Lab: *Bact:* Single swab culture is 100% specif, 75% sens (Ann IM 1987;107:189); smears: males have > 4 polys/hpf by urethral swab even if no discharge; females have 10+ polys/hpf (at 1000×), 17% false pos, 10% false neg (Holmes: Nejm 1984;311:1)

Path: Pap smear detection unreliable

Serol: Enzyme immunoassay method (ELISA) on secretions or urine (Jama 1993;270:2065) can be done in < 30 min; 80% sens, 98% specif (Ann IM 1987;107:189); use to screen.

DNA amplification assay of urine very accurate; 89% sens, 99% specif (Nejm 1998;339:739,768; Ann IM 1996;124:1) and routine.

Rx: Prevent w:
- In adults: Barrier methods
- At birth: Povidone iodine 2.5% soln gtts OU is more effective, less toxic, and cheaper (Nejm 1995;332:562) than tetracycline, erythromycin, or silver nitrate gtts, which still miss some gc, hence have a 10-20% incidence of ophthalmic disease in newborns of infected mothers (Nejm 1989;320:769)

Screen (p 924):
- All multiple-partnered asx men (Jama 1996;276:1737) and women to reduce PID sterilization rates from 2% to 1%/yr (Nejm 1996;334:1362), or all women < 25-30 yr (Nejm 1998;339:739,768; Ann IM 1998;128:277)
- All pregnant women early and at 36 wk w cultures if expected prevalence > 7% (Ann IM 1987;107:188), or at least lower socioeconomic groups, and rx positives with erythromycin 500 mg qid × 7 d; this strategy decreases postnatal eye and lung infections, when given to asx mothers prepartum, from 50% of infants to 7% (Nejm 1986;314:276)

   of active disease (Ann IM 2002;137:255; Med Let 1999; 41:85): Rx pt and partner (Med Let 1994;36:1; Nejm 1978;298:490) w:

1st:
- Azithromycin (Zithromax) 1 gm po × 1 (Jama 1995;274:545; Nejm 1992;377:921; Med Let 1991;33:119)
- Tetracycline 500 mg qid × 7 d (Ann IM 1982;97:216), 250 qid × 14-21 d, or doxycycline 100 bid × 7 d, or × 2-3 wk for proctitis

2nd (1st choice in pregnancy):
- Erythromycin 500 mg qid × 7 d or × 3 wk after tetracycline failure (Ann IM 1990;113:21), which may be due to tetracycline-resistant ureaplasma, for adults; nonestolated types

ok in pregnancy (Med Let 1991;33:119); 12.5 mg/kg/d po or
iv × 14 d for neonatal pneumonia or conjunctivitis
- Ofloxacin 300 mg po bid × 7 d
- Levofloxacin 500 mg po qd × 7 d

Lymphogranuloma Venereum

Ann IM 1983;98:973; Nejm 1978;298:494

Cause: *Chlamydia trachomatis*, immunotype L

Epidem: Venereally spread. Highest incidence in gay males. Male/
female = 20:1.

Pathophys:

Sx: Painless papule (30%); bubo (70%); long incubation period

Si: Adenopathy, local and distant; fever; erythema nodosum; ulcerative proctitis, in gays (Nejm 1981;305:195)

Crs:

Cmplc: Rectal stricture; cancer develops in 2%

Lab: Rv of dx tests (Nejm 1983;308:1563)
Bact: Culture possible and quite easy
Serol: Comp-fix antibody pos (> 1/16) in 60%; r/o psittacosis

Rx (Med Let 1995;37:117):
Tetracycline × 21 d, often must repeat × 1-2; or erythromycin
500 mg qid × 21 d

Primary Atypical Pneumonia

Rev Inf Dis 1990;12:338, Mayo Cl Proc 1986;61:830; Nejm 1971;
285:374 (Emory fraternity epidemic)

Cause: *Mycoplasma pneumonia* (pleuropneumonia-like organism
[PPLO]; Eaton agent)

Epidem: Probably airborne respiratory droplets. Highest incidence in
young adults; 10% of all their respiratory diseases; 49% attack
rate in single-exposure epidemic. Intimate and prolonged contact, eg, intrafamilial, usually necessary for spread.

Pathophys: Intracellular infection

Sx: Malaise (85%), cough (85%), headache (77%), fever (65%), sore throat (44%), sweats (37%), myalgias (41%), arthralgias

Si: Bronchitis; pneumonia (27%); vesicle on tympanic membrane (bullous myringitis), 12% overall, more common age 5-15 yr; rash

Crs:

Cmplc: Hemolytic anemia with cold agglutinins (Nejm 1977;296:1490); peri- and myocarditis (Ann IM 1977;86:544); Guillain-Barré syndrome (Ann IM 1981;94:15)

Lab: *Serol:* Specific comp-fix antibodies increased. Nonspecific cold agglutinins increased (IgM), 35-75% of pts will be positive after 7 d of illness (Ann IM 1977;86:547); r/o collagen vascular disease, lymphoproliferative disease, mononucleosis.

Xray: Chest infiltrates and/or pleural effusions (in 25%: Nejm 1970;283:790)

Rx: Macrolide drug of choice because effective and also gets pneumo-coccus, eg erythromycin, azithromycin, or clarithromycin; tetra-cycline, but 50% after rx still have nonresistant organisms in respiratory tract (Nejm 1967;277:719) although same may be true for erythromycin

9.8 Rickettsia and Related Organisms

Q Fever

Nejm 1988;319:354

Cause: *Coxiella burnetii*

Epidem: Airborne, eg, in hay; animal reservoirs (stock animals, and cats, especially parturient ones). Tick vector from mouse reservoir; milk from chronically infected cows. Worldwide.

Pathophys: Intracellular in vessel endothelium

Sx: Fever, headache, pains in muscles and chest wall; sudden onset

Si: Cardiovascular: Relative bradycardia, migratory thrombophlebitis
Skin: Papule, then vesicle and eschar after 3-4 wk (rare)
Pulmonary: Patchy pneumonitis, dry cough, pleurisy
GI: Hepatitis (Ann IM 1971;74:198)
Rheumatoid: Migratory arthritis

Crs: 2-4 wk

Cmplc: Endocarditis (rare)

Lab: *Bact:* Fastidious grower, needs high CO_2, low O_2
Serol: Comp-fix antibody elevated; use same antigens used to test for typhus, Weil-Felix negative (r/o rickettsial pox)

Rx: Vaccine: None
of disease: Tetracycline

Ehrlichiosis

Jama 1996;275:199 (HGE); Mmwr 1996;45:798 (HME), 1995;44:593; Ann IM 1994;120:730,736

Cause: *Ehrlichia sennetsu* and *chaffeensis* (human monocytic ehrlichiosis) (HME) (Nejm 1996;334:209); and *E. equi, phagocytophilia,* and *ewingii* (human granulocytic ehrlichiosis (HGE) (Nejm 1999;341:148,195)

Epidem: Tick-borne (*Ixodes scapularis* and *Amblyomma americanum*), common in animals. Two types: HME in SE Asia (where causes a mononucleosis-like, **Sennetsu Fever**), now > 300 cases in southern and central U.S. from deer ticks, eg, Tennessee golf course epidemic (Nejm 1995;333:420); and HGE in midwestern and northeastern U.S. (Ann IM 1996;125:904, 1995;123:277; Jama 1994;272:212).

Pathophys: Intracellular in polys, si and sx same in both types

Sx: ±10 d incubation period from tick bite. Acute self-limited febrile illness, headache, malaise, chills, nausea and vomiting.

Si: Fever; occasionally cough; arthralgias; confusion; papular, rarely macular rash

Crs: Fatalities among elderly pts > 60 yr

Cmplc: Pericarditis (Nejm 1996;334:213); perinatal transmission to newborn (Nejm 1998;339:375)
  r/o RMSF and concomitant or distinct Lyme disease or babesiosis (Nejm 1997;336:15; Jama 1996;275:1657)

Lab: *Chem:* LFTs elevated
  Hem: CBC shows pancytopenia, especially thrombocytopenia, and diagnostic mulberry-like inclusions in polys (morulae; 80%) (Nejm 1995;332:1417) in HGE, rarely seen in HME type
  Serol: Diagnostic IFA acute (often neg) and convalescent titers

Rx: Prevent w insect repellent and other antitick measures
  Doxycycline or other tetracycline; chloramphenicol

Rocky Mountain Spotted Fever

Nejm 1993;329:941

Cause: *Rickettsia rickettsiae*

Epidem: Carried by ticks (large and visible) from wild rodent reservoirs. Endemic in Rocky Mountain rodents; also on Cape Cod and throughout most mid-Atlantic states including Virginia and North Carolina; also seen in lab technicians working with ticks. 700-1000 cases/yr in U.S.

Pathophys: Angiitis due to endothelial infection causing proliferation and thrombosis via activation of kallikrein-kinin system (Ann IM 1978;88:764). Subclinical DIC changes in platelet and clotting system detectable even before sx (Nejm 1988;318:1021).

Sx: Seasonal; 95% of cases between April and August. Tick bite (most recall) or dog contact. Incubation period, 5-7 d. Severe frontal headache (90%) is usually first sx; myalgias (80%), emesis (60%).

Si: Rash (90%), centripetal progression (extremities to trunk), palm and sole involved (in 2/12); toxic with fever leading to confusion (in 10/13); muscle tenderness, especially calf and thigh; diffuse angiitis; skin necrosis regardless of pressure points

Crs:

Cmplc: Mortality without rx = 25%; w rx, 5%. Carditis, cerebral edema, DIC

r/o Babesiosis (p 631); rat bite fever (p 536); **Rickettsial Pox** (Nejm 1994;331:1612) from *Rickettsia akari*, seen all over U.S., initial lesion at mouse mite bite, 1 wk latency then fever, malaise, and chicken pox-like vesicular lesions, not too sick, can rx w tetracycline; other rickettsial pox in other parts of world, eg, **North Asian Rickettsiosis, African Tick Bite Fever** (NEJM 2001;344:1504), **Queensland Tick Typhus, Typhus**

Lab: *Hem:* Thrombocytopenia (Nejm 1969;280:58) and DIC

Path: Skin bx of rash positive on immunofluorescent stain (available from CDC)

Serol: Antibody increased by immunofluorescence or microagglutination by day 15. Weil-Felix test: in Rocky Mountain spotted fever, OX2 and OX19 positive, OXK negative; in rickettsial pox, all neg.

Rx: 1st, tetracycline; 2nd, chloramphenicol

Typhus

Cause: *Rickettsia prowazekii* and *mooseri*

Epidem: Endemic: person to person via human body louse or lab technique (Ann IM 1968;69:731); worldwide; especially winter/ spring in cold climates

Brill-Zinsser disease: Recurrent disease in carriers, perhaps via fleas

Murine type: Human to rat to human

Pathophys: Arteritis by intracellular invasion causing vascular occlusion. Nodules in cortical gray matter.

Sx: Headache; rash

Si: Fever; rash, centrifugal (central body spreading to extremities); pneumonia, atypical; CNS sx; necrotic skin over pressure points

Crs:

Cmplc: May precipitate G_6PD deficiency in blacks, leading to hemolysis and subsequent ATN (Ann IM 1968;69:323)

Lab: *Chem:* LFTs show hepatitis picture (Ann IM 1968;69:731)
Serol: Weil-Felix OX19 positive (r/o RMSF and scrub typhus)

Rx: Prevent by killing lice with DDT; kill rats
of disease: Tetracycline or chloramphenicol; loading dose
2-2.5 × daily dose, then rx × 10 d

Trench Fever

Ann IM 1973;79:26

Cause: *Bartonella (Rochalimaea) quintana*

Epidem: Body louse vector, person to person; alchoholic, homeless (Nejm 1999;340:184), and AIDS pts (Nejm 1995;332:419,424); Europe, USSR, Mexico

Pathophys:

Sx:

Si:

Crs:

Cmplc: Endocarditis; bacillary angiomatosis (Nejm 1997;337:1876, 1888,1916, 1995;332:419,424); cutaneous and deep tissue infections as well as osteolytic bone lesions, esp in AIDS and other immunocompromised pts

Lab: *Bact:* Small pleomorphic gram-neg bacilli
Serol: Comp-fix antibody; Weil-Felix OXK positive ST, 50% never become OXK Weil-Felix positive; fluorescent antibody increased 4× in 100%

Rx: Macrolide antibiotics, tetracyclines, chloramphenicol

Cat Scratch Fever

Nejm 1997;337:1876, 1994;330:1509; Ann IM 1993;118:388

Cause: *Bartonella (Rochalimaea) henselae* (Nejm 1994;330:509; Ann IM 1993;118:331). *Afipia felis*, a closely related organism, may be the cause in some cases.

Epidem: Young cats, infected for a few weeks; transmit via bites, scratches, and fleas; 80% of cases are in pts under age 21

Pathophys:

Sx: Bite or scratch by kitten (90% have had by hx); 7-14 d incubation; then papule at site of scratch. Papule at site of infection; fever (< 50%), adenopathy (40% of nodes suppurate).

Si: As above

Crs: All benign including cmplc

Cmplc: Encephalopathy/encephalitis (10%), conjunctivitis, purpura (suppressed platelets), mesenteric adenitis, endocarditis (Ann IM 1996;125:646); hypercalcemia (Jama 1998;279:532)

in AIDS pts (Ann IM 1988;109:449) and otherwise immunocompromised hosts: Disseminated disease; **Bacillary Angiomatosis** (Nejm 1997;337:1876,1888,1916, 1995;332:419,424), which looks somewhat like Kaposi's sarcoma, cutaneous and deep tissue infections as well as osteolytic bone lesions; **Peliosis Hepatis** (Nejm 1992;327:1625, 1990;323:1573,1581), occasionally also seen in immunocompetent pts (Ann IM 1993;118:363)

Lab: *CSF:* Protein increased; occasionally mononuclear cells in 10%
Bact: Small pleomorphic gram-neg bacilli
Hem: Elevated ESR and white count with left shift; eosinophils elevated modestly
Path: Bx shows organism with Warthin-Starry and silver stains
Serol: Bartonella henselae titers > 1/64 (84% sens, 96%

specif-Nejm 1993;329:8), from CDC, available commercially as well

Skin test: DHS pos in 30 d, homemade from ground-up nodes; no longer used due to AIDS and other viral risks

Rx: None may be indicated in mild disease except aspiration of fluctuant nodes to decrease sx of disease:

- Erythromycin 500 mg po qid or other macrolide, especially for disseminated forms
- Doxycycline 100 mg po bid, especially for disseminated forms if can't tolerate erythromycin
- Ciprofloxacin 500 mg po bid (Jama 1991;265:1563)
- Tm/S for children
- Gentamicin iv × 5 d (West J Med 1991;154:330)

9.9 Miscellaneous

Catheter-induced Phlebitis and Colonization

Tip culture and Gram stain (Nejm 1985;312:1142); plastic Teflon tips no worse than steel (Ann IM 1991;114:845); change over guidewire if no obvious infection, or use new site if obvious infection and culture tip, > 15 colonies is significant (Nejm 1992;327:1062)

Fever: False Negatives

Oral temperature will be ≥ 2°F less than rectal if respiratory rate > 20, difference increases with more rapid respirations (Nejm 1983; 308:945)

Fever of Unknown Origin (FUO)

Arch IM 2003;163:1033

Definition: Fever > 101°F daily 3+ wk and 1 wk hospital or physician w/u (p 1139 for differential when fever associated w polyarthritis)

Table 9.1 Fever of Unknown Origin (% per Petersdorf series)

Infections (36%)	Collagen-Vascular (13%)	Miscellaneous (30%)	Neoplasms (19%)	No Dx (2%)
Tbc (11)	Rheumatic fever (6)	Regional enteritis	Disseminated or localized of pancreas, liver, kidney (9)	
Liver/biliary (7)	SLE (5)	Pericarditis	Lymphoma/ leukemia (8)	
Abdominal abscess (4)	Unclassified (2)	Allergic hepatitis	No histologic dx (2)	
Pyelonephritis (3)	RA (84% present as FUO in children: Nejm 1967; 276:11)	Thyroiditis		
Psittacosis (2)	Polymyalgia rheumatica	Myelofibrosis		
Cirrhosis and bacteremia (1)		Erythema multiforme		
GC arthritis (1)		Panniculitis (Weber-(Christian disease)		
Malaria (1)		Neuroleptic malignant syndrome		
Yersinia		Drug fever (protean nature, rv: Ann IM 1987;106:728)		
Fastidious bug, eg, micro-aerophilic strep		Pulmonary embolus		
SBE		Sarcoid		
Osteomyelitis		FMF		
Cholangitis		Ruptured spleen/ pancreas		
Sinusitis		Factitious self-induced or faked)		

Handwashing

Chlorhexidine (Hibiclens) use is better than soap + isopropyl alcohol (Nejm 1992;327:88)

Penicillin Allergy

Jama 2001;285:2498; Am J Med 1999;107:166; Arch IM 1992;152: 930,1025, Ann IM 1987;107:204; Nejm 1985;312:1229

5-10% have cephalothin cross-reactivity (Ann IM 2004; 141:16; Nejm 2001;345:804), use 2 mg/cc solution and do prick tests followed by intradermal test before using

Penicylloyl-polylysine (Prepen—major determinant skin test positive in 80% of people allergic to benzyl penicillin G, cephalothin, and benzyl penicillinoic acid) scratch (10 U/cc), then intracutaneous; will detect

If tests are negative, proceed; if positive, phenoxymethyl penicillin elixir in progressive po 100-U increments, double q 15 min to 1.3 million U total. Beware: Penicillin IgE allergy attenuates over years so pts may have anaphylaxis and 5 yr later not be allergic by above tests but on reexposure will resensitize fast. Thus must retest every time want to use in pt with positive hx.

Prophylactic Antibiotics

- Bacterial endocarditis (SBE) (Med Let 2005;47:59; Jama 1997;277:1794; Nejm 1995;332:38): Use whenever bacteria-containing mucosa is breached, esp if indication is high risk (h/o SBE, artificial valve, cyanotic heart disease, surgical shunts); or bacteremic risk higher from immunosuppression: For dental procedures that cause bleeding (case-control study finds no benefit? Ann IM 1998;129:761,829), T+A, surgery on gi or upper respiratory mucosa, sclero rx of varices, esophageal dilatation, OB surgery, cystoscopy, urethral dilatation, urethral catheterization if UTI, urinary tract/prostate surgery, I+D of infected tissue, vaginal hysterectomy, infected vaginal delivery

Not for sigmoidoscopy (Ann IM 1976;85:77), other endoscopy w bx, cesarean section, normal vaginal delivery (Ann IM 1983;98:509)

Antibiotic choice:

For dental and upper respiratory tract, give 1 hr po or $\frac{1}{2}$ hr iv before procedure, amoxicillin/ampicillin 2 gm; if penicillin allergic, clindamycin 600 mg iv/po, or cephalexin/cefazolin 2 gm po/iv, or azithromycin 500 mg po

For procedures below diaphragm, give ampicillin 2 gm iv alone or if high risk w gentamicin 1.5 mg/kg (up to 80 mg) $\frac{1}{2}$ hr before + 1 gm amoxicillin/ampicillin po/iv 6 hr later; if penicillin allergic, substitute vancomycin 1 gm iv for amoxicillin/ampicillin

- Immunosuppressed patients, post-splenectomy, on steroids or chemoRx: Phenoxymethyl penicillin 250 mg bid (Med Let 1977;19:3), consider especially if not immunized, or use prn fever

- Surgical (Med Let 1999;41:75): Cephazolin (vancomycin if allergic or lots of MRSA around) for all except colorectal/appendectomy, where use cefotetan or cefoxitin to help with anaerobes. Single iv dose, $\frac{1}{2}$ hr pre-op or at least < 2 hr pre-op (Nejm 1992;326:281) for clean cardiovascular, orthopedic, and cranial surgery; clean or contaminated ENT, gi, and gyn surgery including C/S for PROM and therapeutic abortion. In gyn surgery, antibiotics help most with fast surgery as compared to prolonged surgery, and abdominal more than vaginal hysterectomy (Nejm 1982;307:1661). For dirty wound or ruptured viscus surgery, rx as infected × 7-10 d, ie, not prophylaxis.

- Prosthetic joint patients: Within 2 yr of hip/knee (J Infect 2002;45:243; J Arthroplasty 2000;15:675; J Am Dental Assoc 2003;134:895; ADA/AAOS Joint Advisory @ www.aaos.org/wordhtml/papers/advistmt/1014.htm) w cephalexin/

cephadrine/cefazolin 1 gm, ampicillin/amoxicillin 2 gm, or clindamycin 600 mg po or iv 1 hr prior to dental work

Sepsis/Septic Shock, Gram-Negative Shock

Nejm 2003;348:138, 1993;328:1471; Ann IM 1994;121:1, 1994;120:771, 1990;113:227

Pathophys: Systemic inflammatory response (SRS) define by P > 90, respir > 20, T° > 36-38°C, pCO_2 < 32, wbc > 12,000 or < 4000; progresses to sepsis, which progresses to septic shock (Jama 1995;273:117). Nitric oxide production may be a mechanism that can be rx'd w inhibitors (Jama 1996;275:1192).

Cmplc: Encephalopathy correlates w severity of sepsis and Glasgow coma scale score (Jama 1996;275:470)

Lab: Plasma triggering receptor expressed on myeloid cells (TREM-1) levels > 60 ng/cc, 96% sens, 89% specif for bacterial/fungal infection (Ann IM 2004;141:9)

Rx: In shock, arginine vasopressin drip may work when other pressors don't (Nejm 2004;351:159); steroid support beneficial if pressor dependent and use 5-10 d of 50-75 mg hydrocortisone q 6 hr + 0.05 mg Fluorinef po/ng qd, especially if inadequate cosyntropin stimulation test (Ann IM 2004;141:47,70; BMJ 2004;329:480; Jama 2002;288:862); rx with iv fluids and antibiotics to cover staph and pseudomonas like 3rd-generation cephalosporin + aminoglycoside (Med Let 1999;41:97); NSAIDs help fever but no improvement in survival (Nejm 1997;336:912)

Insulin iv drip to keep BS 80-110; monoclonal antiendotoxins of no help (Jama 2000;283:1723; Ann IM 1994; 121:1); but polyclonal iv immunoglobulins may help (NNT = 7) (ACP J Club 2001;135:82)

Activated protein C (recombinant human) (Xigris) if shock and end organ failure, improves survival by 6% (NNT = 16) but not yet standard of care (Nejm 2002;347:993,1027,1030, 2001; 344:699); $7000/rx

Traveler's Advice

Med Let 2002;44:33; Nejm 2000;342:1716; CDC website: www.cdc.gov, phone info: 888-232-3228

Consider, depending on the destination and length of stay:

- Traveler's diarrhea prophylaxis and/or rx prn (p 399)
- Immunizations for hepatitis A and B as combo vaccine Twinrix @ 0, 1 and 6 mo, cost $92/dose (Med Let 2001;43:67); measles if born after 1956 and haven't had 2 doses of vaccine over age 1, meningococcus, polio, diphtheria/tetanus, typhoid, and yellow fever; possibly for rabies, leptosporosis, or Japanese B encephalitis if going to high-risk environment
- Malaria prophylaxis (p 637)
- Insect repellant: 10% (children) to 35% DEET (higher no help); probably ok in pregnancy. Long-acting forms (6-12 hr): Ultrathon, Sawyer Controlled Release. Plus perhaps long-lasting permethrin (Duranon, Permanone) sprayed on clothing or mosquito net.
- Altitude sickness prevention and rx (p 991)
- Ischemic heart disease ok if stable and $pO_2 > 70$
- DVT prophylaxis (Ann IM 2004;141:148) if high risk and/or age > 50 yr and > 8 hr flights w full-length compression stockings (maybe BK for moderate risk), ? plus sc Lovenox. No evidence to support aspirin.
- In-flight medical emergencies (Nejm 2002;346:1068); cabins pressurized to 2200 meters

    Prevent by prohibiting air travel by pts w cardiovascular, pulmonary, CNS, or otologic significant illess, or within 3 wk of surgery, last 4 wk of pregnancy, newborns under 1 wk age

    Volunteers to assist (not run) are protected by good samaritan laws if stay within normal practice parameters, get pt or family permission, and make notes

Traveler's Illnesses

Nejm 2002;347:505

- Fever: Malaria, dengue, et al (see reference table w incubation periods)
- Diarrhea (p 546)
- Rashes (see reference pictures)

FUNGAL INFECTIONS

9.10 AntiFungals

Med Let 1997;39:86

Azoles

Nejm 1994;330:263

All can cause nausea and vomiting, rashes, and hepatotoxicity; all impair cytochrome 450 enzymes, so impair metabolism of many drugs (Med Let 1996;38:72) like macrolides, nonsedating antihistamines, benzodiazepines, cisapride

- Amphotericin B, 1 mg test dose, 0.3-1 mg/kg iv in D$_5$W over 2 hr qd or qod × wk, or perhaps (is it as effective?) less toxic continuous infusion over 24 hr (BMJ 2001;322:579); as 100 mg/cc oral suspension for AIDS oral candidiasis (Med Let 1997;39:14), or liposomal amphotericin B, lipid complex form (Abelcet) has less renal toxicity (Nejm 1999;340:764; Ann IM 1996;124:921) but costs $300-500/d

  Used vs candida, mucor, cryptococcus, histoplasmosis, blastomycosis, and extracutaneous sporotrichosis; adverse effects: RTA and renal damage especially > 4 gm, chills [rx with meperidine 25 mg iv or prevent with hydrocortisone, ASA, acetaminophen (Tylenol), or antihistamines], hypokalemia, anemia, phlebitis, hypotension, pulmonary toxicity (Nejm 1981;304:1185)

- Caspofungin (Nejm 2002;347:2020) 70 mg load, 50 mg iv qd; as good or bettter than amphotericin in safety and for monilial species
- Fluconazole (Diflucan) (Ann IM 1990;113:183) 100-400 mg po/iv qd; vs candida, cryptococcus; none of H_2-blocker interference or testosterone problems of ketoconazole; adverse effects: alopecia (12-20%) after 2 mo rx (Ann IM 1995;123:354), toxic interactions w nonsedating antihistamines like terfenadine (Jama 1996;275:1339)
- Itraconazole (Sporanox) (Med Let 1993;35:7) 200-400 mg po qd × 6-12 mo; may be less toxic than ketoconazole; used vs histoplasmosis, blastomycosis, invasive aspergillosis; 80-90% effective, but amphotericin still better if life-threatening; $10/d for 200 mg qd; adverse effects: toxic interactions w nonsedating antihistamines (Jama 1996;275:1339), some benzodiazepines, and statins
- Ketoconazole (Nizoral) (Ann IM 1983;98:13) 0.2-1 gm po qd; rarely used vs coccidioidomycosis, candida, cryptococcus, blastomycosis, and histoplasmosis; less toxic than amphotericin but generally a little less effective too; adverse effects: usual as above, Antabuse-like effect, need gastric acid to absorb, antitestosterone synthesis causes impotence and gynecomastia (Nejm 1987;317:812), decreased levels with rifampin (Nejm 1984;311:1681) and H_2 blockers
- Miconazole (Monostat); topical, po/iv; vs monilia, tinea; chronic mucocutaneous candida (Med Let 1986;21:31); adverse effects: increased warfarin and phenytoin (Dilantin) levels, hypoglycemia with oral hypoglycemic agents
- Voriconazole (Vfend) (Nejm 2002;347:308, 2002;346:225; Med Let 2002;44:63) 6 mg/kg iv q 12 hr × 1 d, then 4 mg/kg iv q 12 hr, then 100 mg (< 40 kg) to 200 mg (> 40 kg) po q 12 hr; for invasive aspergillosis, perhaps others; $300/d iv, $100/d po

Echinocandins

Caspofungin (Cancidas) (Med Let 2001;43:58) 50 mg iv qd ×
30+ d for invasive aspergillosis if amphotericin B or itraconazole can't
be used; $10,000/mo

Micafungin (Mycamine) (Med Let 2005;47:51) 50-150 mg iv qd;
similar, used for candida esophagitis; $6000/zid

Fluorinated Pyrimidines

Flucytosine (5-fluorocystine) 50-150 mg/kg/d po divided qid;
with amphotericin for cryptococcus, blastomycosis, and candida; renal
excretion; adverse effects: enterocolitis, dose-dependent leukopenia
resistance development prevents using alone

9.11 Systemic Infections

Aspergillosis

Cause: *Aspergillus*

Epidem: Ubiquitous; environmental, eg, from construction, especially
from bird guano; air conditioners; a pathogen primarily in
immunocompromised pts, esp AIDS pts (Nejm 1991;324:654)

Pathophys: Fungus ball, allergic (Ann IM 1982;96:286), and invasive
types. Invasive type is associated with severe and persistent
leukopenias and AIDS (Nejm 1991;324:654). Enters through
nose in immunocompromised host if nose first sterilized by
antibiotics (Ann IM 1979;90:4), through skin ulcers, or through
iv sites (Nejm 1987;317:1105).

Sx: Hemoptysis with fungus ball type; asthma with allergic type

Si:

Crs: Invasive type has 50% survival if start rx within 4 d of infiltrate
appearing; much worse if wait (Ann IM 1977;86:539)

Cmplc:

Lab: *Bact:* Gram stain shows mycelia in sputum ¹/₃ of time; blood culture shows occasionally positive if systemic; nose culture has 40% false-negative rate, 10% false-positive rate (Ann IM 1979;90:4)

Hem: In allergic type, eosinophilia

Serol: In allergic type, RIA-specific IgG and IgE (Ann IM 1983;99:18)

Skin test: In allergic type, shows immediate wheal and flare (Ann IM 1977;86:405)

Rx: in allergic type: Steroids, itraconazole 200 mg po qd-bid × 16+ wk (DBCT: Nejm 2000;342:756), electrostatic dust-free filters help (Ann IM 1989;110:115)

in systemic invasive types:

- 1st: Amphotericin 1 mg/kg qd until improve, then double-dose qod, then q 1-2 wk × 3-12 mo, or, as good or better, voriconazole (Vfend) (see meds)
- 2nd: Itraconazole (Sporanox)
- 3rd: Caspofungin (Cancidas)

Blastomycosis

Nejm 1986;314:529, 575

Cause: *Blastomyces dermatitidis*

Epidem: Airborne in rotten wood dust. North America especially around the Great Lakes and southeastern U.S.

Pathophys:

Sx: 3-12 wk incubation period. Asx (50%), cough (45%), headache (32%), chest pain (30%), weight loss (28%), fever (25%).

Si:

Crs: Usually self-limited, 3-4 wk (Nejm 1974;290:540)

Cmplc:

r/o **South American Blastomycosis** caused by paracoccidioidomycosis (*Paracoccidioides brasiliensis*), which is transmitted by thorn pricks and causes skin disease that looks like leprosy; rx'd with sulfonamides

Lab: *Bact:* Diphasic but yeast form in tissue; *brasiliensis* has multiple budding in yeast form

Serol: CF antibodies positive in only 10% (Nejm 1974;290:540); immunodiffusion positive in 28% of true positives; enzyme immunoassay positive in 77%

Skin test: Doubtful usefulness, positive in < 40% proven cases (Am Rev Respir Dis 1988;138:1081, Nejm 1986;314: 529,575)

Xray: Positive chest xray if pulmonic

Rx: Amphotericin, or miconazole, or ketoconazole 400 mg qd po × 6 mo (low dose) results in 80% cure; high dose (800 mg qd) results in 100% cure but 60% side effects (Ann IM 1985;103:861, 872); not for meningitis. Perhaps itraconazole.

Alternative for North American blastomycosis: 2-Hydroxystilbamidine iv, if confined to skin or noncavitary in lung; amphotericin is just as good (Nejm 1974;290:320)

Alternative for South American blastomycosis: Sulfonamides

Coccidioidomycosis (Valley Fever)

Nejm 1995;332:1077

Cause: *Coccidioides immitis*

Epidem: Airborne spread (inhalation) of mycelial-stage infective spores; endospore spread in body (description of storm-scattered epidemic in Calif: Nejm 1979;301:358). American Southwest especially Arizona, Texas, and Calif, eg, San Joaquin Valley (Stockton to Bakersfield); worst in wet season, especially in patients exposed to dirt in spring and late fall

Increased prevalence (reactivation?) in diabetics and pts on steroid rx, in AIDS and other immunocompromised pts

Sx: Hemoptysis; granulomatous reactions of face and neck; primary cocci picture (Nejm 1972;286:507) of pneumonitis (Nejm 1970; 283:325), flu-like syndrome with generalized pruritus macular/ papular rash; acute polyarthritis (Nejm 1972;287:1133)

Si: Erythema nodosum, pleural effusion

Crs: Mortality is 1% in Caucasians, 20% in Asians and Mexicans with disseminated disease. Recurrent up to 10 yr after amphotericin rx (Nejm 1969;281:950).

Cmplc: Hypercalcemia (Nejm 1977;297:431); extrapulmonary lesions, onset 1+ yr after primary pulmonary infection, eg, bones, joints, skin, meninges

Lab: *Bact:* Mycelial form (white, fluffy, distinctive) dangerous to lab personnel. Diphasic but no yeast forms in tissue. Urine culture frequently positive if concentrated by lab, even when don't suspect disseminated disease. Prostate secretions culture also often positive in same circumstances (Ann IM 1976;85:34).

Serol: Comp-fix antibody titer > 1/16 suggests disseminated active disease. Positive in 14/15 (Nejm 1970;283:326); decreases with successful rx. Counterimmunoelectrophoresis titer has 8% false-negative rate (Ann IM 1976;85:740).

Skin test: 20-50% false neg but still useful (Am Rev Respir Dis 1988;138:1081); indicates present or past disease

Xray: Nodular pneumonitis; primary pneumonias; coin lesions; thin-walled cavities, r/o rheumatoid nodules and pneumatoceles

Rx: Beware steroids
Meningitis after acute rx must be rx'd w lifelong suppression (Ann IM 1996;124:305)
of acute disease (Nejm 1987;317:334):

- Amphotericin $\frac{1}{2}$ mg/kg iv 2×/wk to total of 30 mg/kg if sick, if comp-fix is increased, or if hx of and on steroids; 20% relapse (4/20: Nejm 1970;283:325); intrathecal for meningitis, many complications especially with reservoir (Nejm 1973;288:186)

- Ketoconazole po is at least static in many moderate pulmonary/skin infections (Ann IM 1982;96:436,440); vs meningitis (Ann IM 1983;98:160)
- Fluconazole 400 mg qd po × years effectively suppresses meningitis (Ann IM 1993;119:28) and treats > 50% of nonmeningeal infections (Ann IM 2000;133:676)
- Itraconazole 200 mg po bid, cures 63% of nonmeningeal infections (Ann IM 2000;133:676)

Cryptococcosis

Rev Inf Dis 1991;13:1163; Ann IM 1981;94:611

Cause: *Cryptococcus neoformans*

Epidem: Ubiquitous fungus. Airborne; birds are probable vectors, especially pigeons, grows well in bird guano. Worldwide. Increased incidence in pts with lymphomas, and/or on steroids, AIDS.

Pathophys:

Sx: Meningitis, pneumonitis (Am Rev Respir Dis 1966;94:236)

Si:

Crs: Without rx, nearly 100% dead in 1 yr; with rx, 70% survival, 18% relapse in 29 mo (Ann IM 1969;71:1079) (rv of good and bad prognosis test results: Ann IM 1974;80:176)

Cmplc: Renal papillary necrosis (Nejm 1968;279:60); resistant prostatitis despite rx (Ann IM 1989;111:125)

Lab: *Bact:* Smear sputum, CSF, urine; round nucleoli, large nonstaining capsule, looks like lymphocyte; India ink preparation (drop of ink to CSF) reveals large clear (large capsules) organisms but 35% can have CNS crypto and neg India ink prep (NIH: Ann IM 1969;71:1079). Culture yeast form on rice/Tween agar at 22°C and 37°C; need large volumes of CSF to find.

Serol: Antigen by latex fixation or comp-fix is the only clinically useful test; antigen in bronchopulmonary lavage fluid has

100% sens, 98% specif (Am Rev Respir Dis 1992;145:226); for antibody, by indirect fluorescent antibody (IFA); 92% of pts are positive for one or the other in CSF and/or serum (Nejm 1977;297:1440); pts with positive antigen levels do more poorly; false-positive IFA in 2% of normals, 6% of blastomycosis, 12% of histoplasmosis. No false-positive antigen tests; hence rx a positive antigen but not a positive IFA (Ann IM 1968;69:1113, 1117).

Skin test: False positive in 31%; interferes with serologic testing (Ann IM 1968;69:45)

Xray: CT scan for mass lesions in head, which will decrease with medical rx (Ann IM 1981;94:382)

Rx: Isolation (Ann IM 1985;102:593)

- Amphotericin B 2-2.5 gm total course, 0.3-0.7 mg/kg iv qd (Nejm 1997;337:15), can rx q 1 wk in OPD. No proven advantage in intrathecal use (Ann IM 1969;71:1079), lots of complications especially with reservoir for intrathecal use (Nejm 1973;288:186).
- 5-Flucytosine 50-150 mg/kg/d po qid (Ann IM 1977;86:318; Nejm 1974;290:320); hematologic toxicity; use with amphotericin to prevent resistance and vs meningeal disease × 6 wk (Nejm 1979;301:126) or occasionally 4 wk in otherwise healthy (Nejm 1987;317:334); in AIDS meningitis rx w amphotericin and flucytosine × 2 wk then fluconazole or itraconazole prophylaxis (Nejm 1997;337:15, 1989;321:794)
- Fluconazole or itraconazole as good as and less toxic than amphotericin in AIDS pts with meningitis (Nejm 1992;326:83, 793); maintenance postepisode prevents recurrence in AIDS pts (Nejm 1997;337:15, 1991;324:580)
- Ketoconazole, or miconazole (Ann IM 1983;98:13, 1980;93:569) if above rx fails (p 613)

Histoplasmosis

Cause: *Histoplasma capsulatum*

Epidem: Bats and birds are vectors via airborne spores. Frequently in rolling green countryside (opposite of cocci), eg, Ohio Valley (100,000-pt outbreak in Indianapolis: Ann IM 1981;94:331)

Pathophys: Intracellular

3 clinical syndromes:

- Acute primary (pulmonary)
- Chronic cavitary (pulmonary)
- Progressive disseminated (Ann IM 1972;76:557)

Sx: Pulmonary, acute immune complex-type polyarthritis

Si: Chorioretinitis, focal, macular choroid inflammation, and hemorrhage without vitreous reaction (present with all other types of chorioretinitis)

Hepatomegaly; erythema nodosa

Crs: Usually benign

Cmplc:

- Fibrosing syndromes of mediastinum and/or retroperitoneum
- Endocarditis
- Adrenal insufficiency in 50% of disseminated form (Ann IM 1971;75:511)
- Meningitis, chronic, like cryptococcus
- Ulcerative enteritis, especially of distal ileum and colon

Lab: *Bact:* Silver stain demonstrates; can't see with H+E or Giemsa. Culture of liver, marrow, nodes; positive in ~20% (Ann IM 1982;97:680). Slow grower, takes > 2 wk; filamentous strands of hyphal sporangia; distinctive chlamydospores when grown at room temperature.

Hem: Anemia, thrombocytopenia; marrow culture and stain positive (all only in disseminated form: MKSAT 1980)

Serol (Ann IM 1982;97:680): Comp-fix antibody titer positive in 96% of pts with active, disseminated disease.

INFECTIOUS DISEASE

Immunodiffusion antibody titer positive in 87%. RIA for antigen positive in urine (90%) and blood (50%) in disseminated disease (Nejm 1986;314:83) and more accurate than antibody titers (Ann IM 1991;115:936).

Skin test: Many false positives and negatives, interferes with serologic testing (Am Rev Respir Dis 1964;90:927)

Xray: "Buckshot" calcifications in lungs, spleen

Rx: Steroids for choroid infections

1st: Amphotericin ½ mg/kg iv × 2/wk to a total of 35-40 mg/kg initial crs (Ann IM 1971;75:511); use prophylactically if past hx and starting steroids (Nejm 1969;280:206), or if pt has AIDS and has been rx'd to cure (Ann IM 1989; 111:655)

2nd: Ketoconazole, 400 mg qd po × 6 mo cures 85% all types (Ann IM 1985;103:861), even cavitary disease but not meningitis; or itraconazole (Sporanox) 200 mg po bid, prevents relapse in AIDS (Ann IM 1993;118:610)

Pneumocystis Pneumonia

Nejm 2004;350:2487

Cause: *Pneumocystis carinii,* reclassified as a fungus from protozoan status in 1988

Epidem: Opportunistic, from other people harboring (epidemics in tumor clinic: Ann IM 1975;82:772)

In pts with depressed immunologic responses, eg, hypogammaglobulinemia, "premies," hematopoietic malignancy, immunosuppression, AIDS (vast majority of pts with pneumocystis have AIDS), elderly (Nejm 1991;324:246)

Pathophys: Diffuse interstitial pneumonitis

Sx: Dyspnea, nonproductive cough

Si: Normal chest exam or rales; thrush often concomitantly

Crs: Die in weeks without rx (50%); with rx, mortality ≈ 3%; pts who require ventilator have 25% survival to hospital d/c (Jama 1995; 273:230)

Cmplc: Osteomyelitis rarely (Nejm 1992;326:999); r/o other opportunistic infections (p 670)

Lab: *Bact:* Hypertonic saline–induced sputum (Ann IM 1988;109:7), stain with Giemsa (72% sens), toluidine blue (80% sens), or indirect immunofluorescence (92% sens) (Nejm 1988;318:589)
Path: Fiberoptic bronchoscopic bx, lavage, brushings

Xray: Chest shows diffuse interstitial infiltrate, starts perihilar, 98% bilateral. Gallium scan shows hot lungs even with neg plain films, but 50% false positives including sarcoid pts (Nejm 1988; 318:1439).

Rx (Med Let 1995;37:87; Nejm 1992;327:1853; Ann IM 1988; 109:280):

Preventive (Nejm 1995;332:693; Ann IM 1995;122:755):
Isolation of infected from other susceptible patients?; under CD_4 of 100, Tm/S better than Dapsone, which is better than pentamidine

- Tm/S DS (Arch IM 1996;156:177, Nejm 1987;316:1627) tiw, qd or bid or SS qd, cheaper but tolerated less well than the other 2 (Nejm 1992;327:1836,1842)
- Atovaquone (Nejm 1998;339:1890) 1500 mg po qd, better tolerated than Dapsone as backup for Tm/S-intolerant pts
- Dapsone 50 mg po bid or qd or biw w pyrimethamine, or perhaps 100 mg po biw (Am J Med 1993;95:573), when Tm/S intolerant, also helps prevent toxoplasmosis
- Pentamidine aerosol neb 300 mg q 4 wk (Med Let 1989;31:91) iv q 2-4 wk, or supine (Ann IM 1990;113:677)
- Pyrimethamine + sulfadiazine (Fansidar) perhaps

Treatment:
- Tm/S 2-15 tab po qd as good as pentamidine (Ann IM 1986; 105:37); iv works too (Med Let 1981;23:102) as 10-20 mg/kg/d;

INFECTIOUS DISEASE

watch rash and marrow. In AIDS pts with severe disease, give w 40 mg methylprednisolone iv or po q 6 hr × 7 d, which markedly improves survival from 20% to 75% (Nejm 1990;323:1445,1451).

- Pentamidine 4 mg/kg/d × 12-14 d (Nejm 1972;287:495), better, less toxic in AIDS pts; watch creatinine
- Tm/Dapsone equally effective and only 30% become intolerant of it, unlike 60% with Tm/S (Nejm 1990;323:776)
- Trimetrexate with leucovorin rescue is equally effective (Med Let 1989;31:5; Nejm 1987;317:978)
- Atovaquone (Meprone) (Ann IM 1994;121:174; Med Let 1993;35:28; Nejm 1991;325:1534), a hydroxynaphthoquinone, 250 mg po tid, which also treats toxoplasmosis, may be reasonable backup to Tm/S

Systemic Candidiasis

Ann IM 1984;101:390

Cause: *Candida albicans* and rare species like *tropicalis* (Ann IM 1979;91:539), *cruzii,* and *glabrata,* which are often fluconazole resistant

Epidem: Associated with immunosuppression, antibiotics, TPN

Pathophys: Normal flora, opportunistic invasion

Sx: Rapid deterioration in a debilitated pt; suppurative peripheral thrombophlebitis (Ann IM 1982;96:431)

Si: Fever, papular/pustular rash like gc

Crs: 36+% mortality (Nejm 1994;331:1325)

Cmplc: Systemic type: Myocarditis, endophthalmitis ("a culture of fungus growing on retina") (Nejm 1972;286:675), hepatosplenic abscess (Ann IM 1988;108:88). Purportedly chronic fatigue syndrome, but doubtful (Nejm 1990;323:1717).

Lab: *Bact:* May grow on blood culture but distinction from benign contamination is difficult (Ann IM 1974;80:605)

Rx (Med Let 1990;32:58, 1988;30:30):

> 1st: Amphotericin or fluconazole (Nejm 1994;331:1325), perhaps
> caspofungin (Nejm 2002;347:2020)
>
> 2nd: Ketoconazole or perhaps high-dose flucytosine but resist-
> ance develops esp in HIV pts

Mucor Infections

Cause: *Mucorales* (*mucor, rhizopus*, etc) (Ann IM 1980;93:93)

Epidem: Skin infections from elastoplast tape (Nejm 1978;299:1115);
or sinusitis. Almost exclusively (25/26) in diabetics, usually in
DKA; occasionally in pts with hematologic tumors.

Pathophys: Pulmonary or CNS; invades vessels, causing infarcts without much inflammation

Sx: Pulmonary; CNS; skin and subcutaneous infections, swelling

Si: Vascular infarcts, "black pus"

Crs: Almost always fatal

Cmplc: r/o other opportunistics (p 670)

Lab: *Path:* Must do bx to diagnose

Rx: Amphotericin iv or topical for cutaneous type
Surgical debridement

Sporotrichosis

Nejm 1994;331:181

Cause: *Sporothrix schenkii*

Epidem: Prick from infected plant, of which many are saprophytes, or
inhalation. Worldwide; gardeners especially prone.

Pathophys: Biphasic fungus, mold in wild, yeast in body

Sx:

Si: Peripheral lesion with nodular lymphangitis or, in inhalation type,
pulmonary or systemic sx (Ann IM 1970;73:23) resulting in suppurative arthritis (Ann IM 1977;86:294), multiple skin nodules

Crs:

Cmplc: Chronic meningitis (Nejm 1987;317:935)
r/o (Ann IM 1993;119:883) tularemia (especially in hunters), nocardia, leishmaniasis, *Mycobacterium marinum*, *Pseudomonas pseudomallei*, histoplasmosis, cocci, blastomycosis

Lab: *Bact:* Diphasic, but yeast form (cigar shape) is arranged in aster-oid bodies in tissue; culture at 22°C results in leathery distinctive mycelial growth
Serol: CF titer ≥ 1/8 in systemic (not cutaneous) disease

Rx: 1st: Potassium iodide (KI) + iodine (I_2) (SSKI) 3 cc qd, increased to 9-12 cc qd (Nejm 1974;290:320); amphotericin B, or perhaps itraconazole
Surgical resection of pulmonary cavities

PARASITOLOGY

9.12 Medications

Antiparasitic Drugs

Many hard to obtain; contact CDC (Med Let 1998;40:1; Nejm 1996;334:1178

- Albendazole (Zentel) perhaps at 400 mg po qd × 5 d to all immigrants (Nejm 1999;340:773); for cutaneous and visceral larval migrans, pinworms, hookworms, hydatid cysts and cysticercosis, whipworms; adverse effects: occasionally reversible alopecia, LFT elevations, abdominal pain; rarely leukopenia, severe alopecia, severely elevated LFTs
- Artemether (Nejm 1996;335:69, 76, 124) 2-4 mg/kg im qd for cerebral falcip malaria; adverse effects: long QT syndrome
- Atovaquone (Mepron) 750 mg po tid × 21 d for pneumocystis, possibly malaria; adverse effects: rash, nausea, diarrhea
- Bithionol (Bitin) 30-50 mg/kg po × 10-15 doses for lung fluke and *Fasciola hepatica*; available from CDC only; adverse

effects: photosensitivity, emesis, diarrhea, urticaria; rarely leukopenia, hepatitis

- Chloroquine HCl, chloroquine phosphate (Aralen) 600 mg base (1 gm) or 10 mg/kg, then 300 mg base (500 mg) or 5 mg/kg at 6, 24, and 48 hr for malaria; 300 mg or 5 mg/kg base po q 1 wk for prophylaxis; also used occasionally in amebiasis; adverse effects: emesis, headache/confusion, pruritus, alopecia, weight loss, worsening of preexisting dermatitis, myalgias; rarely irreversible retinal damage, nail changes, neuronal deafness, peripheral neuropathy, myopathy, heart block, hematemesis

- Crotamiton (Eurax) 10% soln topically for scabies; adverse effects: rash, conjunctivitis

- Dapsone (DDS, diaminodiphenylsulfone) 100 mg po qd to prevent *P. carinii* pneumonia (Ann IM 1995;123:584); adverse effects: rashes, headache, gi, mono syndrome, etc

- Dehydroemetine 1-1.5 mg/kg/d im up to 5 d for severe amebiasis; adverse effects: arrhythmias, muscle weakness; occasional diarrhea, emesis, peripheral neuropathy, CHF, headache

- Diethylcarbamazine (Hetrazan) 50 mg or 1 mg/kg po on day 1, 50 mg or 1 mg/kg po tid day 2, 100 mg or 2 mg/kg po tid day 3, then 9 mg/kg/d divided for 21 d crs for filariasis; adverse effects: allergic/febrile reactions w heavy microfilarial load, gi sx; rarely encephalopathy

- Diethylmethylbenzamide (DEET) (Ann IM 1998;128:934) 35% slow release (HourGuard), or 6.5-10% SR formulations; insect repellant, lasts 3-4 hr, better than Skin-So-Soft, Citronella,or others

- Eflornithine (difluoromethylornithine, DFMO, Ornidyl) for trypanosomiasis; adverse effects: anemia, leukopenia, diarrhea, thrombocytopenia, seizures; rarely deafness

- Furazolidone (Furonone) 100 mg or 1.5 mg/kg po qid × 7-10 d for giardiasis; adverse effects: nausea/vomiting, anaphylactoid reactions, hypoglycemia, headache; rarely hemolytic anemia if G$_6$PD deficient, Antabuse reaction w alcohol, polyneuritis

- Iodoquinol (Yodoxin) 650 mg or 10-12 mg/kg po tid × 20 d for amebiasis and *Dientamoeba fragilis;* adverse effects: rash, acne, thyroidomegaly, diarrhea, anal itching; rarely optic neuritis; optic atrophy, peripheral neuropathy
- Ivermectin (Mectizan) for refractory scabies, onchocercal filariasis; adverse effects: malaise/fever w heavy worm load
- Lindane (Kwell) topically for lice and scabies; adverse effects: rash, headache, conjunctivitis; rarely seizures, aplastic anemia; all increased if skin vasodilated, eg, in warm weather
- Malarone (atovaquone/proguanil) (Med Let 2000;42:109) 250/100 mg po qd, start 1-2 d before arrive and keep up 1 wk after departure
- Malathion (Ovide) 0.5% topically for lice; adverse effects: local skin irritation
- Mebendazole (Vermox), varying doses for pinworm, filariasis, hookworm, whipworm, visceral larval migrans, ascariasis; adverse effects: diarrhea, abdominal pain; rarely leukopenia, hypospermia
- Mefloquine (Lariam) 250 mg or 25 mg/kg × 1; adverse effects: vertigo, gi sx, nightmares, headache, confusion; rarely psychoses, seizures, shock, coma, paresthesias
- Melarsoprol (Arsobal) 2-3.6 mg/kg/d iv × 3 d 1st wk, then 3.6 mg/kg/d × 3 d iv 2nd and 3rd wk for CNS trypanosomiasis/ Chagas' disease; adverse effects: cardiac injury, albuminuria, hypertension, colic, Herxheimer reaction, encephalopathy, emesis, peripheral neuropathy
- Metronidazole (Flagyl), various doses for amebiasis, trichomonas, *Balantidium coli,* tapeworm, giardia, hookworm, whipworm, visceral larval migrans; adverse effects: nausea/vomiting, headache, metallic taste, insomnia, stomatitis, rash, dysuria, paresthesias, Antabuse reaction to alcohol; rarely seizures, coli-

tis, encephalopathy, neuropathy, pancreatitis. No increase in cancer risk (Nejm 1979;301:519).

- Miltefosine (Impavido) (Nejm 2002;347:1739) 50-100 mg (2.5 mg/kg) po qd × 1 mo; for visceral leishmaniasis; 95% cures; adverse effects: emesis and diarrhea < 1-2 d in 20-40%
- Niclosamide (Niclocide) 50 mg/kg up to 2 gm × 1 chewed for fasciolopsis fluke and dwarf tapeworm; adverse effects: nausea, abdominal pain
- Nifurtimox (Lampit) 8-10 mg/kg/d po in qid doses × 120 d, double doses for children × 90 d for *T. cruzi* (Chagas' disease); adverse effects: anorexia, emesis, weight loss, sleep changes, tremor, paresthesias, polyneuritis, memory loss; rarely seizures, fever, pulmonary infiltrates
- Nitazoxanide (Alina) (Med Let 2003;45:29) 500 mg po qd-bid for adults, 100-200 mg bid for children, × 3 d; for giardia, cryptosporidiosis, and maybe many others; adverse effects: HA, gi, but minimal; $60/3 d for 200 bid
- Oxamniquine (Vansil) 15 mg/kg × 1, 10 mg/kg bid × 1 d for children, for *Schistosoma mansoni;* adverse effects: headache, fever, somnolence, diarrhea, rash, insomnia, LFT elevations, orange urine; rarely seizures, psych changes
- Paromomycin (aminosidine, Humatin) 25-30 mg/kg/d in tid dosing × 7 d for amebiasis, *Dientamoeba fragilis,* cryptosporidium; adverse effects: gi sx, VIII nerve damage (hearing), renal injury
- Pentamidine (Pentam) 2-4 mg/kg im/iv qd × 14-21 d for leishmaniasis, pneumocystis; adverse effects: hypotension, hypoglycemia/diabetes induction, emesis, renal damage, gi sx, local injection pain, hypocalcemia, cardiotoxicity, hepatotoxicity, delirium, rash; rarely anaphylaxis, pancreatitis, hyperkalemia because is similar to triamterene (Ann IM 1995;122:103)
- Permethrin (Nix, Elimite) topically 1% for lice, 5% for scabies; adverse effects: local irritation

- Praziquantel (Biltricide) 25 mg/kg tid × 1 d for flukes, schisto-somiasis, tapeworms; adverse effects: malaise, sedation, fever, eosinophilia, abdominal pain; rarely rash
- Primaquine 15 mg base (6.3 mg)/d or 0.3 mg base/kg/d × 14 d, or 45 mg base/wk × 8 wk for prevention of *P. vivax* and *ovale* relapse after leave area; adverse effects: hemolytic anemia in G_6PD pts, neutropenia, gi sx; rare CNS sx, hypertension, arrhythmias
- Pyrantel pamoate (Antiminth) 11 mg/kg (max = 1 gm) × 3 d for hookworm, 11 mg/kg × 1 repeat in 2 wk for pinworm; adverse effects: gi sx, headache, rash, fever
- Pyrethrins + piperonyl butoxide (RID) topically for lice; adverse effects: allergic reaction
- Pyrimethamine (Daraprim) 25-100 mg (1 mg/kg)/d × 3-4 wk w sulfadiazine for toxoplasmosis; adverse effects: folate defi-ciency; rarely rash, emesis, seizures
- Pyrimethamine-sulfadoxine (Fansidar), 3 tabs × 1 on last day of quinine for resistant falcip malaria; adverse effects: folate de-ficiency; rarely fatal Steven-Johnson syndrome, emesis, seizures
- Quinacrine (Atabrine) 100 mg or 2 mg/kg tid × 5 d for giar-diasis; no longer available in U.S.?; adverse effects: headache, emesis, diarrhea, yellow skin, psychoses, insomnia, blue nails, rash like psoriasis
- Sodium stibogluconate (Pentostam; pentavalent antimony) 20 mg Sb/kg/d iv/im × 21-28 d for leishmaniasis; adverse effects: myalgias, arthralgias (90%), LFT elevations (25%), T-wave inversions (30%), weakness, colic, bradycardia, leukopenia; rarely diarrhea, rash, MI, hemoytic anemia, renal damage
- Spiramycin (Rovamycine) 50-100 mg/kg up to 3-4 gm/d × 3-4 wk for toxoplasmosis during pregnancy; adverse effects: gi sx; rarely allergic reactions
- Suramin Na (Germanin) 100 mg test dose then 20 mg/kg up to 1 gm iv days 1, 3, 7, 14, 21 for sleeping sickness; adverse ef-

fects: emesis, urticaria, paresthesias, neuropathy, renal damage, optic atrophy

- Thiabendazole (Mintezol), various doses for angiostrongyliasis, cutaneous larval migrans, dracunculus, strongyloides; adverse effects: nausea/vomiting, vertigo, leukopenia, crystalluria, rash, hallucinations, erythema multiforme, smell changes; rarely tinnitus, cholestasis, seizures, angioneurotic edema
- Tinidazole (Tindamax) (Med Let 2004;46:70) like metronidazole for trichomonas (2 gm po × 1), giardiasis (2 gm po × 1), or amebiasis (2 gm po qd × 3 d) but more expensive

9.13 Protist Protozoans

Babesiosis

CPC: Nejm 2003;349:1168, 1993;329:943

Cause: *Babesia microti*

Epidem: Carried by ticks of cattle, deer mice, and deer (same as Lyme disease); or by transfusion of infected blood (Ann IM 1982;96:601)

> In southern New England, esp Nantucket; Fire Island, NY; Georgia; Mexico; California (Nejm 1995;332:298); Washington State (Ann IM 1993;119:284). Incidence increased in AIDS and splenectomized pts (Nejm 1980;303:1098).

Pathophys:

Sx: Fever, malaise

Si: Fever, lymphoma-like si's (Ann IM 1981;94:327)

Crs: 7 d incubation period. Days of fever; asx carriers, persistent longterm infection unless treated, and subclinical infections all common too (Nejm 1998;339:160). May be fatal.

Cmplc: r/o ehrlichiosis (p 602), Lyme disease (p 587) or concomitant infection w same

Lab: *Hem:* Intra-rbc parasites, look like malaria
  Serol: Indirect immunofluorescence antibody $\geq$ 1/64

Rx:

- Atovaquone + azithromycin, which has fewer side effects (Nejm 2000;343:1454)
- Quinine 650 mg or 8 mg/kg tid po + clindamycin 600 mg or 10 mg/kg po (or iv) tid $\times$ 7 d (Ann IM 1982;96:601), but tinnitus and abdominal distress result in 20% failing to complete crs (Nejm 1998;339:160)

  Exchange transfusion cures acute hemolytic crisis (Nejm 1980;303:1098)

Cryptosporidium Diarrhea

Nejm 2002;346:1723, 1994;331:161

Cause: *Cryptosporidium spp.*

Epidem: Fecal–oral dissemination from humans or cattle (Am J Pub Hlth 1989;79:1528) or contaminated water supplies (Nejm 1994;331:161), even those w filtered water treatment systems (Ann IM 1996;124:459)

  Common cause of traveler's and other self-limited diarrhea, 10% prevalence in developing countries; increased under age 4 yr, especially in day care centers; associated with giardia for that reason. 6% of diarrhea in immunocompetent pts; 24% in AIDS/HIV pts.

Pathophys:

Sx: Usually watery, nonbloody diarrhea (86-93%) $\times$ 12 d on average; occasional abdominal cramps (84%); vomiting (48%); anorexia (20%); fever (12-57%); weight loss (20%); nausea (12%)

Si:

Crs: 7-10 d incubation period, 6-12 d course; all immunocompetent hosts recover (Nejm 1986;315:1643)

Cmplc: Chronic cholecystitis/cholangitis as well as dissemination in AIDS and other immunocompromised pts

r/o similar intestinal spore-forming protozoa (Ann IM 1996;124:429):

Cyclospora cayetanensis, coccidia-like organism (Nejm 1993;328:1308); causes fatigue and malabsorption w chronic infection (Ann IM 1995;123:409, 1993;119:377), water-borne epidemics (Central American imported raspberries: Nejm 1997;336:1548), and especially in AIDS pts; prophylaxis and rx w Tm/S (Ann IM 1994;121:654) or cipro as 2nd choice (Ann IM 2000;132:885)

Enterocytozoon bienensis, intracellular microsporidial protozoan (p 409)

Isospora belli, rx with Tm/S, pyrimethamine (Ann IM 1988;109:474; Nejm 1986;315:87), or cipro (Ann IM 2000;132:885)

Lab: *Bact:* Ziehl-Neelsen acid-fast stain of stool for O+P; 10% false neg; 75% still have present in stool after sx subside (Nejm 1986; 315:1643)

Rx: Preventive: Avoid contaminated water; chlorination not adequate

Supportive; and, if necessary as in AIDS, nitazoxanide (Alina); or alternatively parmomycin 500 mg po tid × 2 wk, 500 mg bid maintenance; spiramycin, azithromycin, or furazolidone

Amebic Dysentery

Nejm 2003;348:1565

Cause: *Entamoeba histolytica*, rarely *Dientamoeba fragilis*

Epidem: Encysted organisms excreted in feces, contaminates water or food; human carriers disseminate. Degree of infestation correlates inversely with sanitation. Increased prevalence in mental hospitals and gay males.

Pathophys: Trophozoite (amoebic form) invades wall of colon, secretes autolyzing enzymes, and lives on necrotic tissue in abscess; multiplies by binary fission

Sx: Fever, bloody stool, alternating diarrhea and constipation

Si:

Crs:

Cmplc: Abscess metastases to liver, lung, brain, pericardium, spleen, skin (ulcers)

r/o the much more benign **Ciliate Dysentery** caused by *Balantidium coli*, and nonpathogenic strains of *E. histolytica*, which are commensals in gay males (Nejm 1986;315:353,390)

Lab: *Serol:* Elevated antibody titers, < 10% false neg (Ann IM 1969;71:983); 95% pos after 7+ d of sx in colitis or liver abscess (Gut 1994;35:1018)

Stool: ELISA fluorescent antibody staining; O+P rarely used now but positive in 90% of pts with severe colonic disease, cysts with 4 nuclei, central nucleolus often overdiagnosed by lab technicians thinking wbc's are ameba (Ann IM 1978;88:89)

Xray: BE shows deformed cecum, narrowed; rarely megacolon

Rx: Prevent w tetraglycine hydroperiodate, kills cysts in 30 min; water chlorination doesn't kill cysts

of asx disease: Iodoquinol 650 mg or 10 mg/kg po tid × 20 d; or paromomycin 8-10 mg/kg po tid × 7 d

of intestinal disease: Metronidazole 10-12 mg/kg or 750 mg po tid × 10 d; or tinidazole (not available in U.S.) 50 mg/kg up to 2 gm/d × 3-5 d followed by paromomycin

of hepatic abscess: Metronidazole as above; or tinidazole (not available is U.S.) 800 mg tid × 5 d

Amebic Meningoencephalitis

Ann IM 1978;88:468

Cause: *Naegleria gruberi* and *Acanthamoeba spp.*

Epidem: Worldwide; natural inhabitant of freshwater; in patients who have been swimming in past week; very rare

Pathophys: Meningoencephalitis with predilection for olfactory, cerebellar, and temporofrontal areas; later develop hematogenous spread and often fatal myocarditis. May invade via nose through cribriform plate and into olfactory bulb.

Sx: Headache, swam within past week, fever (*Acanthamoeba* can also cause ocular keratitis in contact lens wearers)

Si: Parosmia (funny smells), cerebellar ataxia, meningoencephalitis without increased CNS pressure

Crs: Almost universally fatal in 4-5 d

Cmplc: Death

Lab: *CSF:* Purulent meningitis with "bubbly" amoeba on high-power wet mount
Path: Organisms in all organs but gi tract

Rx: A few survivors now (Nejm 1982;306:346; Ann IM 1971;74:923)
Amphotericin B iv and perhaps intracisternally; perhaps ketoconazole, or flucytosine (p 613)
of keratitis: Topical 0.1% propamidine + neosporin; or itraconazole po + topical miconazole

Malaria

Clin Infect Dis 1993;16:449; Nejm 1983;308:875-934

Cause: *Plasmodium vivax, ovale, malariae, falciparum*

Epidem: Sporozoites (in mosquito salivary gland) enter via puncture wound of bite, undergo exoerythrocytic schizogony into merozoites, which evolve into trophozoites (ring forms), then into erythrocyte schizonts or into macro- and microgametocytes, which are then ingested by mosquitoes
Distribution: *Vivax* in SE Asia, S. America; *ovale* in W. Africa; *malariae* in Africa; *falciparum* in Africa, Asia, Oceania, S. America

INFECTIOUS DISEASE

Vector: Anopheles *Aedes culex* mosquito. Patients heterozygous for HgbS, HgbC, HgbE, or G_6PD may be more resistant. Duffy blood group FyFy completely protected vs *vivax* (Nejm 1976;295:302).

Increased susceptibility during pregnancy and 2 mo postpartum (Nejm 2000;343:598), probably due to immunosuppression of pregnancy

Pathophys: 3-4 hr fevers, as endotoxins, including tumor necrosis factor (Nejm 1990;320:1586), are released when schizonts rupture into merozoites synchronously in blood. *Vivax* infects young (retics) rbc's only; *malariae*, old rbc's only. *Falciparum* infects all rbc's and causes "sticky" rbc's that infarct in brain, kidney, lung (Nejm 1968;279:732); no exoerythrocytic phase, hence no late recurrences.

Sx: *Vivax:* 6-15 d incubation, tertian (qod) fever but 2 crops can cause qd fevers; onset of sx can be months after return (Nejm 2003;349:1510)

Malariae: 20-25 d incubation, quartan (q 3 d) fevers

Ovale: Quotidian (qd) fevers; onset of sx can be months after return (Nejm 2003;349:1510)

Falcip: < 30 d incubation, tertian (qod) fevers but variable

Si: Splenomegaly (*vivax* = 25%, *falcip* = 80%). Black water fever is hemoglobinuria from massive hemolysis (*falcip*).

Crs: 3.5% mortality for falcip in children, usually within 24 hr, especially if change in consciousness, jaundice, repiratory distress, or hypoglycemia (Nejm 1995;332:1399)

Cmplc: *Vivax:* Tropical splenomegaly syndrome (Nejm 1984;310:337)

Malariae: Recurrence decades later possible (Nejm 1998;338:367)

Falcip: DIC (Ann IM 1969;70:134); CVA, coma (steroids no help: Nejm 1982;306:313); hypoglycemia correlates with severe *falcip* disease and diminished hepatic gluconeogenesis, associated with severe morbidity and mortality in 50% (Nejm 1988;319:1040)

r/o babesiosis in U.S. (p 631)

Lab: *Hem: Vivax:* Single infections of only young (big) rbc's; circulating older ameboid trophozoites and schizonts; 16 merozoites/schizont; Schüffner's dots (small, eosinophilic) in rbc. *Ovale:* Oval rbc's, often fringed at one end. *Ovale* and *malariae:* "Band-like" trophs; 8 merozoites/schizont. *Falcip:* Multiple infections of each rbc; all ages and sizes of rbc's; only young, small ring trophozoites (older trophs and schizonts in RES): 24 merozoites/schizont; Mauer's dots in rbc (eosinophilic, larger).

Serol: Rapid histidine-rich protein 2 or 3 tests; 94% sens, 97% specif; available in Europe (Ann IM 2005;142:836)

Rx (Nejm 1996;335:800; CDC phone: 770-488-7788):
Prevent w DEET (< 35%) insect repellant, screening, long sleeves; vaccine vs sporozoite, becoming practical (Nejm 1997;336:86)

 Prophylaxis (Jama 1997;278:1767, Med Let 2002;44:33):
for all including resistant falcip (Ann IM 1997;126:963) (all areas except Central America, Carribean, and parts of Middle East):
1st:

- Atovaquone/proguanil (Malarone) (Med Let 2000;42:109) 250/100 mg po qd, start 1-2 d before arrive and keep up 1 wk after departure; $106/14 d; or
- Mefloquine (Lariam) 250 mg po 1 wk before arrival and q 1 wk until 4 wk after departure, but worsening of psych and seizure disorders, and variants of fatigue and malaise limit use (ACP J Club 2001;135:68); $70/14 d; or
- Doxycycline 100 mg qd; $23/14 d

2nd:

- Chloroquine and primaquine 30 mg po qd through the week after departure from area (Ann IM 1998;129:241) + Fansidar (pyrimethamine + sulfadoxine) q 1 wk + proguanil 200 mg po qd; or
- Fansidar tabs to take prn fever (avoids severe allergic reactions: Ann IM 1987;106:714)

for all except resistant falcip:

- Choroquine PO$_4$ 300 mg base (500 mg) q wk, 1 wk prior and 6 wk after leave, +
- Primaquine PO$_4$ 15 mg base (26 mg) with last 2 wk of above to radically cure exoerythrocytic phases
    of active disease (Nejm 2005;352:1565; call CDC or visit website):

For all except resistant falcip:

- Chloroquine 600 mg base (1 gm), then 300 mg at 12, 24, and 36 hr; or in severely ill, 10 mg base/kg iv over 8 hr then 15 mg/kg over 24 hr, or 35 mg/kg im/sc q 6 hr or via NG, +
- Primaquine as above

For resistant falcip:

- Quinine sulfate 650 mg po tid × 3-7 d, followed by Fansidar 3 tab × 1, or
- Tetracycline 250 mg qid × 7 d, or
- Clindamycin 900 mg po tid × 3 d, or
- Mefloquine 15 mg base/kg po then 10 mg/kg 8-24 hr later, or
- Quinidine gluconate 10 mg/kg over 1-2 hr iv then 0.02 mg/kg/min constant infusion until can take po + exchange transfusion if > 10% rbc's infected (Nejm 1989; 321:65)
- Artesunate 4 mg/kg qd × 3 w Fansidar (Lancet 2000;355:352)

For cerebral and severe falcip malaria:

- Quinine 10 mg/kg iv/im q 8 hr after 20 mg initial dose, or
- Artemether 2 mg/kg im q 8 hr after 4 mg/kg load (Nejm 1996; 335:69,76,124)
- Deferoxamine iron chelation speeds recovery in falcip pediatric cerebral malaria by denying organism its vitamins! (Nejm 1992; 327:1473)

Toxoplasmosis

Nejm 1985;313:957, 1978;298:550; Ann IM 1976;84:193

Cause: *Toxoplasma gondii*

Epidem: Cats are primary hosts, usually transmitted via cat feces?, contaminated water (Nejm 1982;307:666), or dust (Nejm 1979; 300:695); also from poorly cooked meat

15-30% of U.S. population have had; especially in wet, hot areas

Immunosuppression can induce. Fetus very susceptible; 40% contract disease when mother gets primary infection between 2 and 6 mo gestation (Nejm 1974;290:110). Increased in AIDS as an opportunistic infection.

Pathophys: Inflammation and scarring in brain, liver, spleen, heart, eye. Cysts are inert. Eye lesions probably are due to delayed hypersensitivity reactions. Congenital form somewhat different clinical pattern than acquired.

Sx: Acquired (Nejm 1979;300:695): fever (90%), headache (85%), myalgia (60%), rash (20%)
Congenital: Rash

Si: Acquired: Lymphadenopathy (85%), rash (20%), chorioretinitis
Congenital: Chorioretinitis (100%), icterus, rash, hepatosplenomegaly, hydrops, hydrocephalus

Crs:

Cmplc: Acquired: Meningoencephalitis (50%); r/o lymphoma (Ann IM 1969;70:514); myocarditis

Lab: *CSF:* Congenital: organisms on Wright's stain and grow in mice
Path: Intracellular blue with red cytoplasm; can look like intracellular "grapes" when multiplying in cell. Do brain bx in AIDS pts w meningoencephalitis if don't respond to pyrimethamine + clindamycin within 2 wk (Nejm 1993; 329:995).
Serol: Indirect fluorescent antibody positive if > 1:1000; comp-fix antibody and Sabin-Feldman dye test (interpretation of various mother–child combinations: Nejm 1978;298: 550). IgM titers now available.

Xray: Acquired: CT of head shows focal encephalitis with enhancing rings (Nejm 1988;318:1439)

Congenital: In utero, cerebral calcifications and bony "white puffs"

Rx:

Congenital: Prevent w screening titer at 1st OB visit, then q 1 mo toxo titers (if elevated but stable, no problem), and in exposed seronegative pregnant women; abort if convert and fetal infection documented, eg, by amniocentesis PCR methods (Nejm 1994;331:695); or rx with spiramycin; or pyrimethamine + sulfa, which results in 13/15 healthy newborns, other 2 had only retinitis (France: Nejm 1988;318: 271). Or screen newborns for IgM toxo titers; this detected 1 case/6000 infants in New England and subsequent rx allows prevention of future eye disease (Njem 1994;330:1858).

Acquired: 1st choice is pyrimethamine 25-100 mg/d or 2 mg/kg/d × 3 d then 1 mg/kg/d up to 25 mg + sulfadiazine 1-2 gm or 25-50 mg/kg qid × 3-4 wk; or pyrimethamine + clindamycin 1200 mg qid (Nejm 1993;329:995; Ann IM 1992; 116:33), which is preferable in AIDS because 40% of such pts can't tolerate sulfa. Alternative is spiramycin 3-4 gm/kg or 50-100 mg/kg/d × 3-4 wk.

of eye involvement: Steroids

9.14 Flagellate Protozoans

Giardia Diarrhea and Malabsorption

Nejm 1978;298:319

Cause: *Giardia lamblia*

Epidem: Encysted form excreted in feces, ingested by new host, resides in duodenum. Animal reservoirs: beaver, dog, muskrat, perhaps deer.

Occurs in areas of poor sanitation with raw rural surface (not ground) water; gay males; SE Asian refugees. Associated with globulin deficiencies, especially of IgA; achlorhydria, nodular lymphoid hyperplasia.

Pathophys: Malabsorption due to mechanical obstruction of duodenum; hence fat absorption is especially hard hit

Sx: Loose, watery stools (93%), malaise (80%), bloating and cramps (75%), fatigue, weight loss (73%); true diarrhea in only 30%

"Traveler's diarrhea" that often doesn't start until return from a trip, ie, delayed onset

Si:

Crs: 10 d incubation period, 10+ wk duration

Cmplc: Malabsorption, upper gi bleed rarely

Lab: *Bact:* Stool O+P, 70% false neg; "2-eyed" (nuclei) flagellated trophozoite, or 4-nucleated cyst. Examination of duodenal aspirate or small bowel bx (< 10% false neg).
Serol: Giardia antigen in stool

Rx: Prevent by avoiding sewage contamination of water supplies; filtration; iodine as 2% soln, 0.4 cc/L of water; or heating to 70°C (158°F) × 10 min (Am J Pub Hlth 1989;79:1633). Chlorination probably inadequate even at 8 mg Cl⁻/L × 10 min.
of active disease:

- Metronidazole (Flagyl), 1st, 250 mg or 5 mg/kg tid × 5-7 d; or tinidazole; or alternatively
- Furazolidone 100 mg or 1.25 mg/kg qid × 5 d; no carcinogenicity
- Nitazoxanide (Alina) (Med Let 2003;45:20) 500 mg po bid (100-200 mg bid in children)

Leishmania: Visceral (Kala-Azar) and Mucosal/Cutaneous

Nejm 1993;328:1383; Ann IM 1993;118:779 (cutaneous), 1990;113:934

Cause: *Leishmania donovani* (Kala-azar); *L. tropica, L. major,* and *L. braziliensis* (mucocutaneous)

Epidem: Sandfly feeds in evening and ingests parasitized cell, ruptures, and becomes leptomonad stage, which reproduces in fly gut, then migrates to mouth parts where is injected with next bite, and, as leptomonad stage, migrates to RES cells, where becomes leishmania form that bursts and invades other cells. Recurrent disease in immunocompromised hosts, eg, HIV pts.

Animal reservoirs (eg, dogs, rodents, sloths); human-to-human contact transmission also possible, skin-to-skin in cutaneous types

Indigenous in Asia (India, Nepal), Africa, Middle East (Gulf War regions), and tropical S. America, where there are 2000 cases/2 million/yr

Pathophys: Organisms in macrophages; suppressor T cells keep delayed hypersensitivity to leishmania antigens turned off (Nejm 1982;306:387). Cutaneous lesions often heal only to develop mucocutaneous disease years later.

Sx: Kala-azar: Long incubation period, weight loss, diarrhea
Mucosal/cutaneous: Slow-healing skin ulcers, nasal mucosa, other areas of oropharynx in severe disease

Si: Kala-azar: Fever, hepatosplenomegaly
Mucosal/cutaneous: Large ulcers, scars

Crs: Kala-azar: Chronic, fatal without rx

Cmplc: Kala-azar: Gi and pulmonary superinfections; rarely amyloid and cirrhosis

Lab: *Bact:* Culture all above
Hem: Depressed wbc counts
Path: Typical, 1-3 μ Leishmania-Donovan bodies in monocytes, lymph nodes, spleen, skin lesions, marrow, liver

Rx: • Pentavalent antimony as sodium stibogluconate (Pentostam) 20 mg Sb/kg/d iv/im × 21-28 d + perhaps

- Miltefosine (Impavido) (Nejm 2002;347:1739,1793) 50-100 mg po qd × 4 wk, cures 95%, adverse effects: gi in 20+%, teratogenic
- γ-Interferon 100 μgm/m^2 im qd × 10 d results in 90% cure of cutaneous and visceral (Nejm 1990;322:16); but not yet clearly 1st choice (Nejm 1990;322:55); 70% cure in mild-moderate mucocutaneous type but only 20% in severe disease (Ann IM 1990;113:934)
- Amphotericin B, or pentamidine possibly
- Allopurinol 20 mg/kg qd in qid doses × 15 d, eg, 300 mg po qid (Nejm 1992;326:741); no help w mucocutaneous form
- Fluconazole 200 mg po qd × 6 wk for cutaneous form (Nejm 2002;346:891); clears 50% by 8 wk

Trichomonas Urethritis/Vaginitis

Nejm 1997;337:1896

Cause: *Trichomonas vaginalis*

Epidem: Venereal; 10-25% of U.S. adult female population carries asymptomatically; present in 30-40% of male partners of infected women

Pathophys:

Sx: Profuse, watery vaginal discharge in women, or urethritis in males (rarer, many asx: Ann IM 1993;119:844); dyspareunia

Si: Erythematous cervicitis

Crs:

Cmplc: PROM and postpartum endometritis
r/o bacterial vaginosis (p 550) and candidal vaginitis (p 191)

Lab: *Bact:* Wet prep shows motile, 20μ flagellate with axostyle undulating membrane, 50-70% sensitivity, 100% specificity (Am J Med 2000:108:301); culture possible; rapid DNA and monoclonal antibody tests are 90% sens and 99.8% specif (Am J Med 2000:108:301)

Path: Pap smear presence has 60% sens, 97% specif (Am J Med 2000:108:301)

Vaginal discharge pH = 5-6, w amine smell on "whiff test"

Rx   (CDC: Ann IM 2002;137:255; Med Let 1999;41:86):

Metronidazole 2 gm × 1 po to pt and partner, 90% cure; or 375-500 mg po bid × 7 d, 85-90% cure; local rx no good; ok in pregnancy but does not decrease prematurity complications (Nejm 2001;345:487)

Tinidazole 2 gm po × 1, 2nd choice

in pregnancy: Can use metronidazole; Betadine douche to control sx suppresses fetal thyroid

Chagas' Disease

Nejm 1993;329:639, 1991;325:763

Cause: *Trypanosoma cruzi*

Epidem: Trypanosome stage in blood ingested by reduviid (triatoma) insect, multiply in insect's gi tract into metacyclic stage. Bug infected for life, no vertical transmission; metacyclic stage in feces near bite, enters wound or transferred manually by host to eye and elsewhere; multiplication only in intracellular form, which then ruptures, leading to trypanosomes in blood.

Animal (rodent) reservoirs. Central and South America. Rarely via blood transfusion (Ann IM 1989;111:849, 851) or congenital if placental defect.

Acute form in children; chronic in adults who had acute form in past

Pathophys:

Acute: Infection of muscle fibers, glial cells, and others; after rupture, fibrosis and granulomas develop

Chronic: Autoimmune reaction leads to cardiac fibrosis; diminished ganglionic cells in gut lead to esophageal and colon dilatation

Sx: Acute: Fever

Chronic: CHF, gi sx of megaesophagous and megacolon

Si: Acute: Hepatosplenomegaly, lymphadenopathy. Chagomas = local tissue swelling in skin, especially in children. Unilateral eye swelling (Romaña's si).

Chronic: CHF, heart block, angina, Vtach, or other cardiac involvement in 30-40% eventually

Crs: Acute: 4-6 wk, 5% mortality

Chronic: Sx appear years later in 10-30%

Cmplc:

Acute: encephalitis, asx CNS disease common (Nejm 1978;298:604); myocarditis, r/o Chagas' disease whenever any appropriately exposed pt has ischemic heart disease or dilated cardiomyopathy

Chronic: Recrudescence w immunosuppression

Lab: *Bact:* Acute: Culture from blood or tissue on NNN (type of blood agar)

Hem: Acute: Organisms in peripheral smear, especially buffy coat; prominent kinetoplast; undulating membrane

Chronic: No organisms

Noninv: Thallium ETTs and EKGs appear like MI

Path: Chronic: Organisms in tissue sections in only 25%

Serol: Acute: Comp-fix titer elevated but hemagglutination titer increased first

Chronic: IgG ELISA titer (sens/specif as yet unspecified); or comp-fix titer (Ann IM 1969;71:983) and others; all have a high false-pos rate

Rx: None very good; nifurtimox (Rev Inf Dis 1986;8:884) 8-10 mg/kg/d po divided qid × 120 d; alternative, benznidazole

Sleeping Sickness

Ann IM 1977;86:633

Cause: *Trypanosoma gambiense, rhodesiense*

Epidem: Via tse-tse fly (*Glossina sp.*) from ungulate reservoir; Africa, occasionally seen in returning U.S. visitors

Inoculation through bite of fly, local multiplication, parasitemia in 3 wk, sucked up by fly, develops in fly gut, then migrates to salivary glands

Pathophys: Vascular cuffing and obliteration in CNS; destruction of lymph nodes leading to fibrosis

Sx: Fever, weight loss

Si: Edema of face, etc; hyperesthesia; splenomegaly; cervical lymph nodes; rash; chancre

Crs: Virulent (fatal in days), to chronic

Cmplc: Encephalitis w apathy and somnolence punctuated by intermittent mania

Lab: *Hem and CSF:* Wet smear shows many polymorphic, squirming organisms

Serol: Comp-fix or agglutination antibody elevations

Rx: Prevent w insecticide, use to clear brush around homes of tse-tse fly; relocation to urban areas

Prophylaxis w suramin or pentamidine, but risk of disease is less than the toxicity of drugs (Ann IM 1972;77:797)

of early disease: Above drugs.

of late disease: Melarsoprol, eflorinthine.

9.15 Cestode Helminths

Tapeworms

Nejm 1992;327:692,696,727, 1984;310:298

Cause: *Taenia saginata* (beef), *T. solium* (pork); *Diphyllobothrium latum* (fish); *Hymenolepsis nana* (dwarf tapeworm)

Epidem: Adult worms in "definitive" carnivore hosts (dog, bears, etc), eggs in feces eaten by humans or herbivorous animals ("intermediate hosts") and then encyst in muscle, etc. In *T. solium* and dwarf, humans can be a definitive host or an intermediate host (muscle encystment) via autoinoculation or fecal–oral transmission, eg, in food handlers or in families; humans are only definitive hosts, ie, worm is in gi tract.

Seen especially in children and the retarded. Dwarf tapeworm is most common in U.S. *T. solium* is endemic in Mexico and in many immigrants, eg, in California.

Pathophys:

Sx: *Taenia* and *D. latum:* Rarely cause sx besides complaints of passage in stool

Dwarf: Diarrhea and occasionally obstructive gi sx

Si:

Crs:

Cmplc: *D. latum:* B_{12} and folate deficiencies

T. solium: Cysticercosis in brain (seizures), muscle, and skin (50%); sx may take 4-5 yr to develop when larva dies (Nejm 1984;311:1492)

Lab: *Bact:* Stool O+ P shows characteristic ova and gravid segments in all but echinococcus

Serol: IHA titers increased with *T. solium* cysticercosis

Xray: In cysticercosis, skull films and CT of head (Nejm 2000; 343:420) show calcifications

Rx: For adult forms, in gi tract, of *Taenia, D. latum,* and dwarf:
- Praziquantel 5-10 mg/kg × 1; 99% effective (Ann IM 1989;110:290); or
- Niclosamide 2 gm (500 mg under age 2, 1 gm age 2-12 yr) once (89% cure), then 1 gm (500 mg age 2-12 yr) po qd × 5 d

For *T. solium* cysticercosis: Surgical excision; albendazole as above or praziquantel + dexamethasone (Nejm 1984;311:1492; Ann IM 1983;99:179)

Echinococcal (Hydatid) Cyst Disease

Nejm 2003;348:447

Cause: *Echinococcus granulosus* and *multilocularis* (hydatid cyst); sometimes *T. solium*

Epidem: Humans are only intermediate hosts, ie, they do not spread eggs in stool, rather have only encysted organisms

Pathophys: Like neoplasms, echinococcal cysts grow over years with the appearance of secondary cysts

Sx:

Si: Mass effects anywhere

Crs:

Cmplc:

Lab: *CSF:* In cysticercosis: Aseptic picture with low sugar; eosinophils
Serol: IHA titers increased (from CDC) are pos in 90% with liver, 75% with lung involvement

Rx: Albendazole 5 mg/kg po tid × 28-56 d + either surgical or percutaneous drainage (Nejm 1997;337:881)

for *T. solium* cysticercosis: Surgical excision; albendazole as above or praziquantel + dexamethasone (Nejm 1984;311:1492; Ann IM 1983;99:179). In cerebral cysticercosis: Rx only w albendazole 800 mg + dexamthasone 6 mg po qd × 10 d, not seizure meds (Nejm 2004;350:249).

9.16 Trematode Helminths

Clonorchiasis, Liver Fluke

Nejm 1984;310:298

Cause: *Clonorchis sinensis*

Epidem: Embryonated egg in feces is ingested by snail, where becomes a miracidium, then a sporocyst, and eventually redia (2nd site of multiplication); then evolves to free-swimming cercaria, which penetrate under fish scales and are ingested, then mature into adults, which migrate to bile ducts

Animal reservoirs, dogs and cats. Common wherever poorly cooked fish are eaten, especially Asia.

Pathophys: Adults survive 30+ yr, causing fibrosing response

Sx:

Si: Mild hepatitis

Crs:

Cmplc:

Lab: *Bact:* Stool smear shows embryonated eggs, also in duodenal aspirates

Rx: Praziquantel 25 mg/kg tid × 1 d (Ann IM 1989;110:290)

Fasciolopsiasis and Paragonimiasis

Cause: Fasciolopsiasis: *Fasciola hepatica* (sheep liver fluke)
Paragonimiasis: *Paragonimus westermani*

Epidem: Similar to clonorchis except metacercaria encysts on water plants (fasciolopsiasis) or crustaceans (paragonimiasis)
Fasciolopsiasis: Worldwide wherever sheep are raised and human manure is used to fertilize salad foods
Paragonimiasis: Mink farms in U.S.; SE Asia

Pathophys: Fasciolopsiasis: In adult, "snowplows" through liver to reach biliary system
Paragonimiasis: Hypersensitivity response to encysted adults

Sx: Fasciolopsiasis: Fever, urticaria
Paragonimiasis: Hemoptysis, seizures (brain cysts)

Si: Fasciolopsiasis: Fever, hepatosplenomegaly

Crs:

Cmplc:

Lab: *Bact:* Stool, sputum, urine show operculated eggs

Rx: Fasciolopsiasis: Bithionol (Nejm 1972;287:995) (adverse effects: pneumonias as organisms killed) or praziquantel
Paragonimiasis: Praziquantel 25 mg/kg tid × 1 d (Ann IM 1989;110:290)

Schistosomiasis

Nejm 2002;346:1212; Am J Pub Hlth 2004;94:738 (swimmer's itch)

Cause: *Schistosoma mansoni, japonicum,* and *haematobium*; swimmer's itch from *S. dermatidis* (Maine Epigram 8/87)

Epidem: Free-swimming cercaria penetrate skin or are ingested, become schistosomula in blood, and mature into adults in blood vessels. They then deposit in body tissues selectively (*S. mansoni* and *S. japonicum* about gi tract, *S. haematobium* about bladder); there they mate and lay eggs that work out to feces or urine, are excreted into water where become miracidium, which invade a snail and reproduce again, and eventually are released as cercaria. Can live 30-40 yr in humans.

In *S. dermatidis* swimmer's itch, only cercarial penetration of skin by nonhuman schistosomes occurs; cycle stopped there

S. mansoni in Caribbean, Africa, Middle East; *S. haematobium* in Africa, Asia, and Middle East; *S. japonicum* in Asia (Nejm 1983;309:1533); *S. dermatidis* in marine or fresh water

Pathophys: Focal granulomas, fibrosis, vasculitis
Swimmer's itch due to allergic reaction to worms on 2nd exposure

Sx: Chills, diarrhea, abdominal pain, weight loss, bloody urine/stool
S. dermatidis: Swimmer's itch

Si: Hepatosplenomegaly (70%), fever (60%), diarrhea (60%)
S. dermatidis: Skin welts or swelling

Crs:

Cmplc: Granulomatous response to eggs anywhere, including brain, skin, liver with cirrhosis and varices, gu tract with obstruction and secondary infections (Ann IM 1971;75:49) and immune complex nephritis (Ann IM 1975;83:148)

in swimmer's itch: r/o sea bather's eruptions from anemone medusae (Nejm 1993;329:542)

Lab: *Bact:* Stool/urine show typical eggs: *S. japonicum*, round; *S. ahematobium*, single-tailed; *S. mansoni*, forked-tailed
Hem: Eosinophils increased
Path: Bx of rectum, liver, bladder may show eggs
Serol: Immunofluorescent antibody titers; skin test pos after 20 wk (10/10)

Rx: Praziquantel 20 mg/kg bid × 1 d; good vs all types; 70% cure (Nejm 1984;310:298)
Swimmer's itch: No rx

9.17 Nematode Helminths

Hookworms

Nejm 2004;351:799

Cause: *Ancylostoma duodenale* and *Necator americanus*

Epidem: Larvae penetrate skin in filariform stage (5 d older than rhabditiform stage), or larvae ingested in feces
Africa, Asia, southern Europe, and U.S.; associated w bare-foot walking and poor sewage

Pathophys: Skin penetration, into circulation, then to lung, into tra-chea, to pharynx, where swallowed and then attach to small intestine, where they result in chronic blood loss

Sx: "Ground itch" rash at entry site, usually feet. Cough and sore throat 10 d later when larvae migrate to lungs to be coughed up and swallowed. Apathy from iron-deficiency anemia.

Si: Anemia, 150-200 cc/d with *Ancylostoma* when severe infestations; *Necator* ¹/₅ as much, ~0.03 cc/d/worm

Crs:

Cmplc: CHF, anasarca

  r/o *Ancylostoma caninum,* dog hookworm, which can infect humans and cause abdominal pain (Ann IM 1994;120:369)

Lab: *Bact:* Stool O+P shows eggs that are same size as ascaris, w thin delicate shell; hatch in 24 hr into rhabidiform larvae, which molt into filariform larvae. Can quantify eggs and estimate number of worms.

  Hem: Hgb as low as 1-3 gm; Fe-deficiency anemia; esosinophilia

Rx: Mebendazole (Vermox) 500 mg po × 1 or 100 mg bid × 3 d; or albendazole 400 mg po × 1; either dosing is for all ages and weights

  $FeSO_4$ for the anemia

Larva Migrans

Nejm 2004;351:799

Cause:

  Cutaneous, "creeping eruption": *Ancylostoma braziliense* and *caninum*

  Visceral: *Toxocara canis* and raccoon ascaris

Epidem:

  Cutaneous: Dog and cat hookworm larvae penetrate skin but never get into circulation; children get when crawl under buildings

  Visceral: Ingestion of dog feces w eggs; 20% of U.S. dogs have it. Eggs survive several winters. 10% of adults in U.S. have serologic evidence of it.

Pathophys:
> Cutaneous: Larvae in skin cause local inflammation; can't penetrate dermal/epidermal junction
> Visceral: Worms invade viscera, where permanent granulomas form

Sx: Cutaneous: Raised itchy areas of skin up to 2 wk after exposure
> Visceral: Age 1-4 yr usually; often asx or erratic fever, anorexia, rash, seizures, wheezing, cough

Si Cutaneous: Rash
> Visceral: Hepatosplenomegaly, tumor-like growths in eye in older children

Crs: Cutaneous: Self-limited, lasts several weeks
> Visceral: Self-limited

Cmplc: Visceral: Eosinophilic meningoencephalitis (Nejm 1985;312:1619)

Lab: *Hem:* Eosinophilia in both types
> *Path:* Visceral: Bx (usually not justified since benign crs) of liver, lungs, CNS, muscle show eosinophilic granulomas
> *Serol:* Visceral: Titer $\geq$ 1/32 (98% sens, 92% spec), get kit from CDC
> *Stool:* No eggs in either type

Rx: Cutaneous: Ivermectin or albendazole
> Visceral: Diethylcarbamazine 2 mg/kg tid × 7-10 d; or albendazole; or mebendazole. Steroids for eye disease.

9.18 Roundworms

Ascariasis and Trichuriasis (Whipworm)

Nejm 1984;310:298

Cause: Ascariasis: *Ascaris lumbricoides*, pig roundworm
> Trichuriasis: *Trichuris trichiura*

Epidem: Highest incidence of both is in tropics, where eggs survive
more easily, and in children, who do more fecal–oral transmission
Ascariasis: Fecal–oral, 2 wk incubation of eggs necessary outside
body before infective
Trichuriasis: Fecal–oral

Pathophys:

Sx:

Ascariasis: Only if abnormal site or so many that they block
gi tract. After ingestion, migrate to lungs, then coughed up,
reingested.
Trichuriasis: Embed in superficial intestinal mucosa, mainly
colon; no tissue reaction, hence occasionally diarrhea

Si:

Crs:

Cmplc:

Ascariasis: Small bowel obstruction; perforated bowel; asphyxia
due to aspiration; biliary obstruction; hepatic abscess
Trichuriasis: Anemia, malnutrition; rectal prolapse; allergic pneumonitis (in 10%) (rx w steroids: Weinstein 1987)

Lab: *Bact:* Ascariasis: Stool shows eggs and adults
Trichuriasis: Stool shows barrel-shaped eggs w mucus plug
at both ends; adults: whip is head end, handle is tail end

Rx (Nejm 1996;334:1178):
Mebendazole (Vermox) 100 mg bid × 3 d, or
Pyrantel pamoate (Antiminth) 11 mg/kg (1 tsp/25 kg), or
Piperazine 75 mg/kg up to 3.5 g qd × 2, or
Albendazole, or
Ivermectin
Avoid reinfection; worms live < 2 yr

Enterobiasis (Pinworms)

Cause: *Enterobius vermicularis*

Epidem: Female lives in colon and lays eggs in perianal region; there
reinfected to same host or others by scratching; no tissue
penetration

30% of U.S. population under age 20 gets it, all socioeconomic classes

Pathophys:

Sx: Anal pruritus, vaginitis

Si: Vaginitis

Crs:

Cmplc: Vaginitis can lead to migration into peritoneal cavity, where granulomas form; rarely appendicitis

Lab: *Bact:* Scotch tape to perianal area early in am, then paste on slide to examine under microscope to see characteristic eggs, flat on one side

Rx: Mebendazole (Vermox) 100 mg × 1, repeat in 2 wk (Nejm 1977; 297:1437); or pyrantel 11 mg/kg (1 gm max) × 1, repeat in 2 wk; or albendazole; rx all family members at same time, even if asx since probably all have

Strongyloides Infections

Arch IM 1987;147:1257

Cause: *Strongyloides stercoralis*

Epidem: Skin penetration by filariform larval form, migrates to blood vessels, then to lung, from there up to pharynx, where is ingested back down the gi tract, where embeds and produces live young, which are released into feces. Can mature in gi tract and auto-reinfect or mature on the ground.

Increased prevalence in institutions for retarded; Southern areas

Pathophys: Much tissue damage in gi tract; perhaps exotoxin release. In severe cases, may develop internal autoreinfection.

Sx: Abdominal pain, midepigastric; nausea, vomiting, and bloody diarrhea (60-100%); perineal pruritus

Si:

Crs: May persist > 30 yr in active stage

Cmplc: Superinfections w secondary gram-neg bacteremias, bowel obstruction, and malabsorption in pts w diminished resistance, eg, on steroids (can cause death if already infected: Nejm 1966; 275:1093), Hodgkin's, leukemia, SLE, leprosy (Ann IM 1970; 72:199)

> Acute pneumonitis due to sensitivity reaction w tissue migration; rx with steroids (L. Weinstein 1987)

> r/o *Angiostrongylus*, rat worm; get in Carribean, Pacific, and SE Asia from raw or undercooked mollusks and crustaceans; causes transient benign eosinophilic meningitis (Nejm 2002; 346:668)

Lab: *Bact:* Stool shows rhabditiform larvae in feces sporadically; must use fresh stool, neg in 25%; duodenal aspirate best and most reliable

Hem: Eosinophilia (50%)

Rx: Prevent by wearing shoes, digging latrines
of disease:
- Thiabendazole 25 mg/kg (3 gm max) bid × 2 d; both tissue and intestinal phases hit; cure in 65%; or
- Ivermectin

Trichinosis

Jama 1983;249:23; Nejm 1978;298:1178

Cause: *Trichinella spiralis*

Epidem: Life cycle: Infection on ingestion of meat w cysts, hatch and reproduce for 6 wk in gi mucosa, living young are born and many get into skeletal muscle, where they grow and encyst, some calcify, and others remain viable for years

> From pigs fed uncooked garbage; polar and other bears

Pathophys: Invasion of skeletal (not heart) muscle by worms, degeneration of invaded fiber causing inflammatory reaction, and finally encysted larvae (in all other tissues, this reaction kills larvae)

Sx: Fever, myalgias all over including tongue, diaphragm, etc; gastroenteritis 24-72 hr after ingestion from worms in gi tract

Si: Eye swelling, conjunctivitis, small conjunctival hemorrhages; splinter hemorrhages in nail beds; skin rashes both urticarial and petechial

Crs: gi sx in 24-72 hr; other sx peak 1-6 wk after ingestion

Cmplc: Myocarditis, CNS inflammation

Lab: *Chem:* CPK, AST (SGOT) markedly elevated
Hem: Elevated eosinophils; may be as high as 50%
Path: Muscle bx shows 10-100 larvae/gm tissue; ≤ 1/gm should not produce sx
Serol: Charcoal flocculation test (Ann IM 1972;76:951)

Rx: Prevent by cooking garbage fed to pigs; cook or freeze pork well of disease (Med Let 1990;32:23):

- Mebendazole 200-400 mg po tid × 3 d, then 400-500 mg po tid × 10 d
- ASA for mild disease, or
- Steroids to decrease inflammation if becomes life-threatening, but they also extend life of adult worms

Filariasis

Cause: *Wuchereria bancrofti* (elephantiasis), *Onchocerca volvulus* (blinding worm: Nejm 1978;298:379), *Loa loa* (eye worm), *Brugia malayi* (elephantiasis), *Dirofilaria spp.* (dog filariasis), and perhaps tropical eosinophilia is also a form of filariasis from an unknown worm (TE: Nejm 1978;298:1129)

Epidem: All transmitted by flies or mosquitoes (*Brugia* and *Wuchereria*); take a long time to mature, hence up to 1 yr for onset of sx. 2-wk maturation in insect; infect via puncture holes; males and females in lymphatics produce microfilarial worms that migrate to peripheral blood in diurnal fashion, where ingested by insect and thus complete cycle.

In tropical areas; *Dirofilaria* occasionally in U.S.

Pathophys: Adults block lymphatics, fibrotic nodules form about them in lymphatics or in sc locations (*Onchocerca* and *Loa*). TE probably is an infection w worms whose microfilaria never get into blood; are in nodes and lung biopsies. The antigen-specific suppressor cells produced cause filaremia (Nejm 1982;307:144).

Sx: Onset may be delayed ≥ 5 yr after leaving area
Local swelling and redness of skin where microfilaria enter; fever
Calabar (*Loa*): A swelling of 2-3 cm sc anywhere but often in areas of trauma

Si: Recurrent lymphangitis especially of extremities, male genitalia; can see worms crawling sc often (*Loa*) especially in loose sc tissue, eg, eye, scrotum, breast, penis

Crs: Chronic

Cmplc: Blindness (*Onchocerca*)

Lab: *Hem:* Eosinophilia; microfilaria in blood sporadically (not in TE or *Onchocerca*), 40% pos thin smears; thick smear better, or spin crit and look at buffy-coat smear under low power
Path: Bx of lymphatics or skin nodules (*Loa, Onchocerca*) shows adults
Serol: Positive

Rx (Nejm 1985;313:133):

Prevent w diethylcarbamazine 300 mg po q 1 wk (*Loa loa:* Nejm 1988;319:752); use with ivermectin po q 1 yr to all over age 5 markedly (90+%) decreases prevalence and even improves morbidity of those w elephantiasis (Nejm 2002;347:1841,1885)
of disease: Diethylcarbamazine po, ivermectin; surgical excision of adult worms

9.19 Arthropods

Lice

Cause: *Phthirus pubis*; *Pediculus corporis* (body lice), *P. capitis* (head lice)

Epidem: *P. pubis*, venereal; *P. corporis* and *P. capitis*, via bedding, clothing, and other fomites

Life cycle: 25 d egg-to-egg. Live exclusively on human blood, can't live > 24 hr without it. Only ~10 adults/pt.

Pathophys: Attach to hair; itch and rashes due to bites and allergies to louse and its feces

Sx: Pruritus with all; *P. pubis* localized to axillary, perianal, pubic areas, and occasionally in eyelashes (blepharitis)

Si: Lice and nits (egg sacks on hairs) evident w magnifying glass or careful inspection; bites

Crs:

Cmplc: r/o bird lice (eg, from pigeons on air conditioner)

Lab:

Rx (Med Let 1997;38:6):

Launder clothes, bedding; hanging them outside for 24 hr will also kill since can't survive > 24 hr away from body

Meds: Rx as below, perhaps repeat × 1 at 7 d

1st:

- Permethrin 1% (Nix); $9/2 oz; 95% cure with 1 rx at 14 d (Am J Pub Hlth 1988;78:978), but resistance appearing

2nd:

- Permethrin 5% (Elimite) overnight, 1st choice for pubic lice (Med Let 1999;41:89), avoid for head lice in children; or
- Malathion 0.5% (Ovide) (Med Let 1999;41:73) lotion × 8-12 hr, then repeat in 1 wk
- Pyrethrins + piperonyl butoxide (Rid, Vonce, A-200, Pronto); 65% cure after 1 rx at 14 d (Am J Pub Hlth 1988;78:978); $5/2 oz

3rd:
- Lindane shampoos (1% gamma benzene hexachloride, Kwell), × 1 usually enough; may need × 3 q 4 d; $5/2 oz, or
- Ivermectin (Mectizan) 200 μgm/kg po × 1

4th: Tm/S po bid × 10 d w permethrin topically (Peds 2001; 107:575) improved cure from 80% to 95%

of eye cmplc: 1/4% eserine ophthalmic ointment to lids with cotton-tip applicator

of school outbreaks: Full guidelines (Maine Epigram 10/86); "nit-free policies unrealistic"

Common and Norwegian Scabies

Ann IM 1983;98:498; Nejm 1978;298:496

Cause: *Sarcoptes scabiei* var. *hominis:* an arthropod mite

Epidem: Norwegian rare in U.S. except in AIDS pts and alcoholics

Pathophys:
Common: Burrows in skin, leading to allergic reaction
Norwegian: No burrowing, but hides beneath skin scales

Sx: Common: Itching, worst at night
Norwegian: No itching

Si: Common: Red papules in intertriginous areas
Norwegian: Hyperkeratotic skin hiding mites

Crs: Common: Even w rx takes 2 wk for sx to subside

Cmplc:

Lab: *Bact:* Mineral oil scraping of burrow shows mite or eggs under low power

Rx (Med Let 1993;35:111):
Launder clothes, bedding; hanging them outside for 24 hr will also kill since can't survive > 24 hr away from body
Meds:
1st: Permethrin 5% (Elimite) cream (Med Let 1999;41:89) × 8-12 hr; 30 gm enough to rx adult; 91% cure; safer than lindane

2nd, Lindane 1% (Kwell) (Med Let 1997;39:6) once, though often may need repeat; 86% cure; crotamiton 10% (Eurax) if above fails; 60% cure

Experimental: Ivermectin 200 μgm/kg po × 1, ii 6 mg tabs for average adult; very effective, esp w crusting type and/or in immunosuppressed pts (Nejm 1995;333:26)

Virology

9.20 Antiviral Antibiotics

Med Let 2000;42:1 (HIV drugs w interactions lists), 1997;39:69 (non-HIV drugs)

Most iv courses cost $1000-4000; rapidly changing field, should check most recent Medical Letter and other journal issues

Reverse Transcriptase Inhibitors

All inhibit reverse transcriptase, which converts viral RNA to DNA so it can be incorporated into nuclear DNA; none touch viral DNA already incorporated. Most of their adverse effects (lactic acidosis, fatty liver, myopathy, neuropathy, pancreatitis) are due to inhibition of tissue DNA, esp mitochondrial DNA (Nejm 2002; 346:811).

Nucleoside Analogs (nRTIs)

All cause few drug interactions; all can rarely cause fatty liver and lactic acidosis

- Abacavir (Ziagen) (Med Let 1998;40:114) 300 mg po bid; adverse effects: drug fever (3%); available when other regimens fail (expanded access protocol: 800-501-4672)
- Didanosine (Videx, dideoxyinosine [ddI]) (Nejm 1991; 324:137) 200 mg po qd-bid; vs AIDS, less toxic than AZT and perhaps as good; interacts w zalcitabine; avoid taking

w food; adverse effects: pancreatitis, peripheral neuropathy; $200/mo

- Emtricitabine (Emtriva) (Med Let 2003;45:90) 200 mg po qd, which makes it better than bid stavudine (Jama 2004;292:180); adverse effects: HA, NVD, rash; occasional hyperpigmentation of palms, lactic acidosis, fatty liver; $10/d

- Lamivudine (Epivir; 3TC) (Jama 1996;276:111; Ann IM 1996;125:161; Nejm 1995;333:1657, 1662) 150 mg po bid; for chronic active Hep B, and w AZT for HIV (Jama 1996;276:111,118); $230/mo

- Stavudine (d4T) (Ann IM 1997;126:355) 40 mg po bid; alternative retroviral drug for AZT and ddI failures; adverse effects: peripheral neuropathy, asx hepatitis, rarely lactic acidosis w elevated LFTs (Ann IM 2000;133:192); $250/mo

- Tenofovir DF po once a day (Ann IM 2003;139:313), which makes it better than bid stavudine (Jama 2004;292:180)

- Zalcitabine (dideoxycytidine [ddC]) 0.75 mg po tid, vs AIDS, often alternating w AZT (Ann IM 1993;118:321); adverse effects: diarrhea, abdominal pain; $207/mo

- Zidovudine (Retrovir, azidothymidine [AZT]) (Ann IM 1992;117:487) 200 mg po tid (Nejm 1995;333:1662) or combined w 3TC (Combivir) (300 mg AZT + 150 mg 3TC) bid; ok in pregnancy (Jama 1999;281:151; Nejm 1992;326:857); adverse effects: macrocytic anemia, helped by iv erythropoietin weekly (Nejm 1990;322:1488) and granulocytopenia (Nejm 1989;321:726), both about 1% at 500-600 mg/d; can rx the thrombocytopenia w interferon-α and continue rx (Ann IM 1994;121:423); acetaminophen (Tylenol) worsens toxicity (Nejm 1987;317:192); myopathy in 5-10% (Nejm 1990;322:1098); $287/mo

Nucleotide Analogs

Adefovir (Preveon) (Jama 1999;282:2305,2355; Med Let 1998;40:114) 120 mg po qd; used mostly for Hep B rx w lamivudine

Non-nucleoside Analogs (nnRTIs)

- Delavirdine (Rescriptor) 400 mg po tid; $222/mo
- Efavirenz (Sustiva) (Med Let 1998;40:114) 600 mg po hs; better than indinavir when used w 2 nRTIs in triple rx (Nejm 1999;341:1865,1874,1925); adverse effects: drowsiness, HA, insomnia, rash, nightmares, drug interactions decrease protease inhibitor and clarithromycin levels
- Nevirapine (Viramune) (Med Let 1997;39:14) 200 mg po qd × 2 wk, then bid; possibly useful in drug combinations (Ann IM 1996;125:1019); adverse effects: rash; $250/mo

Protease Inhibitors

Nejm 1998;338:1281; Jama 1997;277:145)

All cost $4000-8000/yr

- Amprenavir (Agenerase) (Med Let 1999;41:64) 1200 mg (8 pills) po bid; adverse effects: NVD, peranal paresthesias, rash occasionally severe, many drug interactions
- Atazanavir (Reyataz) (Med Let 2003;45:90) 400 mg po qd; adverse effects: reversible jaundice, 1st-degree heart block
- Indinavir (Crixivan) (Med Let 1996;38:35) 800 mg po tid; adverse effects: renal stones, increased indirect bilirubin, Cushingoid changes (Nejm 1998;339:1296), increased DVT and PEs (Am J Med 1999;107:624); $360/mo
- Nelfinavir (Med Let 1997;39:14) 750 mg po tid; adverse effects: diarrhea
- Lopinavir/ritonavir (Kaletra) combo (Med Let 2001;43:1) 133/33 mg pill or 80/20 liquid, iii tab or i tsp po bid w food; adverse effects: NV+D, fatigue, headache, hepatocellular enzyme increases, rare pancreatitis, lots of drug interactions
- Ritonavir (Norvir) (Med Let 1996;38:35; Nejm 1995;333:1528) 300-600 mg po b-tid; adverse effects: NV+D, elevated LFTs, paresthesias; $670/mo

INFECTIOUS DISEASE

- Saquinavir (Fortovase, Invirase) (Nejm 1996;334:1011; Ann IM 1996;125:1039) 600-1200 mg po tid; adverse effects: drug interactions w nonsedating antihistamines; $570/mo

Entry Inhibitors

Enfuvirtide (Fuzeon) (Med Let 2003;45:49; Nejm 2003;348:2175,2186,2171,2228,2249) 90 mg sc bid; a 36 aa peptide; adverse effects: bacterial pneumonia increased 8×, 1/330 hypersensitive reactions, universal local sc nodules at injection site; $20,000/yr

Combination Drugs

Med Let 2005;47:19

- Emtricitabine/tenofovir (Truvada) 200/300 mg po qd
- Zidovudine/lamivudiane/abacavir (Trizivir) 300/150/300 mg po bid
- Zidovudine/lamivudine 300/150 mg po bid

Anti-influenza Drugs

Med Let 2004;46:85; Nejm 2000;343:1778

Neuramidase inhibitors:

- Zanamivir (Relenza) (Jama 1999;282:31; J Infect Dis 1999;180:254; Med Let 1999;41:91) 5 mg pwdr inhalation × 2 (10 mg total) qd for prophylaxis, eg, × 10 d in family members (NNT = 7: Nejm 2000;343:1282,1331), bid × 5 d for rx of both influenza A and B; no resistance, but avoid in asthmatics and COPD where may precipitate bronchospasm; $57/5 d

- Oseltamivir (Tamiflu) (Jama 2000;283;1016, 2000;282:1240; Nejm 1999;341:1336,1387) 75 mg po qd to prophylact × 7 d, or rx bid × 5 d decreases severity and duration if start within 36 hr of sx for influenza A or B; adverse effects: mild nausea and other gi sx, headache (15%); $72/5 d

Other:

- Amantadine 100-200 mg qd (Nejm 1990;322:443), 100 mg qd if creatinine clearance < 50 cc/min or over age 65, during first 48 hr of sx or prophylactically × 7-10 d after single exposure or × 2-3 wk in epidemic; helps vs A strains only; may use in elderly nursing home patients even if have used flu shot; renal excretion; works as aerosol too; adverse effects: CNS (don't drive) especially if renal insufficiency is present (Nejm 1990; 322:447); $6/5 d

- Rimantadine (Med Let 1993;35:109) 200 mg qd or 100 mg po bid × 5 d vs influenza, half-dose like amantadine in elderly or renally impaired; works similarly to amantadine but w much less CNS side effects (Nejm 1982;307:580) esp in healthy adults; rapid resistance can develop during course of rx (Nejm 1989;321:1696); hepatic metabolism; $16/5 d

- Ribavirin aerosol, works vs influenza A and B; not available in U.S.

Other

Med Let 2002;44:9, 1999;41:113; Nejm 1999;340:1255

- Acyclovir (Zovirax) (Med Let 1994;36:97; Nejm 1992;327:782); renally cleared, increase dose interval when creatinine clearance < 50 cc/min; adverse effects: gi sx; renal damage; resistance now appearing in AIDS pts (Nejm 1989;320:313); $125 for 800 mg 5 ×/d × 7 d
  of *Herpes simplex* virus I and II: 1st episode, 200 mg po 5 ×/d × 10 d; of recurrences, × 5 d, or 400 mg po bid × 1 yr for frequent recurrence prophylaxis
  of disseminated forms: 5-10 mg/kg q 8 hr iv
  of zoster: 800 mg po 5 ×/d or × 7-10 d may decrease duration of post-herpetic neuralgia from 120 d to 60 d
  of varicella (chickenpox): 20 mg/kg up to 800 mg po qid × 5 d

- Cidofovir (Med Let 1997;39:14; Ann IM 1997;126:257,264) for CMV retinitis; adverse effects: renal toxicity

- Famciclovir (Famvir) (Med Let 1994;36:87) 500 mg po tid × 7 d for acute (< 72 hr) zoster vs 125 mg po bid × 5 d, 250 mg po bid preventively for chronic Hep B and recurrent *H. simplex*; renal excretion; $130/wk
- Foscarnet (Foscavir), vs CMV retinitis in AIDS (Med Let 1992;34:3; Nejm 1992;326:213)
- Ganciclovir (Cytovene) (Nejm 1996;335:720) iv, or 3000 mg po qd for maintenance (Nejm 1995;333:615); vs CMV in AIDS (Nejm 1986;314:801; Ann IM 1985;103:377) and in marrow transplant pts (Ann IM 1993;118:173,179); adverse effects: neutropenia w more frequent bacterial infections (Ann IM 1993;118:173,179), resistance now appearing in AIDS pts (Nejm 1989;320:313)
- Interferon-α2a, 2b, con-1 (Infergen), and n3, used in AIDS (Ann IM 1990;112:805) and hepatitis B and C (p 356); adverse effects: psych disinhibitions and depression, flu sx, marrow suppression
- Penciclovir (Danavir) 1% cream q 2 hr × 4 d for local herpes
- Ribavirin po/iv/aerosol; vs hepatitis C w interferon, lassa fever, influenza, and perhaps RSV; adverse effects: hemolysis (10%), reversible when stop drug; teratogenesis
- Valacyclovir (Valtrex) 500 mg po bid × 5 d vs 1 gm po tid × 7-14 d (Med Let 1996;38:3) for acute zoster and genital *H. simplex*; for suppression, 250 mg bid vs 500-1000 mg po qd (Med Let 1996;38:3); $100/wk for 1 gm tid

9.21 Viral Infections

Acquired Immune Deficiency Syndrome (AIDS)

Note: Rapidly changing field; identify local consultants and resources

Cause: Human immunodeficiency virus (HIV) type 1 (Nejm 1991; 324:308); rarely in U.S. but commonly in Africa, HIV-2 (Ann IM 1993;118:211); a retrovirus

Epidem: Spread via sex (3% infection rate w HIV-pos semen: Jama 1995;273:854), but no heterosexual transmission when viral loads < 1500/cc (Nejm 2000;342:921); contaminated needles; blood products, eg, screened blood transfusion, 1996 risk = 1/500,000 (Nejm 1996;334:1685), factor VIII concentrates (Nejm 1993;329:1835, 1984;310:69), and breast milk (Jama 2000;283:1167, 1999;282:744; Nejm 1991;325:593); rarely by casual or nonsexual familial contact (Nejm 1987;317:1125), percutaneous inoculation in health care workers, 0.3%/incident, risk increases w increased volume and probably HIV titer (Nejm 1997;337:1485)

12% prevalence in wives of infected hemophiliacs (Ann IM 1991;115:764); 0.2% of women positive at delivery in Massachusetts (Nejm 1988;318:525) and NY state, but NY City rate = 14% (Am J Pub Hlth 1991;81: May suppl); 5% Baltimore ER patients (Nejm 1988;318:1645)

Transmission enhanced by the presence of chancroid or other genital ulcers (Ann IM 1993;119:1150)

Prevalence increased in gay males (67% in San Francisco in 1984: Ann IM 1985;103:210), drug abusers, hemophiliacs (Nejm 1983;308:79), female partners of infected males (Nejm 1983; 308:1181)

90% of persons transfused with HIV-pos blood convert to positive themselves (Ann IM 1990;113:733); but only 0.3% become positive after a needle stick from an HIV-pos pt; < 0.5% of exposed health care workers convert over 1 yr (Nejm 1988; 319:1118); 30% untreated babies of HIV-pos mothers are pos at age 16 mo (Nejm 1992;327:1192; Am J Pub Hlth 1989;79:1662)

Incidence in 1990s decreased in U.S. as did AIDS deaths, probably from preventive maneuvers, drug rx of HIV infection, and prophylaxis and rx of opportunistic infections (Mmwr 1997; 46:861)

Pathophys: AIDS defined by HIV infection and T_4 count < 200

Increased suppressor T_8 and decreased helper T_4 cells (CD_4) (Nejm 1985;313:79); deficient production of interferon-γ (Nejm 1985;313:1504)

Billions of virons produced daily from infection w high viral RNA mutation rate, which allows rapid selection of resistant organisms in face of rx (Ann IM 1996;124:984)

Sx: Primary HIV infection (Nejm 1998;339:33; Ann IM 1996;125: 259) consists of a mono-like syndrome 5-30 d after exposure lasting ~2 wk, rarely seek care; w fever (95%), sore throat (70%), weight loss (70%), myalgias (60%), headache (60%), cervical adenopathy (50%), maculopapular or other rash involving trunk (40-80%); test for w HIV RNA assay (100% sens, 97% specif) (Ann IM 2001;134:25)

AIDS: Diarrhea (60%: Nejm 1993;329:14), malaise, weight loss, fever, adenopathy, dyspnea (pneumocystis pneumonia)

Si:

Early: Lymphadenopathy; oral monilia/thrush (exudative, chelosis, or erythematous diffuse rash types) precedes overt disease often (Nejm 1984;311:354), and multiple other oral manifestations (Ann IM 1996;125:487); dermatoses including warts and shingles; chronic fatigue syndrome

Later: Wasting syndromes, chronic diarrhea, dementias/seizures, FUO, thrombocytopenia, cervical dysplasia, KS, hairy leukoplakia corrugations on sides of tongue due to reactivation of EB virus (Nejm 1985;313:1564)

Crs:

Typical Course of HIV Infection

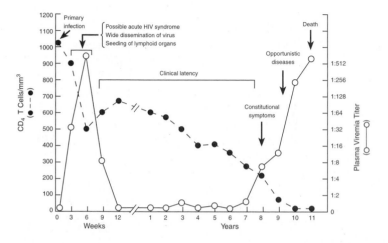

Figure 9.1 Typical course of HIV infection. Reproduced with permission from Pantaleo G, et al. Mechanisms of disease: the immunopathogenesis of human immunodeficiency virus infection, New Eng J Med 1993;328:327-335. Copyright 1993 Mass. Medical Society, all rights reserved.

of HIV infection: Variable RNA viral loads in first 4 mo but worse/faster crs predicted by levels at 5-18 mo from infection and by severity of primary infection sx (Ann IM 1998;128: 613; Jama 1996;276:105); evolution to AIDS 10 yr post-seroconversion varies from 0 to 72%

of AIDS: 1997 mortality figures markedly improving w aggressive multi-drug rx based on viral loads (Jama 1998;279:450), eg, from 29 to 9/100 person-years in pts w CD_4 counts < 100 (Nejm 1998;338:853); Survival worse w increasing age of pt and some HLA MHC types (Nejm 2001;344;1668), but not associated w pre-rx CD_4 and viral load values (Ann IM 2004;140:256), gender, iv drug use, race, or socioeconomic status (Nejm 1995;333:751). Survival improved when co-infection w GB virus C, a hepatitis C-like virus (Nejm 2004; 350:981)

Cmplc:

- Infections with common bacterial pathogens (Nejm 1995;333:845) as well as opportunistic organisms, esp when $CD_4 < 50$ (Ann IM 1996;124:333) including:

  Pneumocystis (in 1980s was presenting sx in 75%, now much rarer w prophylaxis: Nejm 1993;329:1822)

  Atypical tbc (Ann IM 1986;105:184), esp M. *avium/intracellulare*, rarely M. *haemophilum* (Ann IM 1994;120:118)

  Herpes infections including tongue fissures (Nejm 1993;329: 1859); CMV; candida; aspergillosis; strongyloides

  nocardia

  Mucor

  cryptococcus, esp meningitis

  toxoplasma

  legionella

  chlamydia

  monilia, torulopsi

  Penicillium marneffei, a SE Asian dimorphic fungus (Nejm 1998;339:1739)

  Cryptosporidiosis (p 632), *Isospora belli* (p 632)

  Listeria (Nejm 1985;312:404)

  Cat scratch *Bartonella (Rochalimaea) henselae* or *quintana* causing bacillary angiomatosis (r/o Kaposi's by bx) and peliosis hepatitis (p 606)

  Syphilis w rapid (< 4 yr) appearance of neurosyphilis manifested by strokes, meningitis, and cranial nerve palsies and that is only transiently suppressed by penicillin regimens (Nejm 1994;331:1469,1488,1516)

- Tumors including:

  Kaposi's sarcoma (p 693)

Non-Hodgkin's lymphoma, in 15% after 3 yr of AZT rx (Ann IM 1990;113:276)

Burkitt's lymphoma (Nejm 1986;314:874), EB virus associated, in adults

Leiomyosarcoma (Nejm 1986;314:874), EB virus associated, in children (Nejm 1995;332:12)

Cervical cancer due to higher prevalence of HPV infection (Nejm 1997;337:1343); get q 1 yr after 2 q 6 mo Pap smears (Ann IM 1999;130:97)

- Hematologic including ITP (Nejm 1985;313:1375) and aplastic anemias from parvovirus infections (Ann IM 1990;113:926); and from diminished half-life and megakaryocyte infection (Nejm 1992;327:1779)

- Myocardiopathy, dilated type (Nejm 1998;339:1093, 1992;327:1260)

- Neurologic (Ann IM 1994;121:769) including early subtle CNS degeneration (Nejm 1990;323:864) leading to dementia (Nejm 1995;332:934; Ann IM 1987;107:383); progressive multifocal leukoencephalopathy (Ann IM 1987;107:78) associated w papova/polyoma virus, seen in transplant pts as well, cytarabine rx no help (Nejm 1998;338:1345); cord lesions; aseptic meningitis; peripheral neuropathy (Nejm 1985;313:1538); cerebral toxoplasmosis; cerebral lymphomas

- Nephropathy (Nejm 1989;321:625)

- Rheumatologic including Reiter's without conjunctivitis; and psoriasis with arthritis (Bull Rheum Dis 1990;39:5); aseptic necrosis of femoral head 4.5% prevalence (Ann IM 2002;137:17)

- Suicide (Jama 1996;276:1743)

- Diabetes and hyperlipidemia (Nejm 2003;348:702) due to both the HIV infection and its drug rx

r/o HTLV I and II infections—former associated w paraparesis, latter w no disease (Ann IM 1993;118:448); rare idiopathic CD_4 cell lymphopenia syndrome (Nejm 1993;328:429)

Lab:

Immunol: Standard tests:

- Viral load, most important test, positive at $> 50,000$/cc in acute primary disease (Nejm 1998;339:33); RNA by PCR, peripheral mononuclear cell viral mRNA levels predict prognosis (Ann IM 1995;123:641) and treatment success (Nejm 1996; 335:1091, 1996;334:426; Ann IM 1996;124:984); indicates rapidity of disease progression (Jama 1997;278:983); $< 10,000$/cc good, 10,000-100,000/cc moderately ok, $> 100,000$/cc bad

- T_4 (CD_4) < 200/cc defines AIDS now (Mmwr 1992; 41[RR-17]:1) and predicts opportunistic pneumonias (Ann IM 1989;111:223); 200-500 = intermediate risk (Nejm 1989; 321:1141)

- ELISA w Western blot test, only 1.5% false positive in low-risk military population (Nejm 1988;319:961); if indeterminant, repeat in 1 mo and should become pos if really HIV; if persistently equivocal, get viral load and culture (R. Smith 4/95). Tests negative for 4+ mo incubation period (Nejm 1989;321:941).

- P_{24} nuclear antigen detection either of free antigen or dissociated from IgG antibody–antigen complex (Nejm 1993; 328:297); pos usually in early disease including the primary disease syndrome when ELISA still neg in 50% (Nejm 1998; 339:33)

Rapid tests (Med Let 2003;45:54); all require confirmatory Western blot if positive:

- Ora-Sure HIV-1 test from 2 min swab between cheek and gum, as specific as serum by ELISA/Western blot (Jama 1997; 277:254)

- OraQuick, whole-blood fingerstick 20 min test; 99.6% sens, 100% specif; $15

- Reveal rapid HIV-1 test, serum 3 min test; 99.8% sens, 99.1% specif; $15

Path: Bronchoscopic brushings and lavage are 85% specif and sens for specific infections (Ann IM 1985;102:747)

Urine: Proteinuria > 0.5 gm/d in 50%, nephrotic syndrome in 10% (Ann IM 1984;101:429)

Rx:

Preventive maneuvers:

Hospital isolation (guidelines: Ann IM 1986;105:730); risk is very low even with needle sticks (Nejm 1985;312:1)

Screen the general population q 3-5 yr? (Nejm 2005;352:570, 586,620); blood donors with ELISA (Nejm 1989;321:917, 941,947,966), perhaps others, eg, high-risk spreaders like dialysis staff, psych patients (no: Ann IM 1995;122:641,653; yes: Nejm 1986;315:1562), or perhaps all pts age 15-54 in hospitals w 1 case of AIDS/1000 discharges (Nejm 1992; 327:445)

Consistent condom use prevents disease; 0/124 conversions in HIV-neg partners over 2 yr, otherwise 5/100 pt/yr convert (Nejm 1994;331:341)

In pregnancy (Nejm 1995;333:298), peripartum scalp electrodes, rupture of membranes > 4 hr (Nejm 1996;334:1617), and episiotomies. Pre- and peripartum AZT no matter what the maternal viral load or CD_4 count (Nejm 1996;335:1621), reduces maternal–fetal transmission from 25% to 8% (Jama 1995;273:977; Nejm 1994;331:1173) and decreases to a lesser extent w peri- or postpartum rx within 1st 6 mo of age (Nejm 1998;339:1409); so rx mother beginning at 28 wk gestation through delivery and infant for 1st 6 wk of life (Nejm 2004;351:217,229, 2000;343:982). Rx of prepartum mother viral load to < 20,000 (Jama 1996;275:599) or < 1000 (Nejm 1999;341:394) or < 500 (Nejm 1999;341: 385) yields infant infection rate = 0, and is safe for infant (Jama 1999;281:151). Elective C/S reduces infant infection to < 1% (Jama 1998;280:55) and w postpartum antibiotics reduces infant infection to 2% (Nejm 1999;340:977). Avoid breast feeding, which has a 6-10% transmission rate over 1-1.5 yr (Jama 2001;285:2413, 2000;283:1167). All these efforts have decreased neonatal AIDS in U.S. by 67% (Jama 1999;282:531).

Prophylaxis immediately (< 24-48 hr) (CDC prophylaxis/ exposure guidelines: Mmwr 1998;47[RR-7]:1) post-exposure × 1 mo w AZT (Nejm 1997;337:1485) 300 mg bid + lamivudine (3TC) (Ann IM 1998;128:306; Jama 1998;280:1769) 150 mg bid; may add indinavir 800 mg q 8 hr or nelfinavir 750 mg tid if exposure substantial; for pregnant women, use nevirapine po

Prevention of AIDS-associated infections (Ann IM 2002;137:239; Nejm 2000;342:1416; Jama 1998;279:130); can stop when CD_4 > 200 for > 6 mo:

- Pneumocystis prophylaxis (Nejm 1995;332:693) w CD_4 counts < 200. Can stop after rx persistently raises CD_4 > 200 (Nejm 2001;344:159,168,222, 1999;340:1301).

    1st: Tm/S SS qd (Arch IM 1996;156:177) or DS tiw, qd-bid; also helps toxoplasmosis

    2nd: Pentamidine aerosol 150-300 mg monthly if CD_4 < 200 (Nejm 1991;324:1079, 1990;323:769; Ann IM 1989; 111:223), least toxic; or atovaquone (Nejm 1998;339: 1895) 1500 mg po qd

    3rd: Dapsone 50 mg po bid or qd w pyrimethamine, also helps prevent toxoplasmosis

- M. *avium* (MAI) prophylaxis (p 584) if CD_4 < 50 w clarithromycin, azithromycin 1200 mg po q 1 wk, or rifabutin; can stop after rx persistently raises CD_4 > 100-200 (Nejm 2000; 342:1085)

- Toxoplasmosis after encephalitis, w sulfadiazine + pyrimethamine folate po qd (Ann IM 1995;123:175); or if positive IgG titer and CD_4 < 200, w Tm/S DS qd or dapsone + pyrimethamine

- CMV infections w ganciclovir 1 gm po tid; if $CD_4 < 50\text{-}100$, decreases rates by $^1/_2$ (Nejm 1996;334:1491)
- Pneumovax immunization
- Chickenpox: Vaccination + VZIG if exposed
- Tuberculosis prophylaxis if ppd is positive w INH, or rifampin + pyrazinamide, or rifabutin + pyrazinamide (Nejm 1999;340:371)
- HPV w Pap smears q 6-12 mo esp if $CD_4 \leq 500$ (Jama 2005;293:1471)

Of questionable benefit:

- Cryptococcus, histo and cocci w chronic fluconazole, but no prolongation of survival (Nejm 1995;332:700)
- Candidal local mucosal and systemic infections w fluconazole 200 mg po q 1 wk (Ann IM 1997;126:689) but no prolongation of survival (Nejm 1995;332:700) and resistance is a problem
- Cryptosproidiosis w careful exposure prevention (see list: Ann IM 1999;131:879)
- Human herpes virus 8 (Kaposi virus) perhaps (Ann IM 1999; 131:891)
- Influenza w vaccine (Ann IM 1999;131:430 vs 1988;109:383)

of acute primary infection: Triple drug rx (Nejm 1998; 339:33)

Rx of disease (Jama 2004;292:251, 2000;283:381): Rapidly changing field, should check most recent Med Let and other journal issues

Drug therapy (p 661) triplet$^+$ for adults and children (Nejm 2001;345:1522)—for all pts w HIV viral load RNA levels > 5000-10,000/cc no matter the CD_4 count?—at doses increased to get RNA load levels < 500; both survival and other measures of disease severity are improved (Jama 2001;286:2560,2568, 1998;280:1497) but must start at $CD_4 < 200$ and adhere to rx (Ann IM 2003;139:810), starting w $CD_4 < 350$ is better. Women run lower viral loads but prognosis is same, so maybe use CD_4 < 500 even if viral loads are higher (Nejm 2001;344:720). Simultaneous initiation of triple rx results in > 80% still adequately suppressed whereas w sequential initiation < 40% are suppressed at 2+ yr (Jama 1998;280:35); tapering to 1-2 drugs after 3-6 mo not as good as continued 3-drug rx (Nejm 1998;339: 1261,1269,1319; Lancet 1998;352:185). Multiple-drug-resistant organisms appearing, > 12% in U.S. (Nejm 2002;347:385; Jama 1999;282:1135,1142,1177; Ann IM 1999;131:502) so sensitivity testing necessary. Avoid combinations of d4T + AZT; or ddC w ddI, d4T, 3TC, and others (table: Jama 2004;292:259).

Triple drug rx w:

- 2 nRTIs + a protease inhibitor or a nnRTI; or
- 2 nRTIs + ritonavir + another protease inhibitor like lopinavir (Nejm 2002;346:2039)
- Most common triple rx combo: zidovudine (AZT) + lamivudine (3TC) + efavirenz (Sustiva) (best: Nejm 2003;349:2293, 2304,2351) or indinavir

of aphthous stomatitis (p 244)

of lipodystrophy: Perhaps rosiglitazone 4 mg po qd (Ann IM 2004;140:786)

of wasting syndrome (p 439)

of diarrhea: Rx primary cause if can be found; octreotide 50 mg sc q 8 hr (Ann IM 1991;115:705), opiates, loperamide (Imodium), or diphenoxylate-atropine (Lomotil)

Overall AIDS Primary Care Strategies:

General: Discuss meaning, definitions, prognosis; risk reduction, avoidance of cofactors; safer sex, birth control; substance abuse issues; community resources, support network, counseling; facilitate dialogue with partner, friends, family; complete and directed physical; build referral network

Asx HIV-positive (usually > 500 T_4 cells): Viral load, T cells, CBC, chemistries q 6-12 mo, q 6 mo cervical Pap smears ×

2 then q 1 yr (Ann IM 1999;130:97) or similar anal cancer
screening in males (Ann IM 2003;138:453); PPD and controls; pneumovax, H. flu vaccine, yearly flu shots; hepatitis B
status, consider vaccine if still at risk; syphilis serology; baseline toxo and CMV titers; dual- or triple-drug rx to decrease
viral load if recent (6 mo) infection but not if asx and
> 6 mo infected

Symptomatic HIV-positive (usually 200-500 T$_4$ cells): Triple rx;
CBC, chemistries q 2-4 wk until stable on AZT, then q 4-8
wk; T cells, viral load q 3-6 mo; appropriate evaluation of sx;
consider experimental rx's

AIDS and serious HIV infection (usually < 200 T$_4$ cells, occasionally only < 300): Triple rx although advantage/benefit
less clear than when CD$_4$ = 200-500 (Nejm 1996;335:
1099); opportunistic organism prophylaxis esp for pneumocystis, MAI, toxo if baseline titer positive, CMV; mental status exams; ophthalmologic evaluation q 6 mo; aggressive
evaluation of sx; appropriate rx of opportunistic infections
and malignancies; consider experimental rx, consultation/
referral; AIDS-defining dx's and reporting

Arbo Viral Encephalitis

Cause: Several types of arboviruses: St. Louis (Ann IM 1969;71:681),
Eastern equine, West Nile (Ann IM 2004;140:545; Jama
2003;290:524; Ann IM 2002;137:173; Nejm 2001;344:1807),
Western equine, and Lacross encephalitis; single-stranded RNA
flaviviruses, closely related to Japanese and Murray Valley encephalitis (rv of all: Nejm 2004;351:370)

Epidem: Culex mosquito and ticks from birds and invertebrates; rarely
via organ transplant (Nejm 2003;348:2196). Incidence highest in
small children and adults age > 50 yr; many inapparent cases, up
to 99%; incidence up after rainy winter; equine types kill horses
by thousands and children age < 10 yr

Pathophys: Humans and horses don't develop enough viremia to transmit these diseases

Sx: Vast majority of at least West Nile virus infections are asx
Fever (90%), Guillain-Barré–type muscle weakness (56% w West Nile type, unlike others), severe headache (47%), nausea, and vomiting (52%)

Si: Altered mental status (46-86%); frontal lobe si's (78%); stiff neck (71%); cranial nerve palsies, especially of III, IV, VI, VII (22%); Babinski's sign (30%); seizures (10%)
West Nile virus neurologic si (Jama 2003;290:511): Meningitis, encephalitis, acute flaccid paralysis (polio-like), tremor, myoclonus, Parkinsonism

Crs: West Nile virus only 3-6 d, rest 10-21 d; 10-36% mortality, higher if seizures; 35-60% of survivors w neurologic morbidity; both predicted by CSF wbc counts and serum hyponatremia (Eastern equine type: Nejm 1997;336:1867). West Nile virus pts recover well except those w flaccid paralysis (Jama 2003;290:511).

Cmplc: SIADH
r/o tick-borne Powassan encephalitis, which has similar clinical presentation (Mmwr 2001;50:761)

Lab: *Serol:* ELISA for IgM antibodies; reverse transcriptase PCR identification of viral RNA in CSF
CSF: 1-500 wbc's, 50% lymphs; protein 40-500+ mg %

Xray: MRI shows basal ganglia and thalamic focal lesions (Nejm 1997; 336:1867)

Rx: Prevention: Spray to eliminate mosquito population; kill pigeons and other birds, or use them as sentinels and test for antibody titer changes (Nejm 1967;277:12)
of disease: Supportive

Chickenpox (Cpox) and Herpes Zoster (Shingles)

Nejm 2002;347:340, 2000;342:635 (zoster); Ann IM 1999;130:922

Cause: *Varicella*, a herpesvirus

Epidem:

> Zoster: More common in the elderly and pts w HIV and cancer but not a si of occult malignancy; 10-20% of all persons will have in lifetime

> Cpox: < 10% repeat infections, probably quite rare (Jama 1997;278:1520); dramatic drop in U.S. mortality after 10 yr of universal chiildhood vaccination (Nejm 2005;352:450)

Pathophys: Same organism causes first chickenpox, and later shingles (Nejm 1984;311:1362)

Sx: Cpox: 14 d incubation period; fever, centrifugal rash (on face and trunk 1st, then extremities)

> Zoster: Shingles rash; pain often, may precede and sometimes rash never appears

Si: Cpox: Fever < 102°F (38.8°C); herpetic rash various ages, trunk first and worst. New lesions appear for 4 d.

> Zoster: Classic herpetic lesions in dermatome distribution w hyperesthesia and pain; cranial and other neuropathies

Crs: Cpox worse w increased age, so adolescents and adults suffer more than children

Cmplc:

> Cpox:
> - Anterior horn cell myelitis
> - Encephalitis leading to cerebellar ataxia
> - Pneumonia especially in adults
> - Group A β strep cellulitis and toxic shock
> - Reye's syndrome (p 887)
> - Rare (1/11) congenital abnormalities if infected in 1st trimester (Nejm 1986;314:1542)
> - Embryopathy, rate is 2% if infected between weeks 8 and 20 (Nejm 1994;330:901); in pregnancy, 85% of women are immune even if don't recall having had the disease

> Zoster:
> - Secondary bacterial infections
> - Dissemination

- Chronic postherpetic neuralgias and neuropathies (Nejm 1996; 335:32); incidence increases w age, 27% at age 55, 47% at 60, 73% at 70; as is duration, so over age 70 yr lasts > 1 yr in 50%; British study found over age 69, 3 mo prevalence = 20%, 12 mo prevalence = 10%; under age 60, 3 mo prevalence = 2%, 12 mo prevalence < 1% (BMJ 2000;321:794)
- Guillain-Barré
- Encephalitis/myelitis
- Keratitis, heals well unlike *H. simplex*
- Cerebrovasculitis presenting as TIA/CVA (Nejm 2002;347: 1500) weeks to months after an episode of zoster; reversible w iv acyclovir

Lab: *Path:* Skin bx or Tzanck prep shows intranuclear inclusions and giant cells, enhanced by direct immunofluorescent staining assay

Serol: Antibody level to determine past immunity

Rx: Preventive:

Cpox: Vaccine, live attenuated (Varivax-MSD) (Med Let 1995;37:55) 0.5 cc sc × 1 for age 1-12 yr, × 2 1-2 mo apart if age > 13 yr (Mmwr 1995;44:264), must keep frozen until reconstituted, then use within 30 min; 100% effective, 86% in field use (Nejm 2001;344:955) vs only 45% against all disease, although 86% against moderate–severe disease w significant attenuation of protection > 3 yr out (Jama 2004; 191:851; Nejm 2002;347:1909), or 84% effective after 95% in 1st year, although cases milder; more failures if RAD (Jama 1997;278:1495); safe (Jama 2000;284:1271); may decrease later zoster incidence (Jama 1997;278:1529; Nejm 1989;320:892, 1988;318:573). Avoid in immunocompromised and pregnant pts.

Isolation, children may return to day care or school as soon as lesions are crusted (Nejm 1991;325:1577)

Zoster: V-ZIG (varicella-zoster immune globulin) 125 U/10 kg im; expensive; use if immunosuppressed and exposed, perhaps use-

ful in exposed healthy adult? (Ann IM 1984;100:859)
of disease:

Cpox:

- Acyclovir (Zovirax) 800 mg or 20 mg/kg po qid × 5 d ameliorates course modestly (Ann IM 1992;117:358; Nejm 1991;325:1539) if started in first 24 hr but costs $32/d; or 800 mg 5 ×/d × 7 d (Med Let 1994;36:87) speeds healing by 2 d; $125
- Famciclovir (Famvir) (Med Let 1994;36:87) 500 mg po tid × 7 d, similar in all respects including cost of $130/wk
- Valcyclovir (p 661)
- Foscarnet iv q 8 hr for disseminated disease in AIDS pts (Ann IM 1991;115:19)

Zoster: Wet soaks when wet, then topical steroids when dry; antivirals may prevent postherpetic neuralgia? (no: BMJ 1989;289:431; vs do over age 50: J Fam Pract 2000;49:255; or over age 60: BMJ 2000;321:794); but dual rx w steroids and acyclovir × 3 wk does speed healing and comfort? (Nejm 1994;330:896 vs Ann IM 1996;125:376)

- Famciclovir 500 mg po tid × 7 d within 3 d of rash onset speeds healing and decreases neuralgia duration (Ann IM 1995;123:89), use over age 50 or if severe or immunocompromised; or
- Valacyclovir (Valtrex) 1 gm po tid × 7 d (Med Let 1996;38:3); an acyclovir precursor; decreases zoster neuralgia even better than acyclovir
- Acyclovir (Ann IM 1987;107:859) iv or po 10 mg/kg q 8 hr for severe local disease, eg, eye, or disseminated, or at onset in immunocompromised host. 800 mg 5 ×/d × 7-10 d speeds healing and decreases acute neuralgia and neuritis (Am J Med 1988;85:84)
- Prednisone 60 mg → 0 over days/weeks, if over 50, especially if involves head, to speed healing along w above; no decrease in neuralgia

- Amitriptyline 10-25 mg po qd × 3 mo decreases postherpetic neuralgia
  of zoster neuralgia (Nejm 1996;335:32) (see also p 781):
- Oxycodone or other opioid po
- Gabapentin (Neurontin) (Jama 1998;280:1837) 300-1200 mg po tid
- Lidocaine patch 5% (Lidoderm) × 12 hr qd; or gel or cream topically
- Steroid injections (Arch Neurol 1986;143:836; Ann IM 1980; 93:588)
- Dilantin and/or carbamazepine
- Amitriptyline 12-25 mg po hs, increase to q 1 wk; or nortriptyline, or other tricyclic
- TENS
- Phenothiazines
- Nerve block, intrathecal steroid injections (Nejm 2000;343:1514) q 1 wk up to 4 in persistent debilitating disease, dramatically helps > 80%
- Capsaicin topical cream OTC qid 0.075% (Arch IM 1991;151:2225 describes use in diabetic neuropathy); questionable benefit (Med Let 1992;34:61); OTC costs $27/oz

Common Cold

Cause: Rhinovirus, coronavirus, adenovirus, parainfluenza virus, in order of frequency in adults; rarer causes include respiratory syncytial virus (p 896), echo, coxsackie, reovirus, and mycoplasmas

Epidem: Respiratory droplets, most frequently 1-2 d after inoculation, fomites with dried viruses (Nejm 1973;288:1361); hand-to-hand contact (Ann IM 1978;88:463); iatrogenic (adenovirus 8 conjunctivitis: Nejm 1973;289:1341)

Colds occur q 2-4 mo in average adult American; increased attack rates correlate with increasing individual stress levels (Nejm 1991;325:606)

Pathophys: Infection denudes and alters respiratory epithelial cells, especially the cilia (Nejm 1985;312:463) of nasal pharyngeal mucosa. Sinuses are extensively involved as well (Nejm 1994;330:25).

Sx: Upper respiratory tract sx in all

of adenovirus: Acute hemorrhagic cystitis, especially in young males (Nejm 1973;289:344, 373); and conjunctivitis

of reovirus: Exanthematous rash

Si:

Crs: Adenovirus conjunctivitis lasts about 21 d

Cmplc: Severe viral interstitial pneumonia possible with all (Nejm 1972;286:1289)

Adenovirus: Pertussis syndrome; unilateral deafness due to organ of Corti capillary occlusion rarely (Nejm 1967;276:1406)

Lab:

Rx: CDC educational materials to decrease antibiotic use (404-639-2215)

Hot steam (43°C) nasal inhalation speeds recovery (Proc Natl Acad Sci 1982;79:4766); no, new studies disprove (Jama 1994;271:1109,1112)

Ipratropium nasal anticholinergic spray helps nasal sx a little (Ann IM 1996;125:89)

Zinc 13 mg lozenges q 2 hr while awake shorten crs by $\frac{1}{2}$ (Ann IM 2000;133:245, 1996;125:81); but many studies on both sides of use (ACP J Club 1999;131:69), and causes premature and still births in pregnant women (Jama 1998;279:1962; Med Let 1997;39:9)

Questionable: Echinacea OTC preparations but no credible trials find benefit (Jama 2003;290:2825; Ann IM 2002;137:939,1001; Med Let 2002;44:29); vitamin C no help (Nejm 1976;295:973); vitamin E worsens (Jama 2002;288;715)

of rhinovirus: Postexposure interferon-α2a nasal inhalation works (Nejm 1986;314:65, 71)

Coxsackie Diseases

Cause: Coxsackievirus A and B; enteroviruses, eg, enterovirus 71 (Nejm 1999;341:929,936)

Epidem: Fecal–oral spread. Worldwide; summer predominance; very infectious, epidemics.

Pathophys:

Sx: Herpangina causing very sore throat, dysphagia, anorexia, abdominal pain. Hand-foot-mouth disease (HFMD) with URI sx. Acute infectious lymphocytosis (AIL) with diarrhea, weakness, and URI sx. Pleurodynia (Bornholm's disease), a pleural pericarditis causing pleuritic thoracic and abdominal pain. Headache; aseptic meningitis.

Si: Herpangina with red, vesicular lesions in pharynx. HFMD has red macules with vesicles on hands, feet, and stomatitis. AIL has documentable muscular weakness. Pleurodynia has fever, and pericardial or pleural rub. Meningitis si.

Crs: Herpangina = 1-4 d; HFMD = 4-5 d; pleurodynia = 2-14 d

Cmplc: Polio-like syndromes, pulmonary edema, Guillain-Barré syndrome, encephalitis, chronic myocarditis

Lab: *Serol:* Culture and PCR

Rx: Supportive only

CMV Infections

Nejm 1985;313:1270; Ann IM 1983;99:326

Cause: Cytomegalovirus (CMV), a herpesvirus

Epidem: Congenital via transplacental transmission; newborn via vaginal infection at birth (Nejm 1973;289:1); blood products and organ transplantation

Congenitally infected children spread for years (Nejm 1973; 288:1370); so do many others with asx recrudescence (Nejm 1980;303:958); semen and vaginal carriers (Nejm 1974;291:121).

Pregnant mothers with children in day care are at high risk (Nejm 1986;314:1414). Most fetal damage occurs due to primary infections during pregnancy, leading to 10% damaged offspring; but can occur in immune mother from infection w different strains (Nejm 2001;344:1366), although damage is minimal (Nejm 1992;326:663).

No increased incidence in female health workers (Nejm 1983;309:950)

Increased incidence in gay males (90% positive by serology: Ann IM 1983;99:326)

Pathophys:

Sx: Adults: Mononucleosis-like syndrome; rarely sore throat, unlike mono

Si: Adults: Fever, splenomegaly, mild hepatitis in 100%; cervical adenopathy is rare, unlike mono

Congenital/newborn: Jaundice, hepatosplenomegaly, hemolytic anemia, ITP

Crs: Adult: 2-4 wk

Cmplc:

Congenital: Deafness and mental retardation (Nejm 1976;295:469), now ahead of rubella

Adult: AGN in transplant patients (Nejm 1981;305:57); Guillain-Barré (Ann IM 1973;79:153); retinitis (Nejm 1982; 307:94; Ann IM 1980;93:655,664); if immunocompromised, pneumonitis (Ann IM 1975;82:181) and encephalitis (Ann IM 1996;125:489)

Lab: *Hem:* Atypical lymphs (Nejm 1969;280:1311); anemia (50%) with positive Coombs in 20% (Ann IM 1970;73:553)

Serol: Rapid urine DNA hybridization detection method, accurate and fast, is possible (Nejm 1983;308:921). Specific antibody by neutralization, comp-fix, and indirect fluorescent antibody.

Xray: Congenital, skull xrays show periventricular calcifications

Rx: Preventively screen women before pregnancy and perhaps in future immunize them? (Nejm 1992;326:663); screen blood products (Nejm 1986;314:1006); and isolate immunosuppressed pts from susceptible pts who spread it for weeks

Prophylaxis of immunocompromised pts with:

- Acyclovir (Nejm 1990;320:1381)
- Interferon × 14 wk (Nejm 1983;308:1489)
- CMV immune globulin iv (Nejm 1987;317:1049)

of disease in immunocompromised hosts:

- Ganciclovir (Nejm 1999;340:1063, 1991;325:1601; Med Let 1989;31:79), which kills CMV but patients still die and resistance to it now developing (Ann IM 1990;112:505; Nejm 1989; 320:289); helps retinitis (Ann IM 1985;103:377) if continued in suppressive doses, 3000 mg po qd after iv rx (Nejm 1995; 333:615) or given prophylactically if $CD_4 < 50$ (Nejm 1996; 334:1491); can stop if CD_4 count up and 0 RNA loads after rx (Jama 1999;282:1633). Also available as intraocular implant (Nejm 1997;337:83); but neutropenia is a problem (Ann IM 1993;118:173,179).
- Valacyclovir prevents CMV in renal transplant (Nejm 1999; 340:1462) and is as effective and easier (po drug) than ganciclovir for rx in retinitis AIDS pts (Nejm 2002;346:1119)
- Foscarnet × 2-3 wk, qd iv maintenance gives better survival rates than ganciclovir but costs more ($24,000 vs $7500) (Med Let 1992;34:3; Nejm 1992;326:213)
- Cidofovir iv (Med Let 1997;39:14; Ann IM 1997;126:257, 264); adverse effects: renal toxicity

Erythema Infectiosum (Fifth Disease)

Nejm 2004;350:586

Cause: Parvovirus B19

Epidem: Endemic and epidemic; spread primarily by respiratory secretions, esp in infected young children (Jama 1999;281:1099).

Nosocomial epidemics in nursing staffs caring for children in aplastic crisis (Nejm 1989;321:485). 2-yr-olds are 75% seropositive (Nejm 2005;352:768). In adults, > 50% are seropositive, indicating past infection.

Pathophys: P antigen on rbc is prime cellular receptor for the virus; hence the rare pt who is pp (homozygously P antigen negative) is immune from infection (Nejm 1994;330:1192). Anemias and CHF occur because infection of erythroid progenitor cells results in their lysis acutely, and these conditions then develop if there is already chronic hemolysis for some other reason, or if no antibodies are formed at all, as in AIDS (Ann IM 1990;113:926).

Sx: 7-10 d incubation period. 20% of adults and children may be asymptomatic. In children, it presents as rash; in adults, it presents as polyarthritis and malaise.

Si: In children, "slapped cheek" may develop into diffuse exanthematous, pruritic rash lasting 5-7 d (picture: Nejm 1994;331:1062). In adults, acute arthritis; rash on neck, extremities, trunk, but not face.

Crs: Arthritis is usually self-limited although it can be chronic and recurrent; rash may recur over weeks or months.

r/o other childhood exanthems: Chickenpox, rubeola, scarlet fever, rubella, and roseola

Cmplc: Aplastic crisis in patients with underlying chronic hemolysis and occasionally chronic marrow failure (Nejm 1987;317:287)

In pregnant women, spontaneous abortion in 1-3% exposed in first 20 wks of pregnancy (Nejm 1986;315:77); other fetal anomalies (Nejm 1987;316:183, 1985;313:74), including hydrops fetalis from anemia and CHF (Ann IM 1990;113:926)

Lab: *Hem:* Marrow has giant pronormoblasts and/or multiple nucleoli in pronormoblasts

Serol: IgM, IgG antibody titers by ELISA (Jama 1999;281:1099); or, in immunosuppressed pts, by DNA dot-blot hybridization studies of serum (Ann IM 1990;113:926)

Rx: Isolation may be unnecessary. In cases of persistent infection and marrow aplasia, IgG im qd (Nejm 1989;321:519) or iv (Ann IM 1990;113:926).

German Measles

Cause: Rubella virus

Epidem: Carrier is newborn infant, excretes for > 1 yr postpartum. Maternal infection in first 7 wk causes 50% fetal death, 25% malformation rate at birth, premature delivery in 25%, and no problem in 20%; infection at 20 wk gestation and beyond results in no teratology and < 10% prematurity rate.

Incidence is down to a few hundred/yr in U.S. (Jama 2002;287:464)

Pathophys: A mild virus, hence damages without killing the fetus

Sx: Malaise; rash

Si: Exanthematous rash, usually; face first, spreads in 3 d; macular-papular; in infant with congenital syndrome as well; r/o other childhood exanthems: roseola, rubeola, scarlet fever, erythema infectiosum (5th disease)

Lymphadenopathy, posterior cervical, 98%; postauricular, 90%; suboccipital, 90%; preauricular, 50%

Conjunctivitis; splenomegaly (25%); fever < 102°F; sore gums

Crs: 12-21 d incubation period

Cmplc: Encephalitis (0.01%), myelitis; thrombocytopenia; RA-like syndrome (Nejm 1985;313:1117)

Congenital syndrome: Rash, low birth weight, platelets < 140,000 (91%), hepatosplenomegaly (75%), congenital heart disease (70%) especially PDA and VSD, cataracts (50%), mental retardation (100%), deafness (55%: Nejm 1968;278:809)

Lab:

Bact: Culture possible but not clinically practical

Serol: Latex, fluorescent antibody, ELISA

Rx: Rv of hospital epidemic control (Nejm 1980;303:541)

Vaccine, live attenuated 1 cc sc; rarely spreads to other family members; although spreads to fetus (25%) if pt is pregnant, no fetal damage reported in 683 documented CDC cases (Mmwr 1989;38:289). Give to all childbearing women unless h/o previous immunization beyond age 1 yr or titer is positive; may cause transient but not chronic polyarthropathy (Jama 1997;278:551).

Herpes, Types I and II

Nejm 2004;350:1970 (type II), 1986;314:686,749; Ann IM 1985; 103:404

Cause: *Herpes simplex*

Epidem: Both types may be venereally spread, ²/₃ of the time when active lesions are present, but even when no active lesions (Nejm 1986;314:1561) ¹/₃ of the time (Nejm 1995;333:770)

Type I: At age 14, 25% of whites and 70% of blacks are seropositive (Nejm 1989;321:7). ²/₃ of new cases are symptomatic; 50% are oral and 50% genital (Nejm 1999;341:1432). Associated with tic douloureux, and appears in those patients when operated on (Nejm 1979;301:225). Epidemics (herpes gladiatorum) among wrestlers (Nejm 1991;325:906).

Type II: About 20% seropositive prevalence in U.S. adults (Nejm 1997;337:1105); higher in women and blacks (Nejm 1989;321:7). ²/₃ of new cases are asx (Nejm 1999;341:1432) and shed virus as much (83%) as symptomatic pts (Nejm 2000;342:844).

Pathophys: Type I tends to be orolabial and have complications of encephalitis; type II tends to be genital and neonatal with complications of meningeal involvement; but clinically both have full overlap. The two types are distinguishable bacteriologically by serotyping and genotyping (50% different).

Sx & Si: Primary infections are sicker; have fever, tender adenopathy, gingivostomatitis (looks like aphthous stomatitis), pharyngitis, cervicitis, external genital lesions, paronychia (herpetic whitlow, primary and recurrent infection with lymphangitis)

Zoster-like syndrome in newborns (Nejm 1971;284:24)

Recurrent type manifests as classic cold sore, or genital sores

Crs: Type I: Recurs less frequently than type II (Nejm 1987;316:144)
Type II: Primary infection lasts 10 d, recurs 1-2×/yr lasting 4 d
(Nejm 1978;299:237)

Cmplc: Ocular keratitis by self-inoculation; colitis; aseptic meningitis especially with vulvovaginitis, or recurrently as **Mollaret's Meningitis** proven by PCR CSF studies (Ann IM 1994;121:334; Nejm 1991;325:1082); urinary hesitancy and sacral paresthesias especially with colitis (Nejm 1983;308:868) or vulvovaginitis; disseminated, systemic forms and encephalitis (p 692); neonatal HSV infection w 50% mortality if infection occurs < 6 wk prior to delivery (Nejm 1997;337:509)

r/o erythema multiforme, hand-foot-mouth disease (base is not erythematous), tanapox (Nejm 2004;350361) and African monkey pox herpes in monkeys (Ann IM 1990;112:833) and rodents (Wisconsin prairie dog pet epidemic: Nejm 2004;350:342)

Lab: *Bact:* Culture, can read in 2-3 d; 77% sens in primary herpes (Nejm 1992;326:1533)

Path: Skin bx shows inclusions and giant cells; scraped Tzanck prep of skin lesion very sens/specif

Serol: by western blot or glycoprotein G immunodot (HerpeSelect) methods; use PCR for CSF

Rx: Prevention:

Keep people with cold sores away from newborns and immunosuppressed pts; good handwashing technique, condom use (Jama 2001;285:3100);

In pregnancy (Jama 2003;289:203), asx shedding is common so unclear how to handle (Ann IM 1993;118:414). C-section only if clinical lesions when goes into labor because risk of infection in infant is < 8% if recurrent disease, ~50% if pri-

mary disease (Nejm 1986;315:796, 1986;316:240), but
< 10% of mothers who cultured herpes at delivery have a
h/o herpes lesion (Nejm 1988;318:887).

Vaccine, glycoprotein D adjuvant type at 0, 1, and 6 mo, 75% effective in women seronegative for both types I and II (Nejm 2002;
347:1652) but no help if seropositive for either, or in men.

Prophylaxis w valcyclovir (Nejm 2004;350:11) 500 mg po
qd, or perhaps acyclovir bid (C. Crumpacker: Nejm 2004;250:67)
in couples discordant for HSV-2 (NNT-1 = 38)

of disease (CDC: Ann IM 2002;137:255; Med Let 2002;
44:95):

Oral:

- Acyclovir (Zovirax) (Med Let 1994;36:1) 200-400 mg po 5×/d
  × 7-10 d for primary; or × 5 d for recurrent episode, then 400
  mg po bid prophylaxis reduces recurrences by > 50% long term
  (Nejm 1993;118:268); for all neonatal (iv), whitlow, primary,
  or frequently recurrent herpes progenitalis, or oropharyngeal
  stomatitis; renal excretion, dialyzable; resistance appearing in
  immunocompetent and incompetent now (Nejm 1993;329:
  1777); $0.50/pill

- Famcyclovir (Famvir) 125 mg po bid × 5 d at 1st sx of recurrence decreases shedding and duration/severity of sx (Jama
  1996;276:44); or 500 mg po tid × 7 d for primary or severe infection; 250 mg po bid long-term prophylaxis decreases recurrence at 6 mo from 75% to 25% and is safe (Jama 1998;280:
  887); 500 mg po bid preventively in AIDS pts w pos serology
  perhaps (Ann IM 1998;128:21)

- Valacyclovir (Valtrex) bid × 5-7 d (Arch IM 1996;156:1729);
  2 gm po q 12 hr × 2 for recurrent type I shortens crs by 1 d;
  500 mg po qd for long-term suppression, cheapest regimen
  (Med Let 1999;41:90)

Topical (recurrent type I rx only):

- Ducosanol (Abreva) (Med Let 2000;42:108) OTC 10% cream
  5×/d shortens duration by 1-2 d, works by blocking cell

entry—not viral synthesis like others—so may help if used w 1st si of recurrence

- Penciclovir 1% cream q 2 hr × 4 d; speeds healing and end of shedding by 1 d (Jama 1997;277:1374; Med Let 1997;39:57) vs no help at least in genital herpes (Med Let 1999;41:90)
- Acyclovir 5% ointment 6×/d shortens crs by ½ d
    Herbal: Avoid Herp-Eaze (chaparral shrub), which is hepatorenal toxic (Arch IM 1997;157:913)

Herpes: Disseminated, Systemic, or Encephalitis

Nejm 1986;314:686,749; Ann IM 1985;103:404

Cause: *Herpes simplex* types I and II

Epidem: Occurs in babies < age 3 mo born of mothers with active disease (Nejm 1991;324:450, 1985;313:1327) or to asymptomatic but viral shedding mothers (56/15,000) (Nejm 1991;324:1247); immunosuppressed pts; atopics (eczema)

    Asx shedding when no lesions in 10-20% w type I or II genital herpes in 1st yr after primary infection (Ann IM 1992;116:433)

Pathophys:

Sx & Si: Encephalopathy: Olfactory sensations, focal seizures and si, low-grade fever, often no skin lesions

    Disseminated type has classic herpes vesicular rash all over body

    Systemic type has fever, malaise, etc

Crs: Encephalopathy: Rapid crs of early rx helps, otherwise 70% mortality

Cmplc: Myelitis, hepatitis, pneumonitis, meningitis (Nejm 1982; 307:1060); encephalitis may look like temporal lobe mass lesion, r/o similar **Lacrosse Viral Encephalitis** (Nejm 2001;344:801) for which no approved rx is available, mostly in children, 15% have permanent residual defects.

Lab: *Bact:* Culture eye, blood, pharynx

CSF: Tzanck prep has a 50% false-negative rate

Path: Brain bx is abnormal

Serol: Diagnostic in 57% (Ann IM 1983;98:958,977: K. Holmes); most helpful in primary infections, not recurrences

Rx: Prevent by keeping people with cold sores away from newborns and immunosuppressed pts; good handwashing technique; in pregnancy, culture weekly, C section only if clinical lesions when goes into labor because risk of infection in child is < 8% if recurrent disease, ~50% if primary (Nejm 1986;315:796, 1986;316: 240), but < 10% of mothers who cultured herpes at delivery have a h/o herpes lesion (Nejm 1988;318:887). In sexually active pts, about 10%/yr transmit to their partners even when being careful (Ann IM 1992;116:197). Vaccine eventually? of disease:

- Acyclovir for all (Med Let 1994;36:1; Ann IM 1987;107:859), including neonates (Nejm 1991;324:444), 5 mg/kg q 8 hr iv × 5-7 d; renal excretion, dialyzable, resistance now appearing (Nejm 1989;320:313) in 5% of cases (Ann IM 1990;112:416); or, if acyclovir-resistant,
- Foscarnet (Ann IM 1989;110:1710), which is better than
- Vidarabine (Nejm 1991;325:551), although often recurrence within 6 wk of rx completion

Kaposi's Sarcoma

Nejm 2000;342:1027

Cause: Human herpes 8 virus (HHV-8) coinfection w HIV (Nejm 1999;340:1863, 1998;338:948, 1997;336:163, 1996;334:1168, 1292; Jama 1997;277:478)

Epidem: HHV-8 is transmitted venereally and perhaps more importantly orally by saliva as it commonly is in children in developing countries (Jama 2002;287:221,1295; Nejm 2000;343:1369), and by needle sharing (Nejm 2001;344:637) at least among gay males and other immunosuppressed pts; some endemic pockets in Africa and Near East; also induced? by immunosuppression for transplants (Nejm 2000;343:1378) like kidney most commonly

Pathophys:

Sx & Si: Violaceous skin eruptions, ulcers on legs, r/o angiomatosis

Crs: 80% mortality if immunosuppressed; not bad otherwise

Cmplc: r/o bacillary angiomatosis by bx

Lab: *Path:* Spindle-shaped tumor cells

Rx: Intralesional HCG (Nejm 1996;335:1261); interferon-α helps 50% (Nejm 1983;308:1071; debatable: Ann IM 1990;112:582) given w antiviral rx; vinblastine 4-8 mg iv q 1 wk (Ann IM 1985;103:335); topical alitretinoin (Panretin), $2000/60 gm

Radiation helpful for localized disease

of post-renal transplant type: Sirolimus (Rapamune) very effective (Nejm 2005;352:1317)

Influenza

Cause: Influenza virus, types A (most common), B (very young and very old), and C (rare); a myxovirus

Epidem: Worldwide; spread by respiratory droplets. Incidence higher in pts with elevated pulmonary artery pressures, eg, mitral stenosis, pregnancy. School absenteeism increases from 6% to 20% within 2 d of epidemic, best way to monitor. Frequency and severity of A > B > C. 2 types of external antigens: hemagglutinin and neuraminidase; both can undergo antigen shifts; they occur infrequently; there may be a finite and predictable nature to shifts, eg, 1978 A2 variant was similar to 1889–1890 type (Nejm 1978;298:587).

Pathophys: Ulceration of tracheobronchial tree can cause secondary bacterial infections

Sx: Cough invariably, fever, malaise

Si: Cough, usually nonproductive at first

Crs: 1-2 d incubation period; sx last 5-6 d, malaise may last 2 wk

Cmplc: Secondary bacterial pulmonary infections acutely or during convalescent stage; fulminant viral infection leading to death in 1st 48 hr, myocarditis, parotitis (Nejm 1977;296:1391)

r/o RSV, 2nd most common winter respiratory infection in nursing homes (Nejm 2005;352:1749; J Am Ger Soc 2003;51:761)

Severe acute respiratory syndrome (SARS) (Nejm 2003;349:2431; Ann IM 2004;141:3331, 2003;139:715; Jama 2003;289:2801), a coronavirus community-acquired pneumonia; 12% mortality, worst over age 60; 16% transmission rates on airplanes; fever (99%), nonproductive cough (44%), HA (33%), myalgia/malaise, elevated LDH and CRP, die of renal and respiratory failure

Lab: *Serol:* Rapid diagnostic tests have 73% sens, 95% specif; $20 (Med Let 1999;41:121). Comp-fix, FA, or hemagglutination antibodies to types A, B, or C.

Rx (Med Let, yearly update in Sept; Nejm 2000;343:1778):
Vaccine, 0.5 cc im or 0.1-0.2 cc intradermal is just as good in young (< 60 yr) pts (Nejm 2004;351:2286,2295,2330), trivalent usually, annually in October if health care worker, child ½-2 yr old, over age 50, or chronically ill. New combination each year based on best guess from previous year's new organisms; usually two A strains and one B strain. 50% effective (reduction in incidence) in the elderly (Jama 1994; 272:1661), mortality NNT = 300, 25% reduction in elderly mortality if given annually over several years (Jamam 2004; 292:2089); 25-50% reductions in pneumonia and CHF (Nejm 1994;331:778); in young healthy adults, vaccination reduces illness incidence by 25% and workday losses by 40% (Nejm 1995;333:889) and probably worth it (Ann IM 2002; 137:225); in health care workers caring for elderly,

mortality of their pts is decreased (J Infect Dis 1997;175:1). Adverse effects: generally no different from placebo except sore arm (Nejm 1995;333:889), hepatic metabolism of many drugs decreased by 50% for 1 wk, eg, theophylline, warfarin (Nejm 1981; 305:1262; questionable: Med Let 1985;27:81). Can give at same time as pneumovax at different site. In children, split virus under age 4 into 2 0.25-cc doses if 1st immunization was 1 mo earlier (Nejm 1977;296:567); debated if worth using in elderly (Jama 1990;264:1139). In cancer pts, diminished response so try to give between chemoRx courses (Ann IM 1977;87:552); diminished response in nursing home patients. Not protective in HIV-positive pts (Ann IM 1988;109:383).

FluMist (MedImmune) (Med Let 2003;45:65) ¼ cc each nostril × 1, live attenuated lA vaccine, effective in children as well (Nejm 1998;338:1405); avoid in pregnancy, immunocompromised pts, within 48 hr of antiviral drugs, and in children on chronic ASA rx; adverse effects: transiently worsened asthma, egg allergies, ? Bell's palsy reported in Swiss version (Nejm 2004; 350:896); $50/dose

Drug prophylaxis and rx of disease (p 664) w rimantadine (cheapest), oseltamivir, amantadine, or zanamivir (Relenza)

Lassa Fever

Nejm 1990;323:1120,1139, 1986;314:20

Cause: Lassa fever virus, an arenavirus

Epidem: In western Africa, endemic in Sierra Leone. Perhaps a flea vector from African rat reservoir; also from blood exposure like hepatitis B and HIV; respiratory exposure has minimal risk.

Sx: 7-18 d incubation. Fever, sore throat, back pain, cough, headache, abdominal pain

Si: Pharyngitis, often exudative; conjunctivitis

Crs: 1-4 wk, 15-20% mortality; 53% without rx, 5% with rx

Cmplc: gi hemorrhage, hypovolemic shock; ARDS; encephalopathy; pericarditis, CHF; sensorineural deafness

r/o similar syndrome produced by southwestern U.S. **Hantavirus**, transmitted by deer mouse fleas/ticks and experimentally rx'd w ribavirin as well (Nejm 1994;330:949); perhaps also the cause of medieval "sweating sickness" in England (Nejm 1997;336:580)

Lab: *Chem:* Aspartate aminotransferase (AST = SGOT) ≥ 150 IU/L; other hepatocellular enzymes are also up

Serol: IgM antibody titers

Urine: Proteinuria

Rx: Call CDC; quarantine

Ribavirin iv or po helps if given prophylactically after exposure or within 6 d of sx onset

Measles

Cause: Rubeola, a paramyxovirus

Epidem: Spread by direct contact with pt in day 2 or more of incubation period. Worldwide, common. Mortality up to 50% in developing countries, highest (0.1%) in rural infants over age 1 (Am J Pub Hlth 1980;70:1166); higher in vitamin A–deficient pts (Nejm 1990;323:160).

Pathophys: Respiratory tract involved, nose to bronchial tree

Viremia within 2 d of contact. Koplik's spots and skin lesions are areas of local intracellular viral replication (Nejm 1970;283:1139).

Encephalitis is hypersensitivity damage, not infectious (Nejm 1984;310:137)

Sx: Fever of infection, with rash, on day 2 after exposure, is rare

4-6 d prodrome of gradually increasing fever to 104°F (40°C), brassy cough, nasal discharge (coryza), photophobia, and then rash

Si: • Koplik's spots on buccal mucosa, white on red base, opposite
molars
 • Conjunctivitis, palpebral only
 • Vascular spiders on soft palate
 • Rash, "brown paint spilled over head and neck," starts around
ears, macular/papular, can be on palms and soles when severe
 • Fever increasing to 105-106°F (40.5-41.1°C) with rash appearance, then decreasing to normal in 24 hr
   Atypical measles in previously vaccinated = lymphadenopathy, pulmonary infiltrates, distal rash including palms and soles,
high fever (Ann IM 1979;90:873-887)

Crs: 12-14 d incubation period. 2-10% mortality in developing countries (Nejm 1985;313:544).

Cmplc:
   Early: Hecht's giant cell pneumonia in adults; secondary bacterial
      infections of lung, ear; thrombocytopenia (rare); encephali-
      tis in 0.1%, 65% of these will have neurologic residua, sub-
      clinical in 15-20% (L. Weinstein 1986)
   Late: Subacute sclerosing panencephalitis 10-20 yr later (Nejm
      1975;292:990), a slow virus effect, associated with dimin-
      ished DHS and IgA levels (Nejm 1985;313:910), cf progres-
      sive multifocal leukoencephalopathy from papovavirus
      (Nejm 1973;289:1278), or AIDS (p 666)
      r/o other childhood exanthems: roseola, rubella, scarlet
   fever, erythema infectiosum (5th disease)

Lab: *Hem:* Wbc decreased, if increased look for bacterial infection,
      encephalitis, or viral pneumonia; platelets depressed usually
   Path: Skin bx of rash shows intranuclear inclusion bodies
   Serol: Antibody by neutralizing, hemagglutination, or comp-fix

Rx: Passive prophylaxis with IgG
      Active immunization with live attenuated virus vaccine, af-
ter age 15 mo; ~15% won't take, these pts later sustain outbreaks
as adults (Nejm 1987;316:771); give after only 9 mo of age in de-

veloping countries (Nejm 1985;313:544); under 2 mo, $< \frac{2}{3}$ respond (Jama 1998;280:527). Continued outbreaks in U.S. preschoolers with low vaccination rates and in schoolchildren because of vaccine failures; revaccinate at age 5 (Nejm 1989;320:75) or 10 (Med Let 1989;31:69); 2-shot series is 98% effective (Jama 1997;277:1156). Safe even if allergic to eggs (Nejm 1995;332:1262).

Vitamin A 200,000 IU × 2 increases survival in developing countries (Nejm 1990;323:160)

of depressed platelets, if bad enough: Steroids

Mononucleosis

Ann IM 1993;118:45

Cause: Epstein-Barr virus (Nejm 2000;343:481), a herpesvirus

Epidem: Spread by intimate contact with carrier. 18% of adults are asx, oral excreters (Nejm 1973;289:1325). Especially in college age adults; only in previously EBV antibody negative; at Yale freshmen class = 75% antibody negative, but only 35% negative after 4 yr; apparent to inapparent infections = 2:1 (Yale: Nejm 1970;282:361).

Pathophys: Lives in only B lymphocytes (Nejm 1979;301:1133) and mouth epithelial cells; replicates only in latter (Nejm 1979;301:1255). IgM antibody response (heterophile) decreased rapidly (Nejm 1966;274:61). EBV antibody (IgG, anti-early antigen) persists for years and correlates with cancer risk (Ann IM 1986;104:331; Nejm 1985;312:750). Diminished DHS transiently (Nejm 1974;291:1149).

Sx: Macular rash; sore throat; fever, low grade with malaise; pain behind eyes helps tell from strep throat, r/o rubella, flu; alcohol worsens malaise

Si: Pharyngitis, purulent sterile tonsillitis; splenomegaly (50%, males; 25%, females); hepatitis, low grade, especially if age > 40 yr

(Nejm 1975;293:1273); eyelid edema; palatal petechial rash,*
lymphadenopathy* (40%), especially postauricular and posterior
cervical (r/o secondary syphilis and CMV). Genital ulcers lasting
30 d (Nejm 1984;311:966).

Crs: Usually benign

Cmplc: Rare encephalitis with residual impairment (L. Weinstein
3/85); Guillain-Barré and Bell's palsy, often EBV positive without
clinical mono (Nejm 1975;292:392); ruptured spleen; hemolytic
anemia; pharyngeal obstruction; rash in 100% if given ampicillin;
nasopharyngeal cancers (Nejm 2001;345:1877); B-cell lymphoma
(Nejm 1983;309:745) and AIDS-associated or post-transplant
lymphoproliferative disease (Nejm 1993;327:1710,1750);
leiomyosarcomas (Nejm 1995;332:19); thymic cancer (Nejm
1985;312:1298); Hodgkin's within 5 yr in 1/1000 young adults
(Nejm 2003;349:1324); hairy leukoplakia in AIDS (S. Sears
8/97); perhaps multiple sclerosis (Jama 2001;286:3083)

r/o mono-like syndrome caused by CMV (p 684) and human
herpesvirus 6 (Nejm 1993;329:168)

Lab: *Chem:* Amylase elevated even without pancreatitis due to salivary source

Hem: Wbc shows > 50% monos and lymphs with > 10% atypical lymphs (serrated where touch rbc, clear cytoplasm, often
vacuolated) (Nejm 1969;280:836); r/o hepatitis A, rubella,
toxoplasma, phenytoin (Dilantin) (Nejm 1981;305:722),
Graves's disease, CMV especially postpump, PAS

Serol: EBV immunofluorescent antibody > 1/80

Heterophile by rapid slide (monospot), which will be
positive if titer > 1/40, but if too high must be diluted 1st;
false positive with serum sickness; or by sheep rbc agglutination by pt serum, with which serum sickness is distinguished
by absorbing sera 1st with guinea pig kidney cells, while
mono still agglutinates, and 2nd by beef cells, after which

*If neither present, no point getting monospot: Ann IM 1982;96:505.

serum sickness still agglutinates. Heterophile goes negative over 6-12 mo.

Rx: Symptomatic, steroids for pharyngeal obstruction, hemolytic anemia, or severe neurologic sx

Acyclovir no help in chronic fatigue syndrome (Nejm 1988;319:1692) or acute mono

Mumps

Nejm 1968;279:1357

Cause: Mumps virus, a paramyxovirus

Epidem: Common; all susceptible exposed pts get neutralizing antibody, 60% get sx

Pathophys: A parotitis

Sx: Nausea and vomiting, fever, pain, and swelling in front of ear and at jaw angle

Si: Parotid enlarged (9/13), unilateral in 15%; ear pushed out, jaw angle obliterated; r/o influenza et al, which can also cause parotitis (Nejm 1977;296:1391). Opsoclonus (dancing nystagmus) and small pupils; fever; aseptic meningitis, 25% have CSF cells, usually benign, can have without parotitis.

Crs:

Cmplc: Pancreatitis, often; meningoencephalitis; orchitis in adult; arthritis, large joint, asymmetric; pneumonia; diabetes induction

Lab: *Chem:* Amylase elevated
CSF: Cells in 25%; glucose diminished, protein increased for a long time, often (Nejm 1969;280:855)
Serol: Antibody titers elevated, reliable index of immunity; skin test not helpful

Rx: Isolation of pts of little value since spreads before sx. Passive immunization with hyperimmune IgG not effective (Med Let 1968;10:14). Active immunization with live virus gives lifelong immunity (Ann IM 1983;98:192).

Polio

Cause: Polio virus, an enterovirus

Epidem: Fecal–oral spread; peak incidence in summer and fall. Paradoxically occurs in countries with good sewage systems; correlates inversely with infant mortality, when < 70/1000, many persons not infected in infancy when protected with maternal antibody and hence are susceptible when older when the disease is much more damaging. Most cases now acquired outside of U.S. in persons immunized as children or as vaccine associated (see below). Global eradication now nearly 90% complete.

Only 0.1-1% of cases show clinical si's, ie, most are subclinical. Increased clinical incidence in pregnant or ovulating females; after T+A bulbar polio is increased, even if T+A was years ago (L. Weinstein 6/67).

Pathophys: Hits anterior horn cells and sympathetic ganglia; starts in gi reticuloendothelial system; inhibits RNA polymerase

Sx: Fever, malaise, drowsy, headache, nausea, diarrhea or constipation, sore throat; may have stiff neck, low-back pain

Si: An aseptic meningitis; meningismus for 2-10 d; flaccid paralysis, maximum in a few days, maximum recovery in 6 mo. Spinal type may be in muscles of lumbar, dorsal, or cervical areas; bulbar type in upper (cranial nerves III-VIII), lower (CN IX-XII), or medullary (immediate threat to life).

Crs: 6-18 d incubation period. Death in 15% if pt > 15 yr old; in 2.5% if pt < 15 yr.

Cmplc: Encephalitis; viral pneumonia
Late post-polio muscular atrophy due to reactivated CNS infection (Nejm 1991;325:749) w partial motor neuron dysfunction and dropout but not total dropout (Nejm 1987;317:7, 1986; 314:959), including dysphagia from bulbar involvement (Nejm 1991;324:1162)

r/o other causes of "viral" meningitis: coxsackie, echo, viral hepatitis, leptospirosis, et al (p 778)

Lab: *CSF:* Aseptic meningitis picture

Serol: Comp-fix and neutralizing antibody titers

Rx (Ann IM 1982;96:630):

Gamma globulin for passive, short-lived protection

Vaccine:

IPV (Salk): Killed virus, primary 3-shot series then boost × 1 in 4-5 yr and on foreign travel; lasts 6+ yr; 70% effective; used in U.S. rather than OPV to avoid no spread to immunocompromised pts

OPV (Sabin) (Nejm 1977;297:249): Live attenuated, 90% effective, spreads to other intimate contacts, elicits gi RES secretory IgA immunity as well as systemic unlike Salk (Nejm 1968;279:893); used now in developing countries where benefit of spreading it seen as offsetting risk to immunocompromised pts

Rabies (Hydrophobia)

Nejm 2004;351:2626; Ann IM 1998;128:922

Cause: Rabies virus, a rhabdovirus

Epidem: From saliva of infected animal, inhaling infected guano in bat caves, or corneal transplants (Nejm 1979;300:603). Bats may be reservoir since not killed by it. Cats are now most commonly affected domestic animal. Most common wild animals affected: bats, foxes, skunks, raccoons; and prey species like rabbits, woodchucks, and goats (Me Epigram 12/95).

Cyclic prevalence q 100 yr, peaked in 1965. 20 cases in U.S. 1960–1980 (Ann IM 1984;100:728); increasing again in U.S.: 22 cases in 1990–1996. Over 20 cases in animals annually in Maine alone (Me Epigram 12/95).

Pathophys: Spreads along nerves to CNS

Sx: H/o animal bite except in bat rabies, where often no h/o bite or even bat contact (Mmwr 1995;44:625)

Pain/paresthesias at exposure site in 50%; difficulty swallowing in 65%; fever; priapism; nausea and vomiting; Guillain-Barré-like syndrome

Si: Encephalitis with tonic contractions of muscles, especially throat on minimal stimulation (hence hydrophobia)

Crs: 15-60 d incubation (depends on nerve length), rarely up to 6 yr later (Nejm 1991;324:205)

Fatal unless rx'd before sx, usually, although some severe cases now recovering with supportive care, ie, respirator (Ann IM 1976;85:44). 2/38 survived 1960–1980.

Cmplc: May be misdiagnosed as Guillain-Barré

Lab: *CSF:* Elevated protein after 1 wk; cells are a mix of lymphs and polys, 6-300/mm^3

Path: Negri bodies in brain at postmortem

Serol: Half positive after 1 wk of sx, $^2/_3$ after 1$^1/_2$ wk, all positive by 2 wk of sx

Rx: See flow sheet: Jama 2000;284:1003

Vaccinate (Med Let 1998;40:64) w human diploid cell vaccine (HDCV) (Imovax); rabies vaccine absorbed, or purified chick embryo cell (PCEC) (RabAvert); all ~$700/5-shot series; chloroquine malaria prophylaxis may prevent adequate immunization (Nejm 1986;314:280)

- Primary series postexposure = HDCV im on day 1, 3, 7, 14, and 28
- Preexposure = day 1, 7, and 28 im, or 1/10 im dose intradermal day 1, 7, 21, or 28
- Booster

  Post repeat exposure after previous primary series w shots day 0 and 3

  Q 2 yr to veterinarians and other high-risk people

For acute single exposure: Vaccinate as above + HRIG (immune globulin) 20 IU/kg, ½ in wound, ½ im in deltoid in adult, thigh in child, not gluteal area (Nejm 1987;316:1256,1270); use liberally even if no bite in bat exposures (Mmwr 1995;44:625)

of disease: Supportive care, like respirator

Roseola (Exanthem Subitum, 6th Disease)

Cause: Human herpesvirus 6

Epidem: 14% of febrile children under age 2 in ER have it, cause of ⅓ of febrile seizures under age 2 yr (Nejm 1994;331:432, 1992;326:1145)

Pathophys:

Sx: High fever to 105°F (40.5°C) for 3-4 d, defervesce, then rash in 10%

Si: Viral exanthem, fever

Lab:

Rx: Symptomatic

Yellow Fever

Jama 1996;276:1157

Cause: Yellow fever virus, an arbovirus

Epidem: Vector is the mosquito, *Aedes aegypti* in urban type, *A. hemogogus* in jungle type. Humans are only reservoir in urban type, monkeys in jungle type. Increasing problem is Africa and S. America; could reappear in U.S.

Pathophys: Viremia and hepatitis

Sx: Malaise and jaundice

Si: Icterus; tender liver; fever > 105°F (40.5°C); minimal tachycardia r/o salmonella, gram-negative shock, psittacosis, and Q fever

Crs: 3-6 d incubation; 10-15% mortality, 50% mortality if reach toxic icteric phase

Cmplc: Hepatic or renal failure, myocarditis
r/o malaria; leptospirosis; viral hepatitis; typhus; ebola virus
r/o **Dengue** (Jama 1997;277:1546; Nejm 1989;321:957),
mosquito-transmitted febrile illness often with exanthematous
rash, usually benign course, possibly helped by vaccination vs
Japanese encephalitis (Nejm 1988;319:808)

Lab: *Chem:* Elevated LFTs
Path: Liver bx shows viral hepatitis picture but more irregular
necrosis and Councilman bodies that are questionably distinguishable from Mallory's bodies?
Serol: IgM antibodies

Rx: Prevent by spraying to kill mosquitos if > 5-10% homes
have *Aedes*
Vaccine, live virus; effective in 1 wk; use in endemic areas,
eg, S. America and Africa; $^1/_2$ cc sc; lasts 10+ yr; egg base (Ann
IM 1969;71:365); available at special distribution centers in U.S.

Chapter 10

Neurology

D. K. Onion

10.1 Vascular Disease

Transient Ischemic Attack

Nejm 2002;347:1687

Cause: Carotid or aortic arch (Nejm 1992;326:221) plaque and/or platelet emboli, cardiac emboli, vascular spasm, hypercoagulable states, and idiopathic

Epidem:

Pathophys: Plaque ulceration correlates poorly with TIA and it is hard to accurately make that dx (Curr Concepts Cerebro Dis 1987;22:19); occasionally is vasospastic and can rx w calcium-channel blocker (Nejm 1993;329:396)

Sx: Lateralized neurologic sx, usually lasting < 5-10 min but by revised (Nejm 2002;347:1713) definition always < 1 hr w no evidence of CVA by imaging

Anterior circulation sx: Amaurosis fugax (Stroke 1990;21:201), weakness of arm > face > leg paresis (middle cerebral artery pattern), leg > arm > face paresis (anterior cerebral artery pattern)

Posterior circulation sx: Bilateral blindness, diplopia, numbness in face and mouth, slurred speach, quadriplegia

Si: Carotid bruit, but correlates poorly with symptomatic disease (Ann IM 1994;120:633); in elderly pts, asx bruit present in 10% and does not correlate with CVA rate in or out of affected carotid distribution; 60% disappear over 3 yr (Ann IM 1990;112:340)

Flow reversal through supraorbital artery (feel, then occlude preauricular artery; if lose pulse, then flow is reversed) indicates significant carotid stenosis or occlusion

Crs: Subsequent stroke, 5% within 2 d (Jama 2000;284:2901), 8% in 1st mo, 5%/yr for 3 yr, 3%/yr thereafter; 41% will die of MI

Cmplc: r/o tumor, can mimic exactly (Arch Neurol 1983;40:633); r/o carotid or vertebral dissections (see below); post zoster cerebral vasculitis (Nejm 2002;347:1500) if zoster within weeks to months ago, reversible w acyclovir rx iv

Lab: *Noninv:* All about 85% sens and 90% specif (Ann IM 1995; 122:360, 1988;109:805,835)

Not substitutable for angiography unless local comparisons made (Nejm 1998;339:1415, 1468; Stroke 1995;26:1747) but still is often done (Stroke 2003;33:2003)
- Carotid Doppler or duplex US
- Magnetic resonance angiography

Xray: CT to r/o bleed or MRI to r/o stroke (Neurol 2004;62:S29); carotid angiography, if ready to operate; % stenosis denominator is normal carotid, not bulb or poststenotic dilated area; Europeans calculate differently (Nejm 1998;339:1415)

Rx:

of asx carotid bruit: (see below)
Meds:
- ASA 30 mg qd after 300 mg load as good as higher doses and has fewer side effects (Nejm 1991;325:1261); or as Aggrenox (Med Let 2000;42:11) 25 mg ASA + 200 mg dipyridamole po bid; not clearly better than ASA alone; $90/mo
- Clopidogrel (Plavix) 75 mg po qd (Lancet 2004;364:331)

- Ticlopidine (Med Let 1992;34:65) 250 mg po qd but not as good as ASA (Jama 2003;289:2947) but causes gi side effects often and agranulocytosis in 1%; $80/mo
- Warfarin for pts > 60 yr w Afib and intrinsic heart disease, hypertension, LVH, or previous TIA (Ann IM 1994;121:41,54) (p 709); or ASA or ticlopidine if bleeding risk w warfarin judged too high (Ann IM 1994;121:45)

Stenting w post-op ASA and clopidogrel (Plavix) in high-risk pts (and maybe others?) as good as open endarterectomy (Nejm 2004;351:1493)

Surgical endarterectomy (Jama 1992;268:3120) of stenosis > 70% (Nejm 1995;332:238), in pts with TIA or mild CVA, reduces strokes by 17% (NNT = 6) (Nejm 1991;325:445); stenosis of 50-70% in symptomatic pts equivocally helped (Nejm 1998; 339:1415). If asx carotid stenosis > 60-70%, NNT-5 = 16 (Nejm 2000;342:1743; Jama 1995;273:1421,1459 vs Lancet 2004;363: 1491; ACP J Club 2004;141:31; Nejm 2000;342:1693), and clearly if > 80% (Ann IM 1995;123:720 vs 723; ACP J Club 1995;123:2; Lancet 1995;345:209); but still debatable if asx (S. Kolkin 5/97) since NNT-3 = 36 (ACP J Club 1999;130:59), and cost per stroke avoided = $500,000 (Ann IM 1997;126:338). No help if stenosis is < 50% (Lancet 1996;347:1591); presumes a combined cmplc rate of angiography and surgery of < 3%; often much higher morbidity in community hospitals, but only 1+% in big centers (Ann IM 2004;140:303).

Aspirin + dipyridamole no help postendarterectomy to prevent recurrence (Ann IM 1992;116:731)

Carotid or Vertebral Artery Dissection

Nejm 2001;344:898; Neurol 1995;45:1517

Cause: Spontaneous, or trauma that is often trivial ("hairdresser's stroke"), or spinal manipulation (Med Let 2000;44:50)

Epidem: 1/100,000/yr for vertebral and 2.5/100,000/yr for carotid. 2% of all ischemic CVAs but 10-25% of those age < 50; peak in 40s.

Increased in Ehler-Danlos, Marfan's, osteogenesis imperfecta, polycystic kidney disease, and w positive family hx

Pathophys: Intimal tear in extracranial portions of the vessels

Sx: Age 35-55 yr

> Carotid: Sometimes h/o minor neck twist or trauma; facial pain (50%), unilateral headache (66%) often hemicrania, cerebellar ischemic sx (63%), retinal ischemia w amaurosis fugax, cranial nerve palsies (10%), dysgeusias, tinnitus (35%) that is often pulsatile

> Vertebral: Posterior neck pain (50%) or headache (66%); cerebral, cerebellar, brain stem ischemic sx (90%), eg, lateral medullary plate syndrome (p 713)

Si: Horner's syndrome (46%) (p 776); bruit (24%) (Nejm 1994;330:393; Arch Neurol 1986;43:1234; Neurol Clin 1983;1:155)

Crs: Contralateral dissection in 2%, usually within 1 mo; rarely in same artery

Cmplc: Raeder's neuropathic pain (p 776); CVA; blindness

Lab:

Xray: MRI/MRA (Nejm 1996;335:1368) usually diagnostic; or angiography

Rx: Heparin followed by warfarin × 3 mo; surgery sometimes if progresses

Embolic Stroke

Nejm 1992;326:1672

Cause: Atherosclerotic plaque, esp carotid, and protruding atheromatous plaque > 4 mm in thoracic aorta (Nejm 1996;334:1216); mitral stenosis; SBE and atrial myxoma; cardiac valve prostheses; from silent DVT (Ann IM 1993;119:461) paradoxically through ASD, may be silent (Ann IM 1986;105:695); 40% of pts < 55 yr old with CVA have patent foramen ovale (Ann IM 1992; 117:461; Nejm 1988;318:1148); post-MI mural thrombus, 5% of pts with big anterior MI develop a mural thrombus, most in first 10 d (Nejm 1989;320:392); chronic Afib (Arch Neurol 1984; 41:708); billowing mitral valve (Nejm 1980;302:138)

Also from fat emboli (p 995), and air emboli esp in divers (Ann IM 2001;134:21)

Epidem: 31% of all strokes; incidence increased 5× in atherosclerotic Afib, 17× in rheumatic Afib (Neurol 1978;28:973); 35% lifetime incidence of stroke in Afib, ¾ are embolic (Curr Concepts Cerebro Dis 1986;21:5). Associated with homocystinuria (p 317), hypertension, and smoking (Nejm 1986;315:717).

Pathophys:

Sx: Very abrupt onset; seizures with onset occasionally, unlike thrombotic CVA

Si: Occlusion patterns like thrombotic stroke

Crs: 15% 30-d mortality

Cmplc: Like thrombotic strokes

Lab: *CSF:* Protein may be slightly elevated and may have some (< 1000) rbc's

Noninv: Echo cardiogram, 2-D with contrast to find ASD at least in young pts without obvious cause (Ann IM 1992;117:922, 1986;105:695) or LV thrombus (80+% sens); or TEE, 100% sens, 99% specif for LA thrombus (Ann IM 1995;123:817)

Rx (Nejm 1994;121:41):

Prevent by:

ASA prophylaxis po qd (Am J Med 2000;108:205)

Modifying risk factors like HT and smoking (Nejm 1995;333:1392)

Surgical endarterectomy

Anticoagulate all pts w chronic or intermittent Afib w warfarin (Nejm 1992;327:1451), at least those > age 60; or, if bleeding risk of warfarin seems too high, perhaps ASA (Nejm 1990; 322:863) although some studies suggest no help (Ann IM 1995; 123:649 but counted angina and MIs as well?) or, if that fails, ticlopidine; doing so decreases CVA rate by 2.5% on average, but at 2 yr, rate with rx is 1% compared to 7% on placebo, ie, number needed to rx (NNT-2 yr = 16) (Nejm 1990;323: 1505); PT of 1.2-1.5 by control is adequate (Nejm 1992;327: 1406); no need to anticoagulate if age < 60 yr, no h/o TIA, no valve disease, normal echo, and no hypertension (Ann IM 1994; 121:41,54); annual bleeding risk ~ 2.5% (Ann IM 1992;116:6). Anticoagulate anterior MIs with therapeutic heparin doses in first 10 d (Nejm 1989;320:352,392).

Thrombotic Stroke

Nejm 1992;326:1672

Cause: Atherosclerosis; hypotension; migraine; estrogen (Jama 2000; 284:72) birth control pills; arteritis caused by radiation, collagen vascular diseases, drug use (Ann IM 1972;76:823); infection leading to venous thrombosis or carotid occlusion especially in children with tonsillitis; trauma to carotid or head, which may cause spasm, most often seen in pts with migraine hx; hematologic causes like polycythemia, sickle disease, TTP, DIC, dysproteinemias; inherited clotting factor abnormalities, like factor V (Leiden) and prothrombin gene position 20210 mutation, cause venous thrombosis incidence to increase especially w bcp use (Nejm 1998;338:1793)

Epidem: Large-vessel ($\frac{1}{2}$ are carotid) type = 34% of all strokes; lacunar = 19% of all strokes. 3% are in pts < 40 yr old (Curr Concepts Cerebro Dis 1982;17:15).

Incidence decreased by 1+ drinks/wk (Nejm 1999;341: 1557) or < 2 drinks qd (Jama 1999;281:53)

Associated with "crack" cocaine use (Nejm 1990;323:699), homocystinuria (p 317), HT, smoking (Nejm 1986;315:717,

1988;318:937), immediate postpartum period (Nejm 1996; 335:768)

Pathophys: Carotid type usually a watershed distribution in anterior circulation; vertebral basilar syndromes (Curr Concepts Cerebro Dis 1980;15:11)

Sx: TIA hx (80%); nocturnal onset (60%)

Si: Specific occlusion patterns:

Middle cerebral: Face and arm motor; expressive aphasia (Broca's)

Carotid watershed: Parietal aphasias, weakness of arm > face > leg

Posterior cerebral: Homonymous hemianopsia, hemisensory loss, memory loss (Curr Concepts Cerebro Dis 1986;21:25)

Lateral medullary plate syndrome (posterior inferior cerebellar artery: Curr Concepts Cerebro Dis 1981;16:17): Ipsilateral pain and temperature loss on face, contralateral for rest of body, hoarseness, swallowing dysfunction, Horner's, hiccups, ipsilateral cerebellar si's

Supraorbital/preauricular artery test (see TIA) is positive if carotid occlusion

Crs: 15% 30-d mortality; < 15% return to work (Nejm 1975; 293:955); survival (as well as incidence) correlates inversely with systolic BP prior to stroke (Ann IM 1978;89:15)

Cmplc: Pulmonary embolus, pneumonias, UTIs, poststroke depression (probably physiologic, not psychological phenomenon) (Stroke 1994;25:1099) in 70% in dominant hemisphere CVA and 30% in nondominant stroke @ 2-3 wk (UCLA 9/02); swallowing dysfunction in 45% (Stroke 1999;30:744), rx w thickened liquids and pureed foods w/o swallowing studies (UCLA/Brummel-Smith 9/02)

Lab: CSF: Normal

Xray: CT scan normal first 2-4 d, positive later; MRI abnormal within hours (rv: Curr Concepts Cerebro Dis 1989;24:13)

Rx: Prevent (Nejm 1995;333:1392) by same maneuvers mentioned for embolic stroke; plus by HT control; smoking cessation; eating fish 1-2×/mo (Jama 2002;288:3130); i ASA qd (Arch IM 1999;159:1248; Lancet 1999;353:2179; Ann IM 1991;115:885), better than warfarin (Nejm 2001;345:14444); perhaps HMG-COA statin rx of elevated cholesterol (Nejm 2000;343:317; Ann IM 1998;128:89) or lower HDL w fibrates (gemfibrozil) (Circ 2001;103:2828)

Supportive care (Curr Concepts Cerebro Dis 1989;24:1): Keep pCO_2 at 25-30 mm Hg if on respirator; monitor; give 100-125 cc/hr of Ringer's or D_5S; rx diastolic BP > 140 or systolic BP > 230 acutely with iv nitroprusside, if diastolic BP persists > 105 or systolic BP > 180 for hours then rx with labetalol iv or po and/or nifedipine sl or po; mannitol 25-50 gm as 20% soln over 30 min q 3-12 hr and/or furosemide iv; ASA po qd improves outcome (Lancet 1997;349:1569,1641). Acute care in designated stroke units in England dramatically improves mortality/morbidity (BMJ 1997;314:1151).

Rehab helps 80% and can keep out of nursing home. Speech rx of aphasia of questionable help (Lancet 1984;1:1197 vs Arch Neurol 1986;43:653). Heparin sc if hemiparesis acutely to prevent DVT, which occurs in 70% (Ann IM 1992;117:353). Sinemet × 3 wk increases benefit of rehab (Lancet 2001; 358:787).

Acute rx:

- Thrombolysis w alteplase (Jama 2004;292:1831,1839,1883; Nejm 2000;343:710) within 3 hr of and maybe even up to 48 hr after onset (Jama 2004;292:1862), even basilar system and even if CT shows early changes of CVA (Jama 2001;286:2830); ok if BP < 185/110 and no ASA or heparin for at least 24 hr. But benefit/risk ratio marginal and worse w increasing age, altered mental status, and hospital inexperience. Perhaps w enhancing "mixing" of TPA into the clot, 50% lysis vs only 30% w TPA alone, and 5% major stroke risk same with both (Nejm 2004;351:2170).

TPA 0.9 mg/kg up to 90 mg max, given 10% as bolus, 90% over next 60 min; better results in 20% (NNT = 5) evident at 3 and 12 mo, not acutely, 2-10% bleed into CVA (Nejm 1999;340:1781, 1995;333:1581 vs Jama 2000;283: 1151, 1995;274:1017)

Streptokinase; ? no benefit w harmful CNS bleeding (European SK trial: Nejm 1996;335:145) vs borderline helpful if given in tertiary care stroke center w 3+% risk of fatal CNS bleed and 12% better outcome at 3 mo (Jama 1996; 276:961, 995)

Urokinase intra-arterial (Jama 1999;282:2003) possibly up to 6 hr after onset

Ancrod (Jama 2000;283:2395,2440) iv × 72 hr adjusted to fibrinogen level may be as good as TPA w same 5% bleed risk; available in Canada

- LMW heparin sc qd-bid × 10 d improves 6-mo function and survival (NNT = 5) (Nejm 1995;333:1588) vs no help over long term (Jama 1998;279:1265). iv heparin for "stroke in progress" is no help (Ann IM 1986;105:825) although ASA may be worth trying.

- ASA alone may be as good as thrombolysis (ACP J Club 1996; 124:58; Lancet 1995;346:1509)

- Unsuccessful experimental treatments: Nimodipine, a calcium-channel blocker (ACP J Club 2000;133:20; Lancet 1990;336: 1205); warfarin anticoagulation (Nejm 2005;352:1305). Surgical extraintracranial bypass no help (Nejm 1985; 313:1191).

Of poststroke depression: SSRIs (Stroke 1994;25:1099) and/or ritalin, tapering after 1 mo

Hemorrhagic Stroke

Nejm 2000;342:29 (SAB), 1997;336:28, 1992;326:1672

Cause: Subarachnoid: Aneurysm or AV malformation (Nejm 1983; 309:269)

Hemorrhage into brain substance (Nejm 2001;344:1450):
Cerebrum, cerebellum, or brain stem

Epidem: Risk increased by use of α agonists for nasal congestion or
weight loss (Nejm 2000;343:1826,1886; Med Let 2000;42:113)
Subarachnoid: 7% of all strokes; 1% of all adults have an
aneurysm. 2% of all w subarachnoid hemorrhage and
aneurysm have polycystic kidneys. Associated w iv (not
"crack") cocaine use (Nejm 1990;323:699); sometimes familial; also w Ehlers-Danlos and Marfan's syndromes, and type I
neurofibromatosis.
Brain: 9% of all strokes. Increased in smokers (Nejm 1986;315:
717) and "crack" cocaine users (Nejm 1990;323:699). 50%
are due to hypertension, 17% from amyloid angiopathy, 10%
from anticoagulation rx, 5-10% from brain tumors, 5% from
smoking, 5% from "crack."

Sx:

Subarachnoid: Headache, severe—often "worst in life," thunder-
clap-like (Nejm 2000;342:29), usually w emesis (r/o colloid
cyst of 3rd ventricle: Nejm 1995;332:1267); may have loss of
consciousness; low back pain
Brain: With cerebellar: severe vertigo (unable to walk or stand),
headache, and vomiting. With cerebral: decreased level of
consciousness, sudden onset, headache, and vomiting

Si:

Subarachnoid: HT, stiff neck, **Parinaud's Si** (upward-gaze paralysis), subhyaloid retinal hemorrhages. Specific patterns:
pons = Horner's si, cranial nerve nuclei, pyramidal tract.
Brain: With cerebellar: Awake, alert even w ophthalmoplegias;
acute hypotonia; conjugate gaze paresis, skew deviation
With cerebral: Motor and always sensory deficits; seizure (13%)
w onset or within 48 hr
With brainstem: Early loss of consciousness, brainstem si's,
quadriplegia

Crs:

Cmplc: Subarachnoid: Secondary cerebral vessel thrombosis; r/o "hereditary" cerebral hemorrhage w amyloidosis (Nejm 1984; 311:1547)

Lab: *CSF:* Some intracerebral bleeds and all subarachnoid bleeds show bloody tap (protein $>$ 1 gm %; rbc's (100% sens, 80% spec); xanthochromia present in immediately spun CSF in 90% but also in 30% traumatic taps; w traumatic tap, rbc's decrease $\geq$ 10-fold from 1st to 3rd tube (80% sens, 60% specif: Ann IM 1986; 104:880)

Noninv: EKG shows abnormal anterior MI patterns w SA bleeds (Nejm 1974;291:1122; J Neurosurg 1969;30:521)

Xray: CT before LP to r/o mass lesion; overall, 25% of subarachnoid bleeds won't show blood on CT so must LP after CT neg. False neg rate by CT varies over time (Nejm 2000;342:29): 2% 1st 12 hr, 8% next 12 hr, 14% day 2, 25% day 3, 42% day 5.

MRI (as good as CT for acute hemorrhage: Jama 2004;292:1823) or MRA to find AVMs, r/o cerebral cavernous malformation, inherited in Hispanics and present w seizures in 3rd-4th decades (Nejm 1996;334:946)

Rx: Prevent SAH by HT control; aneurysm surgery if transient or mild sx, or asx aneurysm $>$ 10 mm (Nejm 1998;339:1725); screening 1° relatives w MRA and operating on even $<$ 5 mm aneurysms causes more harm than good, 11/18 had residual neurol damage (Nejm 1999;341:1344).

of av malformations: Bucrylate embolization, can cause late bleeding (Nejm 1986;314:477); or stereotactic radiosurgery obliteration, 94% successful (Nejm 2005;352:146)

of acute SAH: Transient (5 mo) hemicraniectomy markedly improves outcomes? (Jama 2001;286:2084); calcium-channel blockers (Neurol 1998;50:876) like nimodipine 60 mg po q 4 hr × 21 d (Med Let 1989;31:47; Curr Concepts Cerebro Dis

1989;24:31). Surgery or other ablation of aneurysms before rebleed, 20% will within 2 wk.

of intracerebral bleed: Dexamethasone for cerebral edema no help (Nejm 1987;316:1229); maybe factor VIIa therapy marginally helpful? (Nejm 2005;352:777)

of intracerebellar bleed: Aspiration surgery if > 3 cm diameter (Nejm 2001;344:1455)

10.2 Headache

Migraine Headache

Nejm 2002;346:257, 1992;326:1611

Cause: Genetic?

Epidem: Perhaps autosomal dominant with incomplete penetrance; 80% have pos family hx. Higher incidence in obsessive/compulsives, pts w family hx of epilepsy, after psychologic trauma, and pts who had motion sickness as children.

Common and classic: female/male ratio = 3-4:1; in women on bcp's, incidence increased 9×, 10% have each year, 15% have in lifetime. Cluster: male/female ratio = 10:1.

Pathophys (Nejm 1994;331:1713): Angiographically documented cerebrovascular constriction, shunting; perhaps from 5-HT-induced vascular and neurogenic (Nejm 1991;325:353) changes, perhaps sludging leads to brain ischemia, which causes vasodilatation and pain especially in external carotid distribution. Or all neurologic deficits due to "the spreading depression of Leao."

Sx (Nejm 1982;307:1029):

Common (80%): Slow onset over 4 hr, no scotomata or other aura; prodrome of yawning, euphoria, depression; usually bilateral; lasts 4-72 hr

Classic (10%): Precipitated by bright light, sound, or idiopathic; usually unilateral headache follows 20-30 min scotomata, which spread then recede, or other sensory, speech, or motor aura. Headache lasts 4-72 hr; associated with NV+D, polyuria, and hemiplegias, all on opposite side of headache and scotomata. Consistently on one side 90% of time.

Cluster (10%): "A migraine packed into 1 hr." Clusters of several/week for ~1 mo; precipitated by vasodilators like alcohol, nitroglycerin during cluster period only; sweating, tearing, flush, salivation, runny nose; nocturnal; severe, may precipitate suicide.

Si: Ergotamine trials help most but not all

Common: Eye tearing, face and neck muscle stiffness

Classic: On affected side, small pupil, external carotid pain; carotid sinus pressure temporarily relieves headache

Cluster: Horner's syndrome

Crs: Classic: Relief with illness, steroids; after attack, ~1 wk immunity from recurrence

Cmplc: CVA

r/o glaucoma (distinguished by cupped discs), epilepsy (scotomata last longer with migraine), trauma/tumor (in migraine no permanent scotomata except in very old, varies to opposite side 10% of time, headache not worse with Valsalva); see also diff dx of tension HA

Lab: *Noninv:* EEG shows spike patterns (46%: Nejm 1967;276:23)

Xray: CT/MRI unnecessary if classic sx (Neurol 1994;44:1191,1353)

Rx (Med Let 1995;37:17; Nejm 1993;329:1476):

Prevention:

Cluster: Avoid vasodilators; lithium 300+ mg qd (Med Let 1979;21:78); verapamil 120 mg po tid (Neurol 2000;54:1382)

Common and classic: Stop bcp's; i ASA po qod (Jama 1990; 264:1711); then

1st: • β-Blockers like propranolol, works in 70+%, 80-240 mg in bid doses or long-acting forms qd, or timolol (Blocadren) 10 mg po bid or 20 mg po qd, or metoprolol 100-200 mg qd
   • TCAs like amitriptyline 10-50 mg po hs, or nortriptyline 25-75 mg po hs
   • Valproate (Arch Neurol 1995;52:281) 250 mg po bid, or as Depakote ER 500-1000 mg po qd
2nd: • Calcium-channel blockers like verapamil 40-240 mg po qd, or nimodipine (Ann IM 1985;102:395)
   • ACE inhibitors like lisinopril, or ARBs (Jama 2003;289:65)
   • Topiramate gradually increased to 50-100 mg po bid, reduces HA days by > $1/3$ (DBRCT: Jama 2004; 291:965)
   • Cyproheptadine (Periactin) 2 mg qd–4 mg tid po
Rx of acute attack:
   Cluster: Prednisone 40-60 mg po qd × 7 d (Nejm 1980;302:449); chlorpromazine 100-700 mg qd (Med Let 2005;47:9; Nejm 1980;302:449); sumatriptan (see below)
   Common or classic (Ann IM 2002;137:840; Med Let 1998; 40:97): Stepped care (Jama 2000;284:2599) based on severity or during attack w reevaluation q 2 hr
      1st:
      • Single-agent NSAIDs: ASA, ibuprofen, naprosyn
      • ASA/acetaminophen/caffeine (Excedrin) i-ii tab po × 1; much better than placebo by RCT, NNT = 4 (Arch Neurol 1998;55:210), or
      • ASA 900 mg + metoclopramide 10-20 mg po, as effective as po sumatriptan (Lancet 1995;346:923)
      2nd: Triptans; adverse reactions: drug interactions w MAO inhibitors, ergots, bcp's, cimetidine, and SSRIs that could produce an excessive serotonergic response but rarely do; chest pain, angina, MI, HT, CVA; all po's op-

tions about $20/dose, higher-cost sl/intranasal versions if available

- 1st: Rizatriptan (Maxalt) 5-10 mg po/sl q 2 hr up to 30 mg/24 hr
- 2nd: Sumatriptan (Imitrex) (serotonin [5-HT] analog) 6 mg sc × 1 helps 90% within 2 hr ($58/dose), follow w 50 mg po; or 100 mg po × 1 helps 50% within 2 hr; or as nasal spray 20 mg/dose helps within 15 min ($25/dose)
- 3rd: Zolmitriptan (Zomig) (Med Let 1998;40:27) 2.5-5 mg po, can repeat in 1-2 hr, $13/dose; or as nasal form 5 mg, may repeat × 1 in 2 hr (Med Let 2004;46:7), $25/dose
- Almotriptan (Axert) (Med Let 2002;44:19) 6.25-12.5 mg po
- Eletriptan (Relpax) (Med Let 2003;45:33) 20-40 mg po prn, may repeat in 2 hr
- Frovatriptan (Frova) (Med Let 2002;44:19) 2.5 mg po; long half-life, less effective
- Naratriptan (Amerge) 1-2.5 mg, 4 hr later, may repeat × 1, takes 4 hr to work

Other options:
- Dihydroergotamine 0.5-1 mg iv/im/sc repeat q 1 hr; nasal spray (Migranal) (Med Let 1998;40:27; Neurol 1986;36:995) 1 inhalation each nostril repeat in 15 min; max on all + 3 mg/24 hr; fewer side effects than ergotamine; $15/dose
- Caffeine/ergotamine 1 mg po or 1-2 mg pr < 6 mg/24 hr, < 10 mg/wk, used w Compazine 10 mg im + O_2 often; overdose can cause vascular occlusion (Nejm 1970;283:518) especially when on β-blockers or erythromycin
- Butorphanol (Stadol) 1 nasal spray, may repeat × 1 in 1-2 hr

- Lidocaine 4% intranasally, decreases headache by 50% in 50% of pts within 15 min (Jama 1996;276:319)
- Valproate 300-500 mg iv over 15-30 min

Tic Douloureux; Trigeminal Neuralgia

Nejm 1986;315:174

Cause: Idiopathic

Epidem: Most pts > 50 yr old; may occur as cmplc of multiple sclerosis

Pathophys: Unknown

Sx: Paroxysms of neuralgic, unilateral pain in trigeminal nerve distribution, many pts may identify specific actions that trigger the sx; maxillary and mandibular branches more frequently involved than ophthalmic; precipitated by touch. Occasionally painless sensory neuropathy precedes (Nejm 1969;281:873).

Si: Pain on rotation of tongue blade inside cheek with teeth lightly clenched is diagnostic of syndrome, absence is diagnostic of remission (Trans Am Neurol Assoc 1966;91:163)
   Corneal reflex preserved
   ENT consult to look at posterior nasal space?
   Recheck si's q 2 mo since frequent remissions

Crs: Frequent spontaneous remissions in 50%

Cmplc: r/o cluster headache, postherpetic neuralgia, fifth cranial nerve pressure by tumor, arteritis, syphilis

Lab (Nejm 1969;281:873):
   Hem: ESR to r/o arteritis
   Serol: VDRL

Xray: MRI

Rx (Nejm 1996;334:1123):
   Meds:
   - 1st: Carbamazepine (Tegretol) 100 mg po bid × 24 hr, increase by 100 mg q 12 hr until pain is controlled up to 1200 mg/d;

70% effective over long term; adverse effects: agranulocytosis and aplastic anemia, thus get CBC q 1 wk × 3 mo, then q 1 mo × 3 yr (Med Let 1975;17:76) or more recently weekly × 6 then q 6 mo is acceptable; nausea and vomiting; vertigo; urinary retention; multiple CNS reactions (Ann IM 1971;74:449)

- 2nd: Phenytoin (Dilantin)

Others:

- Baclofen (Lioresal) 10-20 mg po t-qid; a muscle relaxant, effective in 70%, less toxic (Ann IM 1984;100:906), used alone or with above, don't stop abruptly (seizures), taper by 5-10 mg qd q 1 wk (Ann Neurol 1984;15:240)
- Gabapentin (Neurontin) 300-1200 mg po tid
  Surgical microvascular decompression helps > 75% immediately and long term (Nejm 1996;334:1077). Radiofrequency probe destruction of nerve results in 90% success (3% have anesthesia, 10% recur: Nejm 1973;288:680). Other surgical procedures sometimes include nerve section, or alcohol or phenol injection; both cause permanent numbness.

10.3 Seizure Disorders

Nejm 2001;344:1145, 1999;340:1565

Epilepsy: Partial Complex and Absence (Petit Mal) Types

Nejm 2003;349:1257, 1992;326:1671

Cause: Petit mal (PM): genetic autosomal dominant, 10% penetrance

Epidem: Absence seizures onset at age 4-8

Pathophys:
> Partial complex (PC): Seizure stays unilateral; in temporal lobe and inferior optic radiation
> PM: Slow waves in basal ganglia, esp thalamus

Sx: Stereotypic, similar w each attack
> PC: Auras, déja vu, visceral (nausea)

PM: Classically short (seconds) staring lapses with facial (eye blinking, etc) or extremity movement; up to hundreds/day; hence ADD or daydreaming dx's often made

Si: Stereotypic, similar w each attack

PC: Lip smacking and automatic limb movements; change in consciousness, unlike simple partial seizures; last > 1 min

PM: Pt unaware of lapse, no postictal confusion, no lateralizing si's; last < 15 sec, hyperventilation induction

Crs:

PC: Onset in adolescence to adulthood

PM: Onset at age 3-4 yr usually, always by age 11; 50% outgrow in 10 yr especially if IQ > 90, male, and otherwise normal (Neurol 1983;33:559)

Cmplc:

PM: In pregnancy, congenital malformations, infant drug withdrawal (Nejm 1985;312:559); 50% go on to have grand mal seizures as adults

Lab: *Noninv:* EEG in PM shows 3/sec slow waves during and even often between attacks; may be precipitated by respiratory alkalosis (hyperventilation); less often conclusive in PC

Rx:

PC: Meds (Jama 2004;291:615; Nejm 1996;334:165; Med Let 1995;37:37; Ann IM 1994;120:411):

1st:

- Carbamazepine (Tegretol) 400-1200 mg qd po [therapeutic level = 6-8 μgm/cc ≥ 2 hr after last dose and ≥ 3 d after last dose change (Jama 1995;274:1622)]; drug/food interactions: grapefruit increases levels, INH potentiates and is potentiated (Nejm 1982;307:1325); adverse effects: nystagmus, drowsiness, ataxia, nausea, teratogenic, spina bifida in 1% (Nejm 1991; 324:674), agranulocytosis, and aplastic anemia, so get CBC q 1 wk × 6

- Oxcarbazepine (Trileptal) (Med Let 2000;42:33) 300-1200 mg po bid; as effective as carbamazepine and better tolerated, no hematologic hepatic or dermatologic toxicity; causes ataxia, increases phenytoin levels, interferes w bcp's, phenobarb and phenytoin can decrease levels, not affected by erythromycin or cimetidine; $200/mo for 600 mg bid

- Phenytoin (Dilantin) (p 728) and/or
- Valproate 1-3 gm po qd divided (see below)

2nd:

- Phenobarbital 150-250 mg po qd or 0.6 mg/kg at 25-50 mg/min [therapeutic level = 15-30 μgm/cc $\geq$ 3 hr after last dose and $\geq$ 20 d after last dose change (Jama 1995;274: 1622)]; adverse effects: sedation; drug interactions, valproic acid toxicity, in utero intelligence impairment of fetus esp in 3rd trimester (Jama 1995;274:1518); $3/mo; or
- Primidone (Mysoline) 750-1500 mg po qd (therapeutic level = 6-12 μgm/cc); works like and is partly broken down to phenobarbital; or
- Felbamate (Felbatol) (see below)
- Gabapentin (Neurontin) (Nejm 1996;334:1583; Med Let 1994; 36:39) 900-1800 mg po qd divided and increased very slowly to avoid intoxication; renal excretion; no interactions with other meds; adverse effects: few, fatigue, ataxia, gi; $235/mo; or
- Lamotrigine (Lamictal) (Nejm 1996;334:1583; Med Let 1995;37:21) 50 mg po qd gradually increased to 300-500 mg po qd in bid doses; hepatic metabolism; levels decreased by most other seizure meds but increased by valproate; adverse effects: teratogenic, headache, N+V, ataxia, diplopia, rash esp w valproate concomitant use; $175/mo; or
- Levetiracetum (Keppra) (Med Let 2000;42:33) 500-1500 mg po bid; adjunctive to other rx; no drug interactions; adverse effects: anxiety, somnolence; $200/mo
- Topiramate (Topamax) (Med Let 1997;39:52) 200-400 mg po qd; adverse effects: mental slowing; $228/mo; or
- Tiagabine (Gabitril) (Med Let 1998;40:45) 4 mg qd–16 mg tid po, GABA reuptake inhibitor; used as adjunct w others; levels

decreased by phenytoin, carbamazepine, and phenobarbital but their levels unaffected; $206/mo

- Zonisamide (Zonegram) (Med Let 2000;42:94) 100-600 mg po qd, a sulfa; adverse effects: rashes, renal stones, weight loss (p 271); $115/mo

Surgical resection for refractory and special cases, pursue if 1st-line meds don't work (Jama 1996;276:470, 1996;334:647)

PM:

1st:

- Valproic acid (Nejm 1980;302:661) 1-3 gm po qd, eg, as Depakote DR b-tid [therapeutic level 50-100 μgm/cc ≥ 2 hr after last dose and ≥ 3 d after last dose change (Jama 1995;274:1622)]; also helps **Myoclonic Seizures;** adverse effects: spina bifida in fetus (Sci Am Text Med 1984), depressed platelet stickiness, hair loss, essential tremor (Neurol 1983;33:1380), pancreatitis; polycystic ovaries in ~50% of women pts because blocks testosterone-to-estradiol conversion (Nejm 1993;329:1383); $217/mo; or

- Ethosuximide (Zarontin) 750-1000 mg po qd (therapeutic level = 40-100 μgm/cc); adverse effects: gi sx, dyskinesias and psychiatric changes after stopped, fatigue, headache

2nd:

- Clonazepam 0.5-5 mg po tid (also helpful for myoclonic seizures); or
- Lamotrigine (Lamictal) (see above); or
- Felbamate (Felbatol) (Med Let 1997;39:51) 300-900 mg po qid; increases levels of other seizure meds (Med Let 1993; 35:107) and has high incidence of aplastic anemia (Jama 1994; 272:995) and hepatic failure
- Tiagabine as above

Grand Mal Epilepsy

Nejm 1992;326:1671

Cause: 20% idiopathic; 80% due to organic disease; trauma (subdural, scar), infection, neoplasia, vascular (AV malformation, CVA), degenerative disease (MS, Alzheimer's), metabolic (intoxications, anoxia, hypoglycemia, fever, hypo-Na, alkalosis, hypo-Mg, hypo-Ca)

Epidem:

Pathophys: Crosses midline; functional brain transection at midbrain (decerebrate)

Sx: Auras, Jacksonian progression, and postictal Todd's paralysis all indicate focal onset/origin; precipitated by menses

Si: Tonic decerebrate posturing evolving to clonic phase after 1-2 min. Postictal amnesia, confusion, often Todd's paralysis.

Crs: Can stop meds (taper over 6 wk: Nejm 1994;330:1407) in children after 2 yr, especially if EEG has no slowing with or without spikes, 60-75% won't recur (Nejm 1998;338:1715). No decrease in IQ due to seizures (Nejm 1986;314:1085) unless complicated by status epilepticus.

Cmplc: Status Epilepticus (Nejm 1998;338:970), seizures > 5 min or failure to awaken between tonic-clonic seizures, causes brain damage after 1 hr even with normal vital si's (Nejm 1982; 306:1337)

In pregnancy, congenital malformations and infant drug withdrawal (Nejm 1985;312:559)

r/o:

In adults: Migraine, syncope, TIA, Meniere's; **Hysterical/Pseudo Seizures**, which have longer, less precise onset and end, "more pelvis," ie, pelvic thrusting, side-to-side head movements, eyes tightly shut, and alternating movements of limbs

In children: Breath holding, long QT, night terrors, sleep walking, febrile seizures (p 899) (Nejm 1992;327:1122); **Lennox-Gastaut Syndrome**, rx'd w lamotrigine (Nejm 1997;337: 1807) or felbamate

Lab: *Chem/urine:* Drug screen to r/o illicit drug ingestion
Noninv: EEG abnormal in 30-50%; 60-90% with repeated studies

Xray: MRI to r/o organic damage

Rx (Jama 2004;291:615; Nejm 1996;334:168; Med Let 1995; 37:37; Ann IM 1994;120:411): Withdrawal successful in ²/₃ if sx-free after 2 yr (Nejm 1988;318:942) unless focal neurol si's, focal-type seizure, or abnormal EEG; prophylactic rx beyond 1 wk after head surgery/trauma no use (Nejm 1990;323:497); consider surgical rx if 1st-line drugs not enough (Nejm 1996;334:647)

Ketogenic (high-fat) diet improves seizure control in children (Peds 2001;108:898) but at atherogenic cost (Jama 2003;290:912) 1st:

- Phenytoin (Dilantin) 300-400 mg qd or fosphenytoin (Cerebyx) 10 mg/kg iv load then 5 mg/kg qd; therapeutic level = 10-20 μgm/cc, ≥ 2 hr after last dose and ≥ 6 d after last dose change (Jama 1995;274:1622); corrected for low albumin = measured level/0.2 × albumin + 0.1) for psychomotor (PC), not petit mal; adverse effects: displaces T_3 and T_4 from TBG, hence lowers levels but TSH ok (Jama 1996;275:1495); rare idiosyncratic mono syndrome with hepatotoxicity due to inherited sensitivity to metabolites (Nejm 1981;305:722); many drug interactions causing elevated levels, eg, with warfarin, disulfiram (Antabuse), INH, chloramphenicol, chlordiazepoxide (Librium), Thorazine, phenylbutazone, methylphenidate (Ritalin), estrogens; interactions lowering levels occur with phenobarbital, primidone, carbamazepine; phenytoin also decreases folate (hence fetal toxicity) and vitamin D levels, and increases theophylline levels (Nejm 1982;307:1189); drug intoxication leads to a drunken state, cerebellar si's, gingival hyperplasia, rashes, hirsutism; $22/mo
- Carbamazepine (p 724), or
- Valproic acid (p 726)

2nd:

- Phenobarbital (p 725), or
- Primidone (Mysoline) (p 725), or
- Felbamate (Felbatol) (p 726), or
- Lamotrigine (p 726)

  Of status epilepticus (p 6):

Table 10.1 Comparison of Traditional and Newer Antiepileptic Drugs

Antiepileptic Drug	Protein Binding (%)	Metabolism	Advantages	Disadvantages
Traditional Agents				
Carbamazepine	80	Hepatic	Extensive patient exposure	Drug interactions, hyponatremia
Phenobarbital	50	Hepatic	Inexpensive, once-daily dosing	Sedation, cognitive effects
Phenytoin	90	Hepatic	Inexpensive, once-daily dosing	Nonlinear kinetics, drug interactions
Valproate	95	Hepatic	Broad spectrum	Weight gain, tremor, hair loss
Newer Agents				
Felbamate	25	Hepatic	Broad spectrum	Risk of aplastic anemia, hepatotoxicity
Gabapentin	< 10	Renal	No drug interactions, rapid titration	Sedation, weight gain
Lamotrigine	55	Hepatic	Broad spectrum, favorable adverse effect profile	Slow titration, rash
Topiramate	15	Hepatic/renal	Broad spectrum	Slow titration, cognitive effects, kidney stones
Tiagabine	95	Hepatic	Novel mechanism of action	Multiple doses per day, tremor
Levetiracetam	< 10	Renal	No drug interactions, rapid titration	Rare behavioral changes
Oxcarbazepine	50	Hepatic	Less neurotoxic adverse effects than carbamazepine	Hyponatremia risk
Zonisamide	40	Hepatic	Broad spectrum, once-daily dosing	Slow titration, anorexia

Reproduced with permission from LaRoche SM, Helmers SL. The new antiepileptic drugs: clinical applications. J Am Med Assoc. 2004;291:617. Copyright 2004, American Medical Association, all rights reserved.

Table 10.2 Dosing and Cost Comparison

Antiepileptic Drug	Starting Daily Dose (mg)[1]	Daily Dosing Interval	Average Daily Maintenance Dose (mg)	Titration Schedule[2]	Monthly Cost ($)[3]
Traditional Agents					
Carbamazepine	400	3 times	1200	Slow	91.80
Phenobarbital	60	Once	150	Slow	2.70
Phenytoin	300	Once	300	Rapid	21.60
Valproate	750-1000	3 times	2000	Rapid	217.20
Newer Agents					
Gabapentin	900	3 times	2400	Rapid	235.80
Lamotrigine	50	Twice	400	Slow	176.71
Added to valproate	25 (every other day)	Twice	100-200	Slow	
Topiramate	25-50	Twice	400	Slow	228.28
Tiagabine	4	2-4 times	48	Slow	206.40
Levetiracetam	1000	Twice	1500	Rapid	164.58
Oxcarbazepine	600	Twice	1200	Slow	193.20
Zonisamide	100	Once	200	Slow	113.40

1. As recommended by each manufacturer's package insert.
2. Rapid titration indicates maintenance dose achieved in less than 2 wk; slow titration, an average of 2-12 wk required to achieve maintenance dose.
3. Brand-name prices from the 2002 *Drug Topics Red Book*. Retail prices may be higher or lower depending on the pharmacy and patient's insurance coverage.
Reproduced with permission from LaRoche SM, Helmers SL. The new antiepileptic drugs: clinical applications. J Am Med Assoc. 2004;291:617. Copyright 2004, American Medical Association, all rights reserved.

10.4 Sleep Disorders

Obstructive Sleep Apnea

Nejm 2002;347:498; 1996;334:99

Cause: Obesity; genetic component since often familial (Ann IM 1995;122:174)

Epidem: Associated with alcohol use, which worsens apnea, and with HT in obese older males; are they cause or effect? (Ann IM 1985; 103:190); CHF (Ann IM 1995;122:487); testosterone rx worsens (Nejm 1983;308:508). 1-5% of men > 60 yr old; 4% of men age 30-60; 2% of women (Nejm 1993;328:1230).

Pathophys: Anatomically smaller pharynx predisposes (Nejm 1986;315:1327)

Sx: Daytime somnolence (in 80%) due to disturbed sleep; hx of deep snoring and apneic episodes from roommate; but such hx is only 65% sens/specif for sleep apnea (Ann IM 1991;115:356); and HT and/or obesity; if 2 of 3 present, sleep apnea will be documented (> 5, 10+ sec apneas/hr sleep) w 86% sens, 77% specif in general adult primary care population (Ann IM 1999;131:485)

Si: Hypertension (90%) (Jama 2000;283;1829; Nejm 2000;342:1378; Ann IM 1994;120:382)

Crs:

Cmplc: Cor pulmonale; car accident incidence increased 6× (Nejm 1999;340:847, 881), ASHD and CVAs (Am J Med 2000; 108:396)

r/o

- Narcolepsy (p 733)
- Restless leg syndrome (see below)
- Normal elderly sleep patterns (Nejm 1990;323:520)
- REM sleep disorder; failure to have full muscle atonia during dreams; rx w clonazepam

- **Central Sleep Apnea**, rare, rx with protriptyline 10-25 mg po hs or other tricyclic to suppress REM sleep especially if apnea occurring during REM, or progesterone as a central stimulant, or theophylline in CHF (Nejm 1996;335:562)

Lab: *Noninv:* Polysomnography (sleep) studies are definitive and probably best 1st test (Ann IM 1999;130:496), positive if > 5, 10+ sec apneas/hr sleep; if not available, overnight O_2 sat monitoring to determine respiratory disturbance index may be helpful

Rx: Avoid sleep meds and alcohol
Weight loss, even modest (eg, 20 lb), helps (Ann IM 1985;103:850)
Nasal CPAP (Ann IM 2001;134:1015,1065; Lancet 1999;353:2100) helps daytime drowsiness and function if impaired, but not if pt has no complaints even w 30+ apneic spells/hr of sleep
Mandibular/tongue advancement devices if CPAP fails
Rarely tracheostomy or uvulopalatopharyngoplasty (Ann IM 1985;103:190), and/or maxillofacial surgery
Perhaps atrial pacing (Nejm 2002;346:404,444)

Restless Leg Syndrome (Periodic Limb Movement Disorder)

Nejm 2003;348:2103; Practical Neurol 2003;3:204; ACP J Club 2000;132:24; NIH Mar 2000 pub #00-3788

Cause: Primary cause: Autosomal dominant on chromosome 12q
Secondary causes: Iron deficiency, diabetes, drug-induced (TCAs, lithium, SSRIs), uremia, cord and peripheral nerve diseases, transiently in pregnancy (20%)

Epidem: Common; 2-5+% prevalence; increases w age, but 35% of adults w severe disease have onset in childhood; strong familial association esp if onset < 40 yr old. Increased incidence in pts on hemodialysis and those w iron deficiency. Females > males.

Pathophys: Dopamine deficiency; iron is a cofactor for tyrosine hydroxylase needed for tyr → dopamine

Sx: Creepy-crawly leg (usually) paresthesias/akithsias relieved by movement. Positive family hx. Sleep interference.

Si: Normal neurologic exam; may have involuntary periodic jerking limb movements, esp when asleep (nocturnal myoclonus) as well as semirhythmnic leg movements during sleep (periodic limb movements) but which are nonspecific

Crs:

Cmplc: r/o nocturnal muscle cramps

Lab:
> *Chem:* r/o secondary causes w iron and TIBC, ferritin, BUN/creat, FBS

Rx (Nejm 2003;348:2106):
> 1st:
> - $FeSO_4$ especially if ferritin < 50; plus
> - Dopaminergics like Sinemet and Sinemet 0.5-I tab of 25/100 CR hs or 2 hr before (20 min onset)
> - Dopamine agonists (2 hr onset) like pergolide 0.10-0.75 mg po hs (Neurol 1999;52:944), bromocriptine, pramipexole (Mirapex), ropinirole (Requip)
>
> Other:
> - Anticonvulsants: Valproate, gabapentin (Neurontin) (maybe: ACP J Club 2003;139:17)
> - Opiates: Propoxyphene, Tylenol #3 hs, oxycodone, methadone
> - Clonidine, baclofen, or clonazepam (Klonopin), carbamazepine

Narcolepsy

Nejm 1990;323:389; Ann IM 1987;106:434

Cause: Genetic in 15%; autosomal dominant; associated with $HLA-DR_2$ in 100%

Epidem: Males and females equally affected; prevalence = 1-10/10,000 population; incidence increased by 60× in other family members; associated with SIDS families (Nejm 1978;299:969)

NEUROLOGY

Pathophys: Drop directly into REM sleep, which causes paralysis, dreams, and loss of postural tone, all of which can also occur inappropriately when awake

Sx: Positive family hx; onset usually in teens, 80% by age 30 yr, all < 40 yr

Periodic inappropriate drowsiness 30 sec–15 min, awake refreshed

Cataplexy: REM-type episodic loss of postural tone precipitated by excitement, laughter, surprise, nostalgia; lasts usually < 1 min; 30% have when 1st present, 50% have eventually

Hypnagogic hallucinations: Vivid dreams at onset of, or coming out of, sleep

Sleep paralysis (60%): Can't move as going into sleep or coming out but latter not diagnostic; lasts up to 10 min

Si:

Crs: Onset usually between age 15 and 35; benign usually, doesn't progress after first 3-4 yr

Cmplc: Accidents, especially with cars; secondary psych problems, especially depression

r/o familial sleep paralysis on awakening (benign), sleep apnea hypersomnolence

Lab: *Noninv:* EEG shows immediate REM sleep or at least slow-wave sleep very abbreviated (1-2 min); not true in all narcoleptics and amphetamines can mask

Rx: Nap 15-20 min at least 1-3×/day

1st: Methylphenidate (Ritalin) up to 200 mg qd; must give drug holidays 1/12 mo or increase doses to levels that cause severe dependence; worse during these holidays

2nd: Amphetamines like methamphetamine 10-60 mg qd, or dextroamphetamine 5-50 mg qd

Others:
- Modafinil (Provigil) (Med Let 1999;41:30) 200-400 mg po qd in am; many drug interactions; comparable to 2 cups of coffee?; $150/mo

- Imipramine or desipramine 25 mg tid for cataplexy (decreases REM) but beware increased BP when used with amphetamines

of cataplexy: Gamma-hydroxybutyrate (Xyrem) (Med Let 2002;44:103) po hs and 2-4 hr later; date-rape drug, so schedule III and special rules

10.5 Movement Disorders

Friedreich's Ataxia

Nejm 1996;335:1169

Cause: Genetic, autosomal dominant or recessive on chromosome 9, causing multiple GAA after 1st intron

Epidem: Prevalence = 1/50,000

Pathophys: Basic process is neuronal decay. Symmetric degeneration of posterior columns, spinocerebellar tracts, posterior roots, and corticospinal tracts.

Sx: Onset before puberty in most, all by age 25. Weakness.

Si: Ataxia w dysarthria, chronic peripheral neuropathy, pes cavus (high-arched feet)

Crs: Die by age 30-40 yr of infections and cardiac causes

Cmplc: Optic atrophy and myocarditis with heart block and fibrosis late in course; diabetes

r/o other causes of ataxia (p 780)

Lab: *Noninv:* EKG shows arrhythmias

Path: Absence of neurons in posterior root ganglia, anterior horns, posterior horns, motor and cerebellar cortices

Rx: None available

Hereditary Ataxia Telangiectasia

Ann IM 1983;99:367; Nejm 1979;300:702

Cause: Genetic, autosomal recessive (Nejm 1995;333:662)

Epidem: 80% lack IgA and thymus; a form of dysgammaglobulinemia type III with decreased or absent IgA, IgE, and two subsets of IgG. 1-7% gene prevalence in the U.S.

Pathophys: Diabetes due to defective insulin receptors (Nejm 1978;298:1124). Ataxia due to damage to posterior columns and anterior horn cells. The immunodeficiency is caused by a failure of a DNA "glue" enzyme in both T and B lymphocytes to switch from acute responses (eg, IgM) to chronic immune defense (eg, IgG) (Nejm 1990;322:124).

Sx: Amenorrhea (no ovaries); recurrent sinopulmonary infections (no IgA)

Si: Oculocutaneous telangiectasias, impaired delayed-hypersensitivity problems, progressive neurologic dysfunction, ataxia, acanthosis nigrans (Nejm 1978;298:1164)

Crs: Onset usually as learn to walk w subsequent choreoathetosis, dysarthria, abnormal eye movements, etc

Even carriers have an 8-yr shortened life expectancy (Ann IM 2000;133:770)

Cmplc: Increased incidence of many neoplasms, especially of the immune tissues, and especially of T-cell origin (Nejm 1979;300: 700); and breast cancer, in pts with HAT as well as in heterozygous carriers; represents 9% of all U.S. breast cancer cases (Nejm 1987;316:1289); exposure to radiation, eg, mammograms, may markedly increase incidence in both HAT pts and heterozygotes (Nejm 1991;325:1831). Also increased colon, lung, prostate, and pancreatic cancers.

Insulin-resistant diabetes

Lab: *Serol:* IgA, IgE, IgG_2, and IgG_4 usually are absent; increase in IgM and α_1-fetoglobulin (r/o embryonal cell cancers and CEA)

Rx: Avoid xrays and radiation rx (Nejm 1991;325:1831) in these pts and close blood relatives

Huntington's Chorea

Nejm 1986;315:1267

Cause: Genetic, autosomal dominant, on chromosome 4; senile type rarely genetic

Epidem: Origin in England; brought here by colonists; may have been the etiology of several Salem witches; "Woody Guthrie disease" Equal racial incidence

Pathophys: CAG triplet repeats (36-121) on chromosome 4 (Nejm 1994;330:1401) somehow cause degeneration of caudate and lenticular nuclei, as well as frontal lobe; γ-aminobutyric acid (GABA) is deficient in these areas (Nejm 1973;288:337)

Sx: Onset usually around age 35 yr
Chorea of arms, legs, face; pediatric onset often has no chorea and looks like Parkinson's

Si: Chorea and dementia with preservation of memory longer than problem-solving skills

Crs: Live about 15 yr after diagnosis of the disease

Cmplc: Suicide common (~7%)
r/o inherited cerebellar ataxia, myoclonus in Alzheimer's, Creutzfelt-Jakob disease, Wilson's disease a-beta lipoproteinemia/acanthocytosis, tardive dyskinesia, and infarction of basal ganglia

Lab: L-dopa evocation trial: Gradually increase from 250 mg to 1 gm qd, usually increases chorea (reversibly) at least in pts with barely perceptible, questionable si (Nejm 1972;286:1332; Lancet 1970; 2:1185)
DNA restriction fragment length methods can identify asx pts in at least $\frac{1}{2}$ of cases (Nejm 1988;318:535); this information provided with counseling decreases anxiety in both high- and low-risk groups (Nejm 1992;327:1401)

Xray: CT and MRI characteristically show caudate atrophy
PET scans in asx pts show decrease in glucose metabolism in caudate nucleus (Nejm 1987;316:357)

Rx: Prevent by genetic counseling
of disease: Phenothiazines like haloperidol (Haldol) or other
ancillary drugs like reserpine to decrease chorea

Parkinson's Disease (Paralysis Agitans)

Nejm 2005;353:1021

Cause: Idiopathic, vascular, or postencephalitis lethargica (1918 flu);
some genetic component, rare autosom dominant (Jama 1999;
281:341)

Epidem: Male/female ratio = 1.5. Present in high % of U.S. elderly:
15% by age 65-75, 30% by age 75-85, 50% over age 85 (Nejm
1996;334:71). Early-onset type associated w genetic mutations
(Nejm 2000;342:1560).

    Increased incidence in Guam of a variant with more demen-
tia, where is associated with ALS (O. Sacks, *Island of the Color
Blind,* A. Knopf, 1996; Nejm 1970;282:947)

    Decreased incidence in coffee and other caffeine users (Jama
2000;283:2674) and smoking ($^1/_2$ risk)

    Increased incidence w pesticides and welding

Pathophys: Relative dopamine deficiency in basal ganglia with concomitant increased inhibitory GABA activity

Sx (Jama 2003;289:347): Tremor, akinesia, drool, characteristic stoop-
ing posture, rigidity

Si: 4 major sx; dx if at least 2 present:
- Tremor, 3-4/sec, "pill rolling" at rest; asymmetric onset
- Bradykinesia, with masked facies; a paucity of movement; slow
finger tapping; can still respond to true danger easily
- Rigidity, cogwheeling muscle type
- Gait disturbance: Forward falling, shuffling; diminished arm
swing, prolonged turning

    Also seborrhea; low-volume voice, micrographia, failure to
extinguish blinking w glabellar tapping

Crs: Progressive; risk of death (Nejm 1996;334:71) 2× that of pts w/o, worse if gait disturbance

Cmplc: Inanition, late dementia (30%), upper airway obstruction due to tremor and stiffness of upper airway muscles (Nejm 1984; 311:438); postural hypotension (p 753) from autonomic insufficiency (Ann IM 2000;133:338); drowsiness and "sleep attacks" (Jama 2002;287:455,509), constipation

r/o (BMJ 1995;310:447) Parkinsonism induced by phenothiazines, metoclopramide (Reglan) (Jama 1995;274:1780), Wilson's disease, reserpine (Nejm 1976;295:816), manganese toxicity (Nejm 1970;282:5), carbon monoxide toxicity, drug impurity in heroin addicts (Nejm 1985;312:1418)

r/o "Parkinsonism plus" syndromes like Lewy-body dementia (p 426), normal-pressure hydrocephalus (p 431), **Progressive Supranuclear Palsy** w paresis of downward gaze, and multisystem atrophy subtypes like **Olivopontine Cerebellar Atrophy, Striatonigral Degeneration**, **Shy-Drager Syndrome**, and **Cortical Basal Ganglionic Degeneration** (Nejm 1993;324:1560)

Lab: *Noninv:* Evoked potentials (Nejm 1982;306:1140,1205)
Path: Substantia nigra and locus coeruleus have lost
melanin-containing neurons; remaining neurons have lacy
bodies with eosinophilic inclusion bodies in cytoplasm

Rx (Ann IM 2003;138:651; Med Let 1993;35:31; Nejm 1993; 329 1021):
Avoid metoclopramide (Reglan), a CNS dopa antagonist
to slow progression:
- Dopamine agonists?
- Exercise programs?
- Coenzyme Q-10 600 mg po qd (UCLA 9/02); multivitamins and vitamin E 400-800 U po qd
- Selegiline (L-deprenyl, Eldepryl) (Nejm 1993;328:176; Neurol 1992;42:339); a MAO B inhibitor, weak effect often not worth cost and side effects; adverse effects: may increase mortality

(BMJ 1995;311:1602; ACP J Club 1996;124:57); interactions with meperidine (Demerol) (Can J Psych 1990;35:571) causing sedation and/or hallucinations, and w tricyclics and SSRIs causing severe agitation; insomnia; depression

Rx of major sx:

1st, esp if over age 70 or demented; 80% end up on: L-dopa with carbidopa, a decarboxylase inhibitor, = Sinemet 25/100 or 250 (not 10/100), or as Parcopa, a more expensive immediate-release formulation (Med Let 2005;47:12); w up to 100 mg carbidopa qd and as little L-dopa as can get away with (2-8 gm qd); Sinemet CR 50/200 mg sustained-release version may be preferable and save money, but it takes 30% more than other forms since less bioavailable, start ½ po bid fasting, may need plain Sinemet to jump-start in morning (Med Let 1991;33:92); $40/mo; adverse effects (drug holidays no help):

- Postural hypotension, due to diuretic effect (Nejm 1971;284:865), nausea, and vomiting (Ann IM 1970;72:29) most frequently

- Mental changes, especially hallucinations in older pts (Neurology 1983;33:1518)

- On–off phenomena, most commonly in pts < 60 yr old; including wearing off too soon, and start hesitation, especially after 5 yr of use; rx w apomorphine (Apokyn) (Med Let 2005; 47:7) 2-10 mg sc up to qid, a dopamine agonist esp good for "off"; $3/mg

- Dyskinesias, dystonias, and athetosis always within 5 yr (rx with lowering dose and adding bromocryptine, antihistamine, amantadine, or baclofen); the major reason for waiting to add L-dopa (Nejm 2000;342:1484); the therapeutic window gets narrower over time

- Peripheral adrenergic effects that lead to loss of weight and appetite (use higher doses of carbidopa to prevent, and pretreat 2-3 d before starting L-dopa);

- Overall, decreased effectiveness after 5 yr

2nd (first if < 70 yr): Dopamine agonists (Med Let 2001;43:59), which delay onset of motor sx and are neuroprotective. No effect of food in absorption; all can cause edema, sedation, there are hallucinations, nausea, dyskinesias, and all these worse w increased age; unclear if fewer side effects but lesser motor improvements than L-dopa make them preferable (Jama 2000;284:1971):

- Pergolide (Permax) 0.25-1.5 mg po bid up to 8 mg tid; dopamine agonist like L-dopa and bromocriptine; $60/mo

- Ropinirole (Requip) 3-5 mg po tid, slowly increase dose; hepatic metabolism; adverse effects: nausea, syncope, drowsiness, headache; increased levels w cipro, decreased levels w antipsychotics and metoclopramide

- Pramipexole (Mirapex) (Jama 2000;284:1931) 0.125-1.5 mg po tid; renal clearance; adverse effects: hallucinations, nausea; increased levels w cimetidine; $170/mo

- Bromocriptine (Parlodel) 5-10 mg po tid alone or with L-dopa, or if L-dopa fails; not as good as other dopamine agonists; adverse effects: orthostatic BP changes, sweating, mental status changes; $240/mo

Ancillary meds:

- Amphetamines like dexedrine 5 mg po b-tid help akinesia and psych depression

- Anticholinergics (inhibit the dopamine-uninhibited acetylcholine neurons) (ACP J Club 2004;140:15) like antihistamines, eg, diphenhydramine (Benadryl) 50 mg tid po, or benztropine (Cogentin), or trihexyphenidyl (Artane) (Nejm 1971;284:413), help tremors; lots of side effects

- Amantadine 100 mg po bid, effect diminishes in 6 mo, helps 64% (Jama 1972;222:792), helps rigidity and bradykinesia, used late in disease crs for L-dopa dyskinesias

- Estrogen replacement therapy

COMT (catechol-O methyl transferase) inhibitors, block DOPA breakdown in brain:

- Tolcapone (Tasmar) (Med Let 1998;40:60) 100-200 mg po tid; works as L-dopa booster; helps w early "wearing-off" phenomenon; use when other drugs fail; adverse effects: significant hepatotoxicity, pulled off Canadian mkt; $162/mo for 100 mg tid
- Entazapone (Comtan) (Med Let 2004;46:39) 200 mg po w each 50, 100, or 150 L-dopa dose, esp for "wearing off"; less hepatotoxicity; $180/mo

Rehab: Strength training and front-wheeled walker

Surgical:

- Pallidotomy? (Nejm 2000;342:1708, 1997;337:1036, 1996;334:114; Med Let 1996;38:107) for bradykinesia and tremor; unilateral thalamotomy, or continuous uni- or bilateral subthalamic nucleus electrical stimulation (Nejm 2000;342:461) for severe tremor unresponsive to meds; or
- Electrical stimulation of subthalamic nucleus (Nejm 1998;339:1105), occasionally causes severe acute depression w left substantia nigra placement (Nejm 1999;340:1476); or
- Fetal dopa-producing brain cell implants to caudate nucleus or putamen perhaps (Nejm 2001;344:710, 1995;332:1118)

Of dementia: Rivastigmine (Exelon) and other anticholinesterases effect a modest improvement but cause nausea, vomiting, and tremor (Nejm 2004;351:2509)

10.6 Muscle Weakness

Guillain-Barré Syndrome (Acute Infectious Polyneuritis)

Nejm 1992;326:1130; Ann Neurol 1990;27:s21

Cause: Often viral, probably several types including Epstein-Barr virus (7/24 children: Nejm 1975;292:392) and *Campylobacter jejuni* (Nejm 1995;333:1374), ⅓ cases have a h/o such as a precedent.

Occasionally/rarely follows flu shots (Nejm 1998;339:1997, 1981;304:557), CMV, and HIV.

Epidem: All ages, both sexes equally; 1-2 cases/100,000/yr

Pathophys: Allergic polyneuropathy leads to demyelination and decreased conduction velocity especially at root exit on cord dorsum (hence areflexia); must get ventral root too, although pathologically unimpressive. Can experimentally mimic by sensitizing animals with injections of dorsal root homogenates and Freund's adjuvant.

Sx: URI, mild, precedes by 1-3 wk. Vague sensory losses, including, often early on, paresthesias of toes and fingers, which then extend proximally; deep aching at onset is very characteristic; proximal muscle weakness evolves over 24 hr.

Si: No sensory losses; afebrile; diminished reflexes always; proximal weakness >> distal involvement; always symmetric; no mental changes; facial nerve palsies (60%): cranial nerves X, XI, XII often; V occasionally; II, III, IV, VI rarely

Crs: Deteriorate after admission; start improving within 3 wk; back to normal in 16 mo, although slight decrease in reflexes and foot drop may persist; no relapses. Campylobacter type has worse outcome w 60% of pts at 1 yr still w moderate to severe disability, compared to only 25% of pts from other causes (Nejm 1995; 333:1374).

Cmplc: Insidious respiratory paralysis, monitor by having count to 20 in 1 breath; glomerular nephritis (Ann IM 1973;78:391)
r/o cord compression, especially if CSF protein ≥ 2.5 gm %; collagen vascular disease; diabetic neuropathy; multiple sclerosis; polio; diphtheria; myasthenia; heavy metal toxicity; infectious mono; amyloid; rabies (Nejm 1979;300:603); botulism; red tide disease; Lyme disease; HIV; CNS neoplasia; sarcoid meningitis; chronic, HLA associated; tick paralysis (Nejm 2000;342:90), rapidly ascending paralysis, rx'd by finding and removing tick;

chronic inflammatory demyelinating polyneuropathy (Nejm 2005;352:1343)

Lab: *CSF:* Increased protein to 120-300 mg % by end of 1st wk; wbc < 5000-6000

Noninv: Nerve conduction velocities profoundly decreased; if normal several days into course, find another dx

Rx: 1st: Supportive care including respirator; iv steroids no help (Lancet 1993;341:586)

2nd: Immune globulin iv high dose, eg, 0.4 gm/kg/d × 5 d if can't walk and < 2 wk of sx; will help ½ of pts in 1 mo (Nejm 1992;326:1130); or plasmapheresis/exchange at a tertiary care center for pts who can't walk or are progressing rapidly; both equally effective although combination use is not (Neurol 2003;61:736; Lancet 1997;349:225)

Myasthenia Gravis

Jama 2005;293:1906

Cause: Autoimmune

Epidem: Especially in young females, and in males age 65-75 yr; female/male = 3:1 overall. Associated with:

- Thymomas, especially in older males; 30% have; 30% of pts with thymomas have myasthenia
- Thyrotoxicosis, especially Hashimoto's
- Collagen vascular disease, especially SLE
- HLA B_8
- Penicillamine (BMJ 1975;1:600)

Pathophys: Antibodies to neuromuscular junction acetylcholine receptors (Nejm 1977;296:125); measured antibody doesn't correlate with disease severity; some pts have more lethal antibody function than others (Nejm 1982;307:769)

Sx: Precipitated by thyrotoxicosis, muscle-paralyzing anesthesia, antibiotics like streptomycin, quinine (including gin and tonic), quinidine, perhaps Dilantin, procainamide, propranolol (Ann IM 1975;83:834)

Diplopia and other ocular sx (6090), muscle fatigue with repetitive use

Si: Increased weakness with repeated use, often in extra-ocular muscles first, or pharynx; reflexes intact

Crs: Prognosis much poorer if thymoma present (Neurol 1966;16:431); remissions during times of stress often, eg, pregnancy

Cmplc: Respiratory failure; transmission to fetus, normalizes within 6 mo as maternal IgG decreases

r/o botulism; Guillain-Barré; polio; ALS; Graves' disease; curare poisoning; **Snake Bite** (Nejm 2002;347:347), acetylcholine receptor blockade, rx with edrophonium (Tensilon) (Nejm 1986;315:1444) or sheep/horse antivenom Fab fragments iv within 6 hr (Med Let 2001;43:55); **Eaton-Lambert Syndrome**, a similar disease associated with cancer especially of lung and pancreas (Nejm 1989;321:1267) and caused by antibodies to calcium channels responsible for neurotransmitter acetylcholine release (Nejm 1995;332:467)

Lab: *Noninv:* EMG shows fatigue with > 2/sec stimulation; post-tetanic facilitation present; Tensilon (edrophonium) test can be diagnostic, do double blind with saline, 2 mg then 8 mg iv causes no side effects (tearing, increased sputum, cramps) if myasthenia rather than cholinergic crisis

Serol: Acetylcholine receptor antibody (80$^+$% sens in full blown disease but only 50% if only ocular Sx)

Rx (Nejm 1973;288:27): Avoid neomycin-like drugs; maintain K$^+$
1st: Anticholinergics:
- Pyridostigmine (Mestinon) 30-60 mg po qid; or
- Neostigmine (Prostigmin) 0.5-1.5 mg im q 1-6 hr or 15+ mg po qid long-release type
2nd: Immunotherapy:

- Prednisone ~100 mg po qod alone, magically good results at NIH (Ann IM 1974;81:225; Nejm 1972;286:17); start low, work up to avoid crisis (Nejm 1974;290:81);
- Azathioprine (Imuran);
- Cyclosporine 6 mg/kg/d po helps (Nejm 1987;316:719); short-term option;
- Plasmapheresis (Nejm 1984;310:762), with prednisone and/or azathioprine if thymectomy and anticholinergics not enough (Med Let 1979;21:64; Nejm 1977;297:1134); or
- Immunoglobulin high dose 400 mg/kg/d × 5 d (Nejm 1992;326:107; Acta Neurol Scand 1991;84:81); and
- Thymectomy, for severe disease in all groups, but especially for pts with onset between puberty and age 60 yr; 2% operative mortality

10.7 Degenerative CNS Diseases

Multiple Sclerosis

Nejm 2000;343:938; 1997;337:1604

Cause: Perhaps autoimmune; perhaps precipitated by EB virus infection (Jama 2005;293:2496, 2003;289:1533, 2002;286:3083). Genetic component indicated by 25% concordance with monozygotic twins but only 2% with dizygotic twins and siblings (Nejm 1986;315:1638).

Epidem: Transmissible somehow (Faroe Island epidemic after WWII troop occupation); increased incidence with birth and/or childhood distance from equator; equal sex ratios, although females get at younger age; onset at age 10-50 yr, bell-shaped curve; 1/1000 of population have disease (probably tip of carriers)

Pathophys: Autoimmune attack of myelin basic protein by T cells (Nejm 1987;317:408) or by tumor necrosis factor-α which is measurable in CSF (Nejm 1991;325:467); or of neuronal glia

(Nejm 1977;297:1207); decreased suppressor T cells (Nejm 1987;316:67). Axonal demyelination and ultimately transection (Nejm 1998;338:278).

Sx: Motor (most often ataxia), nearly always hyperreflexia and positive Babinski's; and sensory tract (most often visual) sx, confusion, depression

Si: Diagnose by 2 or more attacks of neurologic deficits in different parts of CNS that last > 24 hr, not by CSF or MRI lesions (Nejm 1993;329:1764, 1808)

Loss of abdominal reflexes early, in contrast to ALS

Lhermitte's si: Electric shock sensation to extremities with neck flexion (posterior column stretch); r/o any disease involving cervical or thoracic cord

Crs: Worse with hot climate, late onset; slightly fewer relapses in pregnancy and slightly more relapses postpartum (Nejm 1998;339:285); 25% are benign with 1-2 episodes and minimal disability

Types:

- Acute attack
- Initially remitting/relapsing (80-90%), but many evolve to progressive; M/F = 1/2
- Initially progressive (10-20%); M = F; superimposed subsequent relapse/remit cycles don't improve prognosis (Nejm 2000;343:1430,1486)
- Stable (Nejm 1987;317:442)

Cmplc: Pain, neuralgia including trigeminal (Nejm 1969;280:1395)

Optic neuritis; 40% of MS pts will have it sometime; up to 75% of women and 34% of men with isolated optic neuritis will develop MS up to 15 yr later (Neurol 1988;38:185; Nejm 1973;289:1103,1140); r/o Sjögren's syndrome, which can mimic (Ann IM 1986;104:323)

Lab: CSF: Oligoclonal bands (90%), present throughout disease; IgG/albumin ratio elevated (70%); positive antimyelin antibodies (2 types) 77% sens, 95% specif when both pos (Nejm 2003;349:139)

Noninv: Brainstem-evoked potentials, no false positives except
for other similar diseases like Friedreich's ataxia; ~10% false
negatives in early MS

Xray: MRI, 25% false negatives (Neurol 1993;43:905; Jama
1993;269:3146), and many false positives

Rx: Avoid flu shots in pts w definite MS
of remitting/relapsing (not chronic progressive):

- Interferon-β1b (Betaseron) 250 μgm sc qod or interferon-β1a
  (Avonex, Rebif) 30-44 μgm im/sc qd or tiw for years, decreases
  relapse rate and severity by 50%; $1000/mo (Lancet
  1998;352:1491,1498; Ann Neurol 1996;39:285; Neurol
  1995;43:641, 1993;43:641,655,662; Med Let 1996;38:63,
  1993;35:61). Weekly im Avonex for years w 3 d of iv then 11 d
  of po steroids, given on 1st demyelinating si/sx and UBOs on
  MRI, decreases MS by $\frac{1}{3}$ (Nejm 2000;343:898); NNT = 9
  (Lancet 2001;357:1576).
- Glatiramer (Copaxone; copolymer I) (Med Let 1997;38:61;
  Neurol 1995;45:1268) 20 mg sc qd, reduces recurrences from
  85% to 60%/yr; $1000/mo
- Mitoxantrone perhaps, iv q 3 mo (Lancet 2002;360:2018)

of progressive MS: Mtx, cyclophosphamide, cyclosporine
of acute attack: Hyperbaric and plasmapheresis rx no longer
thought useful

- Cyclophosphamide (Cytoxan) 400-500 mg iv qd × 7-10 d;
  alone, best 1st choice now, but many still disagree with its use,
  eg, Canadian multicenter study (Lancet 1991;337:441); with
  ACTH, decreases morbidity (Nejm 1983;308:173,215)
- ACTH 25 U tapering to 5 U iv qd × 2 wk, then 40 U tapering
  to 20 U im × 1 wk, then stop; or short course of steroids, eg,
  methylprednisolone 1000 mg iv in 3 hr qd × 3, then taper in
  7-14 d

of incontinence (p 435)
of neuralgias: Carbamazepine, phenytoin (Nejm 1969;280:1395)

of muscle spasms (Med Let 1997;39:62; Nejm 1981;304:29,95),
in order of efficacy:

- Baclofen, a GABA agonist, 5-20 mg po tid, or even chronically intrathecally via pump (Nejm 1989;320:1517); or
- Tizanidine (Zanaflex) (Med Let 1997;39:62) 4 mg hs to 6+mg tid; adverse effects: dry mouth, sedation, dizziness, hypotension, rare visual hallucinations and hepatitis; or
- Diazepam (Valium), but makes sleepy; or
- Dantrolene 300 mg qd, but causes weakness

of fatigue: Amantadine, methylpenidate (Ritalin), modafinil (Provigil)

Amyotrophic Lateral Sclerosis

Nejm 2001;344:1688

Cause: Genetic in 10%, autosomal dominant, on chromosome 21 at least half the time (Nejm 1991;324:1381)

Epidem: 1/250,000 persons in U.S. will die of it; 50× increased prevalence in Guam (Nejm 1970;282:947) along with a unique dementing variant of Parkinson's; both associated with a specific HLA genotype and decreased delayed hypersensitivity (Nejm 1978;299:680)

Pathophys: Degeneration of anterior horn cells and motor Betz cells of cerebrum progressively up from caudad portion of body. Can start anywhere in cord. Circulating antibody inhibits protein stimulation of axonal sprouting secreted by denervated muscle, primary or secondary effect? (Nejm 1984;311:933). Perhaps defective glutamate transport systems permit neurotoxic levels to build up (Nejm 1992;326:1464) or autoimmune IgG against calcium channels (Nejm 1992;327:1721).

Sx: Paresis and leg weakness

Si: Marked muscle atrophy, usually upper extremity, accompanied by asymmetric fasciculations of many muscle groups including tongue, and hyperreflexia of the atrophic muscles; paraplegia; and no sensory abnormality or sx, which distinguishes it from cervical disc disease

Crs: Fatal over 3-5 yr

Cmplc: Dysphagia, respiratory paralysis, dysphonia, and dysarthria
With paraplegia, r/o mass lesion, syphilis, B_{12} deficiency, parasagittal meningioma, Shy-Drager syndrome (p 739, 752), postpolio muscular atrophy (Nejm 1986;314:959)

Lab: *Path:* Muscle bx shows neuronal degenerative changes; cord shows atrophy with decreased anterior horn cells and lipofuscin in degenerated corticospinal tracts

Rx: Riluzole (an antiglutamate) 50-200 mg po qd slows progression minimally (Lancet 1996;347:1425), perhaps in pts w bulbar onset but not with limb-onset disease (Med Let 1995;37:113; Nejm 1994;330:585,636)

10.8 Neuropathies

Bell's Palsy

Nejm 2004;351:1323

Cause: *H. simplex* (majority) (Ann IM 1996;124:27); ? EB virus (Nejm 1975;292:392); sarcoid, usually bilateral; Lyme disease (Nejm 1985;312:869); Swiss nasal influenza vaccine (Nejm 2004; 350:896)
Other causes of facial nerve paralysis: *H. zoster* (10%; called the Ramsay-Hunt syndrome), basilar skull fracture (5%), otitis media (2%), birth (2%), other including syphilis (1%)

Epidem: Increased incidence in diabetics (Nejm 1982;307:348), or are those diabetic nerve infarcts?

Pathophys:

Sx: Facial weakness, acute onset, may also be painful; increased noise sensitivity from diminished stapedial reflex

Si: Cranial nerve VII weakness. Decreased taste on anterior tongue (helpful if absent taste because it distinguishes from primary motor disease, eg, polio); only true occasionally, since often the process is more distal and chorda tympani is spared. Diminished ipsilateral salivation and lacrimation from lesions proximal to geniculate ganglion.

Crs: 80% recover completely, only 50% if Ramsay-Hunt syndrome. If there is some residual motion on affected side, pt always recovers (Nejm 1975;292:748).

Cmplc: Corneal ulceration, prevent by taping lid, especially hs. Misregeneration of the nerve, causing "jaw winking" of orbicularis ori with orbicularis oculi, and vice versa; parasympathetics regenerate incorrectly sometimes leading to eye tearing when taste good food ("crocodile tears").

Lab: *Noninv:* EMG at 2 wk if still fibrillation; consider decompression of nerve then

Rx: Protect eyes w Lacrilube gtts and hs taping
Steroids, such as prednisone 60 mg po qd tapered over 10 d to 5 mg (Nejm 1972;287:1268,1298), double-blind study shows results in less denervation (Laryngoscope 1993;103:1326); consider especially if no motor function at all
Valcyclovir or famicyclovir (p 661) w steroids (Ann IM 1996;124:63) probably helpful
Surgery no help? (Nejm 1975;292:748), perhaps decompression if flat EMG at 1 wk; physical therapy program no help (Nejm 1982;307:348)

Dysautonomias

Ann IM 2002;137:753

Cause: Primary degeneration of autonomic system, alone in Bradbury-Eggleston syndrome (BES), or combined w multisystem atrophy in Parkinson's disease (Ann IM 2000;133:382), olivopontine cerebellar atrophy (prominent Parkinsonian si), striatonigral degeneration (prominent cerebellar si's), Shy-Drager syndrome (SDS; acquired), and Riley-Day syndrome (RDS; congenital).

Secondary causes: CNS injury from spinal cord injury esp above T_6, amyloid neuropathy, Guillain-Barré syndrome, diabetic neuropathy, cancer, HIV, porphyria, pernicious anemia, tabes dorsalis from syphilis, drug toxicity like alcoholic neuropathy

Epidem: RDS in Eastern European Jews

Pathophys: RDS from decreased dopamine → norepinephrine conversion; BES and SDS from autoimmune antibodies to ganglionic Ach receptors (Nejm 2000;343:847) causing multineurosystem degeneration; diminished or no sympathetic CNS stimulation on standing

Sx: Postural hypotensive sx; heat intolerance; constipation (occasional diarhea), dysphagia; nocturia, frequency, urgency, incontinence, urinary retention; erectile and ejaculatory failure; stridor, apnea; Parkinsonism, ataxias
RDS: Absent taste; intermittent skin blotching
SDS: Mix of autonomic failure, Parkinson's type sx, and sometimes cerebellar sx

Si: Postural hypotension; anhidrosis; anisocoria, Horner's syndrome; stridor, apnea; Parkinsonism, cerebellar si's
RDS: Loss of anterior tongue papillae; poor coordination; absent deep-tendon reflexes; paroxysmal hypertension; defective temperature control and sweating; absent corneal reflexes
SDS: Dementia, tremor

Crs:

Cmplc: Autonomic dysreflexia = hypertensive crisis precipitated in quadriplegics by distended viscus (NE Rehab Hosp lecture 10/89)
r/o vasovagal syncope; carotid hypersensitivity; postural tachycardia syndrome (Nejm 2000;343:1008), increased pulse w/o decreased BP in young women w partial sympathetic denervation of legs

Lab: In RDS and SDS, methacholine sc causes eye tearing, transiently improved taste; in eye, i gtt methacholine causes potentiated miosis (denervation supersensitivity). Histamine intradermally causes no flare.

Noninv: Measure with expiratory-inspiratory respiratory variation in sinus rates; if < 10, suspect neuropathy present (BMJ 1982;285:559)

Rx:

of postural hypotension: Avoid diuretics, vasodilators, and tricyclics, increase salt intake; or try

- Dihydroergotamine 6.5-13 μgm/kg sc in am (Ann IM 1986;105:168), w
- Caffeine 250 mg po ½ hr ac (Ann IM 1986;105:168; Nejm 1985;313:549)
- Fludrocortisone (Florinef) 0.1+ mg po qd (Nejm 1989;321:952)
- β-Blockers
- Anticholinergics like disopyramide (Norpace) (Jama 1995;274:961)
- Midodrine 10 mg po tid (an α agonist) (Med Let 1997;39:59; Jama 1997;277:1046)
- Ibuprofen (Motrin) ir indomethacin (Indocin) (Sci Am Text Med, 1986)

of SDS: L-dopa + above

if anemic (hct < 40%), old or young, rx w erythropoietin (Ann IM 1994;121:181; Nejm 1993;329:611)

Peroneal Muscular Atrophy (Charcot-Marie-Tooth Disease)

Cause: Genetic, gene on chromosome 17 (Nejm 1993;329:96); autosomal dominant usually

Epidem: Male/female = 3-5:1

Pathophys: Peripheral neuropathy w spinal cord changes in some types

Sx: Onset in 1st or 2nd decade (as late as 6th decade occasionally), may sometimes start before age 5

Pains, paresthesias, and muscle cramps especially in cold weather; club feet; usually starts in lower legs and progresses, or may start in hands; trunk and girdle always spared

Si: Occasional muscular fibrillations; no nerve tenderness; diminished sensation; diminished vibratory and position sense in feet nearly always; diminished pin-prick frequently; ankle jerks gone at start; knee jerks last until quadriceps affected; arm and abdominal reflexes stay; absent plantar responses. Hammer toes, high-arched feet (pes cavus).

Crs: Slow, usually not incapacitating, death rarely due to it

Cmplc:

Lab: CSF: Usually normal, occasionally increased protein

Rx: None except palliative, eg, footdrop braces

Refsum's Disease

Cause: Genetic, autosomal recessive

Epidem:

Pathophys: Phytanic acid (simple lipid with branches, 16 carbons) pile up in serum; can drop to normal in 1 yr on no-chlorophyll diet. Phytolic acid, a fatty side chain of chlorophyll, is major source of phytanic acid in humans; there is no endogenous source. Block is in initial decarboxylation to pristanic acid. Heterozygous relatives metabolize to $\frac{1}{2}$ normal rate; diseased patients at 3% of normal by cultured fibroblasts.

Sx: Night blindness (100%), often 1st sx; sensorineural deafness (88%), begins in early adult life; anosmia (75%); muscular hypertrophy in some cases

Si: Cerebellar ataxia (100%); retinitis pigmentosa (100%), r/o syphilis and a-beta lipoproteinemia (p 376); tunnel vision, narrow fields

(95%); lenticular opacities (cataracts) (82%); epiphyseal dysplasia (53%); ichthyosis (67%); muscular atrophy, especially of peroneal and intrinsic hand and foot muscles

Crs: Appears in childhood, earliest onset at age 3 yr; may be precipitated by acute illness; relapses and remits

Cmplc: Cardiac arrhythmias and block are the most frequent cause of death

Lab: *Chem:* Serum phytanic acid > 2 μgm/cc
CSF: Protein increased as high as 450 mg %
Noninv: EKG abnormal (57%)
Path: Nerve and brain biopsies show 15% of fatty acids in myelin are phytanic acid

Rx: Diet low in chlorophyll (no milk, vegetables)
Plasmapheresis if sx develop (Nejm 1984;310:762)

Metachromatic Leukodystrophy

Nejm 1991;324:18, 1984;310:445

Cause: Genetic, autosomal recessive; at least 3 types of genetic mutations

Epidem: 1/40,000; gene frequency = 1/200

Pathophys: Lysosomal storage disease; metachromasia of myelin of CNS and peripheral nerves as well as deposits of intracellular metachromatic lipid in gallbladder and kidney. A failure of cerebroside sulfatase, which converts cerebrosulfatide to cerebrosides like arylsulfatase A (Nejm 1970;282:1336).

Sx: Onset at age 1 yr to adulthood, depending on severity of genetic deficiency. Gait disorder (1st sx in children); schizophrenia and other psychiatric sx (adult presentation); seizures.

Si: Weakness, ataxia, progressive spastic tetraparesis; peripheral neuropathy; dementia; decreased hearing; abnormal fundi; optic atrophy; gray-brown perimacular changes

Crs: Fatal in a few years in children, many years in adults

Cmplc:

Lab:

> *Chem:* Urine arylsulfatase, 24-hr sulfatide (Nejm 1971;284:739); metachromasia by dry slide test
>
> *CSF:* Elevated protein
>
> *Noninv:* Nerve conduction velocities always abnormal
>
> *Path:* Nerve (sural) bx shows metachromasia and myelin degeneration; rectal bx shows metachromasia of nerves. Fibroblast tissue culture assay of arylsulfatase: half normal in heterozygote, absent in homozygote; r/o "pseudodeficiency" seen in 1% of the normal population.

Xray: Gallbladder series shows no uptake (false-positive results in 50% of normal children, however)

Rx: Perhaps marrow transplant before severe damage (Nejm 1990;322:28)

Lipidoses (Niemann-Pick, Gaucher's, Tay-Sachs, and Wolman's Diseases)

Nejm 1991;325:1354 (GD); Ann IM 1975;82:257 (all)

Cause: Genetic, autosomal recessive
Gaucher's disease (GD) on chromosome 21

Epidem: Niemann-Pick disease (NPD): Children age 2-5 yr
GD: Children and adults, especially in Jews (1/850)
Tay-Sachs (TSD): Jews only; gene prevalence 1/30 Ashkenazi Jews

Pathophys: Neurologic disorder due to distention of neuron with lipid, displacement of nucleus toward axon hillock. All cause enlargement of RES organs, bone involvement, etc. General increase in brain size. All have a defective catabolic enzyme.
NPD: Cholesterol and sphingomyelin foam cells
GD: Enzyme defect at glucosylceramide (a glucocerebroside) → sphingosine + folic acid (Nejm 1971;284:739)

TSD: Ganglioside foam cells due to hexosamidase A deficiency (Nejm 1970;282:15)

Wolman's disease (WD): Cholesterol foam cells exclusively in RES

Sx: Bone pain, fractures, failure to thrive, and seizures

Si: Pathologic fractures; neurologic si's, large head, seizures, amaurosis; cherry-red macular spot; splenomegaly, anemia, bleeding; pingueculae

Crs: NPD and GD: Most die before age 5 yr

TS: Die before age 5 yr, although one gene type presents in adolescence

WD: Die by age 3 mo

Cmplc: GD: Pulmonary HT (Ann IM 1996;125:901)

r/o carnitine deficiency, presents as Reye's syndrome (Nejm 1980;303:1389)

Lab: *Chem:* GD: Elevated acid phosphatase, nonprostatic portion, increased B_{12} binding proteins (Nejm 1976;295:1046)

TSD: Increased AST (SGOT), hexosaminidase A absent in homozygote, intermediate levels in heterozygote (Nejm 1970;283:15)

Hem: GD: Low platelets (hypersplenism)

Path: NPD: Nerve biopsy shows foam cells

GD: Marrow shows foam cells, spindle-shaped with eccentric nuclei

WD: RES bx shows foam cells

Urine: 24-hr collection analyzed for glycoceramide (Nejm 1971; 284:739)

Xray: Erlenmeyer flask–like lesion, lucent, often in lower femur

Rx: NPD: Genetic counseling by detecting heterozygote (Nejm 1974; 291:989)

GD: Genetic counseling; splenectomy helps CBC but may speed course; marrow transplant (Nejm 1993;328:745, 1984;311: 84,1606); or iv enzyme, alglucerase (Ceredase) (Ann IM

1994;121:196; Nejm 1992;327:1632, 1991;324:1464), which costs $250,000-500,000/yr, or recombinant type (Cerezyme) (Ann IM 1995;122:33)

TSD: Screen serum or tears with hexosaminidase-based test (Nejm 1973;289:1072), confirm with DNA-based test (Nejm 1990;323:6)

Fabry's Disease

Ann IM 2003;138:338, 1975;82:257l; Nejm 1991;324:395

Cause: Genetic, sex-linked "partially recessive," ie, appears in males always and occasionally in female heterozygotes

Epidem:

Pathophys: Normal metabolic pathway is globoside → ceramide trihexoside (via the enzyme that is deficient in Fabry's disease, α-galactosidase A) → glucosylceramide (a glucocerebroside) → (via the enzyme missing in Gaucher's disease) sphingosine and folate. Thus there is a failure of a catabolic enzyme system to degrade the lipid, which accumulates in vascular endothelium, smooth muscle cells, renal tubular cells, nervous system, etc.

Sx: Febrile episodes; burning pain in extremities ("acroparesthesias")

Si: Macules and papules (angiokeratomas), multiple, small, dark, especially in umbilical and scrotal areas; the most frequent si in young men. Ocular corneal opacities (by slit lamp, in carriers too), cataracts, retinal edema. Hypohydrosis.

Crs: Death in 4th-5th decades from renal failure

Cmplc: Renal failure; CNS sx; gi sx's; cardiac including CHF, MI, mitral insufficiency, angina (Nejm 1991;324:395), and idiopathic hypertrophic aortic stenosis (Nejm 1982;307:926)

Lab: *Noninv:* EKG has short PR interval (Nejm 1973;289:357) Echo cardiogram shows LVH, only finding in heterozygous men; Fabry's present in 3% of all men w LVH (Nejm 1995;333:288)

Urine: Proteinuria, may be only clue or si (Nejm 1971;284:233); elevated 24-hr trihexasylceramide (Nejm 1971;284:739)

Rx: Agalsidase beta (Fabrazyme) (Med Let 2003;45:74; Jama 2001;285:2743; Nejm 2001;345:9,25) 1 mg/kg; α-gal A enzyme iv q 1-2 wk × 6 mo helps neuropathic pain, renal function, weight gain, and cardiac conduction in adults; adverse effects: rigors, fever w infusion; $70,000-150,000/yr depending on size

Organ transplant doesn't work (Nejm 1972;287:1215)

10.9 Myopathies

McArdle's Disease (and Other Glycogen Storage Diseases)

Ann IM 1994;120:218

Cause: Genetic, half are spontaneous mutations, half are autosomal recessive gene on chromosome 11 (Nejm 1993;329:241)

Epidem:

Pathophys: A glycogen storage disease; intramuscular phosphorylase deficiency prevents breakdown of muscle glycogen. Contrast with von Gierke's disease, in which glu-6-phosphatase deficiency in liver and kidney causes an inability to form glycogen in those organs. In McArdle's disease, all muscle energy must come via blood glucose; therefore painful muscle paralysis occurs during exercise, with muscles in contraction without EMG activity. Since glycogen is formed in muscles but not broken down, muscle size increases.

Sx: Static contraction with exercise, painful

Si: Tourniquet worsens; pseudohypertrophy

Crs:

Cmplc: ATN (Nejm 1972;286:1237)

r/o similar enzyme deficiencies causing pain, fatigue, cramps, and myoglobinuria, eg, phosphofructokinase deficiency (Nejm

1991;324:364), carnitine palmityl transferase deficiency, etc (Nejm 1985;312:370); other types of glycogen storage diseases in which patients die of cirrhosis by age 4 yr and can be rx'd with liver transplants (Nejm 1991;324:39); myofibrillar myopathies, esp desmin myopathy w associated cardiomyopathy (Nejm 2000;342:770)

Lab: *Chem:* K$^+$ and lactates w and w/o tourniquet before and after exercise (lactate doesn't increase with ischemia as it normally should)

Path: Muscle bx shows large blebs of glycogen beneath sarcolemma

Urine: Myoglobinuria (Ann IM 1978;88:610) (p 762)

Rx: Pre-exercise high-protein diet provides amino acid fuel to substitute for glycogen when need anaerobic metabolism (Nejm 1985;312:355), or oral corn starch (Nejm 1990;323:590), or sucrose solutions (Nejm 2003;349:2503); all markedly improve exercise capacity

Dyskalemic Myopathies (Familial Periodic Paralysis; Normo- or Hyperkalemic Myopathy; and Hypokalemic Myopathy

Cause: Familial periodic paralysis (FPP) is inherited; unknown cause in other two

Epidem: FPP is more common in Asians and associated with hyperthyroidism

Pathophys: "Channel-opathies." Hyperkalemic myopathy (hyperK) may be mediated through an aldosterone-like steroid intermittently secreted.

Sx: Paralysis, intermittent, periodic, often precipitated by exercise or, in hyperK, insulin

Si: Flaccid paralysis

Crs: Most occur throughout life

Cmplc: Death due to cardiac arrhythmias and respiratory impairments especially; PVCs and ventricular tachycardia (Nejm 1972; 286:253)

if K^+ elevated, r/o rare hypoaldosterone syndrome probably due to absent renin (Nejm 1972;287:573)

Lab: *Path:* Muscle biopsy shows clear vacuoles throughout muscle, intracellular "focal hydropic changes," often PAS-positive (glycogen)

Renal bx shows similar vacuoles at base of tubular cells

Rx: of FPP: Rx of hypo/hyperK+

of normo- or hyperkalemic myopathy: Acetazolamide 125-250 mg po bid (Ann IM 1977;86:169) probably works by increasing K^+ loss by blocking H^+ secretion

of hypoK: K^+ iv, or po acetazolamide 125-250 mg po bid, which works by causing acidosis and thereby driving K^+ up; or, more likely, inhibits an aldosterone-like steroid (Ann IM 1970;73:39; Nejm 1968;278:582)

Paroxysmal Myoglobinuria (Meyer-Betz Polymyopathy)

Am J Med 1963;39:49

Cause: Acquired or genetic

Epidem: Acquired type seen with heavy alcohol use, heroin OD, high fevers, ischemia, crush injuries, infections, and iv amphetamine use (Ann IM 1977;86:381)

Genetic type seen in carnitine palmityl transferase deficiency (Nejm 1985;312:370) and McArdle's disease (p 759)

Pathophys:

Sx: Mild exercise-induced muscle weakness, swelling, and tenderness

Dark urine (r/o alkaptonuria [Nejm 2002;347:2111], porphyria, and hemoglobinuria)

Si:

Crs:

Cmplc: Acute tubular necrosis (Ann IM 1976;85:23), respiratory paralysis, infection, hyperkalemia

      r/o rhabdomyolysis w myoglobinuria (see ATN, p 1027)

Lab: *Chem:* Serum benzidine, if negative, means myoglobinemia; if positive, means hemoglobinemia; elevated AST (SGOT), LDH, CPK, and aldolase

    Path: Muscle bx shows segmental necrosis of muscle fibers; extensive regeneration, with basophilia of muscle cytoplasm

    Urine: Dark; positive benzidine (or guaiac); if becomes negative after addition of 80% NH_4SO_4, then diagnosis is hemoglobinuria; if stays positive, then diagnosis is myoglobinuria caused by paroxysmal myoglobinuria, or muscle trauma; negative benzidine (or guaiac) means cause is alkaptonuria or porphyria

Rx: Prevent by avoiding exertion; supportive care of sx

Pseudohypertrophic Muscular Dystrophy (Duchenne's Muscular Dystrophy)

Rv of all muscular dystrophies: Am J Med 1963;35:632

Cause: Genetic, sex-linked; occasionally autosomal recessive

Epidem: Mostly males; most common of all muscular dystrophies

Pathophys: Decreased calcium uptake, but normal muscle efficiency early in course of disease affecting both fast and slow fiber bundles (Nejm 1969;280:184); deficient dystrophin, a muscle protein (Nejm 1988;318:1363)

Sx: Aggressive: Onset at age 1-5 yr. Calf hypertrophy early, later may decrease; symmetric pelvic involvement, w waddle gait and Gowers' si.

    Benign: Onset usually at age 6-18 yr, but can be 2-35 yr. Calf, deltoid, infraspinatus hypertrophy; pelvic 1st, then shoulder in pts age 5-10 yr.

Si: As above

Crs: Aggressive: Relentless, often rapid progression, in bed by age 10 yr

Benign: Able to walk 25-30 yr after onset; life expectancy into 4th-5th decades

Cmplc: Progressive skeletal deformities; death due to wasting, inanition, infection; pseudo-gi obstruction and gastric dilatation due to smooth muscle involvement (Nejm 1988;319:15); myocardopathy in both pts and female carriers (83%), gradually progressive (Jama 1996;275:1335)

r/o metabolic myopathies: acid maltase deficiency; carnitine deficiency (Nejm 1985;312:370); other sex-linked muscular dystrophies: Becker's dystrophy, and Emery-Dreifuss muscular dystrophy (Ann IM 1993;119:900)

Lab: *Chem:* Elevated CPK (also in carrier females), aldolase, and AST (SGOT); all elevated early before clinical sx and si, decrease later with burnout

Path: Muscle bx shows dystrophy before clinical sx and si's, ie, random-sized fibers; lipomatosis; increased connective tissue in interstitium; degenerative changes like hyalinization, vacuolization; nuclear shrinkage; basophilic staining of some fibers

Rx: Prevent by prenatal dx at age 18-20 wk in utero via amniotic CPK (Nejm 1977;297:968); or DNA probe techniques via amniocentesis sample of early pregnancy (Nejm 1987;316:985) or by activation of myogenesis (Nejm 1993;329:915)

Prednisone 0.75 mg/kg qd $\times$ 6 mo increases strength (Nejm 1989;320:1592)

Myotonic Dystrophy

Cause: Genetic, autosomal dominant on chromosome 19

Epidem: 1/8000

Pathophys: Abnormal insulin fasting levels and increased response to stimulation (Nejm 1967;277:837). In vitro the sarcoplasmic reticulum shows increased rapidity of calcium uptake initially and normal total uptake, suggesting fast but not slow fibers most affected (Nejm 1969;280:184) and may thus explain some of the myotonia.

Sx: Onset at age 20-25 yr

Si: Weak jaw, weak sternocleidomastoids, ptosis; early frontal balding; myotonia (unable to release grasp); cataracts; gonadal atrophy. Muscle percussion (thenar eminence) with reflex hammer causes localized myotonic contraction.

Crs:

Cmplc: Diabetes mellitus; flaccid esophagus with secondary reflux and strictures; billowing mitral valve (Ann IM 1976;85:18), Vtach and heart block (Jama 1995;274:813) contribute to 15-30% incidence of sudden death (Ann IM 1991;115:607)

r/o other myotonic syndromes (Nejm 1993;328:482) including cold myotonia (autosomal dominant) and excitement myotonia (autosomal dominant), both of which respond to quinidine; "stiff man syndrome" (p 577); hyperkalemic periodic paralysis (p 760)

Lab: *Chem:* Flat glucose tolerance test with normal FBS; decreased urinary ketosteroids

Noninv: EMG has a diagnostic pattern

Serol: IgG low (increased catabolism), without other globulin changes. Southern blot analysis w DNA probe detects the abnormal gene 90+% of the time (Nejm 1993;328:471).

Rx: Acetazolamide rx helps sx but causes severe muscle weakness of quads (Ann IM 1977;86:169)

Limb-Girdle Muscular Dystrophy

Cause: Genetic (60%), autosomal recessive (rarely dominant); or sporadic (40%)

Epidem:

Pathophys:

Sx: Onset as child (rarely in 20s or 30s)

Si: Pelvic girdle weakness causes waddle and Gower's si; upper shoulder girdle and face muscles affected later and less often

Crs: Progressive, spreads upward over ~20 yr; usually can't walk by age 20-30. Prognosis is between that of Duchenne's and facioscapulohumeral muscular dystrophies.

Cmplc: Myocardiopathy

Lab: *Chem:* CPK and aldolase high-normal or increased; never as high as in Duchenne's; these enzymes distinguish the disease from neurogenic atrophy

K^+, total body, decreased in pts and carriers (Nejm 1967;276:1349)

Rx:

Facioscapulohumeral Muscular Dystrophy

Cause: Genetic, autosomal dominant (rarely recessive)
Epidem:
Pathophys:

Sx: Onset in childhood to middle age, usually adolescence

Si: Expressionless face with "transverse smile." Facial, scapular, and humeral muscles involved. Pelvic girdle and proximal legs involved later after 20-30 yr, causing waddle and Gower's si. Pseudohypertrophy of calves infrequently.

Crs: Slow, insidious, leading to moderate disability and skeletal deformity, rarely unable to walk. Death from nondystrophic causes.

Lab: *Chem:* Enzymes normal, occasionally slightly increased CPK
Path: Muscle biopsy shows same changes as in Duchenne's
Rx:

Reflex Sympathetic Dystrophy Syndrome (Complex Regional Pain Syndrome, Causalgia, Shoulder-Hand Syndrome)

Bull Rheum Dis 1986;36:3

Cause: Previous injury/arm pain

Epidem: Up to 25% of pts with locally painful organic disease

Pathophys: Diminished sympathetic tone leads to increased vascular responsiveness to adrenergic stimulation (Ann IM 1993;118:619)

Sx: H/o painful organic injury, eg, MI, trauma, CVA, or cervical disc disease. Burning pain with tenderness in an extremity usually; swelling; dystrophic skin changes; vasomotor dysfunctions; bilateral in 40%; hot/cold sensations.

Si: Tenderness, dystrophic skin changes, vasomotor instability, edema

Crs: Progressive leading to atrophy over 1+ yr

Cmplc: r/o rheumatoid arthritis, septic joint, SLE, Reiter's, peripheral neuropathy

Lab:

Xray: Local osteoporosis; bone scan positive over affected joints

Rx: Prevent w early mobilization
       Rx of sx (Nejm 2000;343:654): Local hot/cold; prednisone 15 d tapering rx po 60 mg to 0 mg qd divided; intensive PT; sympathetic ganglion blocks, eg, stellate; surgical sympathectomy; TENS unit; implanted spinal cord stimulator (Nejm 2000;343:618); chronic intrathecal baclofen infusion (Nejm 2000;343:625)

10.10 Tumors

Subdural Hematoma, Chronic

Cause: Head trauma, in older pts, may be mild (eg, sitting down hard) if also volume depleted

Epidem: Predominantly in pts age < 1 yr or > 50 yr

Pathophys: Vein wall tear; no sx's until > 50 cc; forms semipermeable membrane that absorbs fluid and thus becomes a tumor; ipsilateral upper motor neuron si's from contralateral cerebral peduncle being pressed against the tentorium, and ipsilateral 3rd cranial nerve deficit from herniating temporal lobe tip pressure especially dilated nonreactive or poorly reactive pupil before abnormalities of extraocular movements, but later as hematoma expands opposite pyramidal tract also becomes compressed

Sx: Headache and confusion (essential, to consider dx)

Si: Progression over days to weeks, from confusion and equivocal contralateral hyperreflexia, to severe headache and ipsilateral hyperreflexia and pupillary dilatation, to varying contralateral pupillary changes (Neurol 1990;40:1707), and finally to bradycardia, hypertension, coma, and fixed dilated pupils

Crs: Chronic > 15 d-6 mo (7.5% mortality)

Cmplc: Chronics are bilateral 20% of time, hence no lateralization r/o much more obvious acute < 3 d (55% mortality) and subacute 3-15 d (15% mortality)

Lab: LP dangerous to do without CT first, but often will show increased pressure and xanthochromia

Xray: CT scan, rarely need arteriogram. Skull films to look for fracture.

Rx: of acute: Rapid craniotomy and decompression within 4 hr helps prognosis (Nejm 1981;304:1511); plus steroids and osmotic agents

of subacute and chronic: Craniotomy and decompression

Pseudotumor Cerebri

Nejm 1983;308:1077

Cause: Idiopathic

Epidem: Associated with anemia; vitamin deficiencies and intoxications, especially vitamin A toxicity, eg, acne rx with isotretinoin and tetracyclines (Neurol 1984;34:1509; FDA Bull 1983;13:21); chronic hypoxia; post-head trauma; post-otitis media; hypoparathyroidism; start of thyroid replacement in myxedematous pts; steroid administration and withdrawal (Addison's); lateral sinus thrombosis. Mostly in young, overweight women.

Pathophys:

Sx: Headache, visual field losses; no impairment of consciousness

Si: Enlarged blind spot, central vision losses; later, inferior quadrantic defects/visual field constrictions. Papilledema without hemorrhages or exudates.

Crs:

Cmplc: Visual loss, monitor rx w quantitative visual perimetry

Lab: *CSF:* High pressures (> 200 mm), normal CSF

Xray: CT shows small or normal ventricles

Rx: Repeated LPs; 2-6 wk of steroids
　　　Surgical shunt rarely needed

Meningioma

Nejm 2001;344:114

Cause: Neoplasia; chromosome 22q deletions and thereby associated w neurofibromatosis type 2

Epidem: Peak incidence between age 50 and 70 yr; rare in pts < 20 yr; 20% of all brain tumors, 25% of all cord tumors. Increased in irradiated children (Nejm 1988;319:1033) and pts with breast cancer. Female/male = 2:1.

Pathophys: Most commonly over hemisphere convexities; also deep in cleft (parasagittal), over sphenoid ridge, olfactory groove, spinal cord. Slow growing with few si of brain damage. Often have estrogen and progesterone receptors. 2% are malignant.

Sx: Headache, seizures (often 1st sx)

Si: Of subtle mass lesion

Crs: Very slowly progressive. After resection, 10-20% recurrence at 10 yr if thought to have been completely resected, 80% if obviously could not get all.

Cmplc:

Lab: *Path:* Uniform-sized cell whorls; these may calcify to form psammoma bodies

Xray: Skulls show hyperostosis or radiolucency of underlying bone, large feeding vessel impression, foramen spinosum enlarged due to middle meningeal enlargement, 33% are calcified (Fraser, Edinburgh 1968)

CT scan usually is diagnostic; often do not show up on MRI unless use gadolinium-enhanced imagery

Rx: Surgery

Radiation as adjunctive rx if unresectable or only partially resectable

Perhaps hormone rx in future

Medulloblastoma

Nejm 1994;331:1505, 1991;324:464

Cause: Neoplasia

Epidem: Usually in children; 20% of all pediatric brain tumors; usually cerebellar (70% of all childhood tumors are in posterior fossa)

Pathophys: Often starts in vermis of cerebellum; increased pressure due to hemorrhage, gliosis, and both local and diffuse edema due to increased venous pressure from increased intracranial pressure

Sx: Truncal ataxia, sx of increased intracranial pressure like headache, vomiting, etc, over weeks

Si: Papilledema

Crs: Highly malignant; 30-70% 5-yr remissions, 92% 5-yr survival; and perhaps 50% cure, 60% in girls vs 25% in boys (Jama 1998;279:1474)

Cmplc: Metastases down spinal cord; hydrocephalus from aqueductal stenosis; uncal and cerebellar foramen magnum herniations (p 766, 777)

Lab: *Path:* High nuclear/cytoplasmic ratio, round oval nuclei, scant stroma, many mitoses, small cells, pseudorosettes

Xray: CT/MRI useful for initial dx but not much help as surveillance for recurrence; hx and PE pick up 83% of recurrences (Nejm 1994;3330:892)

Rx: Combinations of surgery, craniospinal irradiation, and chemotherapy iv and introthecal (Nejm 2005;352:978) yield 90% survival if full surgical resection, 33% if mets; but cause diminished IQ, as does radiation

Astrocytoma

Grade I (astrocytoma); grades 2 (glioma) and 3 (astroblastoma) = anaplastic astrocytoma; grade 4 (glioblastoma)

Nejm 2001;344:114, 1991;324:1471,1555

Cause: Neoplasia; chromosome 10 deletion, etc

Epidem: 50% of all brain tumors (pediatric: Nejm 1991;324:463). Occasionally associated w both types of neurofibromatosis and Turcot's syndrome.

Pathophys: In children, in cerebellum and pons; in adults, in spinal cord (most common spinal cord tumor), cerebrum and cerebellum

Sx: Seizures, CNS mass lesion sx's including headache

Si: Depends on location

Crs: Without rx, < 6 mo for grade 4 glioblastoma, 5% 2-yr survival; others are low-grade tumors compatible with survival for many years, eg, 50% 2-yr survival for anaplastic astrocytoma

Cmplc:

Lab: *Path:* Biopsy to be sure is not lymphoma, abscess, etc

Xray: MRI

Rx: Radiation; chemoRx 1st in very young children, allows brain maturation (Nejm 1991;324:463), in adults w temozolomide (Temodar) (Nejm 2005;352:987, 997); surgical resection

Craniopharyngioma

Nejm 1994;331:1506, 1991;324:1555

Cause: Neoplasia

Epidem: Mainly in children

Pathophys: Suprasellar tumor arising from pharyngeal epithelium

Sx: Adults: Headache; bitemporal hemianopsia; hypothalamic dysfunction including personality changes, obesity, diabetes insipidus, sleep changes
Children: Growth failure

Si:

Crs: Slow growing, with rx live at least 15 yr

Cmplc: Panhypopituitarism post-op (80-90%)

Lab:

Xray: MRI or CT shows calcification in 95%

Rx: Surgery difficult in floor of 3rd ventricle, 70% able to be completely resected, 90% cured w post-op radiation
Radiation is quite sensitive, gives 5-10 yr of asx life; often used postsurgery

10.11 Miscellaneous

Aphasias

N. Geschwind; Curr Concepts Cerebro Dis 1981;16:1; Nejm
    1971;284:654

> Definition: Unable to name an object

Nonfluent: Broca's area; associated with hemiplegia, arm > face
    > leg

fluent:

- Wernicke's; posterior superior temporal; can't comprehend or
  repeat
- Conduction; parietal lobe above Sylvian fissure; comprehends
  but can't repeat
- Anomic; angular gyrus; comprehends and repeats
- Isolation of speech area; above and below Sylvian fissure; can't
  comprehend but repeats

Caloric Stimulations (Calorics)

With ear canal irrigation, normally fast nystagmus component to
same side as warm stimulation and opposite side of cold stimulation.
No fast component if cortex out (coma); good way to distinguish
feigned coma. Patterns (measure seconds duration and/or inverse of
onset lag): right ear end-organ damage = Warm L + Cold L > WR +
CR; central (brainstem) = WL + CR > WR + CL.

Coma Prognosis

In medical, nonoverdose, nontraumatic coma (Jama
2004;191;870; Ann IM 1981;94:293) 0% if 3 d out fewer than 2 of 3
eye si's (corneal, pupillary, doll's eyes). Somatosensory-evoked potentials 24 hr into medical coma is 100% sens and 42% specif for nonre-
covery (ACP J Club 2004;140:24). Persistent vegetative state
prognosis: ~50% become conscious after 6-12 mo if traumatic, only
~10% in nontraumatic types (Nejm 1994;3330:1572).

Glasgow coma scale (best efforts) (Nejm 1991;324:1477); ≤ 8, needs ICU and intubation; scoring:

Opens eyes: Spontaneously (4); to speech (3); to pain (2); none (1)

Verbal: Oriented (5); confused (4); inappropriate (3); incomprehensible (2); none (1)

Motor: Spontaneous/obeys (6); localizes pain (5); withdrawal (4); flexion to pain (3); extension to pain (2); none (1)

Rx: Hypothermia to 33°C (91.4°F) × 24 hr may help in traumatic coma (Nejm 1997;336:541); postarrest thiopental (Nejm 1986; 314:397) and calcium-channel blockers (Nejm 1991;324:1225) are no help.

CSF Eosinophilia

Helminths or lymphoma (Ann IM 1979;91:70)

CSF, Increased Protein

Usually < 100 mg %; medical causes: (1) diabetes, (2) hyperparathyroidism, (3) myxedema, (4) rheumatoid arthritis (Ann IM 1979;90:786)

Delirium (Organic Brain Syndrome)

Ann IM 1990;113:941; Nejm 1989;320:578

Cause: Drugs, long list (Med Let 1993;35:65); primary intracranial diseases; systemic diseases secondarily affecting the brain; withdrawal from alcohol/sedatives; metabolic like hypo/hyperNa, hypoglycemia, and UTI in pt with atonic bladder leading to elevated NH_3 levels (Nejm 1981;304:766); infectious, eg, syphilis, crypto; brain mets; status epilepticus, petit mal or partial complex seizures (Neurol 1983;33:1545)

Epidem: High incidence in elderly; eg, 50% of pts with hip fx develop it; 15% of elderly pts develop it after general surgery; higher rates in those with dementia

Sx: Hallucinations, often visual as well as auditory

Si: Acute onset and fluctuating course; transient (days-weeks; unlike permanent dementia), global (unlike acute psychosis) disorder of cognition and attention. Loss of attention span is most prominent deficit; test by serial 7's; serial digits up to 7, eg, phone numbers; spell "world" backward. Disorganized thinking and/or altered level of consciousness; typically "sundown," ie, worsen at night.

Rx: Prevent in hospitalized elderly (Nejm 1999;340:669) by programs directed at cognition, sleep, immobility, hearing, vision, and dehydration; reduces incidence from 15% to 10%

Find and rx primary cause

Haloperidol (Haldol) 0.5-1 mg po/im prn (J Am Ger Soc 2003;51:234); higher doses in younger pts

Dermatomes and Cutaneous Nerves

Fragile X Syndrome

Nejm 1991;325:1673,1720

Epidem: 1/1000 males, 1/2000 females; X-linked, 80% penetrance in males, 65% in heterozygote females due to triplet repeats (Nejm 1996;335:1222); most common inherited form of mental retardation after Down's syndrome

Sx: Mental retardation

Si: Long face, large testicles, big ears, big chin

Rx: Prenatal dx

Frontal Lobe Si's

Gegenhalten (paratonia), snout, suck, palmomental, grasp, pathologic laughing and weeping; rx latter with low-dose (25-75 mg) amitriptyline (Nejm 1985;313:1480)

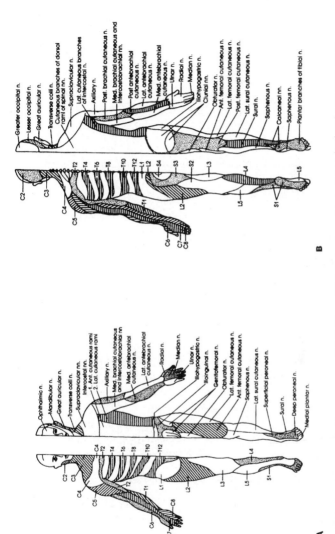

Figure 10.1 Dermatome and cutaneous nerve distribution. (A) Anterior view of dermatomes (*left*) and cutaneous areas supplied by individual peripheral nerves (*right*). (B) Posterior view of dermatomes (*left*) and cutaneous areas supplied by individual peripheral nerves (*right*). Reproduced from Carpenter MB and Sulin J. Human Neuroanatomy, 8th ed. Baltimore: Williams and Wilkins, 1983 (www.lww.com)

Head Injuries (Concussion)

In sports, many systems, some w 3 categories; latest just breaks into simple and complex concussions, but rx has become more conservative (Clin J Sport Med 2005;15:48; Jama 2003;290:2549,2556,2604, 1997;277:1190); recurrence within 7 d in almost 15%; computer-based systems to compare results/progress over baseline (www.cogsport.com, www.impacttest.com)

Dx: Grade 1 (15%): Confusion < 15 min without amnesia
Grade 2 (70%): Confusion > 15 min without amnesia; or any amnesia
Grade 3 (15%): Loss of consciousness

Rx: Return to play guidelines—applies to both types of concussion. Once asymptomatic, proceed to next level. If sx recur, then rest 24 hr and drop back 1 level.
1. Complete rest 48 hr.
2. Light aerobic exercise.
3. Sport-specific exercise, add resistance training.
4. Noncontact drills.
5. Full-contact training.
6. Game play.

in ER: CT if loss of consciousness or amnesia for event w any of the following sx/si: headache, vomiting, > 60 yr old, drug or ETOH intoxication, short-term memory deficit, trauma evidence on physical exam above clavicles, seizures. Otherwise CT not necessary, no false negs (Nejm 2000;343:100:138); no benefit from hypothermic rx (Nejm 2001;344:556) or iv steroids (Lancet 2004;364:1321).

Horner's Syndrome (Oculosympathetic Paresis)

Ipsilateral ptosis of eyelid, decreased facial sweating, and miosis of pupil unresponsive to cocaine 10% gtts because is denervated (Nejm 1997;337:1359); all due to interruption of sympathetics either at apex of chest (eg, Pancoast syndrome) or w carotid diseases like aneurysm or dissection; r/o Raeder's paratrigeminal syndrome (Acad EM 1996; 3:864), which manifests as Horner's w/o loss of sweating and w neuralgic pain, seen w carotid dissection

Immune Globulin Iv Rx

Ann IM 1997;126:721

May help several autoimmune neurologic diseases; very expensive, $6,000-12,000/mo

Innervations

Table 10.3   Innervations

Reflex	Innervation
Biceps	C_{5-6}
Supinator	C_{5-6}
Triceps	C_{6-7}
Abdominal	T_{8-12}
Cremasteric	L_1
Quadriceps	L_{3-4}
Ankle	L_5-S_1
Extensor pollicis longus	S_1

Intracranial Mass Effect Treatment

1st, hyperventilation; if that fails, mannitol 0.5 gm/kg iv or furosemide 1 mg/kg. Brain masses, tumors, subdurals, hemorrhage, and CVA all produce diminished mental status due to lateral brain shifts (Nejm 1986;314:953).

Meningismus si's

Kernig's = hamstring spasm with straight leg raising; Brudzinski's = neck flexion causes hip flexion

Meningitis, Definitions and Causes

Aseptic meningitis (predominant lymphocytes in CSF; if polys in first LP, redo in 6-12 hr to look for change to lymphs: Nejm 1973;289:571)

- Treatable: Tuberculosis, SBE,* fungal (crypto), tumor, Listeria, *H. simplex,* NSAIDs (Ann IM 1983;99:343), syphilis, subdural* or epidural* abscess (eg, in spine due to disc abscess), cysticercosis (*T. solium:* Nejm 1984;311:1492), leptospirosis, partially rx'd bacterial, RA (Ann IM 1979;90:786), rickettsia, Lyme disease, HIV, cat scratch fever, *Borrelia* (relapsing fever), high-dose immunoglobulin rx (Ann IM 1994;121:254)
- Untreatable: Sarcoid, viral including enteroviruses* (polio, coxsackie, echo), mumps,* mono,* rabies, lymphocytic choriomeningitis* in lab worker, arbovirus,* rarely CMV (infants)

Septic meningitis: CSF sens/specif numbers (Ann IM 1986; 104:880): glucose < 40 mg % (40% false neg), <$\frac{1}{3}$ of blood glucose (30% false neg), antigen studies (10-40% false neg)

*Normal CSF glucose

Movement Disorders

Chorea (irregular joint movement):
- Rheumatic Sydenham's chorea (distal)
- Hemiballismus, from vascular damage from ASCVD or in SLE [if proximal, rx with Haldol (Nejm 1976;295:1348)]
- Huntington's chorea

Athetosis (writhing):
- Huntington's chorea, can't keep tongue extended
- Tardive dyskinesia after phenothiazine rx (Ann IM 1981;94: 788); lip smacking, tongue and perioral/periorbital tics; rx with perhaps clozapine, which has cmplc of seizure and agranulocytosis (Nejm 1991;324:746) (p 940), or vitamin E 1600+ U/d

Asterixis (failure of postural tone) in hepatic or other (eg, CO_2 retention) metabolic encephalopathy

Torticollis: Basal ganglia disease; the most common focal dystonia; inherited (Nejm 1973;288:284); rx with botulinum
toxin (Med Let 2001;43:63) q 3 mo; expensive

Myoclonus: Muscle contractions of CNS origin; all movements
but palatal type (central tegmental tract lesion) disappear
with sleep; rx with barbiturates or L_5-HT + carbidopa
(Nejm 1980;303:782), r/o myoclonic epilepsy (Nejm 1986;
315:296)

Tics:
- Simple benign
- **Tourette's Syndrome** (Nejm 2001;345:1184; Jama 1995;
273:498)

Cause: Genetic, autosomal dominant (Nejm 1986;315:993) but incomplete penetrance so male/female = 4:1

Epidem: 3-5/10,000; associated w ADHD (p 882)

Sx: Motor tics; vocal tics, usually sniffs or grunts but may be swears or
echoes of own or others' speech; obsessive touching of hazardous
things, eg, stove burners

Si: Above plus often obsessive compulsive counting, checking
rituals, etc

Crs: Onset around age 7 yr, progressive into adulthood

Cmplc: ADHD in 60% (Jama 1998;279:1100)

Rx: 1st: Haloperidol (Haldol) augmented w nicotine gum (Am J
Psychiatry 1991;148:793), or pimozide (ORAP) 1-16 mg qd
(Med Let 1985;27:3)
2nd: Clonidine (Lancet 1979;2:551)
3rd: Benzodiazepines

Tremor ("involuntary motion back and forth about a point")
(Ann IM 1980;93:460; M. Samuels 3/85)
- Parkinsonism tremor (at repose, better with action/intention)
3/sec

- Constant tremor (at repose, increases with action/intention, 9/sec, all "soluble in alcohol"):
  1. Exaggerated physiologic tremor from hyperthyroidism, coffee, tea, theophyllines, adrenergic stimulation, lithium, drug withdrawal; rx with propranolol 10-40 mg or others, β-blockers (Nejm 1975;293:950), peripheral effect within minutes
  2. **"Essential" Tremor**, idiopathic and familial; can coexist with parkinsonism or other degenerative neurologic disease; rx with propranolol (best of β-blockers), which helps 50%, takes weeks to work (probably CNS effect); primidone 50-250 mg bid; gabapentin (Neurontin); rarely clozapine
  3. Wilson's disease (Nejm 1978;298:1347)
- Coarse intention (cerebellar) tremor, peripheral and/or truncal ataxia; rx with limb weights, INH 600-1200 mg qd helps perhaps via GABA; causes:
  1. Multiple sclerosis
  2. Tumor, primary or metastatic; or paraneoplastic syndromes seen with breast or gyn tumors (Nejm 1990;322:1844)
  3. Alcoholic degeneration, only in legs
  4. Vascular diseases of cerebellum: Cerebellar hemorrhage or thrombotic medullary plate syndromes
  5. Foramen magnum syndrome from short neck or Paget's disease by compression of vertebral artery
  6. Genetic ataxias: Friedreich's ataxia, hereditary ataxia telangiectasia (p 735), diminished pyruvate oxidation (Nejm 1976; 295:62), olivopontine cerebellar ataxia, vitamin E deficiency (Nejm 1995;333:1313)

Vocal tremor; stuttering/cluttering; worsened by tricyclics and other anticholinergics; helped by bethanechol 5 mg po tid (Nejm 1993;329:813)

Muscle Weakness

Motor neuronal disorder, eg, ALS
Polyneuropathy

Neuromuscular transmission: Myasthenia, Eaton-Lambert, lithium or β-blockers; curare, snake bite (Nejm 1986;315:1444)

Myopathy:

- Electrolyte abnormalities, eg, low K or PO_4
- Endocrine: Hyperthyroid or hypothyroid, Cushing's, acromegaly, vitamin D deficiency, hyperparathyroid
- Infections: Toxo, trichinosis, cysticercosis
- Immune: Poly/dermatomyositis, sarcoid, amyloid
- Drug/toxin: Alcoholic, steroids, colchicine, rifampin, chloroquine, clofibrate, emetine, β-blockers, diuretics

Neuropathy, Peripheral

Nejm 1979;300:546

Diabetic, uremic, myxedemic, alcoholic, idiopathic, familial, amyloid (diminished pain and temperature; associated with autonomic neuropathy), leprosy (diminished pain and temperature especially in vitiligo patches), toxic (N-hexane: Nejm 1971;285:82)

Pain, Chronic

Rx of neuropathic types (Nejm 2003;348:1243):

Medications:

NSAIDs, including tramodol

Narcotics, eg, oxycodone and oral morphines

Psychoactive agents:

- Anticonvulsants:

Carbamazepine (esp for tic douloureux) 400-800 mg po qd

Phenytoin (for tic or peripheral neuropathy) 300-400 po qd

Gabapentin (Neurontin) (Med Let 2004;46:29; Jama 1998;280:1831,1837,1863) 300-1200 mg po tid, but increase slowly to avoid intoxication; renal excretion;

adverse effects: somnolence, dizziness, confusion; study of use w morphine suggests pain improved by $\frac{1}{3}$ more than w either drug used alone (Nejm 2005; 352:1324)

Oxcarbazepine
Lamotrigine
Clonazepam
Topiramate

- Antidepressants/antipsychotics: Imipramine, desipramine, amitriptyline (not helpful in HIV neuropathy: Jama 1998; 280:1590), haloperidol, fluphenazine, chlorpromazine, SSRIs (J Gen Intern Med 1997; 12:384), venlafaxine, bupropion
- Antiarrythmics: like lidocaine 5% topical patch; or mexiletine (Mexitil) 200 mg po qd to tid, last resort, related to lidocaine; adverse effects: arrhythmias

Electrical stimulation (TENS)
Acupuncture (not helpful in HIV neuropathy: Jama 1998;280:1590)
Neurosurgical ablation
Injections
Biofeedback
Hypnosis
Cognitive/behavioral programs; coping strategies

Paraplegia Causes

Treatable:
- B_{12} deficiency (subacute combined degeneration)
- Syphilis (general paresis of the insane)
- Mass lesion including trauma, disc, cervical spondylosis, metastatic cancer (Nejm 1992;327:614)
- Parasagittal meningioma
- Shy-Drager syndrome (p 739, 752)

Untreatable:
- Multiple sclerosis
- ALS
- Syringomyelia
- Chronic progressive myelopathy due to HIV infection (Nejm 1988;318:1195)

Pupillary Abnormalities

Argyll-Robertson pupils: React to accommodation, not to light; caused by syphilis or diabetes

Adies pupils: Dilated unilaterally (80%), slow (5 min) reaction to light and accommodation; idiopathic cause

Horner's syndrome (p 776)

Uncal herniation (p 766)

Cranial nerve III palsy from aneurysm of internal carotid

Sleep

Circadian sleep cycles and work (Nejm 1983;309:534; Sci 1982; 217:460); bright lights at beginning of work and dark rooms to sleep in, very effective (Nejm 1990;322:1253)

Insomnia, review of causes and rx (Nejm 1990;322:239); medications (p 937) used 50-90% of time in hospital and probably no help (Ann IM 1984;100:441); in elderly pts, aerobic exercise 3-4 ×/wk helps (Jama 1997;277:32)

Third Cranial Nerve Palsies

Eye deviates laterally; diabetic type spares pupil; aneurysm of internal carotid does not (p 858 for innervations of eye movements)

Transient Global Amnesia

Curr Concepts Cerebro Dis 1983;18:13

Perhaps bilateral temporal lobe ischemia; lasts minutes to hours (< 24 hr); usually in pts > 50 yr old, no associated neurologic deficits, no permanent damage, rarely recurs

Vertigo/Dizziness

Past pointing with finger-to-nose testing with closed eyes, vestibular not a cerebellar sign

Causes of dizziness:

Primary care practice (Ann IM 1992;117:898):

- Vestibular (54%) ("an illusion of motion"), of which ⅓ are benign positional vertigo
- Psychiatric (16%)
- Presyncope (6%)
- Dysequilibrium (2%), imbalance when moving, sense of falling; usually from musculoskeletal and/or sensory deficit
- Hyperventilation (1%)
- Multiple other causes (13%)
- No cause found (8%)

Elderly pts: Present in 25% over age 72; may be a syndrome (Tinetti: Ann IM 2000;132:337) like delirium or falls in which elements of several of these causes contribute: anxiety, depression w or w/o medications, impaired balance (test by turning circle in < 4 sec), post-MI, postural BP drop (mean BP decreases by > 20%), 5+ meds, hearing impairment

Causes of acute vestibular syndrome (Nejm 1998;339:680, 1984; 310:1740):

Labyrinthitis/Vestibular Neuritis (Nejm 2004;351:322,354)

Cause: Perhaps viral, like *H. simplex*

Crs: Better in 2-3 d, residual mild sx for up to 2 yr

Rx: With small doses of iv diazepam (Valium), or dimenhydrinate (Dramamine) po, or scopalomine as Transderm (Ann IM 1984;101:211); steroid taper × 3 wk from 40 mg tid mg po prednisone, especially if see within 1st 24 hr + perhaps valcyclovir × 7 d

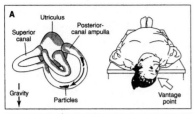

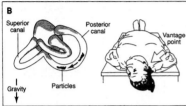

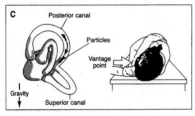

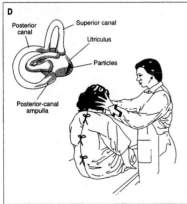

Figure 10.2 Bedside maneuver for the treatment of a patient with benign paroxysmal positional vertigo affecting the right ear. The presumed position of the debris within the labyrinth during the maneuver is shown in each panel. The maneuver is a three-step procedure. First, a Dix–Hallpike test is performed with the patient's head rotated 45° toward the right ear and the neck slightly extended with the chin pointed slightly upward. This position results in the patient's head hanging to the right (A). Once the vertigo and nystagmus provoked by the Dix–Hallpike test cease, the patient's head is rotated about the rostral–caudal body axis until the left ear is down (B). Then the head and body are further rotated until the head is face down (C). The vertex of the head is kept tilted downward throughout the rotation. The maneuver usually provokes brief vertigo. The patient should be kept in the final, face-down position for about 10-15 seconds. With the head kept turned toward the left shoulder, the patient is brought into the seated position (D). Once the patient is upright, the head is tilted so that the chin is pointed slightly downward. Reproduced with permision from Furman C. Benign paroxysmal positional vertigo. New Eng J Med 1999;341:1594. Copyright 1999 Mass. Medical Society, all rights reserved.

Benign Positional Vertigo (Nejm 1999;341:1590): Move pt from sitting to supine with first one, then other ear down (Hall-Pike head-hanging test), appears after a 5-20 sec delay and will pass in 1-2 min; rarely lasts > 1 yr. Caused by canalithiasis; best rx'd (80% successful) w canalith repositoning w Epley maneuvers (Otolaryng Clin NA 1996; 29:323; Otolaryngol Head Neck Surg 1995;112:154). Meclizine (Antivert) 25 mg po q 12 h or prn of modest help; surgery also possible.

Cerebellar Hemorrhage (p 715) or stroke; sudden onset, severe, associated w other brainstem findings, lasts weeks, needs acute CT/MRI to r/o neurosurgically reversible cerebellar bleed and/or brainstem swelling

Cerebellar-pontine angle tumor (p 231)

Temporal bone fracture, usually with severe hearing loss although not always (Nejm 1982;306:1029)

Floccular-nodular or insular seizures

Meniere's disease with tinnitus and diminished hearing although both may not start at once

Inner ear hemorrhage, acute, w hearing loss

Rx all types w repetitive exercises that habituate pt to unstable positions, will speed recovery (Ann IM 2004;141:598,641)

Chapter 11
Obstetrics/Gynecology

D. K. Onion and R. DeJong

11.1 Breast Diseases

Breast Cancer

Nejm 1998;339:974; 1992;327:319,390,473

Cause: Neoplasia; genetic component in some (esp Ashkenazi Jews) when have BRCA-1 or-2 gene, mutations of p53 area of chromosome 17; BRCA-1 present in 10% of women w cancer onset before age 35 (Nejm 1996;334:137,143), women w gene have 85% lifetime risk for breast and 20-40% risk for ovarian Ca while BRCA-2 women have same breast cancer risk and a 10-20% ovarian Ca risk, but environmental factors may ameliorate (Nejm 1997;336:1448)

Epidem: Incidence = 100/100,000 women, 37/1000 women die of it; 45,000 die/yr in U.S.; 12% of women will get in their lifetime; 0.5% of all male cancers (Ann IM 2002;137:688, 1992;117:771) especially in undescended testicles or Kleinfelter's syndrome, which is found in 20% of men w the dx

Increased incidence with obesity; infertility; smoking in postmenopausal women who are slow acetylators (Jama 1996; 276:1494); late motherhood (age > 30 yr); uterine cancer; h/o breast cancer in 1st-degree relatives (×3-10); post-irradiation, eg, Hiroshima, fluoroscopy, even thymus radiation in childhood

(Nejm 1989;321:1281), and mammography over age 40 causes 40 cases/1 million women after a 20-yr lag (Nejm 1989; 321:1285); moderate alcohol use (Ann IM 2002;137:799), linear increase w increased use (Jama 1998;279:535); hereditary ataxia telangiectasia heterozygotes who may represent 9% of all U.S. breast cancer (Nejm 1986;316:1289), and in whom radiation from mammograms, etc, may increase incidence a lot (Nejm 1991;325:1831); generally in women exposed to more estrogen, eg, peri-menopausal users of estrogen and/or progesterone where relative risk increased × 1.7 (Jama 1999;281:2091 vs 2141; Nejm 1995;332:1589, 1989;321:293), ductal less increased by ERT than lobular (Jama 2003;289:1421); low dietary vitamin A intake (Nejm 1993;329:234); fibroadenomas of breast before age 24 yr (Nejm 1994;331:10); in males with gynecomastia

No increase with abortions (Nejm 1997;336:81); bcp use (Nejm 2002;346:2025); high dietary fat consumption (Nejm 1996; 334:356, 1987;316:22); low fiber intake (Jama 1992;268: 2037); thyroid hormone rx (Ann IM 1977;86:502); silicone breast implants (Nejm 1995;332:1535); exposure to PCBs or DDT (Nejm 1997;337:1253); "fibrocystic disease" except in the ⅓ w proliferative or atypical pathology who are at increased risk (Nejm 1985;312:146)

Lowered incidence in women with 1st pregnancy before age 30-35, ⅓ fewer if 1st pregnancy before age 23, although pregnancy transiently increases risk for ~15 yr or until 2nd pregnancy, especially if over 35 w 1st pregnancy, but protects long term (Nejm 1994;331:5); nursing (more is better) protects against premenopausal type only (Nejm 1994;330:81, 1987;316: 229 vs Lancet 1996;347:431); women who regularly exercise

Sx: Breast mass, usually nontender; nipple discharge or bleeding sometimes. Self-exam helps when combined with regular clinical exams? (Nejm 1979;301:315, 1978;299:265,271 vs Jama 1987;257: 2197); silicone model practice helps (Ann IM 1990;112:772).

Si: Breast mass, nontender, single, firm, in upper outer quadrant in 60%. Sometimes bloody breast discharge. **Paget's Disease of Breast** an areolar dermatitis, if present is strongly correlated with cancer.

Crs: 55% 5-yr survival; with adjuvant CMF, 95% 2-yr survival with positive nodes compared with 70% without CMF (Nejm 1976; 294:405); survival worse with increasing age (Nejm 1986; 315:559)

Cmplc: Metastases to skeleton have prognosis better than those to viscera. Cancer in opposite breast in 7-12%.

r/o **Fibrocystic Disease** (Nejm 1985;312:146, 1982;307: 1010), present clinically in 50% of women, histologically in 90%. **Ductal Carcinoma In Situ** (Nejm 2004;350:1430), 5-10% prevalence in autopsy series, $> \frac{1}{2}$ progress to invasive cancer over 5-8 yr, represent 20% of mammographically detected cancers because often cause microcalcifications; rx'd w mastectomy or lumpectomy and radiation, + tamoxifen if ER+; relatively benign w local resection and irradiation (Jama 1996;275:913, 948) as is lobular Ca's.

Lab: *Chem:* Screen pts in high-risk families for breast and ovarian Ca w BRCA-1 and -2 testing (Jama 1996;275:1885); cost = $2000; beware of overenthusiastic application (Nejm 1997;336:1448)

Path: Aspiration cytology for invasive cancer with experienced pathologists, 95% sens, 98% specif. Breast bx; estrogen receptors (ER) crucial to f/u rx; must freeze tissue within 30 min to $-70°F$; progesterone receptors (PR) now also used. Cyclin E levels predict metastases (Nejm 2002;347:1566).

Xray: Mammograms (p 915); maybe MRI w contrast esp in BRCA/ other high-risk women (Nejm 2004;351:427); not helpful as f/u of mammography findings (Jama 2004;292:2735)

Rx (Nejm 1998;339:974; Jama 1995;273:142): Classified by TNM (lesion size, nodes, mets) system

Prevent perhaps w ASA or other COX inhibitors daily (Jama 2004;291:2433); or by various screening strategies including self-exam, clinical exam, mammography (p 915), aspiration of lesions (Ann IM 1985;103:79,143)

for BRCA-1 and -2 mutations: See table (Jama 1997;277:999); prophylactic mastectomy (Nejm 1999;340:77,141, 1997;336:1472) reduces risk by 90%, NNT = 33

for high-risk women:

Estrogen receptor blockers, which suppresse ER+ tumors effectively (Jama 1999;281:2189):

- Tamoxifen 20 mg po qd × 5 yr (Med Let 1999;41:1; Nejm 1998;339:1609) decreases incidence by 60% in BCRA-2 but not BCRA-1 women since they lack ER (Jama 2001; 286:2251); also helps lipids and osteoporosis although increases risk of thromboembolic disease and endometrial Ca.
- Raloxifene (Evista)

Surgical prophylactic mastectomy, eg, w BRCA-1 or -2 mutations (Nejm 2001;345:159; Jama 2000;284:319); and/or oophorectomy post childbearing (decreases risk by 75%) for BRCA-1 and -2 (Nejm 2002;346:1609,1616,1660)

Surgery, if < 4-5 cm, lumpectomy, sentinel node (Nejm 2003;349:546) dissection, and radiation (Nejm 1995;332:907); total mastectomy no better long term (Nejm 2002;347:1227, 1233,1270)

Post-op prophylaxis:

Antiestrogen rx:

- Tamoxifen, if age > 50 yr, ER+, and positive nodes, 10 mg po bid × 5 yr as well as helping lipids (Ann IM 1991; 115:860) and bone density (Nejm 1992;326:852); adverse effects: endometrial cancer and thromboembolic risks increased; $120/mo
- Anastrozole (Arimidex) (Med Let 1996;38:61), aromatase inhibitor that prevents peripheral adrenal androgen conversion to estrogens but w/o endometrial or thromboembolic cmplcs;

also used in ER+ postmenopausal women after 5 yr of tamoxifen (Nejm 2003;349:1793); $250/mo

- Exemestane (Aromasin) (Med Let 2000;42:35) 25 mg po qd, aromatase inhibitor used × 3 yr after 2-yr post-op tamoxifen improves recurrence and survival better than continued tamoxifen (Nejm 2004;350:1081); adverse effects: diarrhea; $250/mo
- Letrozole (Femara) (Med Let 1998;40:43), aromatase inhibitor; $250/mo
- Fulvestrant (Faslodex) (Med Let 2002;44:65) 250 mg im q 1 mo; estrogen receptor antagonist; $1000/mo

Adjuvant chemoRx, if axillary nodes positive and especially if premenopausal, w TAC (docetaxel, doxorubicin, cyclophosphamide) × 6 cycles (Nejm 2005;352:2302) or FAC (cytoxan, doxorubicin, 5-FU); or others. All improve 5 yr survival to 80-90%, but all also have significant adverse effects (Nejm 2001;344:1997), like weight gain, ovarian failure, fatigue, cognitive dysfunction, and cardiac toxicity in doxorubicin regimens.

Radiation along w adjuvant chemoRx improves survival (Nejm 1997;337:949,956); node-negative ER+ women age 50-70 have 6% absolute risk reduction of local recurrence but by age 70 is only 3%, ? when to stop offering radiation (Nejm 2004;351:963,971,1021)

Post-op f/u for metastatic disease: Routine PEs and annual mammogram enough, no survival benefit in annual bone scans, labs, chest xrays, or liver imaging done on asx pts (Jama 1995;273:142, 1994;271:1587,1593)

Of metastatic disease:
- Radiation good for local recurrences and bone pain
- Chemotherapy first if ER− w CMF or adriamycin + vincristine, paclitaxel (Taxol) (Nejm 1995;332:1004); trastuzumab (monoclonal antibody) or capecitabine (Med Let 1998;40:106)

- Antiestrogen rx as above, first if ER+ or over age 50
- Surgical oophorectomy in premenopausal women, or medically w leuprolide, an FSH inhibitor; adrenalectomy, surgically or medically with aminoglutethimide + dexamethasone (as good as surgical: Nejm 1981;305:545); androgens; pituitary ablation
- Autologous hematopoietic stem cell transplantation + high-dose chemoRx? (Nejm 2003;349:7,17,80)
- Biphosphonates, if bone mets, to prevent sx: Pamidronate (Nejm 1996;335:1785) iv q mo, or clodronate (Nejm 1998;339:357) po qd

11.2 Vaginal/Uterine/Tube Disorders

Vaginal Carcinoma

Nejm 1987;316:514

Cause: Clear cell and squamous cell types; latter from human papillomavirus infection chronically (Nejm 1986;315:1052)

Epidem: Clear cell type increased by maternal estrogen (especially DES) use during 1st trimester; 1/1000 in utero-exposed females get clear cell type; DES exposure does not increase risk of any other cancers (Jama 1998;280:630). 30-50% of squamous type occur in women who have had a hysterectomy for human papillomavirus disease.

Pathophys: In clear cell type, adenosis (uterine cervical columnar cells) is present in vagina, then 2nd carcinogen hits this susceptible tissue and the cells undergo malignant degeneration? May also start in cervix.

Sx: Irregular menses or spotting in young female in clear cell type; peak onset at age 19, 91% are age 15-27 yr; h/o maternal estrogen use in 72%

        Squamous type, occurs usually in postmenopausal female

Si: Carcinomatous mass in both types

In clear cell type, poor I_2 staining of vaginal mucosa = adenosis

Crs: Clear cell type is very malignant, survivals to date only in lesions < 1 cm^2; recurrences can be late

Cmplc: Clear cell, distant mets; squamous cell, local invasive disease

Lab: *Path:* Pap smear in clear cell type shows adenosis present in 11% of cervical, 27% of vaginal pool specimens. In squamous type, 20% false-negative Pap smear; Pap smear post-hysterectomy probably should be done if h/o HPV but otherwise useless (Nejm 1996;335:1559,1599).

Biopsy areas that stain poorly with I_2, bleed, or feel funny

Rx: Preventive (description of New York state clear cell screening program: Nejm 1981;304:47)

Surgery for both types as primary rx; radiation is equally effective and used for advanced invasive disease

Cervical Carcinoma

Nejm 1996;334:1030; Ann IM 1990;113:214

Cause: Human papillomavirus (HPV; venereal wart) (p 195), esp types 16 and 18 plus, less frequently, 31, 33, 35, and many others (Nejm 2003;348:518)

Epidem: Sexual intercourse transmits the virus, hence also associated with genital herpes of cervix and vulva (Nejm 1981;305:517, 483). HPV incidence in college-age women is high (> 40%), resolution and recurrence are common (Nejm 1998;338:423).

Most common cancer in women after breast and lung. 65% of all female genital cancers; 95% are over age 30 yr. Incidence = 20/100,000, 16,000/yr in U.S. women; CIS = 120/100,000; 5000 deaths/yr in U.S.

Increased incidence with early onset of sexual activity, number of sexual partners, h/o other STDs esp HIV (Jama 2000;283: 1031; Nejm 1997;337:1343) and chlamydia (Jama 2001;285:47), smoking, bcp use (slight), and asx macular and raised warty lesions on male partners (Nejm 1987;317:916)

Pathophys: HPV genome becomes integrated into cellular DNA and causes malignant transformation. Squamous dysplasia may resolve, or untreated, may evolve to invasive carcinoma.

Sx: Usually none; may have vaginal bleeding, especially postcoital; vaginal discharge; pelvic pain, when invasive

Si: Cervical erosion and mass
Stage 0: Carcinoma in situ
Stage I: Confined to cervix only
Stage II: Not to pelvic wall and not in lower third of vagina
Stage III: To pelvic wall
Stage IV: Rectum or bladder involvement

Crs: 5-yr survival 50% overall (old data); 100% with CIS; 25% in stage IV with surgery

Cmplc: Ureteral obstruction; lymphatic mets, usually local; pregnancy worsens; post-op sexual dysfunction in 25% (Nejm 1999; 340:1383)

Lab:

Path (Jama 2002;287:2114,2120, 2001;285:1506):
- Conventional cervical Pap smear:
  q 1 yr if < 35 yr old and/or multiple partners;
  q 6-12 mo if HIV pos and CD_4 < 500 and HPV positive (Jama 2005;293:1471);
  q 5 yr if > 35 yr old and < 8 lifetime partners (Canadian Walton Rept: Can Med Assoc J 1982;127:581) and no h/o abnormal Pap or STDs in pt or partner; or
  q 3 yr at age 30-65 (Nejm 2003;349:1501);
  In elderly > 65 yr old, get 2-3 Paps 3 yr apart if not previously done then stop (Ann IM 1992;117:520).

Unnecessary if s/p hysterectomy for benign disease (Nejm 1996;335;1559,1599; Jama 1996;275:940). 5-10% false neg rate in best labs.

Atypical squamous cells of uncertain significance (ASCUS) should be < 5% of Paps; about 25% will turn out to be serious higher-grade lesions; check for HPV DNA (Jama 1999;281:1605,1645) or follow Pap q 6 mo × 2-3 yr after rx of any infection and colpo if + HPV DNA or repeat ASCUS Pap

Atypical glandular cells (AGCUS) over age 35 or under age 35 w irregular bleeding have a higher correlation w occult Ca than LSIL or ASCUS

- Monolayer technologies (Papnet, Autonet, and Thin Prep) have improved sensitivity, not clearly better (BMJ 2003; 326:733); their use for rescreening of 10% unnecessary (Jama 1998;279:235,240) and much more expensive than manual rescreening (Jama 1998;279:235,240)

Colposcopy with bx if Pap shows ASCUS 3 or more times in a row, HPV, or if see a lesion. Looking for cervical intraepithelial neoplasia (CIN) I (mild dysplasia, or low-grade squamous intraepithelial lesion) (LSIL), CIN II (moderate dysplasia), CIN III (severe dysplasia), and carcinoma in situ (CIS); high-grade squamous intraepithelial lesion (HSIL) includes CIN II/III and CIS. Should also do for AGCUS over age 35 or adenocarcinoma in situ.

HPV DNA screening (Jama 2000;283:81,87,108; Nejm 1999;341:1633,1687); may be best used as f/u of equivocal Paps (ACP J Club 2003;139:79); SIL usually develops within 2 yr of infection if at all

Rx:

Prevention: Male circumcision halves rates (Nejm 2002:346, 1105); barrier methods of birth control

Vaccination of sexually active women (p 195)

of low-grade SILs: F/u Paps since most regress and resolve, especially in young women (Nejm 1998;338:423)

of high-grade lesions: CryoRx, laser Rx, loop excision, or occasionally cone bx; latter two increase risk of subsequent PROM and preterm delivery (Jama 2004;291:2100)

of carcinoma stage I and early II: Radiation and surgery equally effective with 80% stage I and 50% stage II cures of advanced stage II, as well as stages III and IV: radiation; w advanced local disease even stage IB, cisplatin chemoRx w radiation improves survival (Nejm 1999;340:1137,1144,1154,1198)

Endometrial Carcinoma

Nejm 1996;335:640

Cause: Prolonged, unopposed (by progesterone) estrogen (estradiol especially) exposure from many possible sources including:
- Estrogens given for menopausal sx (Nejm 1979;300:9,218), risk persists 10+ yr after cessation (Nejm 1985;313:969)
- Polycystic ovary/metabolic (Stein-Leventhal) syndrome
- Granulosa/theca cell tumors (100× incidence)
- Anovulation, especially perimenopausal
- Turner's syndrome
- Tamoxifen use
  Genetic syndromes w breast and right-sided colon cancers

Epidem: 20% of all female genital cancers; 4th most frequent cancer in women; 34,000 cases/yr, 6000 deaths/yr in U.S.; rare before age 40 unless ovarian pathology, median age at dx = 63, only 25% occur in premenopausal women. Lower incidence in smokers, because of smoking's antiestrogen effect (Nejm 1986;315:1305).

U.S. incidence has been decreasing since the early 1980s, perhaps due to the increased use of progesterone (Am J Pub Hlth 1990;80:935) in ERT

Pathophys: Continuous estrogen stimulation causes hyperplasia and eventually can convert to carcinoma; rarely metastasizes distantly

Sx: Postmenopausal vaginal bleeding, r/o atrophic uterine mucosa, bacterial endometritis, polyp; or premenopausal metrorrhagia; or intermenstrual bleeding

h/o infertility, irregular menses, late menopause, obesity, estrogen replacement, hypertension, diabetes

Si: Pelvic/uterine mass

Stage I: Confined to fundus

Stage II: In cervix and fundus

Stage III: Extension beyond uterus

Stage IV: Extension to pelvis

Crs: With rx, 70+% overall 5-yr survival; 75% stage I, 60% stage II, 30% stage III, and 10% stage IV; estrogen supplementation-induced type is less malignant? (Ann IM 1978;88:410)

Cmplc: Metastases, usually local. Increased risk of subsequent colorectal Ca (Ann IM 1999;131:189).

Lab: *Noninv:* Transvaginal ultrasound, w endometrial thickness > 5 mm is 90% sens, 48% specif (Nejm 1997;337:1792) vs 96% sens and 92% specif if not on HRT; and 77% specif if on HRT (Jama 1998;280:1510), perhaps do before bx and skip bx if neg?

Path: Pap smear positive in only 18% (Nejm 1974;291:191); endometrial aspiration bx in office or D + C w tumor grading 1-3

Endo: Hysteroscopy (Jama 2002;288:1610)

Rx: Prevent by always withdrawing at least q 3 mo with progesterone, eg, medroxyprogesterone (Provera) 10 mg qd × 10 d when using estrogen for menopause or osteoporosis, or if obese and having irregular menses, or other chronic estrogen stimulation situation (Obgyn 1984;63:759)

Surgery, TAH + BSOO, pelvic node dissection; for stages I and II, with or without pre-/post-irradiation; for stages III and IV, individualized rx including radiation, surgery, as well as hormonal w progesterone (as Megace), and chemoRx w cyclophosphamide, 5-FU, adriamycin

Endometriosis

Nejm 1993;328:1759

Cause: Ectopic uterine mucosa, unclear why; various theories include embryonic residua, transtubal transport of endometrial fragments and implantation, coelomic metaplasia, "retrograde menstruation," and lymphatic, surgical, or vascular metastases?

Epidem: 10% prevalence in menstruating women

Pathophys: Ectopic foci of functioning endometrium cause pain when bleed into confined, nonuterine areas. Commonly on ovaries but also beneath peritoneum of bladder, tubes, bowel, pelvic scars post-op. Can result in tubal or ovarian sterility. Sx severity correlate poorly with anatomic findings.

Sx: Acquired premenstrual or menstrual pain, dyspareunia, pain on defecation; sterility; but often asx

Si: Tenderness on pelvic exam; retroverted fixed uterus; pelvic mass

Crs: Progressively worse until menopause or pregnancy

Cmplc: Infertility
r/o pelvic inflammatory disease, adenomyosis, ovarian tumor

Lab: *Endo:* Laparoscopy, usually diagnostic, shows hemorrhagic spots or cysts, often scarred

Xray: Ultrasound may show irregular pelvic mass; but is a poor test except to r/o other causes of pelvic pain; frequent false negatives
MRI is 90% sens/specif for endometriosis in women w pelvic pain

Rx (Nejm 2001;345:266):
NSAIDs for pain
Birth control pills, typically high-progesterone-content ones; either cyclic or continuous

Danazol 200-800 mg po qd, a weak androgen; 200-mg pill costs $1 (Ann IM 1982;96:625); adverse effects: androgenic side effects

GnRH (gonadotropin-releasing hormone) analog, nafarelin 400 μgm nasal spray qd (Med Let 1990;32:81; Nejm 1988;318: 485) or leuprolide (Lupron) 3.75 mg im depot q 1 mo for up to 6-mo crs; cost: $300+/mo; adverse effects: estrogen deficiency sx including bone loss, which can be prevented w qd sc PTH (Nejm 1994;331:1618)

Progesterone: Medroxyprogresterone 20-100 mg po constantly × 6-12 mo or cyclic 20 d rx; DepoProvera 150 mg im q 3 mo; levonorgestrel implant (Norplant) q 5 yr (Med Let 1991; 33:17)

Surgical: Laparoscopic electro- or laser cautery helps fertility in mild to moderate cases improve from 18% to 30% and is better than hormonal manipulation (Nejm 1997;337:217); TAH + BSOO is 90% successful in relieving pain

Uterine Leiomyoma (Fibroids)

Cause: Mechanical stress?; estrogen stimulation?, eg, from birth control pills

Epidem: Premenopausal women primarily affected, usually appear age 30-50 yr; fibroids shrink in postmenopausal women and rarely cause sx. Increased prevalence and incidence in blacks.

Pathophys: Intramyometrial stress causes localized smooth muscle proliferation? Estrogens increase rate of formation. Bleeding is from overlying endometrium stretched? and/or poor uterine contractions during menses hence spiral arteries bleed. Pain due to contractions against mass during menses.

Sx: Menorrhagia; pain; sense of fullness; urinary frequency; obstipation; but often asx

Si: Anemia, pelvic mass

Crs: Benign

Cmplc: Infertility; anemia from menorrhagia; ureteral compression and blockage; sudden bleed into fibroid with pain and enlargement; necrosis and calcification (10%); benign metastasizing type (Nejm 1981;305:204); leiomyosarcomas (< 1%)

Lab: *Hem:* Iron-deficiency anemia
Path: Intramural, 90% in fundus, 8% in cx, rarely in round or broad ligaments

Xray: Incidental fining on KUB, calcified in 10%, especially in older women
Ultrasound usually diagnostic, though can't r/o cancer

Rx: Wait for sx; cyclic bcp's low in estradiol to decrease bleeding, although may still stimulate growth; gonadotropin-releasing hormone agonists like leuprolide (Nejm 1991;324:97) (p 1056) decrease estradiol by feedback inhibition, shrink fibroids and cause medical menopause, may be used presurgically
Surgical hysteroscopic resection of submucous types; or myomectomy ("shelling out") may allow future pregnancies; hysterectomy, or subtotal hysterectomy (Nejm 2002;347:1318)
Uterine artery embolization 90% effective (Met Let 2005; 47:31)

Ectopic Pregnancy

Nejm 1993;329:1174

Cause: Implanted conceptus outside uterine cavity; intraabdominal fertilization

Epidem: 2+% of all pregnancies; 89,000/yr in U.S., increasing incidence (Mmwr 1995;44:46), multiple reasons including antibiotic rx of PID before sterility results. 95% are tubal; but also can be ovarian, cervical, or abdominal (0.5%).
Post tubal ligation rate is 1/1000 over 10 yr, higher (30/1000) after electrocoagulation tubals (Nejm 1997;336:762)

Pathophys: Scarred tubes (rarely uterus) slow transfer and as a result the blastocyst implants wherever it is on day 6. Chorionic villous trophoblasts perforate basement membrane and muscle layers of tubes. If death of embryo occurs first, endometrium is shed, which results in brownish, modest vaginal bleeding; if trophoblast erodes first, results in massive intraperitoneal bleeding.

Sx: Nearly all in 1st trimester; missed period, although withdrawal bleed may mask; most occur at about 8 wk gestation, earlier for isthmus, later for cornual

Abdominal/pelvic pain similar to menstrual/uterine pains; vaginal bleeding; shoulder pain from diaphragmatic irritation by blood

"Funny period, funny pain, funny pregnancy," followed by "syncope in the bathroom"

Si: Abdominal/pelvic mass (present in < 50%) and tenderness; cervical tenderness if blood in pelvis; shock

Crs: Without surgery, death in 186/102,000 population (Obgyn 1984; 64:386)

Cmplc: Shock, surgical sterility

r/o PID, ruptured ovarian corpus luteum or follicle cyst, endometriosis cyst, appendicitis

Lab: *Chem:* Serum HCG positive in all, repeat in 48 hr, should double in normal pregnancy, decrease if abortion, rise slowly if ectopic. Progesterone level < 25 ng/cc.

Paracentesis or culdocentesis: May show blood in peritoneum

Urine: Pregnancy test positive in all with β-HCG > 50 U and 90+% are therefore positive at first missed period

Xray: Ultrasound of pelvis w vaginal probe; if see intrauterine pregnancy, then dx is essentially ruled out, although the very rare circumstance of twins with one ectopic does occur

Rx (Nejm 2000;343:1325):

Methotrexate 50 mg/M^2 im × 1 (Nejm 1999;341:1974), 91% successful overall, best if HCG <15,000 mIU/cc, follow w HCG levels post rx on days 4, 7, and q 1 wk until < 15 mIU, usually takes 35 d; or

Laparoscopic salpingostomy
Laparotomy for rupture w hemoperitoneum

Pelvic Inflammatory Disease

Nejm 1994;330:115

Cause (Med Let 1999;41:86): Chlamydia causes over half of mild cases (Ann IM 1981;95:685; Nejm 1980;302:1063) (p 596), maybe most; *Neisseria gonococcus* (15%), anaerobes, mycoplasma. All via sexual intercourse, especially with multiple partners; IUD use previously thought to increase risk (Nejm 1985;312:937, 941,984; Med Let 1980;22:87), now felt to have minimal effect.

Epidem:

Pathophys: Lower genital tract infections ascend cervical canal usually just before or during menses, to tubes and ovaries

Sx: Pain in lower abdomen, constant or colicky; dyspareunia; dysuria; tenesmus; dysmenorrhea; nausea and vomiting; anorexia

Si: Adnexal mass (20%) and tenderness or pain on cervical motion ("Chandelier si"); fever; cervical discharge

Crs:

Cmplc: Infertility (15+% with each episode); ectopic pregnancy; pelvic abscess; septic thrombophlebitis; surgical excision of reproductive organs

r/o endometriosis, adenomyosis, ectopic pregnancy

Lab: *Bact:* Gc culture, chlamydia screens
Hem: Wbc elevated; ESR elevated in ⅓; the higher the ESR, the more likely sterility
Noninv: Laparoscopy if dx unclear or improvement slow

Xray: Pelvic ultrasound; CT scan for possible abscess

Rx: Prevent w condom use (Am J Pub Hlth 1990;80:964); bcp's help (Jama 1984;251:2553)

Screen asx women for chlamydia if expected prevalence > 7%, reduces PID by ½ (Nejm 1996;334:1362); or perhaps all women and maybe men under age 25 w PCR techniques (p 924) (Nejm 1998;339:739,768)

of disease (Med Let1999;41:86): Pain and tenderness are adequate indication to initiate rx (Mmwr 1993;42:76)

Outpatients:

  1st: Cefoxitin 2 gm im + probenecid 1 gm po, or ceftriaxone 250 mg im × 1 then doxycycline 100 mg bid × 14 d

  2nd: Ofloxacin 400 mg po bid + metronidazole 500 mg po bid × 2 wk

Inpatients: Hospitalize if

- Dx is unclear,
- Mass is present,
- Unable to keep po meds down,
- Peritoneal si's present,
- Outpt rx failure, or
- If expect poor compliance
- Rx w:

  1st: Doxycycline 100 mg q 12 hr iv + cefoxitin 2 gm iv q 6 hr ("FoxyDoxy") or cefotetan 2 gm iv q 12 hr until better, then doxycycline 100 mg po bid × 14 d

  2nd: Gentamicin 2 mg/kg iv × 1 then 1.5 mg/kg iv q 8 hr + clindamycin 900 mg iv q 8 hr until better, then f/u w po doxycycline × 14 d

  3rd: Levofloxacin 500 mg pd iv/po, or ofloxacin 400 mg po q 12 hr + metronidazole 500 mg iv 8 hr; amp/sulbactam 3 gm iv q 6 hr + doxycycline100 mg iv q 12 hr; all followed by doxy × 14d

Rx of partners for gc if culture is positive, otherwise just for chlamydia

11.3 Ovarian Disorders

Polycystic Ovary Syndrome (Stein-Levinthal Syndrome)

Nejm 2005;352:1223; Ann IM 2000;132:989

Cause: Probable genetic autosomal dominant

Epidem: Present in 1.5% of infertile pts, 75% of anovulatory women, 87% w hirsutism; only 2.8% of pts with polycystic ovaries by laparoscopy have the syndrome. Increased prevalence in obesity, seizure pts, especially those on valproic acid, 50% of whom have it (Nejm 1993;329:1383); and in IDDM often w insulin resistance.

Pathophys: Hyperandrogenism + anovulation

Obesity induces and/or exacerbates by increased conversion of androstenedione to estrone in fatty tissues, which causes pituitary FSH suppression and increased LH; this leads to ovarian LH-stimulated androgen production, which in turn causes follicle atrophy and further stimulation of peripheral fat conversion to more estrone. More common in insulin-dependent diabetes because insulin resistance stimulates ovarian conversion of steroids to androgens (Nejm 1998;338:1876, 1996;325:617,657; Ann IM 1982;97:851); or IDDM may cause the syndrome by deficiency of a D-chiro-inositol–containing phosphoglycan, which mediates insulin action (Nejm 1999;340:1314).

Abnormally high LH levels induce ovarian thecal cell synthesis of 17-hydroxylase and C-17,20-lyase, (see Figure 5.1) causing increases in 17-OH progesterone, estrone, and androstenedione, which in turn cause further LH surges and masculinization (Nejm 1992;327:157, 1989;320:559)

Sx: Syndrome onset at menarche. Oligo- or amenorrhea (80%); infertility (35-75%); obesity (37%); hirsutism (65%); acne (25%); visual acuity sx. Dysfunctional uterine bleeding.

Si: Withdrawal bleeding with progesterone; large ovaries, palpable if not too obese; hirsutism usually without masculinization. Astigmatism, myopia, hyperopia? Obesity.

Crs:

Cmplc: Endometrial cancer; possibly higher incidence of coronary artery disease (Ann IM 1997;126:32) and ASCVD in general; HT; diabetes; infertility

Lab: Usually unnecessary; diagnose clinically
   Chem: Androstenedione, testosterone (> 2 SD above mean), and LH elevated, or high normal; glucose intolerance, increased lipids
   Path: Ovaries 2-3× normal size, cystic follicles; microscopically show variable theca cell hyperplasia and luteinization

Xray: Pelvic ultrasound may show polycystic ovaries

Rx: Weight reduction, if obese
Meds:

- Birth control pills, especially those w minimally androgenic progesterones like norgestimate and desogestrel
- Spironolactone or similar, drospirenone
- Metformin 500-850 mg po tid (Nejm 1996;335:617,657), if insulin-resistant diabetes present, as it often is
- Glitazones, which lower insulin levels and thus drive conversion of peripheral estrogen to androgen
- Medroxyprogesterone 10 mg qd or other progesterone × 10 d q 1-3 mo to prevent endometrial cancer
   of hirsutism (p 842)
   of infertility (p 844): Clomiphene; insulin secretion inhibition w metformin 500 mg po tid (Nejm 1998;338:1876); human menopausal gonadotropin/menotropins (Pergonal); rarely wedge resections or laser drill holes of ovary done

Ovarian Carcinoma

Nejm 2004;351:2519; Jama 1995;273:491

Cause: Neoplasia; 5-10% familial association w breast cancer chromosome 17 BRCA-1 and BRCA-2 gene deletions (Nejm 2002;346: 1609,1616,1660, 1997;336:1125, 1996;335:1413)

Epidem: 5th-ranking fatal female cancer in U.S., ahead of cervical and uterine; 1/70 lifetime risk, is 1/20 if a 1st-degree relative has had ovarian cancer; 16,000 deaths/yr in U.S.; 25,000/yr incidence in U.S.

Increased risk w low parity, mumps, perineal talc use, ERT users 2× esp after 10 yr (Jama 2001;285:1460), BRCA- 1 or 2-gene carriers

Decreased incidence (40%) with birth control pill use, even 3 mo of rx protects for 15+ yr (Nejm 1987;316:650); w high FSH levels postmenopausally and w low androgen levels (Jama 1996; 274:1926)

Usually affects postmenopausal women age 50-60 yr; 5% of cases are familial

Pathophys: Epithelial type cancer, 35-50% serous, 6-10% mucinous

Sx: Often asx until widespread; or (Jama 2004;291:2705) back pain (45%), fatigue (34%), abdominal pain (22%), pelvic or lower abdominal mass, pelvic discomfort, urinary pain (16%), bowel bloating (27%) and/or constipation (24%); upper abdominal sense of fullness and increasing abdominal girth

Si: Abdominal or pelvic mass, often (50%) bilateral; may be huge (largest = 148 kg); ascites. Occasionally unique polyarthritis, palmar fasciitis syndrome (Ann IM 1982;96:424), hypercalcemia, multiple seb keratoses.

Table 11.1   Ovarian Cancer Staging and Survival

Stage	5-Yr Survival (%)
I	
Ia: Confined to 1 ovary	90+
Ib: Both ovaries	90+
Ic: 1-2 ovaries, w ascites + positive peritoneal cytology	80
II: 1-2 ovaries w local pelvic extension	
IIa: Confined to uterus and tubes	51
IIb: Other pelvic tissues	42
IIc: Ascites or positive abdominal cytology	42
III: 1 or 2 ovaries and peritoneal or retroperitoneal mets	
IIIa: Microscopically out of pelvis	
IIIb: Peritoneal mets < 2 cm^2	All ~20
IIIc: Retroperitoneal nodes or mets >2 cm^2	
IV. Distant mets	10

Cmplc: r/o common, benign ovarian corpus luteum cyst by rechecking
pelvic during a different part of menstrual cycle, getting ultrasound if increasing in size, doing surgery if > 5 cm; germ cell or
sex cord struma types (p 809), 13-20% of ovarian cancers, very
treatable; mets from elsewhere (Krukenberg's tumors); Meig's
syndrome (p 809)

Lab: *Chem:* Ca-125 monoclonal antibodies elevated in 80% but not
useful as screening test (Nejm 1992;327:197) unless 2 1st-
degree relatives w same type of ovarian cancer (Jama
1995;273:491); serum inhibin levels elevated in many, especially mucinous cyst-adenocarcinomas, like Ca-125, not useful for screening but helpful post-op tumor marker (Nejm
1993;329:1539)

    Path: "Borderline malignant" cell types of both serous and muci-
nous have much better prognosis than numbers shown
above, eg, 85-95% 5-yr survival

Xray: Pelvic ultrasound; screen w vaginal probe if positive family hx as
above

Rx: Prevent in BRCA-1 and -2 w prophylactic oophorectomy (BSOO) after childbearing, reduces ovarian and breast Ca risk by 75% (Nejm 2002;346:1609,1616,1660); maybe bcp's decrease incidence by 50+%? (Nejm 1998;339:424 vs 2001;345:235)

Preventive screening w tumor markers ineffective primarily due to low prevalence (Ann IM 1994;121:124, 1993;119:901), and w pelvic exams because fast growing and usually already spread when palpable

Staging laparoscopy/laparotomy to fully judge extent of metastases, eg, often on diaphragm

Debulking surgery after initial chemoRx (Nejm 1995;332:629) but a 2nd debulking surgery after chemoRx no help (Nejm 2001;351:2489)

ChemoRx for most except good-histology stage Ia, especially for stages III and IV (Med Let 1996;38:96): Cisplatin (Nejm 1996;335:1950), or carboplatin (Med Let 1993;35:39) + paclitaxel (Taxol) (Med Let 1993;35:39; Nejm 1996;334:1)

Ovarian Teratoma (Mature Cystic Dermoid)

Cause: Benign transformation of germ cell after first meiotic division (Nejm 1975;292:61)

Epidem: Most common in young reproductive females; 15% of all ovarian tumors, 20-40% of all ovarian tumors of pregnancy

Pathophys: Contain ectodermal, mesodermal, and endodermal elements

Sx: Pain with hemorrhage into tumor, with torsion, or rupture; usually asx

Si: Pelvic mass; 10-20% are bilateral

Crs:

Cmplc: r/o ovarian cancer; dysgerminoma similar to male seminoma (p 1051); thyrotoxicosis from proliferation of thyroid elements (struma ovarii); carcinoid sx also possible but rarer

Lab: *Path:* Bone, teeth, etc (all 3 layers of embryonal tissues)

Xray: KUB may show bone, teeth, etc
Ultrasound usually diagnostic

Rx: Surgery; any teratoma with mature elements can be assumed to be benign and rx'd with simple ovarian cystectomy so both ovaries are preserved

Granulosa-Theca Cell Tumor

Cause: Neoplasia; idiopathic and perhaps radiation induced

Epidem: In women and girls; 60% are postmenopausal; 10% of all ovarian cancers (Nejm 1989;321:790); incidence is 1/100,000 women > 19 yr old; 1/54,000 women age 50-65. The only pediatric functional ovarian tumor.

Pathophys: Arises from cortical stroma or wall of involuting follicle, especially in aging ovaries. It is curious that it presents as an estrogen-producing tumor, yet granulosa cells or corpus luteum produce mainly progesterone. Estrogen production is never more than that during a normal menstrual cycle.

Sx: Abdominal pain, tumor; secondary amenorrhea and menometror-rhagia. Precocious puberty (vaginal bleeding), r/o trauma/abuse, exogenous estrogen, craniopharyngioma, luteoma.

Si: Abdominal mass

Crs: High survival rates; can recur decades later; benign in children except for the precocious puberty

Cmplc: Meigs's syndrome (ascites and hydrothorax) with benign types as well as more common benign fibromas of ovary
Malignancy, in < 40% of pts; endometrial carcinoma, especially in those over age 50

Lab: *Chem:* Inhibin levels correlate with tumor presence and bulk (Nejm 1989;321:790)
Path: 12% are microscopically bilateral

Rx: Surgery; radiation is very good for recurrences

11.4 Pregnancy-Related Conditions

Spontaneous Abortion (Miscarriage)

Cause: Idiopathic usually; autoantibodies; or structural (eg, uterine septum, fibroids)

Epidem: 15-20% of all pregnancies. Most at 10 wk (Nejm 1988; 319:189). ⅓ have chromosome abnormalities, ½ are blighted ova. Late (> 20 wk) associated w Leiden factor V, prothrombin gene mutations (Nejm 2000;343:1015), and antiphospholipid antibodies (Lupus anticoagulant, anti-β_2 glycoprotein I antibodies, or anticardiolipin antibodies) (p 147) (Nejm 2002; 346:752).

Increased risk (1.4-1.8×) w smoking and cocaine use (Nejm 1999;340:333); w coffee use (Nejm 2000;343:1839, 1999;341: 1688); w video display terminals (Nejm 1991;324:727); w NSAIDs esp in 3rd trimester; w low folate levels (Jama 2002; 288:1867)

Pathophys:

Sx: Crampy pain, spontaneous vaginal bleeding, passage of tissue means fetal death

Si: Open cervical os and/or tissue means inevitably will abort

Crs: When threatened (bleed), 50% will eventually lose pregnancy

Cmplc: Sepsis, uterine necrosis leading to myoglobinuria and ATN, DIC; significant depression (Jama 1997;277:383), onset within 1 mo, esp if childless (20+% incidence) or PMH/o depression (50%) incidence

r/o ectopic, molar pregnancy, self-induced abortion

Lab: Chromosomal studies if ≥ 3 spontaneous abortions looking for balanced translocation

Rx: Emotional support
D + C if
- Heavy bleeding;
- > 8 wk gestation, since will bleed longer and more heavily;

- Is 2nd SAB, to r/o intrauterine anatomic abnormalities; or
- if infected.

   In lupus anticoagulant pts, heparin (Nejm 2002;346:752); ASA + prednisone prophylaxis no help (Nejm 1997;337:149)

Induced ("Therapeutic") Abortion

Cause:

Epidem: No, or minimal, increased risk of spontaneous abortion in future pregnancies after an abortion (Nejm 1979;301:677)

Pathophys:

Sx:

Si:

Crs:

Cmplc: Septic abortion if not done medically (Nejm 1994;331:310), but even then infection occurs in 1% (prophylactic tetracycline 500 mg po qid × 5 d decreases to 0.25%); uterine perforation; re-tained products of conception; **Postabortal Syndrome:** bleeding, in absence of retained tissue, which spontaneously resolves or is rx'd with methergine

   No increase in breast cancer risk (Nejm 1997;336:81; Jama 1996;275:283,321)

Lab: *Path:* Confirm gestational tissue and r/o mole

Rx: of 1st-trimester pregnancy (Nejm 2000;342:946):
- Mifepristone (Mefeprex, RU-486) (Med Let 2000;42:101; Nejm 1993;329:404), an antiprogesterone, in 1st 2 mo of preg-nancy, 200-600 mg po followed in 1.5-2 d with misoprostol (Cytotec) 400 μgm po (Nejm 1998;338:1241) or 800 μgm vaginally (Jama 2000;284:1948; Nejm 1995;332:983); causes 95+% to abort completely (Nejm 1998;338:1241, 1993;328: 1509, 1990;322:645; Med Let 1990;32:112); adverse effects:

Möbius Syndrome (facial paralysis and limb defects) if fail to abort (Nejm 1998;338:1881); cost: $100/200 mg

* Suction evacuation; or
* Misoprostol (Cytotec) (Nejm 2001;344:38,59) 200 μgm vaginally q 12 hr; a prostaglandin that causes 90% to abort within 2 d; 55% need subsequent D + E; adverse effects: fever (11%), abdominal pain (57%), emesis (4%), diarrhea (4%); cost $1; or
* Methotrexate 50 mg/m^2 im, followed in 3-7 d by misoprostol 800 μgm vaginally × 1 and repeated in 1-7 d if no abortion; 90+% complete abortions, 4-9% require vacuum extraction w or w/o dilatation (Med Let 1996;38:39; Nejm 1995;333:537; Jama 1994;272:1190)
* Epostane (prevents progesterone synthesis) 200 mg qid × 7 d at 5-8 wk causes 84% to abort within 2 wk, usually at 5 d (Nejm 1988;319:813)

of 2nd-trimester pregnancy:

* Prostaglandin E$_2$ (Nejm 1994;331:290) 20 μgm vaginally q 3 hr; aborts 80% within 2 d, 70% will need D + C as well; adverse effects: fever (63%), pain (67%) and abdominal cramping, emesis (33%), diarrhea (30%); cost: $300
* D + E up to 18+ wk

Pregnancy

Cause:

Epidem: 20% abort before clinically apparent, another 10% abort later (Nejm 1988;319:189)

Pathophys: Ann IM 1984;101:683

Sx: Early: nausea and vomiting (50%); breast engorgement; missed period. Quickening at 20 wk, 1-2 wk earlier in experienced multiparous women.

Si: Soft uterine neck, blue cervix by 6 wk. Fetal heart by Doppler at 9-12 wk; by feto- or stethoscope at 18-20 wk.

Crs: 39-42 wk for maximal perinatal survival in singleton births, 37-38 wk for twins (Jama 1996;275:1432)

Cmplc: Adverse outcomes are not increased by long hours or stress (residents: Nejm 1990;323:1040)

- Asthma management is nearly the same as in the nonpregnant, but be aware that β agonists like terbutaline inhibit labor (Nejm 1985;312:897), iodides induce fetal goiter (Lancet 1990;1:1241); tetracyclines stain fetal teeth
- Bleeding and/or contractions (pain):
  1st trimester: Ectopic or threatened abortion, mole, septic abortion
  2nd trimester: Mole, pyelonephritis, placenta praevia, incompetent cervix, or bicornuate uterus
  3rd trimester: Premature labor, previa, or abruption that can be caused by trauma (Nejm 1990;323:1609)
- Cardiac disease rx (Nejm 1993;329:250), generally stenotic lesions (AS, MS) a greater problem than insufficiency lesions (MR, AI) because of increased cardiac output during pregnancy (J. Love 12/94); rare (1/10,000) MI (Ann IM 1996; 125:751)
- Diabetes: Increased C/S rates because of increased rates of toxemia, macrosomia, and congenital malformations (Nejm 1986; 315:989)
- Gi (Ann IM 1993;118:366): Esophageal reflux, nausea and vomiting, bloating/constipation from diminished LES pressure and motility; gallstones (2%) and sludge (present by ultrasound in 31% of pregnancies) occur but often revert to normal postpartum (Ann IM 1993;119:116)
- Hyperemesis gravidarum, usually in 1st trimester; for rx, see below
- Liver disease, various types including acute fatty liver of pregnancy, intrahepatic cholestasis, et al (Nejm 1996;335:570)
- Low birth weight (p 894)

- Premature rupture of membranes, if before 32 wk gestation, rx for group B strep (p 535) w ampicillin/amoxicillin 250 mg + perhaps erythromycin for chlamydia (Jama 1997;278:989)
- Rheumatologic disorders: Safe medications (Bull Rheum Dis 1992;41:1)
- Stroke risk not increased during pregnancy but is increased for 1st 6 wk postpartum (Nejm 1996;335:768)
- Thyrotoxicosis (Nejm 1985;313:562) more commonly when high HCG levels from gestational trophoblastic disease since HCG structurally close to TSH (Nejm 1998;339:1823); more common postpartum in IDDM pts (10%) (Ann IM 1993; 118:419)
- Toxemia of pregnancy (p 824)
- Urologic: Pyelonephritis from physiologic dilatation or ureters and/or decreased motility and/or compression; proteinuria associated w toxemia; nephrogenic diabetes insipidus in 3rd trimester (Nejm 1984;310:442); chronic renal failure (Nejm 1985;312:836)

Lab: Routine initial prenatal package: UA and culture, hgb/hct in 1st and 3rd trimesters, ABO and Rh type, VDRL, chlamydia antigen, gc culture, Pap smear; rubella titer (if neg, advise on avoiding exposure during pregnancy and offer postpartum immunization: Nejm 1992;326:663,702); HIV test w informed consent since AZT rx will decrease fetal transmission from 25% to 8% (Jama 1995;273:977); perhaps toxoplasmosis titer? (Nejm 1994; 331:695) and TSH (Nejm 1999;341:549 vs 601)

at 16-20 wk: Quadruple markers (AFP, HCG, inhibin, and estriol) for Down's syndrome

at 24-28 wk: Screen with 50 gm glucose, nonfasting, if 1-hr blood sugar > 130-140 mg %, get full GTT; full GTT = 100 gm glucose, FBS < 105, 1-hr < 190, 2-hr > 165 (but problems even if 120-165), 3-hr < 145; dx gestational DM by ≥ 2 values too high (Nejm 1986;315:989,1025) at 35-37 wk: Group B strep culture (Nejm 2000;342:15)

Chem: Serum β-subunit tests positive within 2 wk of conception

Hem: Hgb drops by midtrimester from an average of 13.7 gm to 11.5 gm, then usually rises to 12.3 gm in 3rd trimester; if stays up, indicates plasma volume decrease and decreased fetal weight (Ann Obgyn Scand 1984;63:245). Platelets average 322,000 in 1st trimester, 275,000 in 2nd, and 300,000 in 3rd (Jama 1979;242:2696).

Urine: Pregnancy tests now sensitive down to β-HCG of 50 U and hence 90% positive by 1st day of missed mense, 97% by 7th day (Jama 2001;286:1759)

Xray: Ultrasound at 4-6 wk for gestational sac, at 8-12 wk for crown/rump length, or at 14-20 wk for biparietal diameter, if dates unclear; routine ultrasound for congenital anomalies not helpful? (Nejm 1993;329:821 vs 874)

Rx: Avoid teratogens, including antibiotics (list: Med Let 1987; 29:61); safe meds list (Nejm 1998;338:1135); spina bifida caused by maternal vitamin A ingestion of ≥ 10,000 IU qd esp in 1st trimester (Nejm 1995;333:1369)

Table 11.2 Selected Drugs That Can Be Used Safely during Pregnancy, According to Condition

Condition	Drugs of Choice	Alternative Drugs	Comments
Acne	Topical: erythromycin, clindamycin, benzoyl peroxide	Systemic: erythromycin, topical tretinoin (vitamin A acid)	Isotretinoin is contraindicated
Allergic rhinitis	Topical: glucocorticoids, cromolyn, decongestants, xylometazoline, oxymetazoline, naphazoline, phenylephrine, systemic diphenhydramine, dimenhydrinate, tripelennamine, astemizole		
Constipation	Docusate sodium, calcium, glycerin, sorbitol, lactulose, mineral oil, magnesium hydroxide	Bisacodyl, phenolphthalein	
Cough	Diphenhydramine, codeine, dextromethorphan		
Depression	Tricyclic antidepressant drugs, fluoxetine	Lithium	When lithium is used in first trimester, fetal echocardiography and ultrasonography are recommended because of small risk of cardiovascular defects
Diabetes	Insulin (human)	Insulin (beef or pork)	Hypoglycemic drugs should be avoided
Headache Tension	Acetaminophen	Aspirin and nonsteroidal antiinflammatory drugs, benzodiazepines	Aspirin and nonsteroidal antiinflammatory drugs should be avoided in third trimester

Migraine	Acetaminophen, codeine, dimenhydrinate	Limited experience with ergotamine has not revealed evidence of teratogenicity, but there is concern about potent vasoconstriction and uterine contraction
	β-adrenergic-receptor antagonists and tricyclic antidepressant drugs (for prophylaxis)	
Hypertension	Labetalol, methyldopa	Angiotensin-converting enzyme inhibitors should be avoided because of risk of severe neonatal renal insufficiency
	β-adrenergic receptor antagonists, prazosin, hydralazine	
Hyperthyroidism	Propylthiouracil, methimazole	Surgery may be required; radioactive iodine should be avoided
Mania (and bipolar affective disorder)	Lithium, chlorpromazine, haloperidol	If lithium is used in first trimester, fetal echocardiography and ultrasonography are recommended because of small risk of cardiac anomalies; valproic acid may be given after neural-tube closure is complete
	β-adrenergic receptor antagonists (for symptoms)	
	For depressive episodes tricyclic antidepressant drugs, fluoxetine, valproic acid	

(continues)

11.4   *Pregnancy-Related Conditions*   **817**

Table 11.2 continued

Condition	Drugs of Choice	Alternative Drugs	Comments
Nausea, vomiting, motion sickness	Diclectin (doxylamine plus pyridoxine)	Chlorpromazine, metoclopramide (in third trimester), diphenhydramine, dimenhydrinate, meclizine, cyclizine	
Peptic ulcer disease	Antacids, magnesium hydroxide, aluminum hydroxide, calcium carbonate, ranitidine	Sucralfate, bismuth subsalicylate	
Pruritus	Topical: moisturizing creams or lotions, aluminum acetate, zinc oxide cream or ointment, calamine lotion, glucocorticoids; systemic: hydroxyzine, diphenhydramine, glucocorticoids, astemizole	Topical: local anesthetics	
Thrombophlebitis, deep-vein thrombosis	Heparin, antifibrinolytic drugs, streptokinase		Streptokinase is associated with a risk of bleeding; warfarin should be avoided

Reproduced with permission from Koren G, et al. Drugs in Pregnancy. New Eng J Med 1998: 228:1135. Copyright 1998 Mass. Medical Society, all rights reserved.

Folic acid 1 mg qd and iron 325 mg qd supplements throughout pregnancy prevent deficiencies; folate periconception at 0.4 mg qd × 1 mo decreases neural tube defect risk by 71% (Peds 1993;493:4), 4 mg po qd if pos family hx

Prenatal visits q 1 mo to 36 wk then q 2 wk if low risk, more if high risk (Jama 1996;275:847) to monitor fetal growth and maternal BP and education

of **Hyperemesis Gravidarum**: Small feedings, stop Fe pills, give vitamin B_6 (pyridoxine) 25 mg po tid × 3 d (Obgyn 1991; 78:33); antihistamines like diphenhydramine (Benadryl) 25-50 mg po q 4-6 hr, or trimethobenzamide (Tigan) 200 mg rectal suppos; or phenothiazines like prochlorperazine (Compazine) 25 mg po or pr qid, or 5 mg im, or promethazine (Phenergan) 25-50 mg po or pr qid, or chlorpromazine (Thorazine) 25-50 mg im q 4 hr, or metoclopramide (Reglan) 5-10 mg po/im/iv; iv fluids and hospitalization for volume depletion and ketosis. Bendectin (contains pyridoxine) no longer available in U.S. but sold as diclectin in Canada, and as Unisom sleep aid (pyridoxine + doxylamine) in U.S. ½ tab po bid, and probably is safe (Nejm 1998; 338:1128).

of seizure disorders in pregnancy: Seizure meds increase risk of congenital malformations (Nejm 2001;344:1132); cleft palate and spina bifida increased w all, least w phenobarb, more w valproate, and most w carbamazepine (Am J Pub Hlth 1996;86: 1454) vs only carbamazepine? (Nejm 1991;324:674); phenobarb, esp if given in last trimester, impairs subsequent intelligence (Jama 1995;274:1518); for phenytoin, one can predict which fetus will be deformed by an enzyme assay of amnion (Nejm 1990; 322:1567)

of depression in pregnancy: TCAs and SSRIs probably ok (rv: Jama 1999;282:1264)

of hypothyroidism: Monitor TSH, often need higher thyroid dose in pregnancy

of valvular heart disease in pregnancy (Nejm 2003;349:52)

of gestational diabetes w diet, BS monitoring, and insulin to keep BS < 150 clearly decreases newborn size and consequent cmplc of macrosomia (Nejm 2005;352:2477)

Labor and Delivery

Cause:

Epidem: 60% go into labor between 39 and 41 wk; rare to go > 300 d unless anencephaly

Pathophys: Nejm 1999;341:660

Sx: Rhythmic pains radiate to small of back; bloody show; ruptured membranes with positive ferning and/or nitrazine paper testing

Si: Cervical effacement and dilatation. Presentations: vertex (96%), breech (4%), transverse lie and mental (< 1%).

Crs: Stage I: Onset of labor to full dilatation of cervix; usually 4-12 hr
Stage II: Complete dilatation to infant delivery, median duration 50 min in nullips, 20 min in multips
Stage III: Infant delivery until placental delivery, usually 5-15 min

Cmplc: Many, especially preeclampsia, abruption, stillbirth, and fetal growth retardation, associated w undetected clotting factor mutations, eg, factor V (Leiden) (Nejm 1999;340:9)
- Endometritis
- Failure to progress, caused by cephalopelvic disproportion, or overmedication
- Mortality: Maternal = 3-4/10,000; infant/perinatal = 3.5%, 2% stillborn, rates increased 3× in breech
- Perineal lacerations:
  1st degree: Superficial
  2nd degree: Tissue injury sparing rectal sphincter
  3rd degree: Partial or complete separation of rectal sphincter
  4th degree: Tear into rectum; even w good repair, many (> ½) 3rd- and 4th-degree lacerations pts have long-term fecal

incontinence, especially if episiotomy or forceps used (Nejm 1993;329:1905)

- Premature labor, often due to bacterial chorioamnionitis (Nejm 2000;342:1500); due to short "incompetent" cervix predictable by transvaginal US @ 24-28 wk (Nejm 1996;334:567)

- Premature rupture of membranes (PROM) > 1 hr before onset of labor; w/u w sterile speculum exam and tests of vaginal fluid for ferning and nitrazine positivity, check fetal lung maturity (eg, L/S ratio) if < 36 wk, group B strep, chlamydia, and gc cultures; rx (see below)

- Prepartum bleeding in 3rd trimester: Do digital exam of cervix only after ultrasound or set up to do immediate C/S because may be **Placenta Previa**, 1/150 deliveries, increases w maternal age and h/o previous previa; caused by low implantation of placenta so it partially covers cervical os, those discovered in early pregnancy by ultrasound often migrate away by 3rd trimester; **Placental Abruption** (Jama 1999;282:1646), associated w HT and trauma but most are spontaneous, usually painful unlike previa; can cause uterine enlargement and tenderness, fetal distress, maternal shock, rx by delivery; **Vasa Previa**, cord vessels scattered throughout membranes, 1/100 antepartum bleeders, pulsatile vessels at cervical os

- Presentation, abnormal: Breech; rx w external cephalic version after 35 wk; ? moxibustion w herbs and acupuncture (Jama 1998;280:1580) at 33 wk

- Postpartum bleeding in mother: Increased by aspirin use within 5 d of delivery (Nejm 1982;307:909); first examine for laceration or retained placenta, then oxytocin 10 U im or in dilute iv soln, eg, 10-30 U/1000 cc (not iv push), then vigorous bimanual massage of uterus, then methylergonovine (Methergine) 0.2 mg im (not iv), then 15-methyl prostaglandin E_2 (Hemabate) 250 mg im, may repeat in 15-90 min, then hysterectomy or hypogastric artery ligation

- Pulmonary embolus in 1/4000, a 10× increase over baseline
- Shoulder dystocia; for rx, see below
- Urinary incontinence in mother subsequently increased from 10% prevalence in nullips to 16% post-C/S, and 21% post–vaginal deliveries (Nejm 2003;348:900); true for breeches too (Jama 2002;287:1822)

Lab: *Chem:* Amniotic fluid to test for lung maturity, if may be premature; false positives in diabetics

Noninv: Nonstress test (NST) for fetal movement and heart rate; oxytocin challenge stress test or nipple stimulation produces 3 or more contractions in 10 min to measure effect on fetal heart rate

Biophysical profile by ultrasound; calculate by scoring 0 if absent and 2 if present for fetal breathing movements, gross fetal body movements, fetal tone, reactive NST, and amniotic fluid volume in one pocket or total cm in each quadrant (amniotic fluid index) ≥ 2 cm; last 2 most important; 8/10 score is good (Am J Obgyn 1987;156:527)

Fetal monitoring used in most deliveries now, although abnormalities correlate w an already injured fetus and does prevent cerebral palsy (Ob Gyn 1995;86:613); repetitive late decelerations and decreased variability both are associated w 2.5-3.5 increase in incidence of CP but 99.8% false-pos rate (Nejm 1996;334:613); if use in all pts, you increase C/S rate without any improvement in outcome (Nejm 1986;315:615)

Xray: Ultrasound, for gestational age, or for amniocentesis for fetal maturity if premature labor

Rx: Avoid peripartum ASA (Nejm 1982;307:909); and bupivacaine 0.75% for epidural or paracervical blocks since causes cardiac arrests, hard to resuscitate (FDA Drug Bull 1983;13:23)

Analgesia possible w local paracervical blocks, spinal, and/or continous epidural blocks (rv: Nejm 2003;348:319), which may impair ability to walk but can be done before > 4 cm dilatation and does not increase operative delivery rate (Nejm 2005; 352:655)

Episiotomy does more harm than good (Jama 2005; 293:2141)

Spontaneous vaginal delivery; amniotomy (rupture of membranes) at 3+ cm dilatation speeds labor by > 2 hr safely (Nejm 1993;328:1145); walking during early labor has no effect (Nejm 1998;339:76)

Vaginal birth after C/S (VBAC) successful in 60-80% if previous low horizontal incision; but ability to predict in which pts works best is difficult (Nejm 1996;335:689); cmplc: uterine rupture (Nejm 2001;345:3) in 0.8% w/o but 2.5% w prostaglandin induction, compared to 0.15% if do repeat C/S and never goes into labor; infant hypoxic damage rates higher, endometritis and need for transfusions (Nejm 2004;351:2581)

Cesarean sections: Current increase to 25% of all deliveries is fueled to some extent by "repeats" (Nejm 1984;311:887) but also by individual physician practice styles (Nejm 1989;320:706); in Ireland, still only 5% C/S rate and perinatal mortality as good as U.S. (Obgyn 1983;61:1); "active management of labor" by amniotomy within 1st hr and pitocin at 6-36 mU/min to keep q 2 min contractions reduces C/S by 30% (Nejm 1992;326:450) vs no reduction in C/S rate although labor duration decreased by 2 hr plus less maternal fever (Nejm 1995;333:745)

of PROM (pathophys rv: Nejm 1998;338:663), w watching only vs induction w pitocin + protaglandin E (Nejm 1996;334:1005,1053), antibiotics if fever, fetal tachycardia, pos group B strep culture, if lasts > 12-18 hr

of threatened premature delivery from PROM, premature labor, or preeclampsia (Jama 1995;273:413): β-Methasone 12 mg im × 2, 24 hr apart, or dexamethasone 6 mg im q 6-12 hr × 4 once (Jama 2001;286:1581), between 24-34 wk gestation to reduce fetal risk of hyaline membrane disease and intraventricular hemorrhage

of premature labor, < 34 wk (Nejm 1984;311:571, 1984; 310:691):

- 1st: MgSO$_4$ 4 gm iv over 20 min, then 2 gm/hr iv/im and follow Mg levels, 5-7 mg/cc is therapeutic range (Clin Obgyn 1990;33:502), overdose can cause fatal respiratory depression
- 2nd: Terbutaline or isoxsuprine (Ritodrine), but delays delivery by only 24-48 hr w/o improving survival so use to buy time to transport or get steroids on board (Nejm 1992;327:308,349); adverse effects: elevate blood sugar, cardiovascular risks (Med Let 1980;22:89), especially pulmonary edema (Ann IM 1989; 110:714)
- 3rd: Nifedipine 10 mg sl up to 40 mg/hr then 20 mg q 6 hr maintenance, safer than Ritodrine (Am J Obgyn 1990;163:105) but may impair uteroplacental bloodflow; or
- Progesterone? in high-risk women (Nejm 2003;348:2379)
- Indomethacin also works but infant cmplc's not worth it (Nejm 1993;329:1602)

of shoulder dystocia, all within 5 min:

1st: Episiotomy

2nd: Legs up (McRobert's maneuver)

3rd: Suprapubic pressure

4th: Wood's screw maneuver or disimpact anterior shoulder

5th: Remove posterior shoulder, fracture clavicle

6th: Cesarean section

of failure to progress: Risk of neonatal intracranial bleed or other damage elevated by use of forceps, vacuum or C/S so none preferable over the others (Nejm 1999;341:1709)

Pregnancy-Induced Hypertension, Preeclampsia/Eclampsia, Toxemia

ACOG Tech Bull 219, Jan 1996; Nejm 1993;329:1265, 1992;326:927, 1990;323:434,478

Cause: Unknown; genetic component, incidence increases × 2 if maternal or paternal h/o preeclampsia (Nejm 2001;344:867)

Epidem: Incidence 4-6% in primips who represent 85% of all pts with PIH/eclampsia, 1.8% in subsequent pregnancies although risk gradually returns to primip rate as interval between pregnancies increases to 10 yr, not correlated w partner change (Nejm 2002;346:33); 25% in pts with chronic hypertension (Nejm 1998;339:667). 2nd most common cause (15%) of maternal deaths after pulmonary embolus.

Pathophys (Nejm 1996;335:1480, 1991;325:1439):

Sympathetic vasoconstrictor hyperactivity that abates w delivery (Nejm 1996; 335:1480)

Normally, pregnancy induces a decrease in peripheral vascular resistance mediated by increased resistance to angiotensin; somehow this effect is lost via a trophoblast-dependent process w platelet dysfunction (Nejm 1990;323:478). Vasodilating prostacyclin (PGI$_2$) level suppression present even in 1st trimester (Jama 1999;282:356).

CNS sx associated w reversible brain edema and leukoencephalopathy, also seen in immunocompromised and renal failure pts (Nejm 1996;334:494)

Sx: Pregnant, weight gain, edema, headache,* visual changes,* acute onset, abdominal pain* especially epigastric

Si:
- Hypertension, systolic > 140 and/or diastolic > 90 on 2 exams 6 hr apart; before 20 wk = chronic HT, r/o molar pregnancy; after 20 wk gestation = PIH; diastolic > 110* is ominous for eclampsia (seizures)
- Edema
- Proteinuria (= preeclampsia), ≥ 300 mg/24 hr or 1+ proteinuria
- Hyperreflexia incidentally often but without prognostic significance

*predicted by number of findings

OBSTETRICS/GYNECOLOGY

Crs: All sx disappear (in 95%) by 72 hr postpartum; a small percentage may persist for weeks. If occurs in 1st trimester, must be mole or trophoblastic tumor.

Cmplc: Preeclampsia: HT + proteinuria after 20 wk gestation, most in 3rd trimester; associated, when severe but short of eclampsia, w 1% maternal and 10% prenatal infant mortality; when severe, evolves to eclampsia, without rx, in 25-50%

Eclampsia (toxemia; defined by seizures); renal failure; CHF; CNS bleed; DIC; Sheehan's syndrome; fetal demise; hepatic hemorrhage and rupture (Nejm 1985;312:424); HELLP syndrome (p 827); newborn neutropenias, transient in 50%, associated with sepsis (Nejm 1989;321:557)

Fetal growth retardation

r/o other causes of HT in pregnancy: Pheochromocytoma; more benign **Transient Hypertension of Pregnancy**; and chronic HT in pregnancy (Nejm 1987;316:715)

Lab: *Chem:* Uric acid elevated; creatinine elevations*; eventually perhaps measurements of angiogenic factors like tyrosine kinase and placental growth factor (Nejm 2004;350:672), urinary placental growth factor levels significantly low 4-8 wk before onset (Jama 2005;293:77)

Hem: Hemolytic anemia* and thrombocytopenia,* which may be mild; platelet intracellular calcium markedly elevated by vasopressin in susceptible pts (Nejm 1990;323:434); polycythemia indicating hypovolemia

Path: Renal, bx or at postmortem shows ATN, occasionally bilateral cortical necrosis, swollen glomerular endothelial cells with fibrin in them. Placenta shows spotty necrosis with small-vessel disease.

Urine: 24-hr protein > 300 mg, may be > 2 gm*; creatinine clearance decreased (normally in pregnancy is 100-150 cc/min). 24-hr calcium < 100-150 mg, unlike benign hypertensives who excrete more calcium (Nejm 1987;316:715).

*predicted by number of findings

Rx: Preventive w ASA 60-100 mg po qd by wk 12? (BMJ 2000; 322:329 vs Nejm 1998;338:701); perhaps vitamin C 1000 mg qd + vitamin E 400 IU qd; calcium controversial but probably not helpful (Nejm 1997;337:69 vs 1991;325:1399)

of HT during pregnancy (Can Med Assoc J 1997;157:1245): α-Methyldopa (Aldomet) alone; or propranolol (Nejm 1981;305: 1323); or α-methyldopa + hydralazine; or clonidine + hydralazine (Med J Aust 1991;154:378). But rx of PIH, unless severe, does not improve outcome. Avoid ACEIs, which are teratogenic (Jama 1997;277:1193).

of preeclampsia (Can Med Assoc J 1997;157:1245): Bed rest; deliver when fetus mature; hospitalize for failure of home bed rest, diastolic BP ≥ 110, or proteinuria ≥ 2+ by dip or ≥ 500 mg/24 hr; avoid diuretics and salt restriction; hydralazine 5-10 mg q 20 min iv to get diastolic BP < 105; or labetolol 10-20 mg iv q 10 min; or perhaps nifedipine 10 mg sl then po q 6 hr (Obgyn 1991;77:331); follow with po hydralazine, α-methyldopa, or β-blockers. Rx does not improve fetal outcome but does protect maternal CNS (Am J Obgyn 1990;162:960).

of eclampsia (seizures): Stabilize, then deliver within 4-5 hr of onset, may need D + C to get rid of all placenta; $MgSO_4$ 4 gm iv over 20 min, then 2 gm/hr iv, or can give im, eg, 10 gm load then 5 gm q 4 hr (Nejm 1995;333:201); follow Mg levels, 5-7 mg/cc is therapeutic range; continue 12-24 hr postpartum; unknown mechanism of action but better than all other drug options (Nejm 2003;348:275, 304); may cause fatal newborn respiratory depression, helped by iv calcium gluconate gm for gm

HELLP Syndrome (Hemolysis, Elevated Liver Function Tests, Low Platelets)

Jama 1998;280:559

Cause: PIH/preeclampsia

Epidem:

Pathophys: Unknown; overlaps w acute fatty liver of pregnancy (Ann IM 1987;106:703; Nejm 1985;313:367); both may be manifestations of a mitochondrial fatty acid metabolizing enzyme that also lead to liver disease in the infants (Jama 2002;288:2163; Nejm 1999;340:1723)

Sx: Onset after 30th (usually > 35th) week of pregnancy. Usually none but may have any sx of PIH and/or headache, confusion; fatigue, malaise; nausea and vomiting; abdominal pain, diffuse or right upper quadrant.

Si: Edema, hypertension, proteinuria, jaundice, encephalopathy, seizures, coma; small liver; tender right upper quadrant; preeclampsia in all

Crs: 85% mortality without rx. Does not seem to recur in future pregnancies.

Cmplc: Hypoglycemia, DIC and hemorrhage, renal failure, eclampsia, pancreatitis (back pain), fetal and/or maternal death

Lab: *Chem:* AST (SGOT) and ALT (SGPT), uric acid, NH_3 all elevated; bilirubin goes up later; hypoglycemia

Genetic testing: Of family (Nejm 1999;340:1723)

Hem: Wbc > 15,000; microangiopathic anemia/DIC picture w nucleated rbc's, rapidly falling platelet counts; elevated hct, PT, PTT, and fibrin split products, and low fibrinogen levels

Path: Liver bx shows easily missed fat in microvesicles with central (not peripheral) nuclei; r/o Reye's and tetracycline hepatotoxicity

Urine: UA shows proteinuria

Rx: Stabilize, stat delivery, transfuse platelets

Hydatidiform Mole (Molar Pregnancy)

Nejm 1996;335:1740

Cause: Gestational trophoblastic neoplasia; complete from a haploid sperm duplicating own chromosomes and inactivating ovum chromosomes, or partial w haploid karyotype

Epidem: 1/1500 pregnancies; 10% of all spontaneous abortions have mole changes (A. Hertig 1967)

Increased incidence in Asians, women over age 40, and in women w h/o previous spontaneous abortion

Pathophys: Molar changes seen at junction of placenta and chorionic laeve when chorion is undergoing atrophy at 8-12 wk. Embryo portion dies at 3-5 wk; chorionic villi then accumulate fluid in connective tissue spaces from maternal circulation. Fetal circulation is absent, hence fluid accumulation. Invasive mole doesn't follow a normal pregnancy unless a twin was present.

Range of disease exists from benign mole to choriocarcinoma (p 830)

Sx: H/o recent spontaneous abortion; severe morning sickness (hyperemesis gravidarum) lasting into 2nd trimester

Si: Vaginal bleeding in 1st trimester; uterus enlarged beyond dates, although 10% may be small for gestational age

Crs:

Cmplc: Local invasion and/or benign metastases; choriocarcinoma or persistent gestational trophoblastic tumors (20-30%); thyrotoxicosis from a TSH-like protein present in 100% of moles (Ann IM 1975;83:307); pregnancy-induced HT; tumor emboli

Lab: *Chem:* HCG levels very high, does not decrease to normal within 6 wk of removal as a normal spontaneous abortion should

Path: Endometrial bx by D + C shows entire endometrium involved; volumes up to 3 L; translucent villi up to 1 cm diameter, appear like "grapes"; organized trophoblast (benign), to pleomorphic (potentially malignant)

Xray: CT and chest xray to look for mets; ultrasound done for abnormal bleeding detects most

Rx: Rhogam if Rh neg

Benign moles may be rx'd with simple D + E, followed by HCG levels q 2 wk

Invasive types or mets rx'd like choriocarcinoma (see below)
Good birth control to prevent new pregnancy while follow
serial HCGs to 0 to be sure benign course

Choriocarcinoma

Nejm 1996;335:1740

Cause: Fetal chorionic tissues of placenta; teratomas of ovary? (Nejm 1969;280:1439)

Epidem: ⅓ after spontaneous abortions, ⅓ after moles, and ⅓ after normal pregnancies; 500/yr in U.S.; incidence increased 10× in Asians and Hispanics

Pathophys: Local invasion and bloodborne metastases. In 50%, can't find primary lesion because it's so small.

Sx: Bleeding, excessive nausea and vomiting (morning sickness)

Si:

Crs: Without rx, die within 1 yr

Cmplc: Metastases: 80% to lung, 30% to vagina, 25% local, 10% to brain, 10% to liver, 5% to kidney; toxemia of pregnancy in late 1st or early 2nd trimester; perforated uterus; endometritis

Lab: *Chem:* HCG levels very high, > 100,000 IU/24-hr urine (normal pregnancy, even at 28 d peak, is less than this, and later decreases to 5000 IU during most of pregnancy, and drops in last 2 wk at term). T_4 increased via TSH-like substance, and perhaps HCG. Liver function tests elevated if metastases.

Path: Hemorrhagic central necrosis. Ovaries have large thecal cysts from HCG stimulation that will regress. On microscopic, syncytio-cytotrophoblasts with necrosis, hemorrhage, and inflammation.

Xray: Head CT to r/o metastases. Ultrasound shows clumps of placenta.

Rx: Surgical resection

Chemotherapy w methotrexate po or im and/or dactinomycin qd in 5-d bursts; 5-yr survival rates with this rx are nearly
100% for intrauterine, 75% for extrauterine, 50% if CNS mets,
but 0% if hepatic mets

11.5 Miscellaneous

Amenorrhea

Rx all anovulatory pts with medroxyprogesterone 10 mg po × 10
d q 3 mo to prophylact vs uterine cancer (D. Federman 1985)

Primary amenorrhea (no menses by age 16-18) w/u: Physical
exam to look for imperforate hymen, vaginal agenesis, cervical stenosis, endometrial tbc, dwarfism (Turner's, get buccal smear or karyotype), pregnancy, virilized external genitalia (congenital adrenal
hyperplasia, hermaphroditism, mixed gonadal dysgenesis, or
androgen-producing ovarian tumor) (see Figure 13.2).

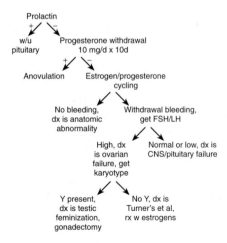

Figure 11.1 Primary amenorrhea w/u.

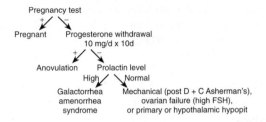

Figure 11.2   Secondary amenorrhea w/u.

Anovulation Causes

Polycystic ovary syndrome, FSH/LH surge failure, eg, at times of menarche or menopause, w anorexia, et al

Birth Control

Med Let 1995;37:9: a rv of all methods, efficiencies, advantages, and disadvantages

25-30% of couples having regular intercourse get pregnant each month (Nejm 1988;319:189)

Medications (Med Let 2000;42:42; Nejm 1993;328:1543):

Estrogen/progesterone shots q 1 mo (Lunelle)

Birth control pills (P. Myers 5/91): Combination pills of estrogen (usually ethinyl estradiol [EE]; or mestranol [ME] [50 μgm = 30 μgm of EE], or ethynodiol diacetate [EDA]); plus a progestin (usually norethindrone [NE], or norgestrel [NG], or levonorgestrel [LG], or norgestimate [NGE], or desogestrel [DG]), all of which suppress LH surge and ovulation, maintain estrogen levels, and mature endometrium regularly. Avoid (Jama 2001; 285:2232) in pts w HT, migraine, DVT/PE, smokers over age 35.

Estrogen side effects: Thrombosis (venous, coronary, CNS) although low-dose (≤ 35 μgm) estrogen pills may not increase CVAs (Ann IM 1997;127:596; Nejm 1996;335:8 vs Jama

2000;284:284:72 meta-analysis) or other manifestations (Ann IM 1998;128:469) unless age > 40 or smoke, no increase in risk after stop smoking, but super-low-dose estrogen pills (~20 μgm) may be slightly worse because of newer progesterones effect; nausea and lactation suppression

Progestin side effects: ASCVD via lipids, risk ends when discontinue pills (Nejm 1988;319:1313); hypertension; glucose intolerance; acne (androgenicity); depression; rarely liver adenomas (Nejm 1976;294:470); gallstones (Nejm 1976;294:189); all seem less w desogestrel as in Desogen 28 or Ortho-Cept 21 (Med Let 1993;35:73) including thromboembolism risks (Nejm 2001;345:1787)

No increase in breast cancer (Nejm 2002;346:2025); no overall adverse effect of bcp's on mortality (Ann IM 1994; 120:821) and may decrease ovarian cancer risk substantially

Androgenicity decreases as go from levoNG > NG > NE > NE acetate > EDA > DG. Triphasic oral contraceptives like Trinorinyl, Orthonovum 7/7/7, and Triphasil all increase, then decrease progesterone dose during cycle to try to decrease ASHD risk; questionable value (Med Let 1985;27:48, 1984;26:93).

Progesterone Only

Medroxyprogesterone (DepoProvera) 25-150 mg im q 3 mo; adverse effects: debatable small increase in breast cancer (Jama 1995;273:799), osteoporosis (? dexascan as start) w prolonged use

Norethindrone (Micronor) 0.35 mg po qd

Norgestrel (Ovrette) 0.075 mg po qd

Low Estrogen

Loestrin 1/20 (NE acetate 1 mg/EE 20 μgm)

Alesse and Levlite (LevoNG 0.1/EE 20)

Mircette (desogestrel 0.15/EE 20-10)

Moderate (30 μgm) Estrogen

Desogen/Orthocept (desogestrel 0.15/EE 30)

Loestrin 1.5/30 (NE acetate 1.5/EE 30)

Lo-ovral/Low-Orgestrel (NG 0.3/EE 30)

Nordette/Levora/Seasonale, Levlen (levoNG 0.15/EE 30)

Yasmin 28 (EE 30 + spironolactone-like progestin: drospiren-
done) (Med Let 2002;44:55)

Moderate (35 μgm) Estrogen

Demulen/Zovia 1/35 (EDA 1 mg/EE 35 μgm)

Genora/Ortho/Norinyl 1/35 (NE 1/EE 35)

Modicon/Brevicon (NE 0.5 mg/EE 35 μgm)

Norinyl/ Orthonovum/Neocon 1/35 (NE 1/EE 35)

Ortho 777 (NE 0.5-0.75-1/EE 35)

Ortho 10/11 (NE 0.5-1/EE 35)

Orthocyllen (NGE 0.25/EE 35)

Ortho Tricyclen (NGE 0.18, 0.215, 0.25/EE 35)

Ovcon 35 (NE 0.4/EE 35)

Tri-Norinyl (NE 0.5-1-0.5/EE 35)

Triphasil and Tri-Levlen (levoNG 0.05-0.75-0.125/EE 30-40-30)

High Estrogen

Demulen 1/50 (EDA 1 mg/EE 50 μgm)

Genora/Ortho/Norinyl 1/50 (NE 1/ME 50) or 1/80 (NE 1/ME 80)

Norlestrin 1/50 (NE acetate 1/EE 50)

Orthonovum 1/80 (NE 1/ME 80)

Ovcon (NE 1/EE 50)

Ovulen (EDA 1/ME 100)

Transdermal/Mucosal

Norelgestromin/ethinyl estradiol 150/20 (Evra [Ortho]) (Med Let
2002;44:8; Jama 2001;285:2347) patch q 1 wk, 3/4 wk; as
effective and better compliance than bcp's

Nuva vaginal ring, 3/4 wk

Maneuvers for Birth Control Pill Side Effects

• Breakthrough bleeding: r/o infection; wait, since decreases
from 30% to < 10% after 3 cycles; increase progestin or go to
monophasic if on triphasic; increase progestin androgenicity;
increase estrogen if early in cycle

- Amenorrhea: r/o pregnancy; increase androgenicity or progestin; increase progestin; perhaps increase estrogen
- Nausea: Take pill with food or at bedtime
- Acne: Change to less androgenic progestin like Desogen 28 or OrthoCept 21 (Med Let 1993;35:73); Ortho Tricyclen is FDA approved
- Fluid retention, mastalgia, depression: decrease progestin; also estrogen?

Table 11.3   Oral Contraceptive/Drug Interactions

Drug	Effect
Antibiotics, especially ampicillin, macrolides, Tm/S, metronidazole, tetracycline, rifampin, griseofulvin, several HIV drugs	Decrease effectiveness of oral contraceptives; use barrier or alternative methods as backup
Anticoagulants (warfarin)	Decreased anticoagulant effect
Antidepressants	Increased antidepressant effect
Benzodiazepines	Variable effects; use caution during inactive cycle
β-Blockers	Possible enhanced β-blocker effect
Corticosteroids	Decreased clearance, increased half-life
Hypoglycemics	Possible diminished effectiveness
Methyldopa	Decreased antihypertensive effect
Theophyllin	Increased theophylline effect
Seizure meds, especially barbiturates, carbamazepine (Tegretol), phenytoin, primodone, topiramate	Decrease effectiveness of oral contraceptives; use barrier or alternative methods as backup and/or higher-dose pill

(Contraceptive Tech 1994)

Other Methods:

Postcoital contraception, "morning-after pill" (Ann IM 2002; 137:180; Nejm 2003;349:1830), decreases pregnancy rate from 8% to < 2% after single episode of intercourse, best within 12 hr but try up to 5 d out, w:

- Oral bcp's, eg, 1 or 2 50 mg estradiol bcp's, or 2-4 35 mg estradiol bcp's po q 12 hr twice, or as Preven emergency kit, $20 (Med Let 1998;40:102) within 72 hr of unprotected intercourse has < 2% failure rate (Med Let 1989;31:93), causes nausea and vomiting in 25-50%; repeat if vomits within 2 hr of dose or see pill in emesis; double doses if on antibiotics or seizure meds; consider giving all women a home supply (Nejm 1998;339:1)
- Levonorgestrel (Plan B) (Med Let 2000;42:10) 0.75 mg po × 2, 12 hr apart within 48 hr; better tolerated than estrogen/progestin combinations; $21
- Mifepristone (RU-486) 600 mg po; antiprogesterone; < 0.1% failure rate (Nejm 1992;327:1041); no nausea
- IUD insertion esp if > 72 hr but < 5 d since intercourse

Propranolol 80 mg vaginally qd (BMJ 1983;287:1245,1247); effective for > 10 hr, inhibits sperm motility; 3 pregnancies/100 women/yr, comparable to diaphragm and IUD; highly absorbed

Mechanical Methods (in order of decreasing effectiveness)

- Vasectomy; reversals possible if vasectomy < 3 yr old, resulting in a 76% pregnancy rate; if > 15 yr old, 30% reversal pregnancy rate
- Tubal ligation; adverse effects: ectopic pregnancy rate = 7/1000 in 10 yr, higher (30/1000) when done by electrocoagulation (Nejm 1997;336:762), no clear post-tubal syndrome (Obgyn 1983;62:673); no increase in mentrual abnormalities (Nejm 2000;343:1681)
- Intrauterine devices (IUDs); Progestasert q 1 yr, Copper-T q 10 yr (Med Let 1988;30:25), or levonorgestrel (Mirena) (Med Let 2001;43:7) q 5 yr $500; cmplc: increased menstrual bleeding, dysmenorrhea, ovarian cysts (12%)
- Diaphragm; cervical caps, no better and may be worse than diaphragms since dislodge (Am J Obgyn 1983;148:604), may increase cervical dysplasia (Med Let 1988;30:93)

- Condoms, male or female polyurethane, which are as effective (2.6 pregnancies/100 women-years) as diaphragm and prevent herpes and HIV infection (Med Let 1993;35:123)
- Vaginal sponge (Med Let 1983;25:78) and/or spermicides; no increase in trisomies or birth defects (Nejm 1987;317: 474,478); spermicides don't help prevent STDs (Nejm 1998;339:504)

Domestic Abuse/Violence

Nejm 1999;341:886,1892,1899; Ann IM 1995;123:774

Epidem: Incidence ~ 5%/yr, 20-33% of women have a pos hx (Jama 1998;280:433; Ann IM 1995;123:737). Highest risk in women whose male partners abuse drugs or alcohol, are unemployed, and have less than a high school education.

Sx: Trauma; functional gi disorders (Ann IM 1995;123:782), anxiety, depression, somatization

Si: Trauma in excess of hx + above

Rx: Screen by asking, "Have you been hit, kicked, punched, or otherwise injured in this past year, and if so by whom?"; 70% sens, 85% specif (Jama 1997;277:1357), but do it sensitively (Ann IM 1999;131:578) and USPSTF rates data indeterminant (Ann IM 2004;140:382,387 vs 399)

Advocate for, offer choices, avoid blaming, assess danger; national hotline: 1-800-799-SAFE

Dysfunctional Uterine Bleeding

Cause: Anovulatory cycles, eg, polycystic ovaries, androgen/cortisol excess, borderline pituitary or hypothalamic failure including menopause and menarche; uterine, eg, PID, cervical ectropion or polyp, cancer, fibroid, pregnancy; other medical illness, eg, bleeding disorder, hypothyroidism; Addison's disease

Sx: Menorrhagia, long and/or heavy periods; metrorrhagia, bleeding between periods

Si: Pelvic exam for mass, ovarian enlargement, fibroid, pregnancy, polyp

Cmplc: Anemia

Lab:

  Chem: Pregnancy test, H + H

  Path: Pap smear, endometrial bx if age ≥ 40 yr, hysteroscopy for failed medical rx after bx

Rx: For acute bleeding: 2-4 bcp's po × 1 or iv premarin 25 mg q 4 hr until stop

Cycle w medroxyprogesterone (Provera) 10 mg qd × 10 d q 1-3 mo, or oral bcp's

Surgical D + C; hysteroscopy; hysteroscopic resection of pathology; endometrial ablation w resectoscope, cautery, laser, or heat; but hysterectomy is treatment of choice by RCT if progesterone fails (Jama 2004;291:1447)

  of anemia: Iron
  of pain: NSAIDs

Dysmenorrhea

Sx: Cramping, nausea, and vomiting with menses

Rx: Ibuprofen 400+ mg, better than ASA (Med Let 1984;26:67); oral bcp's

Estrogen Replacement Therapy

Not helpful to mortality (ACP J Club 2005;142:1), or quality of life, even after hysterectomy (Jama 2004;291:1701) unless c/o hot flashes (Nejm 2003;348:1839; Jama 2002;287:591,2130)

Estrogens:

• Conjugated estrogens from horse urine (Premarin) 0.625-1.25 mg qd (Obgyn 1984;63:759) and debatably even lower doses

(Obgyn 1996;27:163) like 0.3 mg w adequate vitamin D and calcium enough to prevent osteoporosis (Ann IM 1999; 130:897), or

- Estradiol (Estrace) 1-2 mg po qd, both cost ~$20/mo; or patch (Menostar) (Med Let 2004;46:69) 25-50 µgm/d; may help osteoporosis, unknown breast Ca and thromboembolic effects; or as vaginal rings (Femring, or very-low-dose Estring) q 3 mo, uterine Ca risk still so give progesterone q 3 mo and do endometrial bx
- estropipate (Ogen)

  Estrogen adverse effects: In summary (Jama 2002;288:321), for every year 10,000 women take ERT, 7 more have coronary events, 8 more have CVAs, 8 more have PEs, and 8 more have invasive breast Ca
- Cardiovascular disease (Nejm 2003;349:523,535; Ann IM 2002;137:273; Jama 2002;288:321, 2432); increases CVAs by 30% (Nejm 2001;345:1234; Ann IM 2000;133:933) esp in smokers (Nejm 1996;335:453, 1985;313:1038); also increases thromboembolic disease
- Breast Ca risk (Jama 2003;289:3243,3254,3304, 2002;288:321) increases over 4+ yr, esp when combined w progesterone (Jama 2002;287:734, 2000;283:485,534); decreases mammographic sens and specif (Jama 2001;285:171)
- Ovarian Ca (Jama 2003;290;1739, 2001;285:1460) slightly increases
- Venous thromboembolic risk increases, NNT-3 = 256 (Ann IM 2002;136:680, 2000;132:689) including ischemic heart disease and stroke (Jama 2003;289:2673)
- Gallbladder disease increases (Jama 1998;280:605)
- Rate of Alzheimer's disease may worsen and certainly there is no benefit in controlled study by Women's Health Initiative (Jama 2004;291;2947,2959,3005, 2003;289:2651,2663) and does not improve memory when given to elderly (J Am Ger Soc 2004;52:182,269)

- Dry eye syndrome, risk increases by 15-30% esp in older women (Jama 2001;286:2114)

Estrogen benefits:

- Bone loss and fractures, esp of hip, but not worth the cardio-vascular and breast Ca risk (Jama 2003;290:1739)
- Colon cancer rates decrease by 35-40% w concurrent use by RCT (Nejm 2004;350:991) but tumors that do occur have a higher average stage; rates revert after off for 5 yr (Ann IM 1998;128:705)

Plus (if uterus intact)

Progesterone: In woman w uterus (Jama 1996;275:370):

- Medroxyprogesterone (Provera) 10 mg qd last 10 d of each, q 2 mo, or q 3 mo, must bleed 10 or more days after starting progesterone to be effective in preventing uterine cancer; or
- Micronized natural progesterone (Prometrium) 200 mg po 12/30 d or 100 mg po qd; or
- Continuous progestin, eg, 2.5 mg of medroxyprogesterone w continuous estrogen is just as effective and obviates periods (Jama 1996;276:1389,1430); or
- Estrogen/progesterone combination pills; all ~$25/mo Prempro (premarin 0.625 mg + progesterone 2.5 or 5 mg) or FemHRT w 5 μgm estradiol + 1 mg norethindrone

Selective Estrogen Receptor Modulators (tamoxifen-like):

- Raloxifene (Evista) (Jama 1999;282:637, 1998;279:1445; Med Let 1998;40:29; Nejm 1997;337:1641,1686) 60-120 mg po qd, which helps bone (halves fx rates) and cholesterol w/o endometrial hyperplasia, and may decrease breast Ca incidence (Jama 1999;281:2189) NNT-4 yr = 126 (ACP J Club 1999; 131:58) at least in women w higher estradiol blood levels (Jama 2001;287:216), no benefit if undetectable; but increases hot flashes and thromboembolic disease like DVT (1%) NNH-4 yr = 155 (ACP J Club 1999;131:58) but does not increase cardiovascular events (ASHD and CVA) but reduces them in high-risk women (Jama 2002;287:847); cost: $60/mo

- Tibolone (ACP J Club 1999;131:44) helps hot flashes, LDL, and bone density w/o endometrial or breast effects
- Phytoestrogens from soy, black cohosh, red clover, etc; probably cause no harm but efficacy lacking (Jama 2004;292:65; Med Let 2000;42:17)

Gynecomastia

In male or child, 40% are asx (Nejm 1993;328:490)

Cause: In adolescents, vast majority are transient and benign; Graves' disease (increased sex steroid-binding globulin); renal failure on dialysis; Klinefelter's; gonadotropin-producing tumors of lung or testicle (find with testicular ultrasound or abdominal CT/MRI: Nejm 1991;324:334); malignant adrenal tumors; refeeding after starvation; local irritation; cirrhosis. Drugs: alcohol, α-methyl-dopa (Aldomet), amphetamines, captopril and other ACEIs, chemotherapy, cimetidine, diazepam, digitalis, estrogen—minute amounts in foods or on fomites, haloperidol (Haldol), heroin, INH, marijuana, metronidazole (Flagyl), nifedipine, omeprazole (Prilosec), penicillamine, phenothiazines, phenytoin (Dilantin), ranitidine, reserpine, spironolactone (blocks androgen receptors), tricyclics, verapamil.

Epidem: 25% are idiopathic, 25% pubertal, 10-20% drug-induced, 8% malnutrition or cirrhosis, 2% testicular tumor, 2% hypogonadism (Klinefelter's, etc), 1.5% hyperthyroidism, 1% renal disease

Pathophys: Increased estrogen and/or diminished androgens; many drugs cause it by displacing estrogen from binding protein

Lab: *Chem:* HCG, LH, estradiol, testosterone, sTSH

Rx: Antiestrogens like 1st tamoxifen 10 mg po bid; clomiphene, cimetidine
Surgical resection

Hirsutism/Hypertrichosis

Nejm 1990;323:909; Ann IM 1987;106:95

Cause:

Isolated:

- Normal variation (Nejm 1992;327:194)
- Polycystic ovary

W associated masculinization (voice, baldness, clitoromegaly):

- Adrenal carcinoma
- Cushing's syndrome
- Arrhenoblastoma
- Hilar cell adenoma or hyperplasia
- Luteoma
- Incomplete male pseudohermaphroditism
- Transvestitism/iatrogenic
- Mild congenital adrenal hyperplasia, 21OH deficiency as well as 11β-OHase and 3β-OHase deficiencies (p 252), adult onset, HLA B_{14} and Aw_{33} linked (Nejm 1985;313:224), ~12% of adult female hirsutes

Lab: *Chem:* Testosterone and dehydroepiandrostenedione levels to r/o testosterone-producing tumors; if ≥ 200 ng %, do 5 d dexamethasone suppression test (Nejm 1994;331:968,1015); 17-OH progesterone level < 350 ng % in am; if 350-1000 ng %, do ACTH stimulation test, should be < 1000; and/or DHEA > 800 μgm %

Rx: Cimetidine 300 mg 5×/d works by blocking androgen action at follicles (Nejm 1980;303:1042); spironolactone (ACP J Club 2004;140:74) 75-200 mg qd; chronic steroids help 50%; bcp's help 75%; electrolysis speeds responses. Topical eflornithine (Vaniga) (Med Let 2000;42:96) bid, slows hair follicle growth rate, helps hirsutism in women and pseudofollicultis barbae in men, takes 8 wk to help, < 50% response rate; $42/mo (30 gm tube)

Infertility

No rx at all is as good as any of these in idiopathics (Nejm 1983;309:1201)

Male Infertility (Nejm 1995;332:312; Ann IM 1985;103:906): Present in 50% of infertile couples

1st: Physical exam, especially for varicocele (present in 40% of infertile males and 10% of fertile males); and scarred epididymis, vas deferens, and prostate. Avoid sulfasalazine, cimetidine, lead, arsenic, nitrofurantoin, marijuana, anabolic steroids, cocaine, heat exposure, smoking.

2nd: Sperm count (Nejm 2001;345:1388); normal is > 50 million/cc, > 12% normal morphology, > 60% motile; abnormal if < 13 million/cc, and/or < 32% motile, volume < 10 cc, < 9% normal morphology

3rd: FSH, LH, testosterone levels

if FSH is normal, and LH and testosterone are low, dx is hypogonadotropic hypogonadism (p 322); get drug hx, sella MRI views, and prolactin levels; withdraw drug if on any; rx with HCG-HMG or LHRH if both sella and prolactin normal; bromocriptine or surgery if big sella; bromocryptine and repeat films if sella normal and prolactin elevated

if elevated FSH and LH, and low testosterone, dx is primary panhypogonadism; or if FSH elevated, and normal testosterone and LH, dx is isolated germinal compartment failure; rx both with adoption or artificial insemination

if normal FSH, and elevated LH and testosterone, dx is partial androgen resistance; no rx known except adoption and artificial insemination

if normal FSH, LH, and testosterone, and is oligospermic (not azoospermic), dx is varicocele or idiopathic; rx w surgery for varicocele; steroids? for measurable sperm antibodies, male or female (Nejm 1980;303:722); tetracycline for ureaplasma infection? (Nejm 1983;308:505); split ejaculate insemination

if normal FSH, LH, and testosterone, and is azoospermic, get seminal fructose; if positive, get post-ejaculation UA; if sperm present, dx is retrograde ejaculation and needs a neurology w/u; if fructose-negative, get vasograms, bx, and/or exploration looking for obstruction (majority) and rx with microductal surgery; most of such men have idiopathic obstructive azoospermia associated w cystic fibrosis gene defects but lack other CF manifestations (Nejm 1998;339:687); if negative, dx is germinal compartment failure, rx with adoption and insemination, in vitro fertilization

Female infertility (Jama 2003;290:1767):

Cause: Ovulation disorders (25%), tubal disorders (20%), endometriosis (5-10%), et al

  1st: Regular intercourse × 1 yr without birth control if normal anatomy; avoid nitrous oxide and other anesthetic exposures (Nejm 1992;327:993)

  2nd: Do basal body temperature, increases in 2nd half of the cycle if ovulating; can confirm with mid-cycle serum progesterone levels or endometrial bx. Pregnancy occurs from intercourse 6 d prior to ovulation (10% chance) to day of ovulation (33% chance), and day of conception has no effect on fetal viability or gender (Nejm 1995;333:1517).

  3rd: FSH on day 3 of cycle, urinary LH level (perhaps instead of basal body temperature), and uterine cavity assessment by hysterosalpingogram, ultrasound, and/or laparoscopy

  4th: if no ovulation and partner normal by exam and testing, consider ovulation induction drug rx (Med Let 1988;30:91) w intrauterine insemination (Nejm 1999;340:177,224); adverse effects: multiple births, 20% with some regimens; pathologic ovarian enlargement and ovarian cancer if used > 1 yr (Nejm 1994;331:771)

- Clomiphene: Blocks hypothalamic estrogen receptors so human chorionic gonadotropin–releasing hormone (HCGRH) is stimulated, w intrauterine insemination (IUI); 10% pregnancy rate at 6 mo
- Clomiphene + HCG in sequence; w IUI; 10% pregnancy rate within 6 mo

Then perhaps consider:

- In vitro fertilization w 1, not 2, embryos (Nejm 2004;351:2392) to prevent 33% multiple-birth rate
- FSH + LH (Pergonal), then HCG if low basal gonadotropins and estrogens; 25% pregnancy rate, increases to 33% with clomiphene
- HCG and buserelin (LHRH agonist) (Nejm 1989;320:1233)
- Gonadorelin, HCGRH analog, given in q 90 min bursts iv over 3 wk results in a 60% pregnancy rate (Med Let 1990;32:70)

Male or female infertility:

- Adoption help guidelines (Am Fam Phys 1985;31:109)
- Infertility support group: Resolve, Box 474, Belmont, MA 02178
- In vitro fertilization and embryo transfer, after estrogen/progesterone cycling in ovarian failure (Nejm 1986;314:806); cost = $50,000-100,000/delivery (Nejm 1994;331:239). Or intra-oocyte sperm injection. Both associated w very low birth weights, and doubled rates of birth defects by age 1 yr (Nejm 2002;346:725,731).
- Surrogate parenting; in vitro fertilization and uterine transfer

Menopausal Sx/Hot Flashes

Jama 2004;291:1621; Med Let 2004;46:98

Sx: Age, family hx, and menstrual pattern much more helpful in making dx than FSH or inhibin levels (Jama 2003;289:895)

Rx:

- Estrogens (p 838) help hot flashes, osteoporosis, vaginal atrophy, and sleep; contraindicated in uterine or breast cancer or men w prostate cancer on GRH antagonist rx
- Progesterone alone as pills or topically (Pro-Gest) helps hot flashes and sleep; may worsen for 1-2 d before improving in women on tamoxifen; megesterol (Megace) 20 mg po bid (Nejm 1994;331:347); or DepoProvera 150 mg im q 3 mo
- Veniafaxine (Effexor) 12.5 mg po bid
- Fluoxetine (Prozac) 20 mg po qd, or paroxetine (Paxil) 12.5-25 mg po qd (Jama 2003;289:2827
- Clonidine 0.1 mg po qd helps 40% (Ann IM 2000;132:788)
- Gabapentin (Neurontin) 100 mg po hs up to 300 mg tid
- Testosterone transdermally 300 μgm/d improves sexual function significantly in post-BSOO premenopausal women (Nejm 2000;343:682)
- Alternative meds (Ann IM 2002;137:805): Black cohosh, and soy phytoestrogens for 3-6 mo; of questionable value (RDBCT: Jama 2003;290:207)

Nipple Discharge

Nejm 2005;353:281

needs bx, endoscopy, or ductogram to r/o ductal carcinoma, unless multiductal or bilateral and hence is galactorrhea which itself needs w/u

Placenta Acreta

Cause: Unknown

Epidem: 1/1500 deliveries

Pathophys: Invasion into myometrium

Sx: Pain; antepartum hemorrhage

Si: Can't completely extract on manual removal of placenta

Cmplc: Uterine rupture with subsequent pregnancy

Rx: Manual removal of placenta; if fail, D + C; but gravid uterus easily perforated. May need D + C under direct vision (laparotomy) or hysterectomy if extensive.

Premenstrual Syndrome

Nejm 1995;332:829,1534 (RC trials by Hamilton, Ont), 1991;324:1208

Epidem: 3-8% prevalence in all U.S. women

Pathophys: All due to abnormal response to normal estrogen/progesterone changes during menstrual cycle (Nejm 1998;338:209)

Sx: Last 7 d of menstrual cycle; tension, irritability, dysphoria, bloating, edema, emotional lability, headache, breast swelling (imprecisely defined); r/o depression by at least 1 wk/mo without sx

Rx: Exercise works (endorphins)
Pyridoxine (B$_6$) (BMJ 1999;318:1375) 50 mg po qd-bid
Calcium, eg, Tums ii bid
SSRIs (Med Let 2001;43:5): Continuously or just last 2 wk of menstrual cycle
- Fluoxetine (Prozac) 20 mg po qd continuously helps by DBCT, reduces sx by 50%
- Paroxetine (Paxil) (Neuropsycho Pharm 1995;12:169)
- Sertraline (Zoloft) 50-100 mg po qd prevents by RC trial (Jama 1997;278:983)
  Tricyclics: Clomipramine (Anafranil) po qd
  Benzodiazepams: Aprazolam (Xanax) 0.25-1 mg po qid day 18 to 1st day of menses helps modestly (37% better compared to 30% in controls) (Jama 1995;279:51)
  Others often tried: Progesterone (no good evidence that helps: Med Let 1984;26:101); evening primrose? (prostaglandin precursor) 750 mg po bid; bcp's?; spironolactone; danazol; gonadotropin-releasing factor–blocking analog like leuprolide (Nejm 1998;338:209)

Rape Exam

Nejm 1995;332:234

W/u:
- Medical hx
- Evaluate and rx physical injuries; use only saline as speculum lubricant
- Culture for cervix, rectum, throat (gc only) for gc and chlamydia; sperm sample aspirate; test for hep B, syphilis, HIV, pregnancy, blood type
- Clothing, Wood's lamp exam for semen, then ask victim to place in plastic bag; pubic hair combings, subungual samples

Rx:
- Prophylactic antibiotics if indicated or requested:
  Ceftriaxone 125-250 mg im or spectinomycin 2 gm im; plus
      doxycycline 100 mg po bid × 7 d, or
  Azithromycin 1 gm po × 1 plus metronidazole 2 gm po × 1
- Immunize w Hep B vaccine and HBIG unless contraindicated
- Prevent pregnancy if appropriate w:
  50 μgm estradiol bcp's, or
  35 μgm estradiol bcp's po q 12 hr × 2
- Psychiatric support/counseling
- Report to police

F/u: In 2-4 wk

Vaginitis Causes

Nejm 1997;337:1896

Infectious:
- *Gardernella* vaginalis and other bacteria (p 550), 50%
- *Monilia* (p 191) (25%)

- *Trichomonas* (p 643) (20%)
- Foreign body, eg, tampon

Noninfectious:

- Atrophic in postmenopausal women
- Chemical irritant or traumatic
- Allergic, hypersensitiviy or contact

Chapter 12

Ophthalmology

D. K. Onion

12.1 Diseases

Acute Angle Closure Glaucoma

Cause: Genetic predisposition, hyperopia (farsightedness)

Epidem: ~0.2% of population; especially in middle-aged and elderly

Pathophys: Normally, aqueous humor is secreted in posterior chamber by the ciliary body, then goes through the pupil to the anterior chamber and out the trabecular meshwork at the scleral–iris junction. Congenital predisposition of a smaller eye and shallow anterior chamber w close apposition of iris and lens so that fluid is trapped where it is made behind the iris, which bows forward to cover the trabecular meshwork, blocking outflow. Secretion of aqueous humor then causes pressure to build, compressing first the optic nerve where the scleral cribosa is the weak point, leading to cupping and atrophy when chronic.

Sx: Onset usually at age > 50 yr. Precipitated by mydriatics, antacids, anesthesia, darkness. Rainbow halos often first sx, due to corneal edema; eye pain, sudden, often bilateral; headache, nausea and vomiting, scotomas in nasal fields causing blindness.

Si: Red eye, especially circumcorneal; partially dilated fixed pupil. Corneal edema, blistered and hazy; corneal pressure > 30

mm Hg, pressures > 18 mm Hg have a 65% sens/specif (Nejm 1993; 328:1097).

If chronic or recurrent attacks, optic disc is pale and cupped
Tonometry: 8-22 mm Hg = normal; 20-30 mm Hg = probably normal (only 3.5% will go on to glaucoma in 5 yr); > 30 mm Hg, much higher % go on to glaucoma

Crs:

Cmplc: Blindness; other eye affected within 5-10 yr in 40-80%, and use of pilocarpine does not protect

Lab:

Rx: Surgical laser iridotomy under local; may need pilocarpine 1-2% gtts q 5-10 min until relieved + systemic carbonic anhydrase inhibitor (acetazolamide 1 gm iv or 0.5 gm po stat) to lower pressure enough to allow laser rx

Other Glaucomas: Primary Open Angle; Secondary; Congenital

Nejm 1998;339:1298, 1993;328:1097 (open angle)

Cause: Open angle: gene on chromosome 1 (Nejm 1998;338:1022); often precipitated over 2-3 wk by systemic or topical steroids, including high- but not low- or medium-dose nasal or inhaled steroids (Jama 1997;277:722). Some may evolve out of the 10% over age 40 who have intraocular HT.
Secondary: Multiple (see Pathophys)
Congenital: Genetic

Epidem: Open angle: 2% of population age > 40 yr; most prevalent form in U.S.; more frequent in myopics, diabetics, relatives of pts w it, and the elderly; incidence in blacks is 6-8× that in whites (Nejm 1991;325:1418)
Congenital: Associated with big eyes (except microcornea); Sturge-Weber syndrome; neurofibromas; Marfan's syndrome; Pierre Robbin syndrome; tumors of eye; rubella syndrome; oculocerebrorenal syndrome (Lowe's)

Pathophys:
> Open angle: Gradual meshwork occlusion decreases fluid movement
>
> Secondary: Uveitis inflammation; traumatic bleeding in anterior chamber; diabetic neovascular membranes; post-op; exfoliation; elevated venous pressure; pigmentary; tumors; mature lens induced; ghost cells (old rbc's)

Sx: Open angle: Transient visual blurring; slow loss of bilateral visual sensitivity; no pain, no halos
> Secondary: Red eye, pain
>
> Congenital: Photophobia, manifested in child by tears and eye rubbing

Si: Open angle: Tunnel vision; cupped disc w cup/disc ratio > 0.3, usually > 0.7; intraocular pressures may be elevated or normal, high false-neg rates in Caucasians but not blacks
> Secondary: Debris in anterior chamber; red eye; corneal edema
>
> Congenital: Big hazy cornea, frequently bilateral

Crs: Open angle: 1-3% visual field loss/year

Cmplc: Blindness in all if untreated

Lab:

Xray:

Rx: Secondary: Rx the primary disease, eg, steroids for uveitis, laser rx of neovascularization, evacuate clot for acute traumatic
> Congenital: Surgical goniotomy or trabeculotomy by age 6 yr at latest, results in 90% success
>
> Open angle (Med Let 1996;38:100): All meds may have systemic side effects even though delivered locally (Ann IM 1990;112:120)
>> 1st: β-Blockers:
>> • Timolol 0.25-0.5% i gtt bid, or Timoptic XE qd; adverse effects: may have significant systemic absorption and effects, especially if pt is a genetically slow metabolizer or

there is concomitant po drug use like quinidine (Jama 1995;274:1611); $10/mo/eye
- Betaxolol (β-1 selective)
- Levobunolol (Med Let 1986;28:45)
- Metipranolol (Optipranolol) i gtt bid, cheapest (Med Let 1990;32:91)

  2nd: Prostaglandins: Latanoprost (Xalatan) 0.005% i gtt qd; cmplc: local irritation, brown pigmentation of iris; $25/mo/eye

  α-Adrenergic agonists: Brimonidine tartrate (Alphagen) i gtt bid; cmplc: beware in pts w arterial insufficiency

  Cholinergics: Pilocarpine at i gtt qid

  Carbonic anhydrase inhibitors:
- Acetazolamide 500 mg po bid or 250 mg qid
- Brinzolamide (Azopt) 1% i gtt tid
- Dorzolamide (Trusopt) (Med Let 1995;37:76) 2% i gtt tid, for chronic topical rx; or w timolol as Cosopt

  if fail, laser trabeculoplasty; or if not enough, surgerical trabeculectomy

Optic Neuropathies: Ischemic and Neuritis

Nejm 1992;326:634 (neuritis), 1978;299:533

Cause:

Ischemic: Arteritis, and non-urteritic eg rare cmplc of sildenafil (Viagra) and other similar drugs (Med Let 2005;47:49)

Optic neuritis: Half are idiopathic, half are due to multiple sclerosis

Epidem:

Ischemic: More common over age 50

Optic neuritis: Female/male > 2:1, between menarche and menopause; incidence = 6/100,000/yr

Pathophys:

Ischemic: Arteritis of posterior ciliary arteries

Sx:

Ischemic: Sudden blindness

Optic neuritis: Sudden uniocular, visual loss; painful eye on movement

Si:

Ischemic: Edema of disc and predisc, hemorrhages; pale disc later

Optic neuritis: Normal disc becomes pale and edematous but often normal if retrobulbar neuritis only; impaired color plate acumen; diminished pupillary reaction to light (Marcus Gunn pupil)

Crs:

Ischemic: 42% recover in 6 mo (Jama 1995;273:625)

Optic neuritis: 70% recover in 8 wk; up to 60% later develop MS over next 40 yr (Neurol 1995;45:244)

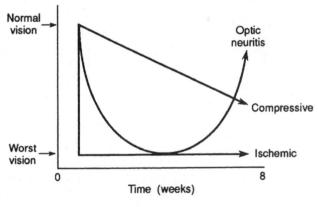

Figure 12.1 Course of optic nerve, compressive, and ischemic neuritis.

Cmplc:

>   Ischemic: 2nd eye often involved days to years later. r/o common
>   nonarteritic type under age 50, associated with diabetes,
>   hypertension
>
>   Optic neuritis: r/o MS (30-50% risk of it); compressive infiltra-
>   tive neuropathies from metastases of pituitary adenoma,
>   meningioma, glioma, internal carotid aneurysm, cranio-
>   pharyngioma, all of which have gradual visual loss and pale
>   disc, shunt vessels

Lab: *Hem:* Ischemic: ESR increased

>   *Path:* Ischemic: Temporal artery bx within 1 wk of starting
>   steroids
>
>   *Noninv:* Optic neuritis: Visual evoked responses decreased

Xray: Optic neuritis: CT of optic canals if no improvement in 6 wk to
r/o compressive nerve lesion

Rx:

>   Ischemic: Stat steroids if ESR elevated or positive temporal artery
>   biopsy; optic nerve surgical decompression may be harmful
>   (Jama 1995;273:625)
>
>   Optic neuritis (Neurol 2000;54:2039): 3 d of q 6 hr iv 250 mg
>   methylprednisolone, perhaps followed by 1 mg/kg po × 10 d,
>   speeds resolution, slightly reduces recurrences, and decreases
>   rate of MS over the next 2 yr (Nejm 1993;329:1764 vs 1993;
>   329:1808) but not over 5 yr and may increase optic neuritis
>   recurrence (Nejm 1992;326:581)

Cataracts

Jama 2003;290:248; Ann IM 1985;102:82

Cause: Age; occasionally steroids, even inhaled types increase risk
slightly (Jama 1998;280:539; Nejm 1997;337:8); diabetes; genetic
predisposition, accounts for 50% of incidence variance (Nejm
2000;342:1786); alcohol use; smoking; chronic lead exposure
(Jama 2004;292:2750)

Epidem: Increased with UVB (320-390 nm wavelength) exposure throughout life (Jama 1998;280:714; Nejm 1988;319:1429). 2nd most common cause of reversible visual loss after refractory error, esp in elderly.

Pathophys: Cortical and nuclear types associated with UVB, posterior types not. Posterior types related to steroid use.

Sx: Blurred vision, impaired near and far vision; glare and/or double vision, esp at night

Si: Opacity in lens seen with naked eye or in red reflex

Crs: Slowly progressive

Cmplc:

Lab:

Rx: UV protection, eg, brimmed hat and glasses (Nejm 1988;319:1429)

Cataract extraction and intraocular artificial lens implantation very successful (Med Let 1982;24:102) and reduces elderly car accidents by 50% (Jama 2002;288:841)

12.2 Miscellaneous

Corneal Burns

Acid/Alkali Burn

Sx & Si: Coagulation of corneal epithelium; acid superficially, alkali deeply

Rx: Irrigate/flush at pH 7 for hours with alkali burn even if looks ok; then long-term lubricants; steroids w ophthalmology consult

Tear Gas: eg, Mace (Nejm 1969;281:413)

Sx & Si: Pain, can cause permanent corneal damage

Rx: Irrigate as above

UV Burn

Sx & Si: Pain, h/o UV exposure; pitted cornea

Rx: Mydriatics, pressure eye patch × 24 hr

Blepharospasm

Rx: Botulism toxin im (Med Let 1990;32:100)

Chalazion (cyst of meibomian gland in eyelid)/HORDEOLUM (inflamed cyst, stye)

Rx: Chalazion w surgical excision; hordeolum (stye) w hot packs and topical antibiotics

Coping with Blindness

Devices available (Nejm 1981;305:458); reading machines (Med Let 1992;34:13); diurnal rhythms may be retained if retinohypothalamic tracts preserved (Nejm 1995;332:6)

Diplopia

Image is displaced maximally in direction of paralyzed muscle's pull. Oculomotor CN innervations; straight up and down are combinations of muscles; pure muscle movements are up and out, up and in, etc. (See Table 12.1.)

Foville's Syndrome

Part of posterior inferior cerebellar artery syndrome; paralysis of horizontal gaze, ipsilateral V impairment including taste on anterior tongue, VII dysfunction, VIII deficits, and ipsilateral Horner's

Internuclear Ophthalmoplegias

Lesions of medial longitudinal fasciculus (MLF), so that conjugate gaze impossible, medial rectus responds only on convergence; seen often in MS

Macular Degeneration

Age-related type (Nejm 2000;343:483)

Cause: Genetic ocular extracellular matrix protein mutations, especially of fibulin (Nejm 2004;351:320,346)

Epidem: Most common cause of severe visual loss in developed countries; present in 30%, 7% symptomatic prevalence over age 75. Associated w smoking (increases incidence 2.4-fold: Jama 1996; 276:1141,1147); obesity; hyperlipidemia; positive family hx; low antioxidant vitamins and zinc intake; Caucasians

Pathophys: Atrophic (90%) and neovascular (exudative; 10%) forms, the latter causes 90% of the severe vision loss. Perhaps an inflammatory element since CRP elevated (Jama 2004;291:704).

Sx: Decreased visual acuity

Si: Drüsen > 63 μM, retinal pigment epithelial atrophy or clumping in macula; loss of central but preservation of peripheral vision

Rx: Prevent perhaps w vitamins C, E, β-carotene, and/or zinc? (Arch Ophthalmol 2001;119:1417)

Laser rx of neovascular lesions; perhaps for neovascular type, marginally beneficial photodynamic rx w verteporfin (Visadyne) (Med Let 2000;42:81); $6000 for 4 treatments

Pegaptanib ocular injections (Med Let 2005;47:55; Nejm 2004;351:2805,2863) q 6 wk × 1 yr; an antiangiogenesis agent, NNT = 8-10 for severe visual loss by DBCTs, $1000/dose, $9000/yr

Table 12.1 Muscles Affecting Right Eye Movements and Their Innervations (Facing Patient)

Lateral	Medial
Superior rectus (CN III)	Inferior oblique (CN III)
Lateral rectus (CN VI)	Medial rectus (CN III)
Inferior rectus (CN III)	Superior oblique (CN IV)

OPHTHALMOLOGY

Myopia

Rv of LASIK, LASEK, PRK, CK, and intracorneal ring surgical techniques and success (Med Let 2004;46:5) and diagrams/illustrations (Nejm 2004;351:472)

Parinaud's Syndrome

Paralysis of upward gaze, convergence retraction, nystagmus, pupillary light/near dissociation, papilledema, lid retraction; seen in lesions of pineal and hydrocephalus

Red Eye, Acute

Nejm 2000;343:345

Foreign body (FB)/Corneal abrasion

Epidem: Most common

Sx & Si: Foreign body under lids or in cornea

Rx: Remove FB, then antibiotic cream × 24 hr; eye patch for comfort but does not change course (Ophthalm 1995;102:1936)

Conjunctivitis (Med Let 2004;46:25)

Cause: Viral especially adenovirus; allergic; bacterial, mostly unencapsulated pneumococcus in colder climates (Dartmouth students: Nejm 2003;348:1079,1112), anaerobic strep, *Haemophilus*, chlamydia, S. aureus, Moraxella

Epidem: 95% of remainder after FB. Viral type highly contagious.

Sx & Si: Feeling of sand in eye, morning secretions; palpebral and bulbar conjunctival injection, PERRLA and normal vision; preauricular lymph node in chlamydial type; itching is predominant sx in allergic type

Crs: Infectious types start in 1 eye, spread to the other; viral type is contagious for > 10 d

Cmplc: r/o gc infection if hyperacute

Rx (Med Let 2004;46:25):

Sulfacetamide 10%, cheap; polymyxin + Tm/S (Polytrim) gtts cidal rather than static and stings less than sulfa but $13 generic and $33 trade; or neomycin/polymyxin qid; or tobramycin or gentamicin 0.3% gtts qid, $7 generic, $30+ trade; or moxifloxacin (Vigamox) ½%, or gatifloxacin (Zymar) 0.3% tid, but both $45. Not chloramphenicol, which can lead to aplastic anemia. Oral tetracycline or macrolide for chlamydial type. Antibiotics do help shorten crs (Brit J Genl Pract 2001;51:473).

For allergic (Med Let 2004;46:35), topical:

- NSAID ketorlac (Acular) 0.5% I gtt qid (Med Let 1993;35: 88); $32/wk; or
- H_1 antihistamine levocabastine (Livostin) (Med Let 1994; 36:35) 0.05% i gtt qid, costs $22/2 wk, or similar emedastine (Emadine) I gtt qid ; or
- Mast cell stabilizers, cromolyn (Crolom) 4% i-ii gtts ou qid, $15/2 wk; or lodoxamine (Alomide) (Med Let 1994;36:26) 0.1% i-ii gtts qid, costs $14/2 wk; or nedocromil (Alocril); or pemirolast (Alamast)
- Mast cell stabilizer/H_1 antihistamine combos: Olopatadine (Patanol) 0.1% i-ii gtts ou bid, $17/wk; or ketotifen (Zaditor) bid, $14/wk; epinastine (Elestat) I gtt bid, $14/wk

Iritis: A form of uveitis

Causes: of anterior and posterior uveitis (Nejm 1978;299:130) (uvea = choroid, iris, and ciliary body): Idiopathic (1st), tbc, syphilis, histoplasmosis (often no bug in lesion), sarcoid, coccidioidomycosis, toxoplasmosis, rheumatoid arthritis especially in children or any inflammatory arthritis, anti-DNA and -RNA antibodies perhaps viral-related (Nejm 1971;285:1502), *H. simplex* and *zoster*, candida, hypermature cataract, trauma, intraocular tumor, Whipple's disease bacterium (Nejm 1995;332:363)

Epidem: 2% of remainder after FB

Sx & Si: Photophobia, eye ache, tenderness, tearing without exudate, visual blurring, turbid aqueous humor (wbc's and protein) or hypopyon, low pressure (5-10 mm Hg), miosis (constricted pupil), circumcorneal injection

Rx: Steroids topically, mydriatics like Cyclogyl to prevent iris–lens synechiae

Keratitis

Cause: *H. simplex* (50%) and other viruses (*H. zoster*, adenovirus), contact lenses especially overnight use (Nejm 1989;321:773,779), exanthems, bacterial, chronic topical anesthetic use (Nejm 1968;279:396)

Epidem: 1% of remainder after FB

Sx & Si: Photophobia, FB sensation; corneal ulcer (dendritic if herpetic), mixed-type injection, PERRLA, corneal wbc infiltrates

Cmplc: Achronic corneal neurotrophic ulcers

Rx: When *H. simplex,* 1st, trifluridine (Viroptic) 1 gtt 1% solution q 2 hr, or 2nd, Ara A; then consider prophylaxis w acyclovir 400 mg po bid × 12 mo, which decreases recurrence rates from 35% to < 20% (Nejm 1998;339:300)

When bacterial, appropriate antibiotics; mydriatics to relax ciliary spasm

In chronic corneal neurotrophic ulcers: Corneal transplant and/or perhaps topical nerve growth factor (Nejm 1998;338: 1174,1222)

Acute glaucoma (p 851)

Epidem: 1% of remainder after FB

Sx & Si: Halo, blurred vision, severe pain, headache and vomiting; steamed cornea, semidilated pupils, circumcorneal injection, hard eye (50-60 mm Hg)

Rx: Miotics, β blockers, and acetazolamide while awaiting surgery to keep angles open. Laser iridotomy.

Retinitis Pigmentosa

Cause: Genetic, autosomal dominant or recessive

Pathophys: Rhodopsin gene on chromosome 3 is mutated (Nejm 1990; 323:1302)

Sx: First night blindness, then tunnel vision. Late loss of color vision, and blind eye by age 50-60 yr.

Si: Optic nerve pallor, pigmentaton of retinal fundus, attenuated arteries

Subconjunctival Hemorrhage

Nejm 2000;343:345

Cause: Trauma (often minor) or coughing/vomiting, bleeding disorders

Sx: Usually just noticed, no pain

Si: Unilateral localized circumscribed hemorrhage obscuring underlying sclera; no conjunctivitis

Crs: Resolves in < 3 wk

Tracoma

Nejm 2004;351:1962

Cause: Chlamydia trachomatis

Pathophys: Chronic keratoconjunctivitis w corneal scarring

Rx: Azithromycin 2 mg/kg up to 1gm po × 1 q 6-12 mo to all, markedly decreases rates
Topical tetracycline ointment bid

Chapter 13

Pediatrics

D. K. Onion

13.1 Newborn Disorders

Erythroblastosis Fetalis

Cause: Maternal antibody, usually vs RhD, but now, w liberal Rhogam use, Kell antibodies account for 10% of all cases (Nejm 1998;338:798); transplacental passage of 7S (IgG) antibody

Epidem: Very rare now with Rhogam rx, better ob outcomes w fewer lower-birth-order children (Am J Pub Hlth 1998;88:209)

Pathophys: Fetal cells cross placenta, mostly at birth, and sensitize mother's immune system; antibody later, during subsequent pregnancies, crosses to hemolyze fetal rbc's although can occur even in 1st pregnancy. Antibody-coated rbc results in hemolysis and elevated bilirubin production, which postpartum, with acidosis and hypotension, can cause kernicterus, since unconjugated bilirubin can cross the blood–brain barrier and is toxic to the brain (Clin Perinatol 1988;15:4). Pre- and postpartum severe anemia causes CHF, called hydrops fetalis prepartum.

Kell antibodies cause not only hemolysis but also blocked erythropoietin effects on rbc precursors (Nejm 1998;338:798)

ABO incompatibility protects against Rh sensitization developing by eliminating incompatible cells quickly before sensitization can occur, ie, a sort of built-in Rhogam injection?

Sx: Spontaneous abortion at 26+ wk in woman with previous sensitizing pregnancy

Si: Postpartum anemia, jaundice, CHF, and hydrops fetalis

Crs:

Cmplc: Intrauterine hydrops fetalis; with kernicterus, spasticity, deafness, and other CNS damage; hypoglycemia, which can cause further CNS damage (Nejm 1968;278:1260)

r/o other neonatal jaundice causes (see below)

Lab: *Chem:* Bilirubin elevated (see Table 13.1, p 869); an indirect > 20 mg % can cause kernicterus (staining of brain); follow q 4 hr postpartum

Blood sugar; keep normal; hypoglycemia can worsen hepatic conjugation of bilirubin too

Amniotic fluid bilirubin elevated (Nejm 1970;282:1163); used to determine need for intrauterine exchanges

Hem: Coombs test positive, direct and indirect; retics low for 3-5 wk, no matter how anemic baby is

Serol: Mother's titer > 1/64 and increases from 1st to 3rd trimester; RhD PCR analysis of fetal DNA in maternal blood is reliable from 2nd trimester on (Nejm 1998; 339:1734)

Xray: Ultrasound detects anemia (Nejm 2000;342:9) and later fetal edema (Nejm 1986;315:430)

Rx: Prevent w Rhogam, about 1 cc within 72 hr of delivery if Rh-positive child or if abortion; adjust dose by Kleihauer-Bettke test of fetal rbc's in maternal circulation; 95% effective; give also at 28 wk gestation to get final 5%

Stop breastfeeding

Exchange transfusions, intrauterine (Nejm 1986;314:1431), or postpartum if cord bilirubin > 6 mg % or serum headed above 20 at > 0.5 mg %/h; cmplc include rare and mild graft-vs-host syndrome (Nejm 1969;281:697)

Neonatal Jaundice

Cause (Nejm 2001;344:581):

Indirect bilirubin elevations:

- Glucuronyl transferase deficiency:

    Normal in premature infant, especially if increased entero-hepatic circulation

    Congenital deficiency (Crigler-Najjar syndrome) rarely; rx w phototherapy, perhaps hepatocyte transplantation (Nejm 1998;338:1422)

- ABO and Rh (see above) incompatibility,
- Breast milk (pregnane-3α, 20α-diol)–induced jaundice, never needs rx no matter how high (Peds 1993;91:470)
- Hypothyroidism (cretin)
- Drug induced, eg, by excess vitamin K, or chloramphenicol (gray baby syndrome)

Direct bilirubin elevations:

- Infections:

    Bacterial sepsis

    Intrauterine infections like syphilis and TORCH (TOxoplasma, Rubella, CMV, Herpes) infections, which typically elevate LFTs and direct bilirubin

    Perinatally acquired infections like herpes, enteroviruses, hepatitis B

- Biliary obstruction

Epidem: Exaggerated physiologic jaundice more common in Asians, males, borderline preterm, poor feeders

Pathophys: More bilirubin production from increased rbc turnover and limited amounts of glucuronyl transferase, which attaches glucuronic acid to unconjugated, poorly water-soluble bilirubin so it can be excreted

Sx: Jaundice in newborn

Si: Icterus

Crs: Usually benign; Crigler-Najjar rapidly fatal although some variants can survive

Cmplc: Kernicterus (brain damage) with retardation and basal ganglia degeneration

Lab: *Chem:* Elevated bilirubin (see Table 13.1, p 869), indirect elevation > direct; up to 17 mg % in term infants in 1st wk of life can be normal

Rx: None at term if under 25 mg % unless prematurity, sick child where should rx > 20 mg % (Peds 1992;89:809, 1983;71:660)

     Feeding on demand, breast or bottle, decreases the enterohepatic recirculation of bilirubin

     Bilirubin lights (fluorescent white, blue, or green) isomerize bilirubin to hepatically excretable benign products (Med Let 1971;13:11)

     Exchange transfusions if lights not enough

Respiratory Distress Syndrome (Hyaline Membrane Disease)

Cause: Immature lungs from premature delivery, often exacerbated by maternal diabetes (Nejm 1976;294:357)

Epidem: Prematurity associated with familial asthma in mother and child (Nejm 1985;312:742)

Pathophys: Surfactant deficiency or inhibition allows collapse of alveoli; plasma exudate forms membrane (Nejm 1971;284:1185)

Sx: Onset at 0-4 hr postpartum

Si: Grunting respirations, tachypnea, intercostal retractions, atelectasis, ductus murmur, flaring

Crs: Worsens over first 24-28 hr, then resolves over 5-7 d

Cmplc: Bronchopulmonary dysplasia chronic lung disease in many from O_2 rx with scarring, and barotrauma (Nejm 1990;323:1793), perhaps helped w inhaled steroids (Nejm 1999;340:1005,1036); pneumothorax; diaphragmatic hernia; patent ductus arteriosus, especially with fluid overload (Nejm 1983;308:743), rx with

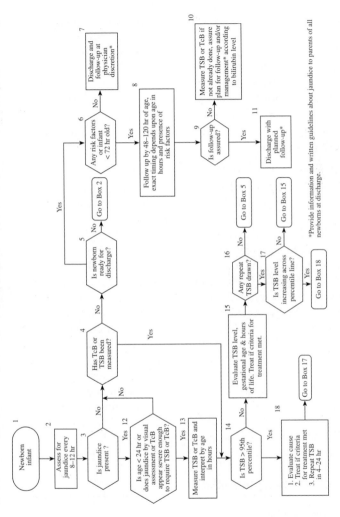

Figure 13.1 Algorithm for the management of jaundice in the newborn nursery. Reproduced with permission from subcommittee on hyperbilirubinemia. Management of hyperbilirubinemia in newborn infants 35 or more weeks of gestation. Peds 2004:114:297.

1. Newborn infant
2. Assess for jaundice every 8–12 hr
3. Is jaundice present?
12. Is age < 24 hr or does jaundice by visual assessment or TcB appear severe enough to require TSB or TcB?
13. Measure TSB or TcB and interpret by age
4. Has TcB or TSB been measured?
5. Is newborn ready for discharge?
6. Any risk factors or infant < 72 hr old?
7. Discharge and follow-up at physician discretion*
8. Follow up by 48–120 hr of age, exact timing depends upon age in hours and presence of risk factors
9. Is follow-up assured?
10. Measure TSB or TcB if not already done, assure plan for follow-up and/or management* according to bilirubin level
11. Discharge with planned follow-up*
14. Is TSB > 95th percentile?
15. Evaluate TSB level, gestational age & hours of life. Treat if criteria for treatment met.
16. Any repeat TSB drawn?
17. Is TSB level increasing across percentile line?
18.
   1. Evaluate cause
   2. Treat if criteria for treatment met
   3. Repeat TSB in 4–24 hr

Go to Box 2
Go to Box 5
Go to Box 15
Go to Box 18
Go to Box 17

*Provide information and written guidelines about jaundice to parents of all newborns at discharge.

indomethacin (Nejm 1984;310:565); retinopathy of prematurity, especially in low-birth-weight (< 1 kg) premies exposed to high light levels in NICUs (Nejm 1985;313:401) or 100% O_2 levels w pO_2 levels > 80 mm Hg for > 12 hr (Nejm 1992;326:1050)

r/o TTN (transient tachypnea of newborn), a benign and common condition; group B strep and other infections; congenital heart disease and other anomalies

Lab: *Chem:* Blood gases show respiratory acidosis, hypoxia; suspect if FiO_2 requirement > 40%

Xray: Chest shows air bronchograms, "ground glass" appearance

Rx: Prevent w steroids between 28 and 32 wk if threatened premature delivery; but not helpful for low-birth-weight infants (Nejm 2001;344:95). Avoid steroids postpartum because diminishes school performance eventually (Nejm 2004;350:1304).

Surfactant prophylaxis endotracheally (Med Let 1990;32:2; Nejm 1988;319:476) at least in infants ≤ 26 wk is better than waiting for sx to start (Nejm 1991;324:867, 1991;325:1696); long term, at 1 yr, use shows no benefit (Nejm 1991;325:1696, 1989;320:959) in morbidity but survival is 30% better and costs less (Nejm 1994;330:1476). Ligation of ductus arteriosus prophylactically if < 1 kg (Nejm 1989;320:1511). Inositol in TPN of premature infants × 5 d helps (Nejm 1992;326:1233).

Support by keeping warm (hypothermia causes bronchoconstriction); $D_{10}W$ at 80-160 cc/kg/24 hr to maintain glucose homeostasis, may need volume infusions to maintain BP or perfusion; continuous positive airway pressure (CPAP) breathing via endotrach tube with surfactant (Nejm 1994;331:1051) or liquid perflubron (Nejm 1996;335:761)

13.2 Congenital Syndromes

Cleft Palate and Lip

Cause: Genetic, but lip alone is separate genetically from isolated cleft palate; plus perhaps in utero environmental factors (vitamin deficiencies cause in rats); autosomal recessive; recurrence in subsequent siblings ~3%, much lower if different father, no change if mother changes town of residence, hence genetic not environmental (Nejm 1995;333:161)

Epidem: 1/1000 Caucasian births, 1/5000 black births; 3rd most common congenital anomaly after club feet and radiologic spina bifida. Increased incidence in inbred populations; associated (25%) with other anomalies too.

    50% are lip and palate, 25% lip alone (male > female), 25% palate alone (female > male)

Pathophys: Failure of maxilla and nasal fusion in midline

Sx: Poor suck

Si: Cleft

Crs:

Cmplc: Social; malocclusion; chronic otitis and hearing loss from eustachian tube dysfunction; mechanical speech problems; FTT from poor caloric intake or associated anomalies

Lab:

Rx: Test hearing and refer to ENT, or government-run cleft lip program available in most states

    Feed with special nipples; speech rx post-op emphasizing hard consonants; blowing exercises through mouth (pinwheel, wind instrument)

    Surgical timing is controversial, some say repair at age 6 wk if lip alone; at age 14 wk if palate involved too; but must repair before start speech

    Dental prosthesis

Down's Syndrome

Cause: Defective chromosome 21; new translocation (3% of all), or congenital trisomy (97%); of the latter, 95% are maternal, 5% paternal (Nejm 1991;324:872)

Epidem: 1/650 live births; increased in mothers age > 35 yr. Associated Alzheimer's disease in families, especially premature Alzheimer's (Ann IM 1985;103:566) and correlates with amyloid A_4 protein excess production and deposition (Nejm 1989;320: 1446).

Pathophys: Usually group G trisomy of chromosome 21 (97% overall, 90% when mother age < 35 yr). Translocations: 50% are chromosome 21 to a D (13-15), associated with parental chromosome abnormalities most of the time, mothers are carrier 95% of time, fathers 5%; or 50% are to a G (20-22) and in that circumstance < 5% of time do parents have abnormal chromosome prep. In mothers age < 35 yr, 10-15% are such G translocations.

Short 5th finger and toe due to middle phalanx failure to calcify normally and late-onset maturation arrest (P. Gerald 1968)

Sx: Mongoloid appearance, floppy, retarded

Si: Findings subtle at birth and become more apparent late: hypotonia; developmental delay; short, brachycephalic with excess skin on the back of the neck; hypoplastic midface bones; single palmar crease, epicanthal fold (50%); Brushfield's spots (white) on iris (present in 10% of normals too); short 5th finger and toes; duodenal obstruction in many, especially from atresia and ring pancreas; low-set, hypoplastic ears; heart murmurs and congenital heart disease, especially atrial septal defect (in 25%); imperforate anus (3%); umbilical hernia; tachycardia and pupillary sensitivity to atropine (Nejm 1968;279:407)

Crs:

Cmplc: Odontoid ligament laxity causing C_1 on C_2 dislocation as in rheumatoid arthritis (Peds 1992;89:1194); leukemia; increased infection rates; increased Hashimoto's thyroiditis (get TSH q 1 yr); increased gluten enteropathy

r/o D-1 (13-15) trisomies with elevated fetal hemoglobin, decreased A_2 hemoglobin, polydactyly, cleft palate, eye defects

(Nejm 1967;277:953); E (17-18) trisomy with many Mongoloid-type changes and associated with congenital biliary atresia; perhaps a viral etiology (Nejm 1969;280:16)

Lab: *Hem:* Chromosome prep shows trisomy or translocation
Serol: SPEP shows diffuse increased globulin

Xray: Hip films show horizontal acetabulum. Skull films, facial and sphenoid views show hypoplasia; bronchogram show "pig bronchus," ie, one ending in a blind pouch.

Rx: Prevention (Nejm 2003;349:1405; Am J Pub Hlth 1998;88:551); many of these tests can be used in combination (Nejm 1999;341:461, 521) to increase sens and specif, positive results < 1/250 chance of trisomy resulting in amnio or chorionic sampling. At 15 wk gestation, 5% sens and 90% specif of first 3 in combo:

- α-Fetoprotein (low in Down's) under age 35 yr, w 2nd trimester, alone, or as "triple test" w
- HCG β subunit and
- Unconjugated estriol
- Protein (inhibin) A levels perhaps combined w above and US of neck, in 1st trimester (Nejm 2003;349:1405, 1998;338:955)
- Karyotype analysis by amniocentesis if over 35 yr or when risk calculated from these results > 1/250 (equivalent to risk at age 35 yr); this strategy equalizes risk of Down's vs abortion from amnio (Nejm 1994;330:1114, 1151)
- Ultrasound in 2nd trimester, which can detect 60-75% by neck skin thickness but specif ~ 25% (Nejm 1997;327:1654) or as low as 0.00015% in normal women or 0.002% in high-risk women! (Jama 2001;285:1044); and by femur length (Nejm 1987;317:1371)
- Chorionic villus sampling now almost as safe as amnio, and abortion can be done much earlier, eg, in 1st trimester (Nejm 1989;320:7), then w 2nd trimester abortion (Nejm 1979;

300:157: useful table of incidence by maternal age); amniocentesis has a 0.3% false-positive rate. Half of fetuses with Down's at 15 wk gestation will spontaneously abort or die perinatally; 1.5% abort after amniocentesis (Nejm 1979;300:118: ethical discussion).

Primary care:

Of newborn: Confirm clinical suspicion w karyotype; cardiac consultation on all; hearing screen, thyroid studies, CBC; early intervention program and parental support group referral

of child: Annual thyroid screen, cervical spine films at 3 and 12 yr prn long tract si's or sx; periodic hearing and ENT assessment; periodic ophthalmologic exam; dental visits begin at age 2 yr

Hirschsprung's Disease

Cause: In familial forms, inactivation mutation in REI proto-oncogene, like type II MEN (Nejm 1995;335:943)

Epidem: Usually in infants; male/female = 1:4

Pathophys: Aganglionic segment of colon, variable in length from a few cm in rectum to all of rectum and descending colon. No sympathetic neurons in this segment, resulting in constant contractions and no relaxation, which is necessary for effective peristalsis, and this results in intestinal obstruction, acute (infants) or chronic (children and teenagers).

Sx: Abdominal pain, chronic constipation without the occasional "huge stools" typical of retentive encopresis

Si:

Crs:

Cmplc: Enterocolitis, most common cause of death
r/o Chagas' disease; chronic idiopathic intestinal obstruction (Nejm 1977;297:233); other malfunction of sphincters with which pts can be operantly conditioned to control stool (Nejm 1974;290:646)

Lab: *Path:* Rectal bx aganglionic

Rx: Surgical excision of affected segments or bypass that segment

Phenylketonuria (PKU)

Nejm 1980;303:1336,1394

Cause: Genetic, autosomal recessive; several different mutations, each with different severity implications (Nejm 1986;314:1276) from mild asx phenylalaninemia to severe PKU

Epidem: 1-7/100,000 newborns (Peds 2000;105:e10); 1.2/100,000 adults (Nejm 1970;282:1455)

Pathophys: Deficiency of hepatic phenylalanine hydroxylase (converts phenylalanine [PheAla] to tyrosine) causes buildup of PheAla in all body tissues, which in turn leads somehow to mental retardation

Sx: Mental retardation; seizures; behavior problems

Si: Retarded, pale, eczema, blond hair; in adult, psychoses often, even if mentally normal (Nejm 1973;289:395)

Crs:

Cmplc: Mental retardation in 100% of offspring of affected women unless level kept < 10 mg % (Jama 2000;283:756; Nejm 1983;309:1269)

Lab: *Chem:* Phenylalanine level > 20 mg % is diagnostic; if > 2 mg %, repeat it; if < 2 mg %, no need for further testing, even if done on 1st day of life and not having eaten yet (Nejm 1981;304:294). Persistent, low (< 12 mg %) elevation has no intelligence-impairing effect (Nejm 1971;285:424).

Rx: Prevent by screening heel blood samples for PheAla once at age 1-3 d (Nejm 1979;300:606); find treated PKU girls at age 12 to counsel about keeping level < 10 during pregnancy to avoid having children with mental retardation (Am J Pub Hlth 1982;72:1386; Nejm 1980;303:1202). Refer all positive screens to tertiary care center.

Diet low in PheAla, commercially prepared; the earlier it is started, the less the retardation; restriction up to age 8 or 10 yr results in higher IQs (Nejm 1986;314:593)

Tetrahydrobiopterin po qd may decrease PKU levels and allow pts w mild form to relax diet (Nejm 2002;347:2122)

Pyloric Stenosis

Cause: Genetic? Sex-linked?

Epidem: Males > females; 10% of affected fathers' offspring will have, 50% of affected mothers' children will have; 1/100-1/600 births. Associated w erythromycin use in infancy? (Lancet 1999; 354:2101)

Pathophys: Concentric muscular hypertrophy of pyloric smooth muscle, in which nitric oxide synthetase deficiency precipitates the disease (Nejm 1992;327:511)

Sx: Well and gaining weight for first 3-5 wk of life, then develop projectile vomiting without bile in it

Si: "Olive" in right upper quadrant by palpation in 70%

Crs: Benign with surgical repair

Cmplc: r/o annular pancreas (rx with duodenojejunostomy); duodenal atresia; Addisonian crisis due to congenital adrenal hypoplasia; antral diaphragm

Lab: *Chem:* Lytes show hypochloremic, hypokalemic alkalosis

Xray: Ultrasound; UGIS only if mass not seen or felt, to confirm dx

Rx: Surgery

Undescended (Cryptorchid) Testicle

Nejm 1986;314:510

Cause:

Epidem: 2-3% of term babies, decreases to 0.7% at age 1 without treatment, then prevalence is flat thereafter

Pathophys:

Sx:

Si: Unilateral in 75%, bilateral in 25%; most have associated inguinal hernia

Crs: Sterility, questionably prevented by early operation

Cmplc: Cancer in affected and contralateral testicles, increased 20-40x; higher with higher inguinal canal location even postop; cellular changes within 6-12 mo of nondescent

   r/o retractile (normal) nonscrotal testicle that can be manipulated to bottom of scrotum; virilized female prepubertally w serum Müllerian inhibiting substance level, which is present in boys but not girls, w 92% sens, 98% specif (Nejm 1997;336:1480)

Lab: (See Figure 13.2, p 878)

Rx: Surgery by age 1 yr
   Hormonal rx with HCG or GnRH not much help (Nejm 1986;314:466,510)
   Educate teenagers to do careful testicular self-exam

Boys with bilateral undescended testes (normal phallus)

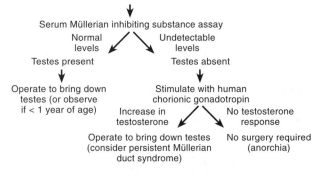

Children with intersexual disorders (ambiguous genitalia)

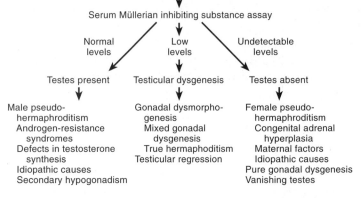

Figure 13.2 Interpretation of the assay of serum Müllerian inhibiting substance in the evaluation of boys with bilateral undescended testes or children with intersexual disorders. Reproduced with permission from Lee MM, et al. Measurements of serum mullerian inhibiting substance in the evaluation of children with nonpalpable gonads. New Eng J Med 1997:336:1480. Copyright 1997 Mass. Medical Society, all rights reserved.

13.3 Orthopedics

Congenital Dysplasia of Hip (Developmental Dysplasia of the Hip)

Peds 1964;34:554

Cause: Perhaps a genetic defect, autosomal dominant

Epidem: < 5/1000 births; female/male = 8:1; winter incidence twice summer incidence by birthdays; positive family hx in $\frac{1}{3}$; increased incidence in Mediterraneans and Scandinavians, in firstborns, and 8× higher if breech delivery

Pathophys: Acetabular defect with shallow, vertically sloping roof and infolded glenoid; weight bearing results in anteversion of femoral neck, which progresses to DJD and eventually to subluxation and/or dislocation

Sx: H/o breech delivery (12-20%). Limp.

Si: In newborn, only finding may be positive subluxation provocation test (Barlow test; subluxation of femoral head with adduction and posterior pressure on femur); Ortolani test, relocates with a "clunk" w hips flexed 90° abducted and anterior pressure up on greater trochanters; telescopic femoral movement with hip at 90° (< 1% false neg, 80% false pos). May have short leg unilaterally; asymmetric buttock folds; wide perineum. Hip abduction often is limited (normal is 90° at birth when hip flexed).

   In walking child, limp and positive Trendelenburg's test unilaterally

Crs: 95% resolved with only conservative rx at 3 yr f/u

Cmplc: Adductor contractures; DJD
   r/o similar hip dysfunctions caused by meningomyelocele and cerebral palsy adductor spasm/contractures

Lab:

Xray: Ultrasound under 3 mo age since no secondary center of ossification yet

Plain films will miss dx in 25%. Femoral epiphysis ossification center smaller, higher, and more lateral relative to acetabular center; acetabular roof obliquity pronounced, > 30°; neck/shaft angle widened, ie, becomes more vertical.

Rx: < 1 mo age: Abduction splint or brace (Pavlok Harness) for weeks or months until xray shows improvement or can no longer dislocate. Best to rx if any doubt; will have 80% false positive by clinical exam. Double diapering inadequate.

Older child: Spica cast in abduction after closed reduction

Adult: Wait until sx's, then crutches, corset, decreased activity, then surgical total hip

Legg-Perthes Disease (Coxa Plana)

Nejm 1992;326:1473

Cause: Unknown

Epidem: Children age 4-9; males > females

Pathophys: Avascular necrosis of proximal femoral epiphysis for unknown reason

Sx: Vague h/o intermittent ache around thigh and/or knee (think of in any child c/o knee pain); limp; avoids running; occasionally bilateral

Si: Internal rotation limited; pain with motion; positive Trendelenburg's test; limp; late, muscle atrophy and leg shortening

Crs: With rx, resolves over many months

Cmplc: DJD of hip; r/o slipped capital femoral epiphysis and other causes of limping child in same age group (p 908)

Lab:

Xray: Widened, irregular epiphyseal line; later increased density of femoral epiphysis; then flattened femoral head ossification center; then sclerotic head with cystic appearance, fragmentation, revascularization; and finally bone abnormalities of coxa magna and flattened articular surface

Rx: In incomplete femoral head involvement, observation and limited activity are usually all that are needed

With whole-head involvement, place in abduction/internal rotation brace while revascularizes

In severe cases, eliminate weight bearing for 2-3 yr while revascularizes. If unilateral, "Perthes sling" = ischial weight bearing with built-up shoe; rarely used now.

Scoliosis

Bull Rheum Dis 1987;37(6):1; Nejm 1986;314:1379

Cause: Genetic, at least in 30% (positive family hx); autosomal dominant; polygenic

Epidem: Female/male = 4:1. 10% of population have minor abnormalities, 1.5% have significant abnormalities, 0.5% need rx. Worldwide. Increased in ballet-trained children (Nejm 1986; 314:1348,1379).

Pathophys: Perhaps due to unequal development of vertebral growth plates, or unequal muscle and ligamentous balance

Sx: Onset at age 9-13, usually asx

Si: Most have thoracic curve convex to R, lumbar to L; hump appears on one side when bent over (razor back deformity) with high, usually R shoulder; asymmetric scapulae; plumb line from posterior neck when standing misses gluteal cleft; when standing, space between arm and body is asymmetric comparing R to L

Screen for lateral hump when bent over using leveling device across back (scoliometer; measures rib rotation); refer to orthopedist if > 15° and still in early puberty; screening efficacy unclear (Jama 1999;282:1427; USPSTF: Jama 1993;269:2667)

Crs: Gradual progression in curvature until skeletal maturity by age 18

Cmplc: Deformity; respiratory compromise
r/o leg length discrepancy

Lab:

Xray: Rarely indicated, can be used to follow care despite radiation

Rx: Minor (< 15-20° by scoliometer): Recheck q 3 mo
Intermediate (20-30°): To prevent increase esp in preadolescent
girls, thoracolumbarsacral orthosis or Milwaukee brace; adverse effects: protrusion of incisors
Severe (30-40°): Surgical placement of Harrington rods

13.4 Infectious/Acquired Diseases

Attention Deficit/Hyperactivity Disorder (ADHD)

Nejm 2005;352:165; Jama 2004;292:619

Cause: Genetic? Multifactorial? 25% of cases have h/o ADHD in a
parent.

Epidem: 3-5% of adults and children; male/female = 2:1 in children,
1:1 in adolescents, 1:2 in adults; high (50%) prevalence in
special-education students (Am J Pub Hlth 1998;88:881), and in
adults w addictions, motor vehicle violations, and life failures
Associated with lead burden, poverty, familial chaos,
Tourette's syndrome (60% of Tourette's have ADHD), and positive family hx

Pathophys: Perhaps metabolic dysfunction in the brain. Decreased
glucose metabolism in brain areas associated with attention and
motor activity by PET (Nejm 1990;323:1361). Neurotransmitter
imbalance? Sugar or aspartame in diet does not correlate w behavioral worsening (Nejm 1994;330:301). Worsened by psychosocial deprivation.

Sx: Inattention, hyperactivity, impulsivity, aggression. In trouble with
peers, parents, and/or school; underachievers in school from poor
self-esteem.

Table 13.1   Diagnostic Criteria for Attention Deficit/ Hyperactivity Disorder*

A. Either (1) or (2):

  1. Inattention: 6 (or more) of the following symptoms of inattention have persisted for at least 6 mo to a degree that is maladaptive and inconsistent with developmental level:

    a. Often fails to give close attention to details or makes careless mistakes in schoolwork, work, or other activities

    b. Often has difficulty sustaining attention in tasks or play activities

    c. Often does not seem to listen when spoken to directly

    d. Often does not follow through on instructions and fails to finish schoolwork, chores, or duties in the workplace (not due to oppositional behavior or failure to understand instructions)

    e. Often has difficulty organizing tasks and activities

    f. Often avoids, dislikes, or is reluctant to engage in tasks that require sustained mental effort (such as schoolwork or homework)

    g. Often loses things necessary for tasks or activities (eg, toys, school assignments, pencils, books, or tools)

    h. Is often easily distracted by extraneous stimuli

    i. Is often forgetful in daily activities

  2. Hyperactivity-impulsivity: 6 (or more) of the following symptoms of hyperactivity-impulsivity have persisted for at least 6 mo to a degree that is maladaptive and inconsistent with developmental level:

    a. Often fidgets with hands or feet or squirms in seat

    b. Often leaves seat in classroom or in other situations in which remaining seated is expected

    c. Often runs about or climbs excessively in situations in which it is inappropriate (in adolescents or adults, may be limited to subjective feelings of restlessness)

    d. Often has difficulty playing or engaging in leisure activities quietly

    e. Is often "on the go" or often acts as if "driven by a motor"

    f. Often talks excessively

    g. Often blurts out answers before questions have been completed

    h. Often has difficulty awaiting turn

    i. Often interrupts or intrudes on others (eg, butts into conversations or games)

B. Some hyperactive-impulsive or inattentive symptoms that caused impairment were present before age 7 yr

C. Some impairment from the symptoms is present in 2 or more settings (eg, at school [or work] and at home

Table 13.1 (continued)

D. There must be clear evidence of clinically significant impairment in social, academic, or occupational functioning

E. The symptoms do not occur exclusively during the course of a pervasive developmental disorder, schizophrenia, or other psychotic disorder and are not better accounted for by another mental disorder (eg, mood disorder, anxiety disorder, dissociative disorder, or a personality disorder)

Diagnostic and Statistical Manual of Mental Disorders, Fourth Edition, code based on type: 314.01 Attention Deficit/Hyperactivity Disorder, Combined Type: if both criteria A(1) and A(2) are met for the past 6 months; 314.00 Attention Deficit/ Hyperactivity Disorder, Predominantly Inattentive Type: if criterion A(1) is met but criterion A(2) is not met for the past 6 months; 314.01 Attention Deficit/Hyperactivity Disorder, Predominantly Hyperactive-Impulsive Type: If criterion A(2) is met but criterion A(1) is not met for the past 6 months. Coding note: For individuals (especially adolescents and adults) who currently have symptoms that no longer meet full criteria, "In Partial Remission" should be specified.
Reproduced with permission from Goldman LS, et al. Diagnosis and treatment of attention deficit/hyperactivity disorder in children and adolescents. J Am Med Assoc 1998; 279:1110. Copyright 1998 American Medical Association, all rights reserved.

Si: Short attention span; poor inhibitory control; aimless restlessness

Crs: Onset usually before school age at least before age 7; 8-10% (Jama 1995;273:1871) continue to have problems in adulthood

Cmplc: Learning disabilities in 25%; conduct (lying, stealing, fights) or oppositional disorders (disobedience, defiance, rule breaking) in 40%, but only if other comorbid dx's; depression/bipolar d/o. Parental discord/divorce.

r/o abuse/neglect, sleep d/o, lead toxicity, learning disability, petit mal seizures, substance abuse, depression, PTSD

Lab:

Rx (Nejm 2005;352:165):

Very complicated teacher/parent/child psychosocial dynamics usually present; best strategy when requested to prescribe meds is to request a school "individual education plan" evaluation that will pay for a multidisciplinary clinic evaluation and result in less unnecessary medication rx (S. Sewall 10/95)

Behavioral modification strategies not clearly helpful (Nejm 1999;340:780). Training in social skills. Remedial education. Parental support systems; sugar intake does not increase hyperactivity in normal or ADHD child (Jama 1995;274:1617).

Medications (Med Let 2001;43:83; Nejm 1999;340:780), clearly help in short term (Jama 1998;279:1100), useful into adulthood; response to meds does not prove dx

1st: Methylphenidate (Ritalin) 2.5-10 mg po q-tid, or as slow-release tabs (Ritalin SR, Concerta, and others) at 10-18 mg po qd under age 10 and 20-36 mg po qd over age 10, $30/mo. Or as dexmethylphenidate (Focalin) (Med Let 2002;44:45) 10 mg po bid 4 hr apart; $55/mo.

2nd: Dextroamphetamine (Dexedrine) 2.5-5 mg po q-tid or as qd spansules, $20/mo. Or as racemic amphetamine mixture (Adderal).

3rd: Atomoxetine (Strattera) (Med Let 2003;45:11) 1.2 mg/kg up to 100 mg po qd; a nonstimulating selective norepinephrine reuptake inhibitor, usually not as effective as the older drugs but can be if pt experiences intolerable side effects or fails to respond to multiple stimulants, so use if they fail (MedLet 2004;46:65); $100/mo

3rd: Bupropion (Wellbutrin) 100-200 mg SR bid in adults; not approved for children; lowers seizure threshold

Last: Pemoline (Cylert) 5-6 mo po qd; rarely used because of unpredictable severe hepatotoxicity even if safely used for years; get consent and q 2 wk LFTs; $40/mo

Other adjunctive meds:

• Antidepressants (tricyclics) like desipramine (Norpramin) but potential sudden death and other cardiac toxicity esp when used w stimulants; or

• Clonidine po or patch (Med Let 1996;38:109); but also has sudden death risk, as well as OD potential in younger siblings w even one 0.1 mg pill

Croup (Acute Laryngotracheobronchitis)

Nejm 1994;331:285, 322

Cause: Parainfluenza virus most commonly, respiratory syncytial virus (p 896), and others

Epidem: Incidence 3/100 under age 6 yr, most age 1-3; 1.3% must be hospitalized; males > females (Jama 1998;279:1630)

Pathophys: Perhaps 2 types, or may be just 2 ends of a spectrum:
- Acute laryngotracheitis follows 2-3 d of cold/cough
- Spasmodic croup, sx without antecedents and probably represents a hypersensitivity reaction to a virus (Am J Dis Child 1983;137:941)

Sx:

Si: Barking cough (seal-like), tachypnea, hoarseness, inspiratory stridor, intercostal muscle retractions; when severe, cyanosis and/or altered level of consciousness

Crs: Vast majority are self-limited

Cmplc: r/o foreign body, epiglottitis, bacterial tracheitis especially diphtheria, congenital anomaly (vascular ring), whooping cough (p 543)

Lab:

Xray: Soft tissue AP of neck shows "steeple sign," a narrowing of air column in trachea as it approaches the larynx

Rx: Mist tent or just humidified O_2, racemic epinephrine by neb or IPPB q 2 hr but watch for rebound

Steroids (BMJ 2000;319:595; Jama 1998;279:1630; Peds 1995;66:220), at least for hospitalized pts or to prevent hospitalization but appears to also speed healing and help even mild cases (Nejm 2004;351:1306)

- Dexamethasone 0.3-0.6 mg/kg im/iv/po single dose
- Budesonide (Pulmicort) 2-4 mg in 4 cc neb; only half as effective as dexamethasone but still much better than placebo (Nejm 1998;339:498)

Kawasaki's Disease

Peds 2004;114:1706; Nejm 1992;326:1246, 1991;324:1664

Cause: Unknown

Epidem: Incidence = 5-8/100,000/yr

Pathophys: A vasculitis of medium-sized vessels and a mucocutaneous lymph node disease

Sx: Prolonged high fever, variety of rashes, red eyes, nodes

Si: Fever in children age 1-8 yr, nonpitting edema, cervical lymphadenopathy, and desquamation of skin especially palms, perineal area, trunk, lips, as well as nonexudative conjunctivitis, and "strawberry" tongue (pictures: Nejm 1995;333:1391)

Crs:

Cmplc: 25% get coronary artery aneurysms later
          r/o measles, scarlet fever, RMSF, leptospirosis, EBV, JRA

Lab: *Hem:* ESR, platelets, and wbc elevated

Rx: IgG to prevent complications (Nejm 1986;315:342,388), 2 gm/kg iv over 10 hr × 1 (Nejm 1991;324:1633)

Reye's Syndrome

Nejm 1999;340:1377, 1984;311:1539, 1983;309:133; Am J Pub Hlth 1983;73:1063

Cause: Unknown; precipitated by salicylates during chickenpox or influenza/URI (Nejm 1985;313:849)

Epidem: In U.S., 555 cases/yr in 1980, now very rare, < 40 with shift away from aspirin use

Pathophys: Perhaps a mitochondrial dysfunction; some cases may be a urea cycle defect

Sx: H/o URI, varicella, or influenza A or B 5-6 d before, or salicylate use (in 15/31). Acute onset, recurrent vomiting with mental status changes (encephalopathy).

Si: Grade I: Sleepy but respond
Grade II: Stuporous
Grade III to IV: Increasing obtundation to coma

Crs: Grade I's survive; 10% of grade II's progress; grade III's and IV's die

Cmplc: r/o other inborn metabolic disorders by liver bx

Lab:

Chem: Elevated ammonia level $\geq$ 100 μgm %; protime > 3 sec, prolonged predicts progression (Nejm 1984;311:1539); ALT and AST; bilirubin normal; glucose low

CSF: Normal except for elevated pressures

Path: Liver bx is diagnostic, shows lipid droplets, decreased succinic acid dehydrogenase, and smashed mitochondria; on EM, SER proliferation

Rx: D_{10} 1/2 S with K^+ at 1500 cc/m^2/d to replete volume and liver glycogen stores; vitamin K

Neuroblastoma and Retinoblastoma

Nejm 1991;325:1608, 1991;324:464, 1985;312:1500

Cause: Retinoblastoma, in 10-15%, is genetic, autosomal recessive; other neuroblastoma is rarely genetic

Epidem: Both, like Wilm's tumor of childhood, associated with in utero radiation exposure (Nejm 1985;312:541)
Other neuroblastoma, male/female = 33:23

Pathophys: Retinoblastoma originates in retina; acts autosomal dominant but really is recessive; develops tumor when normal arm of chromosome 13 is dropped (Nejm 1984;310:550) ("2-hit" theory)
Adrenal medulla origin

Malignancy correlates with the number of N-*myc* oncogene chromosome copies (Nejm 1996;334:231, 1993;328:847, 1985;313:1111) as well as allelic loss of chromosome 1p (Nejm 1996;334:225)

Sx: Positive family hx in 10% w retinoblastoma
In other neuroblastomas, 50% are < age 1 yr; 75% are < 3 yr (75%)

Si: In retinoblastoma, strabismus; "cat's eye" light reflex; bilateral in 30%
In other neuroblastomas, abdominal mass; Horner's syndrome; thoracic mass; hepatomegaly

Crs: In retinoblastoma, peak mortality at age 2-3 yr; 81% survival; rarely metastatic
In other neuroblastoma:
Stage I: Localized to organ of origin
Stage II: Node negative or ipsilateral node positive beyond organ or origin
Stage III: Beyond midline
Stage IV-S: Small primary tumors and mets in liver, bone, skin, often spontaneous regression
Stage IV: Mets to bone or distant nodes, survival <15% (Oncol 1997;11:1857,1869,1875)

Cmplc: In retinoblastoma, osteosarcoma in 30% of genetic type from the same oncogene (Ann IM 1990;113:781); overall 2nd primary incidence is 50% in 50 yr, contrast controls, where 5% in 50 yr (Jama 1997;278:1262)

Lab: *Chem:* Urine VMA and HVA elevation in neuroblastomas if distant mets present often (Nejm 1972;286:1123)
Path: Recombinant DNA studies in retinoblastoma to predict if is in the 40% with chromosome 13 abnormalities who have bilateral recurrent disease (Nejm 1988;318:151, 1986;314:1201)

Xray: MRI helps distinguish neuroblastoma stage IV from IV-S stages

Rx: rv: Ann IM 1982;97:873

of retinoblastoma: If no mets present, surgical excision or radiation; if mets present, partial surgical excision; 6% operative mortality, then radiation rx and chemoRx, eg, with cyclophosphamide, prednisone, actinomycin D, vincristine, and chlorambucil

of neuroblastoma: Screening infants for urinary catechols increases detection rate but not survival rate (Nejm 2002;346:1041,1047,1084)

ChemoRx with "second-look" operations; in stage IV, aggressive radiation, chemoRx and marrow transplant (Nejm 1999;341:1165)

13.5 Miscellaneous

NEWBORNS

Apgar Score

Nejm 2001;344:467

5 min score predicts survival (not neurologic outcome), bad (about $^1\!/_3$ die) if ≤ 3, great if 7-10; score = 0-2 pts for pulse rate, respiratory effort, muscle tone, reflex irritability, and color

Birth Defects

Increased 7× in 2nd child after an affected 1st child; this risk is reduced by changing city of residence (environmental) but not by changing fathers (genetic) (Nejm 1994;331:1)

Increased w organic solvent exposure (13×), esp in 1st trimester (Jama 1999;281:1106); 1st-trimester exposure to folate antagonists (Nejm 2000;343:1608) like Dilantin, primodone, Tegretol, phenobarbital, Tm/S, and triamterene; possibley aspirin? (Nejm 1985;313:347 vs 1989;321:1632)

Breastfeeding: Drugs of Choice

See Table 13.2, p 891.

Cerebral Palsy

Nejm 2003;349:1765

Controversy exists over whether most cases are associated with congenital malformations (Nejm 1996;334:613, 1994;330:188, 1986;315:81,124), or intrauterine exposure to maternal infection (Jama 1997;278:207), or birth asphyxia (but increasing the C/S rate 5× for fetal distress doesn't decrease rate)

20% incidence in infants < 1500 gm at birth, improved if $MgSO_4$ given prepartum, unclear why (Jama 1996;276:1805,1843)

Physical therapy not clearly helpful in rx, at least in infants (Nejm 1988;318:803)

Associated w low T_4 levels in premies (Nejm 1996;334:821)

Circumcision

Debate over utility with minimal benefits, but, probably because is low risk and is tradition, continues to be performed (Nejm 1990;322:1308); some effect on adult sexual practices (Jama 2000;284:1417, 1997;227:1052)

Slightly (2-4×) lower gc and syphilis rates in circumcised adult males (Am J Pub Hlth 1994;84:197) but no decrease in warts or chlamydia

Anesthesia with dorsal nerve lidocaine (Nejm 1987;317:1321, 1347); topical lidocaine-prilocaine (Nejm 1997;336:1197); or circumferential ring block w < 1 cc of 1% lidocaine at penile midshaft is most effective anesthesia (Jama 1997;278:2157)

Diarrhea

Especially rotaviral type (p 406)

Table 13.2   Drugs of Choice for Breastfeeding Women*

Drug Category	Drugs and Drug Groups of Choice	Comments
Analgesic drugs	Acetaminophen, ibuprofen, flurbiprofen, ketorolac, mefenamic acid, sumatriptan, morphine	Sumatriptan may be given for migraines. For potent analgesia, morphine may be given.
Anticoagulant drugs	Warfarin, acenocoumarol, heparin (regular and low-molecular-weight)	Among breastfed infants whose mothers were taking warfarin, the drug was undetectable in plasma and the bleeding time was not affected.
Antidepressant drugs	Sertraline, tricyclic antidepressant drugs	Other drugs such as fluoxetine may be given with caution.
Antiepileptic drugs	Carbamazepine, phenytoin, valproic acid	The estimated level of exposure to these drugs in infants is less than 10% of the therapeutic dose standardized by weight.
Antihistamines (histamine H_1 blockers)	Loratadine	Other antihistamines may be given, but data on the concentrations of these drugs in breast milk are lacking.
Antimicrobial drugs	Penicillins, cephalosporins, aminoglycosides, macrolides	Avoid the use of chloramphenicol and tetracycline.
β-Adrenergic antagonists	Labetalol, propranolol	Angiotensin-converting enzyme inhibitors and calcium-channel blockers are also considered safe.
Endocrine drugs	Propylthiouracil, insulin, levothyroxine	The estimated level of exposure to propylthiouracil in breastfeeding infants is less than 1% of the therapeutic dose standardized by weight; the thyroid function of the infants is not affected.
Glucocorticoids	Prednisolone and prednisone	The amount of prednisolone that the infant would ingest in breast milk is less than 0.1% of the therapeutic dose standardized by weight.

*This list is not exhaustive. Cases of overdoses of these drugs must be assessed on an individual basis.
Reproduced with permission from Ito S. Drug therapy for breast feeding women. New Eng J Med 2000; 343;118. Copyright 2000, Mass. Medical Society, all rights reserved.

Fetal Alcohol Syndrome

Nejm 2003;290:2996

Midface hypoplasia, flattened philtrum (upper lip groove), thin upper lip, widely spaced small eyes; growth retardation, microcephaly, cognitive and social impairment; even low levels of maternal exposure result in increased adverse behavior outcomes by age 6-7 (Peds 2001;108:34)

Fetal Defect Detection

Rv: Nejm 1986;315:305

By ultrasound, and amniocentesis

Fever (T° ≥ 38°C [100.4°F])

Under age 2 mo (Peds 1999;103:843); rectal best, TM temp may be unreliable under age 3 (H. Colt). Incidence of serious bacterial illness has declined w use of HIB and pneumococcal vaccines.

Management (but not followed in >⅓ cases in the real world (Jama 2004;291:1203):

< 28 d: w/u and hospitalize for iv antibiotics

1-3 mo: w/u w blood culture, LP, UA + urine culture, chest xray; and rx w antibiotics, unless looks ok, wbc < 15,000, < 5 wbc in UA; admit and rx if any positive; ok to send home without antibiotics if negative as long as can see q 1-2 d until well (Nejm 1993;329:1437)

3⁺ mo: if nontoxic, w/u only if T° > 39°C (102.2°F)

Rx: Acetaminophen 15 mg/kg q 4 hr; ibuprofen 10 mg/kg q 4-8 hr, although more costly

Hemorrhagic Disease

Am J Pub Hlth 1998;88:203

Gi, dermal, or intracranial; onset at age 5-12 wk; caused by low vitamin K levels, especially in breastfed infants; rx w im vitamin K at birth, perhaps po q 1 mo

Immunizations (p 930)

Low Birth Weight (< 2500 gm)/Very Low Birth Weight (< 1500 gm)

Nejm 1998;:339:313, 1993;327:969

Cause: Small for gestational age (SGA)/intrauterine growth retardation (IUGR), and/or premature birth causes like PROM w chorioamnionitis, idiopathic preterm delivery, HT, abruption, radiation (even dental) (Jama 2004;291:1987), and tobacco, marijuana, or cocaine use (Nejm 1989;320:762); more rarely IUGR, incompetent cervix, cord prolapse fetal distress

Epidem: Increased in (Nejm 1995;333:1737):
- U.S. blacks by 2-3× (13% of deliveries in blacks vs 4-6% for other groups), probably due to poor socioeconomic status and/or shorter (< 9 mo) interpregnancy intervals (Nejm 1995;332:69)
- Teenage pregnancy even up to age 19 (Nejm 1995;332:1113)
- H/o previous preterm (< 37 wk) delivery (Nejm 1999; 341:943)
- Prepregnancy maternal weight < 50 kg
- H/o previous sibling or mother w low birth weight (Nejm 1995;333:1744)

Crs (Nejm 2000;343:378):
Prematurity: At 22 wk gestation, no survival without severe morbidity
At 23 wk, < 10% survive, 5% w/o disability
At 24 wk, 26% survive, 12% w/o disability
At 25 wk, 45% survive, 23% w/o disability
SGA/IUGR: At < 600 gm or < 24 wk gestation, survival ≤ 10-20% although NICU use increases the time to death and morbidity of survivors is severe

At 700 gm or 25 wk gestation, survival = 70-80% (Nejm 1993;329:1597,1649); if no intraventricular hemorrhage, ²/₃ catch up w peers over 10-15 yr (Jama 2003;289:705) vs significant neurobehavioral deficits 10+ yr out (Jama 2003;289:3264)

Cmplc: Stillbirth in subsequent pregnancies as high as 20% (Nejm 2004;350:777) in contrast to baseline 2.5% rate

Rx: Prevent w metronidazole + erythromycin rx of bacterial vaginosis at 24 wk, reduces risk in high-risk women from 50% to 30%? (Nejm 1996;333:1732 vs 2000:342:581)

NICU improves survival of low-birth-weight children if born in NICU hospital from 165 to 128/1000 mortality (Nejm 1982;307:149) vs these rates are no different than survival without NICU use

Indomethacin decreases PDAs and CNS hemorrhage but does not improve 18-mo survival w/o neurologic deficit (Nejm 2001;344:1966)

Ophthalmia Neonatorum

Nejm 1995;332:600

Cause: Gonorrhea, chlamydia

Epidem: Onset in 1st 28 d of life

Pathophys: Conjunctival infection from maternal genital infection

Si: Exudative conjuctivitis in neonate

Cmplc: Blindness, common w gc, rare w chlamydia
r/o *Herpes simplex* if ulcerations

Lab: *Bact:* Gram stain will show gc, not chlamydia

Rx: Prevent w prepartum culture screens and/or prophylaxis at birth w 2.5% povidoine iodone (5% soln diluted 50:50) (Nejm 1995;332:562) which is less toxic and more effective than 1% sil-

ver nitrate, 1% tetracycline ointment, or 14% erythromycin
ointment

of chlamydial disease: Systemic erythromycin (Med Let
1999;41:85), along w topicals

Respiratory Syncytial Virus Bronchiolitis

Epidem: Peak incidence in December–April. Big problem in immunocompromised (Nejm 1986;315:77), premature infants, term infants < 1 mo, and pts w cardiopulmonary disease under age 2 yr

Si: Bronchiolitis w wheezing

Cmplc: Otitis media (Nejm 1999;340:260)
r/o parainfluenza virus (Nejm 2001;344:1917), metapneu-
movirus (Nejm 2004;350:443), asthma, adenovirus, and cystic
fibrosis if recurs

Lab: Nasopharyngeal swab antigen test

Rx: Prevent w isolation, which decreases nosocomial spread
(Nejm 1987;317:329). Monoclonal antibody, palivizumab q 1 mo
(Med Let 2001;43:13) may decrease incidence in high-risk infants. Eventually vaccination (Nejm 2001; 344: 1917;
1999;340:312) when available someday.

of disease (Nejm 2003;349:82): Supportive w O_2; iv fluids,
maybe nasal suction; bronchodilators controversial, no benefit
shown by Australian DBCT (Nejm 2003;349:27,82)

Spina Bifida, Anencephaly, and Other Neural Tube and Ventral Wall Defects

Nejm 1999;341:1509

Cause: Idiopathic usually; seizure medication toxicity (1/100) only
from carbamazepine (Nejm 1991;324:674); maternal vitamin A
ingestion ≥ 10,000 IU q d esp in 1st trimester (Nejm 1995;
333:1369); maternal autoantibodies to folate receptors (Nejm
2004;350:134), may be the most common cause

Epidem: 1/1000 births in U.S.; similar in southern China, but in northern China rate is 6/1000 (Nejm 1999;341:1485). Risk increased 2× w maternal obesity (Jama 1996;275:1089,1093).

Pathophys:

Si: Meningocele, myelomeningocele, etc

Lab: *Chem:* α-Fetoprotein, HCG, and estriol levels at 15-18 wk gestation from last menstrual period; if elevated, then get ultrasound; amniocentesis not needed if ultrasound ok (Nejm 1990;323:557); but maternal AFP elevations are associated w increased fetal loss, levels 2-3× normal w a 2.5× increase, levels > 3× w 10× increase (Nejm 1991;324:662)

Rx: Prevent w folic acid (Med Let 2004;46:17) > 0.4 mg qd periconception, 0/2000 births vs 6/2000 (Jama 1995;274:1698; Nejm 1998;338:1060, 1992;327:1832 vs 1989;321:430); dramatically decreases neural tube defect risk (Nejm 1999;341:1485; Peds 1993;493:4); perhaps 4 mg po qd if pos family hx; now added to all U.S. grain products, eg, flour (Nejm 1999;340:1449) and has decreased overall incidence by 20% (Jama 2001;285:2981)

Consider abortion

In utero repair (Jama 1999;282:1819,1826)

Delivery by cesarean section may result in less motor deficit? (Clin Obgyn 1998;41:393 vs Nejm 1991;324:662)

Sudden Infant Death Syndrome (SIDS) and Near SIDS

Epidem: 1.4 deaths/1000 live births in U.S. Runs in families; no association w DPT immunizations (J Peds 1991;119:411); increased incidence by sleeping prone and by deformable mattress, swaddling, warm room, URIs (Nejm 1993;329:377, 425), and children exposed to passive cigarette smoke (Jama 1995;273:795).

Incidence decreased by 40% to < 1/1000 w public education against sleeping prone (Ped Ann 1995;24:350) but message hardest to get to lower-socioeconomic groups (Jama 1998;280:329, 336,341)

Pathophys: Etiology unknown. URI and nasal obstruction precipitate some events. Some may be associated w long Qtc > 0.44 on EKG (Jama 2001;286:2264; Nejm 1998;338:1709). Correlates w maternal 2nd-trimester α-fetoprotein levels (Nejm 2004;351:978).

Cmplc: r/o trauma/smothering asphyxia (Nejm 1991;324:1858, 1986;315:100,126), Munchausen by proxy

Lab: May be associated with elevated HgbF levels (Nejm 1987; 316:1122 vs 1989;321:1359), and some subset of cases w long QT interval (Nejm 2000;343:262, 1987;317:1501)

Rx: Prevent by positioning children supine (on back; "back to sleep" campaigns) (Jama 2001;285:2244, 1995;273:818, 1994;272:1646) for 1st 6 mo of life (BMJ 1991;303:1209), doing so reduced incidence in Tasmania from 3.8 to 1.5 deaths/1000 (Jama 1995; 273:783) and by 90% in Norway (J Ped 1998;132:340) but no difference found in southern California (Jama 1995;273:790); avoid soft bedding under infant. Apnea monitors not effective (Jama 2001;285:2199,2244).

Temperature Control

In newborn, is poor; higher ambient temperature may precipitate apnea (Nejm 1970;282:461); hypothermia immediately postpartum decreases with plastic swaddle in both newborn premie and term babies (Nejm 1971;284:121)

INFANTS

Diaper Rash

S. Sewall 10/94

Cause: Irritation by stool/urine

Pathophys: Debate over whether ammonia from urea-splitting bacteria plays a role, also about role of stool enzymes and bile salts

Cmplc: Secondary candidiasis, may be associated w oral thrush, and often precipitated by antibiotic use, appears as confluent erythema w 1-3 mm satellite macules/papules

r/o seborrheic dermatitis, well-demarcated fiery-red confluent rash, responds quickly to steroid creams; psoriatic diaper rash w shiny scales, responds slowly to topical steroids; staph infection often causing bullous impetigo lesions that resemble cigarette burns, rx w antibiotics; rarely Jacquet's ulcers of vulva or buttocks, zinc deficiency (acrodermatitis enteropathica), herpes simplex, scabies, and Kawasaki's disease (high fever)

Rx: Frequent diaper change, keeping skin clean and dry; avoid strong soaps; avoid occlusive diapering, put disposables on loosely and/or tear some holes in plastic, omit rubber pants; zinc oxide ointment helps protect skin (Vaseline, A+D ointment, Desitin, Eucerin, etc)

Nystatin cream for monilial type (satellite lesions)

Failure to Thrive W/u

1st look at overall growth curves (p 933). Then CBC, lead levels, UA/culture, lytes, BUN; anti-ttg (p 377) in todders to r/o gluten enteropathy, and TSH if height much less than weight

Febrile Seizures

Nejm 1993;329:79; 1992;327:1122

Epidem: Age of onset usually 6 mo-3 yr. Incidence higher w positive family hx; $\frac{1}{3}$ under age 2 yr caused by roseola? (Nejm 1994;331: 432), but still consider w/u under age 1 w LP etc. 2-4% of children under age 5 have at least one.

Si: $\frac{1}{2}$ are partial complex, $\frac{1}{2}$ are grand mal. Fever usually closer to 101°F than 105°F.

Crs: 33% recur, more often if age < 18 mo; 50% recur within 6 mo, 75% within 1 yr, 90% within 2 yr if going to. No long-term intellectual/behavioral deficits (Nejm 1998;338:1723).

Rx: No prophylaxis; or perhaps, at 1st si of fever, acetaminophen or diazepam (Valium) 0.33 mg/kg q 8 hr (insertion devices: Diastat)

Food Allergies

Including milk allergy (J Allergy Immunol 1999;103:981)

Cause: Proteins in cow's milk, egg whites, peanuts (Nejm 2002; 346:1294), soybeans, fish, shrimp, et al

Epidem: 6% prevalence under age 3, 2% over age 10; $^2/_5$% prevalence of cow's milk allergy alone in children < 2 yr

Pathophys: IgE-mediated types cause classic skin, gi, and systemic histamine reactions

IgA-mediated types cause dermatitis herpetiformis-type skin changes and gastroenteritis

Cell-mediated types cause hypersensitivity reactions, eg, to gluten causing sprue. Peanut allergies may be due to peanut oil–containing skin lotions used on rashes and/or cross-sensitivity to soy protein exposures (Nejm 2003;348:977).

Sx: Histaminic sx including wheezing and rhinitis, or gastroenteritis, or malabsorption, or constipation due to perianal inflammation (Nejm 1998;339:1100)

Crs: 85% "outgrow" most; but peanut allergy lifelong in 80%

Cmplc: r/o nonallergic cow's milk toxicity leading to gi bleeding in children

Lab: RAST test, skin testing

Rx: Elimination diets

Malformations

Rv of all types and causes (Nejm 1983;308:424; K. L. Jones, ed, *Smith's Recognizable Patterns of Human Malformations.* Philadelphia: WB Saunders, 2005)

Metabolic Syndromes

Alport's syndrome (Nejm 2003;348:2543):

Cause: Autosomal dominant, perhaps X-linked recessive

Pathophys: Autoantibodies to type IV collagen destroy basement membrane

Sx: School-age onset of deafness and hereditary nephritis

Cmplc: Occasionally thrombocytopenia (Ann IM 1975;82:639)

Biotinidase Deficiency (Nejm 1985;313:16,43):

Epidem: 2/80,000

Crs: Causes death over months to years

Rx: Easily treated; detect with newborn screen, not mandated in all states

Galactosemia:

Epidem: 1/175,000 newborns

Crs: Die of sepsis, especially *E. coli* (30%) when neonate

Rx: Mass screening program in place in U.S.

Hunter's Syndrome: mucopolysaccharide [glycosamineglycan (GAG)] disorder II:

Cause: X-linked recessive

Pathophys: Increased intracellular chondroitin sulfate (mucopolysaccharide)

Sx: Normal at birth; causes stiff joints, deafness, dwarfism, hepatosplenomegaly, skeletal deformities, progressive mental retardation, death from cardiopulmonary cmplcs, coarse facial features

Lab: Elevated urinary, skin, white cell, or serum mucopolysaccharides

Rx: Recombinant enzyme replacement (Nejm 2001;344:182)

Hurler's syndrome: mucopolysaccharide glycosamineglycan (GAG) disorder I:

Cause: Autosomal recessive

Pathophys: Probably a variant of Hunter's; increased intracellular chondroitin sulfate (mucopolysaccharide); decreased β-galactosidase in skin, brain, liver, spleen, etc, which is normally necessary to cleave terminal gal from the mucopolysaccharides (Nejm 1969;281:338)

Sx: Normal at birth, as in Hunter's; more rapid onset; cloudy cornea; retarded; progressive coarsening of features; hepatosplenomegaly, gingival hyperplasia

Rx: Stem cell transplant w unrelated donor cord blood (Nejm 2004;350:1960)
Recombinant enzyme replacement w α-L-ironidase (laronidase [Alderazyme]) (Med Let 2003;45:88) weekly iv; $3400/wk

Osteopetrosis, Congenital:

Cause: Autosomal recessive

Pathophys: Defective osteoclastic function causes thick bones and nerve compression plus marrow obliteration

Si & Sx: Blindness, deafness, facial palsies, anemia, bleeding

Rx: Marrow transplant; perhaps calcitriol (Nejm 1984;310:409)

Potter's Syndrome of Newborn:

Cause: Genetic

Pathophys: Compression of body and pulmonary hypoplasia from oligohydramnios, which may be caused by renal agenesis or severe dysplasia usually from obstruction or chronic amniotic fluid leak

Sx & Si: Hypoplastic lungs, low-set ears, broad nose with sunken bridge, small jaw

Prader-Willi syndrome:

Cause: Deletion of chromosome 15 segment (Nejm 1992;326:807)

Sx: Infantile hypotonia, poor feeding, and FTT; hyperphagia, extreme obesity in early childhood, hypogonadism, mental retardation, short stature, small hands and feet, albinism (related to oculocutaneous albinism: Nejm 1994;330:529), strabismus, nystagmus due to failure of optic fibers to cross at chiasm (Nejm 1986; 314:1606)

Nutrition

Cow's milk ok after 12 mo if give iron, gi bleeding insignificant (Med Let 1983;25:80); perhaps supplement either breast or cow's milk w $FeSO_4$ from birth to age 2 yr to prevent permanent impairment of school performance from iron deficiency (Nejm 1991;325:687). Breast milk can contain ethanol if mother drinking and can result in psychomotor impairment at age 1 (Nejm 1989;321:425).

Shaken Baby Syndrome

Nejm 1998;338:1822

Cause: Nonaccidental trauma

Epidem: Infants < 3 yr, most < 1 yr; 24% of all trauma in under age 2 children. Associated w poverty and low socioeconomic status.

Pathophys: Subdural and subarachnoid bleeds from torn bridging vessels

Sx: Lethargy, decreased tone, seizures (40-70%), bruises, burns; facial bruises w any nonspecific set of sx under age 3 should prompt queries, CT, and skeletal series (Jama 1999;281:621, 657)

Si: Hydrocephalus

Xray: CT, maybe MRI; plain films (skeletal survey) for fractures

Rx: Hospitalize, child protection

Viral Exanthems

- Measles (rubeola) (p 697)
- Scarlet fever (p 539)

- 5th disease (parvovirus) (p 686)
- Chickenpox (p 678)
- Rubella (p 688)
- Roseola, exanthem subitum, or 6th disease (p 705)

CHILDREN

Ambylopia (crossed eyes)

Rx: Patching or atropine to other eye even up to age 17 may restore visual acuity (Arch Ophthalmol 2005;123:437)

Anesthesia/Sedation

Nejm 2002;347:1094, 2000;342:938

Topical w:
- Lidocaine, epinephrine + tetracaine mixture (LET)
- Tetracaine-adrenaline (epinephrine)-cocaine (TAC) for open wounds; takes 20 min
- LMX (4% lidocaine); takes 60 min to work

Parenteral: Fentanyl iv or ketamine iv/im
Sedation:
- Midazolam (Versed) 0.025-0.05 mg/kg up to 0.4 mg/kg max iv; or 0.1-0.15 gm/kg im; or 0.5-0.75 mg/kg po or pr
- Pentobarbital 1-6 mg/kg iv/im; or 1.5-4 mg/kg po/pr

Autism, Pervasive Developmental Disorders (PDDs), and Asperger Syndrome

Epidem (Jama 2001;285:3093,3141): Prevalence of autism = 17/10,000 and PDDs = 46/10,000 in preschool children; up to 60/10,000 of autism spectrum disorders (Jama 2003;289:49,87)

Pathophys: Severe developmental disorder w delayed language and/or communication skills, social interactions and reciprocity, and imaginative play; all preceded by diffuse brain overgrowth and head circumference in 1st 3 yr of life (Jama 2003;290:337). No association w MMR vaccination (Jama 2003;290:1763; Nejm 2002;347:1477).

Rx: Haloperidol helps but w side effects; risperidone (Risperdal) (Nejm 2002;347:314) helps aggression, tantrums by DBCT; adverse effects: tardive dyskinesia risks

Secretin injection no help (Nejm 1999;341:1801)

Benign Pediatric Murmurs

Table 13.3 Benign Pediatric Murmurs

Murmur	Location	Character	Differential DX
Still's	LLSB to apex	Coarse, vibrating early systolic; S_2 splits and closes normally, murmur diminishes w sitting or deep inspiration	VSD, MVP, IHHS
Basal ejection (pulmonic flow)	ULSB	Base only, no click (unlike real PS), S_2 splits and closes normally	PS (click), ASD, anomalous venous return
Physiologic	UL and RSB	To back and axilla	AS, PS, PDA
Supraclavicular bruit	Supraclavicular area	Teenagers	AS
Venous hum	Neck, USB	Continuous, gone when supine	PDA, AVMs

Echo if systolic murmur radiates to carotids (J. Love 12/94)
(Fam Pract Recert 1986;8:51)

Child Abuse

Nejm 1990;332:1425; Ped Clin N Am 1990;37:791-1012

Physical, sexual in boys (Jama 1998;280:1855) as well as girls, emotional/neglect

Sx: Sleep disorders, nightmares, sexualized play, school problems, phobias, depression

Si: Patterned bruises/burns, fractures, head injuries; in infant, shaken baby syndrome (p 903)

Cmplc: Mortality, greatest in 1st year of life, esp if 2nd or more child of teenage mother (Nejm 1998;339:1211); FTT; in adulthood, more physical sx, depression, drug and alcohol abuse, psych problems (Jama 1997;277:1362)

Xray: Nejm 1989;320:507

Rx: Prevention with home visits (Nejm 1989;320:531)
Hospitalize, report suspect cases
Rx of sexual offenders: Gonadotropin-releasing hormone analog im q 1 mo, medically castrates (Nejm 1998;338:416)

Enuresis (Bedwetting)

S. Sewall 7/98; Med Let 1990;32:38; Ann IM 1987;106:587

Epidem: Male/female = 2:1

Rx: Patient education available (http://www.drynights.com)
Only consider rx after age 6; 15%/yr resolve after age 6 yr
Alarms 75% effective?; compliance tough, although improved w DDAVP given for 1st 3 wk; cost $60-75
Desmopressin (DDAVP) 10-20 μgm in each nostril hs, or 200-400 μgm po hs; may help a little especially when combined with other rx, effectiveness ~ 65% at 6 mo but wears off to 10% at 1 yr; adverse effects: hyponatremia, seizures, and rare sudden death (Med Let 1990;32:53); costs $3-6/night
Imipramine 25-50 mg (75 mg over age 12); helps 25-35%; check QT interval on EKG before starting; cheap but OD risk

Hypertension

Nejm 1996;335:1968

Upper limits of normal (see Table 13.4), or can use limits based on height (Peds 2004;114:555); most HT under age 19 is secondary and a cause can be found (See Table 13.4, p 907)

Table 13.4   95th Percentile of Blood Pressure in Boys and Girls 3–16 Years of Age, According to Height

Blood Pressure	Age yr	Height Percentile for Boys				Height Percentile for Girls			
		5th	25th	75th	95th	5th	25th	75th	95th
		mm Hg				mm Hg			
Systolic	3	104	107	111	113	104	105	108	110
	6	109	112	115	117	108	110	112	114
	10	114	117	121	123	116	117	120	122
	13	121	124	128	130	121	123	126	128
	16	129	132	136	138	125	127	130	132
Diastolic	3	63	64	66	67	65	65	67	68
	6	72	73	75	76	71	72	73	75
	10	77	79	80	82	77	77	79	80
	13	79	81	83	84	80	81	82	84
	16	83	84	86	87	83	83	85	86

The height percentiles were determined with standard growth curves. Data are adapted from those of the Task Force on High Blood Pressure in Children and Adolescents.

Intussception

Epidem: Peak incidence age 1-5; associated w now-discontinued rotavirus vaccine, which may hypertrophy Peyer's patches, which then act as sleeving mass (Peds 1999;104:575)

Sx: Crampy pain and strikingly normal between cramps, although can eventually develop stupor (Peds 1980;65:A1057); bloody "currant jelly" stool

Si: Normal exam between cramps, but often lethargic

DiffDx: Meckel's diverticulum in < 1% of people, usually ulcerates in childhood

Xray: Ultrasound

Rx: Air reduction under fluoroscopy or ultrasound

Limping Child

Am Fam Phys 2000;61:1011

Cause:

> In all: Septic arthritis, osteomyelitis, stress fx, neoplasm
>
> In toddlers: Septic hip, dysplastic hip, occult fx, leg length discrepancy, postviral toxic synovitis
>
> In children: Postviral synovitis Legg-Perthes disease, JRA
>
> In adolescents: Slipped capital femoral epiphysis, avascular necrosis femoral head, overuse, gonococcal arthritis

Sx: Foot pathology if prefers to crawl not walk; rheumatologic if worse in am

Si: Tests:

> Neurologic causes: Reflexes, clonus
>
> SI joint disease: Supine foot on opposite knee w more abduction
>
> Septic: Log roll of hip < 30°; prone flexed-knee hip internal rotation
>
> Slipped cap fem epiphysis: Obligate cross-rotation of hip w flexion
>
> Hip dysplasia: Prone hip internal rotation, asymmetric supine hip abduction, heels to buttocks shows 1 knee lower than other (r/o leg length discrepancy)

Lab: CRP and ESR (> 20); tap joint if suspect sepsis

Xray: Bone scan, "frogs' legs" views of hips

Osteogenesis Imperfecta

Cause: Genetic

Epidem: Prevalence 1/20,000

Pathophys: Genetic defect in collagen matrix (Nejm 1992;326:540)

Si: Blue sclerae (picture: Nejm 1998;339:966), deafness, double-jointedness, cardiac valve degeneration (Nejm 1993;329:1406); fractures decrease with puberty, increase with menopause (Nejm 1984;310:1694)

Rx: Pamindronate 7 mg/kg iv q 6 mo (Nejm 1998;339:947)

Dwarfism (p 299)

Idiopathic short stature (< 3 %tile) (Med Let 2003;45:89; Nejm 1999;340:502, 557) can be rx'd w recombinant HGH sc qd × 5-10 yr to normal adult heights; but expensive (≥ $20,000/yr) and of questionable ethics to do so; or can use LHRH × 4+ yr at cost of osteopenia (Nejm 2003;348:908 vs 942)

Constitutional delay in growth and development in adolescent males can be rx'd without loss of final height with testosterone × 1 yr? (Nejm 1988;319:1563)

Chapter 14

Prevention and Health Maintenance

D. K. Onion

14.1 Screening and Prevention

References

U.S. Preventive Services Task Force's Guide
　　(http://www.ahcpr.gov/clinic/ushsptix.htm)
Ann IM 1997;127:910 (nice historical rv, no recipes)
P. Frame, J Fam Pract 1986;22:341,417,511, 1986;23:29
Jama 1995;273:1030 (Group Health, Seattle; when done over
　　time, decreases death and/or disability, eg, breast cancer,
　　immunizations, bike accidents, smoking)
Ann IM 1992;116:593 (discusses how reasonable people may
　　come to opposite conclusions re a screening strategy)

14.2 General Issues

Types of prevention:
- Primary prevention: Prevention of a disease before it exists, eg, immunization against H. flu
- Secondary prevention: Detection and reversal (cure) of a disease after it already exists but before it is symptomatic

Meta-analysis results agree w subsequent controlled trials only 65% of the time (Nejm 1997;337:536)

Number needed to treat (NNT) (Nejm 1988;318:1728; Ann IM 1992;117:916): The reciprocal of the absolute risk reduction; the number of ps to whom an intervention must be applied over a fixed period, usually 1-5 yr, to confer a benefit for one of them (example of application to finasteride rx of BPH, NNT-4 = 16: Nejm 1998;338:612)

Statistical Calculations (T = true, P = positive, F = false, N = negative):
Sensitivity = TP/TP + FN
Specificity = TN/TN + FP
Positive predictive value = TP/TP + FP
Negative predictive value = TN/TN + FN

Criteria for justifiable preventive intervention (example of application to CHF: Ann IM 2003;138:907)

- For a primary prevention intervention:
  1. Significant disease with a defined and substantial morbidity and/or mortality
  2. The intervention (treatment, education, etc) is:
     Effective, ie, improves prognosis and the result is superior to waiting for the disease to appear
     Acceptable to pts
     Low risk
     Available (financing, facilities, and providers to provide)
- For a secondary intervention, the above must be true, plus:
  1. An asx phase of significant duration must exist
  2. A screening test must be available that is
     Acceptable (financing, comfort, risk) to pts
     Sensitive and specific at the projected disease prevalence and does not detect a lot of subclinical conditions that may never be clinically relevant (Nejm 1993;328:

1237), eg, 40% of men in their 60s may have prostate cancer but less than 1% will ever be clinically affected (Ann IM 1993;118:793,804)

Problems with prevention in primary care practice:
- No or little feedback for a job well done; lots of negative feedback when primary care doctor deals with the complications of preventive rx or works up the false positives
- Without tough rules to follow, primary care doctor may be quickly overwhelmed by off-hand, incorrect, and/or inappropriate specialist recommendations ("if you primary care docs would just screen for UTIs, glaucoma, etc")
- A doctor's sense of responsibility makes him or her assume too much responsibility rather than devolving some onto the community or the individual pt
- Overzealous specialty society (eg, American Cancer Society) recommendations impair our ability to seek informed consent (Nejm 1993;328:438)
- Elimination of wellness through false positives and illness labeling of normal variation (Nejm 1994;330:440)

Goals of the periodic health exam (annual physical, though frequently done, is a waste of time and inconsistently done: P. Frame, J Fam Pract 1995;40:543,547)
- Prevention
- Patient–doctor rapport building to improve future access
- Elicitation of sx (rv of systems) or risk factors that deserve further study and that the pt may have not felt important enough to volunteer
- Maintenance of doctor's skills, eg, Babinski testing, funduscopic exam, thyroid exam, heart sounds, and so forth
- Fulfill patient expectations, eg, of touching, of a heart-lung exam being part of a full exam, and so forth

14.3 Adult Preventive Maneuvers

Reasonable preventive interventions in adults for practicing physicians; * = good evidence for; for others, fair evidence or only expert consensus; alphabetically organized by disease; primary or secondary intervention indicated by (1° prevention) or (2° prevention). In all cases, presumption is of an asx pt; sx should always be investigated.

Abdominal Aortic Aneurysm

Ann IM 2003;139:516; P. Frame, Ann IM 1993;119:411

Group: All age > 65 yr

Screen: Abdominal exam for aneurysm > 5.5 cm q 1 yr; perhaps ultrasound × 1 esp in male relatives over age 60, 18% incidence (Ann IM 1999;130:637), or in males who have smoked (Class B-USPSTF: Ann IM 2005;142:198)

Intervention: Resection (2° prevention)

Issues: Appropriate size to operate on; borderline cost-benefit ratios

Alcoholism

Groups: All

Screen: Take history q 1 yr or with accidents or h/o hypertension

Intervention: AA referral, Antabuse (2° prevention)

Issues: Intervention efficacy; USPSTF class I, insufficient evidence (Ann IM 2004;140:554)

Anemia, Iron-Deficient

Groups: Low socioeconomic status or institutionalized elderly

Screen: Hematocrit

Intervention: Iron po (2° prevention)

Issues: Debatable if efficacious (Ann IM 1992;116:44)

ASHD/CVAs

Groups: All

Intervention 1: *Detect and rx hypertension* (1° prevention) (Ann IM 1995;122:937)

Freq: < q 1 yr

NNT: 3 if diastolic BP > 115 mm Hg; 141 if diastolic BP 90-109 mm Hg

Issues: Treatment goals?

Intervention 2: *Detect and rx elevated cholesterols* (1° prevention), not of value over age 70 (Jama 1994;272:1335,1372) or in women unless established ASCVD (Jama 1995;274:1152)

Freq: < q 4 yr

NNT: In men over 40 w LDL > 150, NNT-5 = 40 (Nejm 1995;333:1301)

Issues: Compliance; risks, morbidity, and costs of medications

Breast Cancer

Primary Prevention: Jama 2001;287:216; ACP J Club 1999;131:58

Groups: Postmenopausal women w detectable estradiol levels

Intervention: Selective estrogen receptor blockers like tamoxifen or raloxifene (Evista) po qd; NNT-4 = 45-126

Issues: Hot flashes, endometrial hypertropy (tamoxifen only), thromboembolic disease. Frame (11/04) points out that such strategies prevent cancer in 8/1000 women under 45 with a positive family hx, but cause 1.5 emboli, 1.5 endometrial Ca's, 1 CVA, and 1.5 DVTs; worse if older.

Secondary Prevention:

Groups (Ann IM 1997;127:1029,1035; Sci 1997;275:1056; Ann IM 1995;122:534,539,550, 1994;120:326): In summary, clearly help-

*good evidence for

ful for age 50-70+, hotly debated for age 40-50 if low risk (nice summary: Jama 1999;281:1470), none promote under age 40. 33% overall false-pos mammogram or clinical breast exam in 5 exams over 10 yr, 50% w 10 mammograms between age 40 and 50 (Nejm 1998;338:1089) or younger (Nejm 1998;339:560)

of elderly women age 65-70+: Screening w mammography q 2 yr (USFSTF: Ann IM 2003;139:835) marginally beneficial up to age 85 if 5-10 yr lifespan likely and esp if have normal bone mineral density (Jama 1999;282:2156; Ann IM 1992;116:722)

of women age 50-70+ yr: Mammography w clinical breast exam clearly increases survival done q 1-2 yr (Rand summary: Jama 1995;273:142,149; Nejm 1992;327:323; Ann IM 1994;120:326 vs Can Med Assoc J 1992;147:1459,1477); Swedish meta-analysis of 5 studies also finds benefit (30% relative risk mortality reduction) between age 50 and 70 yr but not younger (Lancet 1993;341:973); NNT = 270 (Ann IM 1997;127:955)

of women age 40-50 yr: q 1 yr (not q 2 yr), if high risk (positive family hx, cancer in opposite breast [Nejm 1984;310:960; J Fam Practice 1983;16:481], or h/o mammoplasties), clearly benefit

Less clearly helpful if low risk (Ann IM 2002;137:305,347); false-pos mammograms over 10 yr in $1/3$ of the women; mammography saves 2.3/1000, while clinical breast exam alone saves 1.5/1000, so mammography helps 1/1250 in that age group (Nejm 1993;328:438, 1993;329:276), or NNT = 2500 (Ann IM 1997;127:955); discuss risk–benefit ratios w women age 40-50 who frequently think cancer incidence much higher than is, and don't understand risks of f/u of false-pos tests; psychological effects of false-pos mammograms are real, even after all found to be ok (Ann IM 1991;114:657)

Screen:

Physician breast exam* q 1 yr, 54% sens, 94% specif (Jama 1999;282:1270)

Mammography (Ann IM 1995;122:534,539,550), 75% sens, 90% specif; interpretations, 80% agreement intra- and interobserver (Nejm 1994;331:1493) q 1-2 yr (q 2 yr adequate: J Natl Ca Inst 1993;85:1644) over age 50, q 1 yr under age 50 if do at all. Increased sens and specif w age and w increased fatty breast tissue (Ann IM 2003;138:168)

MRI w contrast maybe in BRCA-positive pts (Nejm 2004;351: 427,497; Jama 2004;292:1317); more expensive but 70% sens w 90% specif compared to 40%/98% for mammography in BRCA-positive women since are young w dense breasts, which impairs mammography but not MRI

Intervention: Excise when small (2° prevention)

NNT: Age 40-50 yr, mortality (20 yr delayed) NNT-10 = 1000-2500 w only 4% true pos mammograms; age 50-60 yr, NNT-10 = 400 w 9% true pos mammograms; age 60+, NNT-10 = 150 w 17% true pos mammograms

Issues: Cost/access, test sens/specif, safety, periodicity

Car Accidents

Groups: All

Intervention: Encourage seatbelt use (1° prevention)

Freq: < q 1 yr

Issues: Efficacy of physician intervention?

Cervical Cancer

Nejm 2001;344:1603

Group: Women age 20-70 yr with cervix

Screen: Pap* smear q 1 yr if < 35 yr old and/or multiple partners; q 5 yr if > 35 yr old and < 8 lifetime partners (Canadian Walton

*good evidence for

Rep: Can Med Assoc J 1982;127:581) and no h/o abnormal Paps or STDs in pt or partner; alternatively, at least q 3 yr at age 20-65 (Ann IM 1990;113:214); and in elderly > 65, get 2-3 Paps 3 yr apart if not previously done then stop (Ann IM 1992;117:520). Unnecessary if s/p hysterectomy for benign disease (Nejm 1996;335;1559,1599; Jama 1996;275:940), though still being done in ²/₃ in 2002! (G.Welch: Jama 2004;291:2990). 5-10% false-neg rate in best labs. Atypical squamous cells of uncertain significance (ASCUS) should be < 5% of Paps.

Intervention: Excise, ablate (2° prevention)

Issues: False-negative Paps

Colon Cancer

Jama 2003;289:1288,1297; Ann IM 2002;137:129,132; Nejm 2000;343:1603,1641; Ann IM 1997;126:808; Nejm 1998; 338:1153, 1995;332:861

Groups: All age > 45 or 50 yr; at age 35-40 yr if at higher risk (Jama 1999;281:1611) from IBD, familial polyposis, > 1 1st-degree relative w colon cancer (Nejm 1994;331:1669), or one 1st-degree relative w cancer under age 55

1° Prevention 1: NSAID use, eg, ASA 80-325mg po b-tiw (Ann IM 1994;121:241), or daily (Nejm 2003;348:883,891) but may not be worth the bleeding risk even in high-risk pts

1° Prevention 2: Hormone replacement rx in women decreases risk by 30-40% (Ann IM 1998;128:705)

1° Prevention #3: Calcium 1200 mg po qd as milk or direct supplement (Nejm 1999;340:101; Jama 1998;280:1070)

Screen 1: Stool guaiacs 3× annually by hemoccult (Nejm 2001;345: 555, 1998;338:1153 [nice summary of the debate]; Ann IM 1997;126:808). Rehydration of guaiac cards not recommended (above 2003 references; Ann IM 1997;126:808). Dietary prohibitions around testing impede compliance w no benefit (Eff Clin Pract 2001;4:150).

Intervention: Adenomatous polyp detection and removal, and early cancer excision (2° prevention)

NNT-18: 143 (Nejm 2000;343:1603)

Issues: 24% sens, 94% specif for adenomas > 10 mm (Ann IM 2005;142:81); when colon w/u neg, UGI endoscopy yields ~13% dx's including 1% cancers, esp indicated if anemic (RR = 5×) (Am J Med 1999;106:613). 50-90% sens for cancer and < 30% for polyps; w/u of positives will demonstrate a cancer or polyp in about ⅓ and an upper gi source (benign) in many (~⅓) (Nejm 1998;339:653); false-neg rate increased from 20% to 40% with time (2-8 d) between obtaining and doing the test (Ann IM 1984;101:297). Such annual (not biannual) testing decreases 5-yr mortality by ⅓ (Ann IM 1993;118:1), or from 8% to 5% over 13 yr but overall mortality the same in all groups (Lancet 1996;348: 1467,1472; Minn. guaiac study: Nejm 1993;328:1365,1416).

    Costs, physician skill

Screen 2: Either flex sig or colonoscopy options rational although latter is less clearly cost-effective (Nejm 2002;346:40); under age 50 not worth doing if risk is average (Nejm 2002;346:1781)

    Flexible sigmoidoscopy (Jama 2000;284:1954) q 5-10 yr w guaiacs q 1 yr w colonoscopy if either positive; at 3 yr, 0.8% w cancer or advanced adenomas (Jama 2003;290:41,106)

    Colonoscopy (Ann IM 2000;133:573,647; Nejm 2000;343: 162,169,207) q 10 yr over age 50 since sigmoidoscopy misses 25% of cancers (Nejm 2001;345:555,607); obviates need for guaiacs (D. Hay); misses 10-12% of polyps > 10 mm when compared to virtual colonoscopy (Ann IM 2004;141:352)

Intervention: Polyp (villous, tubulovillous, debatably tubular adenomas: Jama 1999;281:1611) detection and removal w colonoscopy of whole bowel, and early cancer excision (2° prevention)

NNT: 1000

Issues: Costs, physician skill

Screen 3: Virtual colonoscopy (CT colonography) (Nejm
2003;349:2183,2261 vs not yet: Ann IM 2000;142:635; Nejm
2004;350:1148; Jama 2004;291:1713) less invasive, but sens and
specif variable primarily; only 8-14% need f/u colonoscopy (same
day) for lesions > 8 mm

Screen 4: Fecal DNA mutations detection is more sens and specif
than guaiacs but cost ($400-800) and availability of colonoscopy
make use debatable (Nejm 2004;351:2704,2755)

Deafness

Groups: Occupationally exposed

Intervention: Encourage ear noise protection (1° prevention)

Freq: < q 1 yr

Issues: Efficacy of physician education

Dental Caries

Groups: All

Interventions/Freq: *Dental prophylaxis* q 1 yr (1° prevention);
brush/floss qd (1° prevention)

Depression

Ann IM 2001;134:345,418

Screen: Various instruments (Jama 2002;287:1160) like "are you depressed?" and "have you lost interest in things?"; together 95%
sensitive

Intervention: Antidepressants

Frequency: Maybe once

Issues: Cost ($30,000/quality-adjusted life-year); rx efficacy

*good evidence for

Diabetes

USHSPTF: Ann IM 2003;138:212, 215; Jama 1998;280:1757

Groups: Only if sx unless in high-risk ASHD groups w HT (Ann IM 2004;140:689) and/or increased lipids

Screen: FBS > 126 mg %, confirm positives w repeat; less studies is $HgbA_1C > 7.0\%$ (Jama 1996;276:1246, 1261)

Intervention:

Diet and exercise at impaired glucose tolerance stage decreases 5-yr conversion rate to overt DM from 35% to 15% (Nejm 2001;344:1343)

Diet and hypoglycemic agents (1° prevention of cmplc's)

Diphtheria/Tetanus

Groups: All

Intervention: *dT immunization (1° prevention)

Freq: Once ~age 50 yr if had full pediatric series including booster at age 14 (Ann IM 1994;121:540)

Hepatitis B

Groups: High risk (health workers, iv drug users, prostitutes, gay males)

Intervention: Vaccine (1° prevention); HBIG postexposure (1° prevention)

Freq: Once

NNT: 8 in gay males, higher w other groups

Hepatitis C

Groups: High risk (see Hep B)

Intervention: Interferon and ribavirin to prevent cirrhosis/hepatoma

Freq: Not recommended (USPSTF: Ann IM 2004;140:462), class C (D in normals)

*good evidence for

Hypothyroidism

Groups: Women > 50 yr with vague sx (ACP) or > 60 yr (USPTF); or both sexes > age 35-40 (Jama 1996;276:285)

Screen: TSH

Intervention: Thyroid replacement (2° prevention)

Influenza

Med Let discussion annually in Sept

Groups: High risk at least, or all > 65 yr, or over age 50 per CDC 2000; but not usually worthwhile in age 18-65 work forces (RCT: Jama 2000;284:1655). Reduces strokes and cardiac hospitalizations in the elderly (Nejm 2003;348:1322).

Intervention: Immunization (1° prevention)

Freq: q 1 yr

Issues: Immunization efficacy (not bad: Nejm 1994;331:778)

Insect/Tick Bite–Transmitted Diseases

Med Let 2003;45:41

Groups: Exposure to mosquitoes (malaria, West Nile virus, et al) or ticks (Lyme disease, ehrlichiosis, babesiosis)

Intervention: Insect repellants like DEET topically up to 50% solutions; ok in chldren and pregnant women; perhaps picardin in future; plus long-lasting permethrin (Repel Permanone) of clothing

Lung Cancer, COPD, ASHD, Strokes

Group: All smokers

Intervention 1:

Smoking cessation instruction (p 1007) (1° prevention) after asking 3 questions (Ann IM 1991;115:59): (1) What do you know about smoking's impact on your health? (2) Are you ready to quit? (3) What would it take for you to stop? Plus transient nicotine replacement rx (BMJ 1994;308:21).

Intervention 2:

CT; insufficient data that prolongs life (Nejm 2005;352:2714; USPSTF: Ann Im 2004;140:738,740); being studied but unlikely (Jama 2002;289:313; Nejm 2000;343:1627); low-dose spiral CT screening of >20 pack-yr smokers > 60 yr old found 23% w nodules, followed q 3 mo and bx'd ones that grew (10%), and 27/28 were cancer but cost high (Med Let 2001;43:6)

Freq: Smoking cessation try q 1 yr

Issues: Efficacy of intervention? Weight gain of 5-10 lb after quitting a disincentive (Nejm 1991;324:739).

Melanoma

Group: All

Screen: Self-exam q 1 yr?

Intervention: Excision (2° prevention); sun screen use (1° prevention) debatably (Ann IM 2003;139:966)

Issues: Low incidence

Group: Those with family hx of melanoma or atypical (dysplastic) nevus syndrome

Screen: Self-exam q 6 mo? Physician exam q 6-12 mo?

Intervention: Excision (2° prevention)

Neural Tube Defects/Spina Bifida

Folic acid peripartum to prevent (p 896)

Obesity

Groups: All

Screen: Weight q 1 yr?

Intervention: Diet, exercise (2° prevention)

Issues: Intervention efficacy makes screening of questionable value (USPSTF: Ann IM 2003;139:930, 933; Can Med Assoc J 1999;160:513)

Osteoporosis

Of asx pts very debatable—NIH CDC: Jama 2001;285:785, but grade B recommendation of USHSPTF: Ann IM 2002;137:526)

Group: Perimenopausal women and elderly men

Intervention: Calcium + vitamin D po (1° prevention) (Nejm 1997;337:670)

Freq: Continuous

Group: Perimenopausal women

Screen: Bone mineral density by various techniques

Intervention: Estrogen rx (1° prevention) (p 838); alendronate 5-10 mg po qd if low bone mineral density (Jama 1998;280:2077 vs 2119) and esp if can't take ERT and/or have already had fx's

Freq: Continuous

Issues: Risks and cmplc of estrogen rx

Pelvic Inflammatory Disease

Ann IM 2004;141:501,570; Am J Prev Med 2001;20(3S):90

Group: Young (< 25 yr) asx women, and ? male adolescents, esp those w h/o STDs

Screen: 1st-void urine ligase chain reaction test for chlamydial DNA (89% sens, 99% specif)

Intervention: Azithromycin 1 gm po × 1

Freq: q 6-12 mo

Issues: Expensive testing and delayed results

Pneumococcal Infections

Groups: High risk, eg, asplenics; all age > 65 yr, ? > 50 (Ann IM 2003;138:999)

Intervention: Immunization (1° prevention)

Freq: Once, unless 1st dose before age 65, then revaccinate after 5 yr × 1 (Jama 1999;281:243); or once at age 75 (USPSTF 1996)

Prostate Cancer

Unclear if helpful (USPSTF: Ann IM 2002;137:915,917; M. Barry-Nejm 2000;344:1373); most major preventive medicine groups recommend against; may be premature and harmful if undertaken before prospective trials (Jama 1997;277:467 vs ok if life expectancy > 15 yr: Jama 1997;277:497, 1996;276:1976, 1996;275:1976, 1994; 272:773 vs 813; Ann IM 1997;126:394,468,480, 1993;119:914 vs 948; Nejm 1995;333:1401), but is being done more and more without such trial results (Med Let 1992;34:93), now more common than clearly effective colon cancer screening! (Jama 2003;289:1414). Let pt decide after education (Wennberg: J Genl Int Med 1996;11:342).

Group: Males age > 50 yr; ? age 40 and 45 (Jama 2000;284:1399) esp if black and/or positive fam hx @ young age

Screen: Rectal and PSA level > 4 μgm/L (87% sens for aggressive tumors and 55% sens for nonaggressive ones, and 91% specif: Jama 1995;273:289) vs > 2.5 μgm/L in men < 50 yr or if rate of rise is fast (Nejm 2004;350:2239,2292), w f/u transurethral ultrasounds of abnormals? (Nejm 1991;324:1156 vs Ann IM 1993;119:948) vs > 10 μgm/L with ultrasound f/u of abnormals (Med Let 1992;34:93; Nejm 1991;324:1161) q 2 yr if initial level < 2 μgm/L, q 1 yr if 2-4 μgm/L (Jama 1997;277:1460). If free PSA level < 25%, higher cancer risk (Jama 1998;279:1542).

Intervention: Prostatectomy, radiation, or antiandrogen rx; but is unclear that prognosis can be changed (Jama 1992;267:2191) esp if localized disease (Jama 1998;280:969,975,1008), although 1995

data from Mayo Clinic area suggest may be improving incidence (Jama 1995;274:1445) (2° prevention)

Issues: 30% of males age > 50 yr have latent clinically insignificant cancer at incidental postmortem exams and 40% of men in their 60s may have prostate cancer but less than 1% will ever be clinically relevant (Ann IM 1993;118:793,804); need long-term follow-up data; > 25% of tumors found w rectal exam and PSA strategy are small ones found serendipitously so significance unclear (Jama 1997;278:1516)

Rubella Syndrome in Children

Group: All women age < 35 who are potential childbearers

Intervention: Titers and immunization (1° prevention)

Sexually Transmitted Diseases

Group: Prostitutes, gay males, multiple-partner pts, contacts of cases, iv drug users

Screen 1: Culture for gc; enzymatic test for chlamydia; VDRL for syphilis

Intervention: Antibiotics (2° prevention)

Screen 2: HIV serology

Intervention: Counseling re transmission (1° prevention)

Issues: Counseling same whether positive or negative test

Sudden Death in Athletes

Ann IM 1998;129:379

Group: Teenagers and older

Screen: Sports physical, school PE, athletic exam for
Family h/o sudden death or premature heart disease
Personal h/o HT, fatigue, syncope, or DOE

Physical exam for murmurs, supine and standing; femoral pulses; Marfan's stimata; BP

Echocardiogram if abnormalities

Intervention: Avoidance of sports, possible preventive interventions medically or surgically

Suicide/Homicide

Group: All

Intervention: Handgun control via physician support of legislation decreases both by 25% (Nejm 1991;325:1615) (1° prevention)

Testicular Cancer

Group: Men age 15-40 yr

Screen: Self-exam q 1 mo?; or physician exam when see < q 1 yr?

Intervention: Excision (2° prevention)

Issues: Low incidence

Uterine Cancer

Group: Women with an intact uterus especially those with h/o obesity or unopposed estrogen stimulation

Screen: H/o vaginal bleeding, ask q 1 yr; or endometrial sampling in high-risk groups q 1 yr?

Intervention: Hysterectomy (2° prevention)

In Elderly (Age > 65 Yr)

Rv of all issues and literature (J Fam Pract 1992;34:205,320; Am J Pub Hlth 1991;81:1136); must balance benefits w projected life expectancy (NNT estimates: Jama 2001;285:2750)

- Hearing screening by hx, PE, otoscopy for cerumen, and possibly audiometry (w portable Welch-Allyn audioscope: Am J Med Sci 1994;307:40) for presbycusis
- Smoking hx

- BSE instruction, exam, mammogram for breast cancer up to age 75 or to estimated lifespan minus 10 yr (Ann IM 1992;116:722)
- BP for HT
- Visual acuity for refractive error
- Skin exam for cancer, infection, dry skin
- Dental exam
- Pap q 3 yr until 2-3 negatives, then stop (Ann IM 1992; 117:520)
- Immunizations: dT q 10 yr or initial series if not previously done, yearly influenza, debatably pneumovax

Proposed But Not of Proven Help

- Heart disease (USPSTF recommendation = insufficient evidence for all: Ann IM 2004;140:569) by EKG and/or ETT; CRP (Nejm 2004;350:1387, 1450); by calcium in coronaries by CT
- Ovarian cancer by pelvic, ultrasound, or Ca-125, mainly because prevalence so low (Jama 1995;273:491; Ann IM 1994; 121:124, 1993;119:838,901)
- Scoliosis by back exam of early teenagers not clearly effective (USPSTF: Jama 1993;269:2667)
- UTI by UA, urine culture
- Thyroid disease w TSH, even in high-risk groups (USPSTF: Ann IM 2004;140:125) because unclear if rx helps until have sx
- End-stage renal disease by dipstick screening and rx w ACEI/ARB not effective unless pt has HT and/or AODM (Jama 2003;290:3101)
- Inborn errors of metabolism in children by tandem mass spectrometry; unclear if helpful in asx population (Nejm 2003; 348:2304)

Adult Immunizations

Ann IM 1994;121:540; Guide for Adult Immunizations Am College
Phys 3rd ed 1994; Nejm 1993;328:1252; Med Let 1990;32:54

- Td at age 50 yr, perhaps Tdap to control pertussis (Jama
2005;293:3003)
- Pneumococcal vaccine at age 60+ × 1; repeat if given > 6 yr
earlier
- Influenza q 1 yr (see Sept Med Let discussion annually)
- Hep B if at high risk for exposure
- Smallpox (Jama 2003;289:3278,3283,3290,3295); rare transient cmplc, esp myopericaditis, in 5000 U.S. Army administrations; can reduce by use of dilute (<1/10) to revaccinate w
reduced cmplc

14.4 Preventive Maneuvers for Children

Newborns

- Screen for toxoplasmosis, PKU
- Eye prophylaxis vs gonorrhea and chlamydia: Tetracycline 1%
ointment once or erythromycin is better than silver nitrate
(Nejm 1988;318:657)
- Vitamin K to prevent hemorrhagic cmplc; no increase in child-
hood cancers by using it (Nejm 1993;329:905)
- Hearing loss, bilateral screening of questionable benefit
although mandated in 32 states (Jama 2001;286:2000)

Infants/Children

Table 14.1 Lead Screening of All Children, with Serum Lead Levels, at 6–12 Mo and q 6–12 Mo to Age 24 Mo; Screen Older Children Only if High Risk

Level	Plan
< 10 μgm %	Repeat per above schedule
10-25 μgm %	Repeat; improve environment; give po Fe, which decreases Pb absorption
25-45 μgm %	Aggressive rx of environment; po Fe; consider chelation
45+ μgm %	Refer for chelation

Table 14.2 Dietary Fluoride Supplement Dosage Schedule (mg/d)

Age (yr)	Home Water Fluoride Concentration (ppm or mg/L)		
	< 0.30 ppm	0.3–0.6 ppm	> 0.60 ppm
6 mo-3 yr	0.25 mg qd	0	0
3-6 yr	0.50 mg qd	0.25 mg qd	0
6-16 yr	1.0 mg qd	0.5 mg qd	0

Scoliosis (p 881): Screening in schools in preteens is controversial

Immunization Schedules

Jama 1995;273:693; Nejm 1992;327:1794

General rules:

Give when due, as long as temperature ≤ 100°F (37.7°C) (debatable: Jama 1996;275:704, 1991;265:2095); slight increase in febrile seizures w MMR w/o long-term sequelae (Jama 2004;292:351)

Give dT, DPT, Hib, and Hep B im; give MMR sc

Hib in protocol below is for MSD 3-shot series; other types require additional dose at 6 mo but using any of the 3 available Hib vaccines at 2, 4, 6, and 12-15 mo is ok (Jama 1995;273:849)

Egg allergies no contraindication to measles vaccination (Nejm 1995;332:1262)

Conjugate pneumococcal 7-valent vaccine in children debatably now being recommended routinely (Med Let 2003;45:27; Jama 2004;291:2197, 2000;283:1460)

Routine at age:

Birth: Hep B #1 (Jama 1995;274:1201), perhaps eventually in combo w Hep A vaccine

2 mo: DTaP #1 (Nejm 1995;333:1045) +
> Hib #1
> Hep B #2
> IPV #1 (or all as Pediarix: Med Let 2003;45:37)
> Pneumo #1

4 mo: DTaP #2
> Hib #2, or all 4 (DTaP + Hib) as TriHIBit
> IPV #2 (or all as Pediarix)
> Pneumo #2

6 mo: DTaP #3
> Hib #3, or all 4 as TriHIBit
> IPV #3 (or all as Pediarix)
> Pneumo #3

15 mo: DTaP #4
> Hib #4, or all 4 (DPT + Hib) as Tetramune (Med Let 1993;35:104)
> MMR #1
> Hep B #3
> Varicella vaccine (Varivax) (Jama 1997;278:1529) 0.5 cc
> sc × 1

4-6 yr: DTaP #5
> IPV #4
> MMR #2

11+ yr: dT q 10 yr
>MMR #2 if not given at age 4-6
>Hep B #4
>Possibly varicella vaccine if no previous immunization or h/o chickenpox (Jama 1997;277:203)

Catch up under age 7:

1st: DTaP #1
>OPV #1
>MMR
>Hib #1 if < 5 yr
>Heb B # 1, ped dose
>Pneumo #1

2 mo: DTaP #2
>OPV #2
>Hib #2 if < 15 mo when started
>Heb B # 2
>Pneumo? #2 if < 2 yr

4 mo: DTaP #3
>Heb B # 3

6-12 mo: OPV #3

Catch up over age 7:

1st: Td #1
>OPV #1
>MMR #1
>Heb B # 1, 2, 3 q 1 mo pediatric doses, or if over age 10, 2 adult doses 6 mo apart

2 mo: Td #2
>OPV #2
>MMR #2 (optional)

6 mo: Td #3
>OPV #

Growth Charts

Source: National Center for Health Statistics; and the National
Center for Chronic Disease Prevention and Health Promotion
(2000) (http://www.cdc.gov/growthcharts)

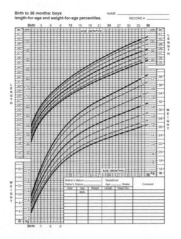

Figure 14.1 Birth to 36 months: Boys length-for-age and weight-for-age percentiles.

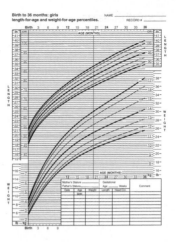

Figure 14.2 Birth to 36 months: Girls length-for-age and weight-for-age percentiles.

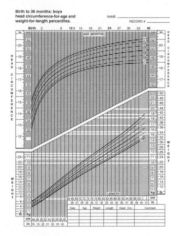

Figure 14.3 Birth to 36 months: Boys head circumference-for-age and weight-for-length percentiles.

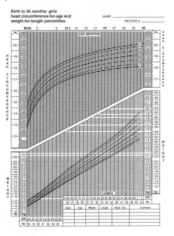

Figure 14.4 Birth to 36 months: Girls head circumference-for-age and weight-for-length percentiles.

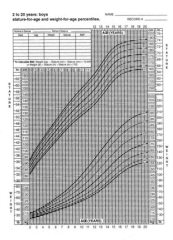

Figure 14.5 2 to 20 years: Boys stature-for-age and weight-for-age percentiles.

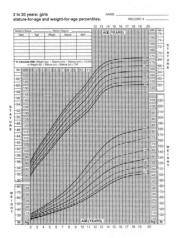

Figure 14.6 2 to 20 years: Girls stature-for-age and weight-for-age percentiles.

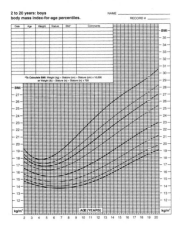

Figure 14.7 2 to 20 years: Boys body mass index-for-age percentiles.

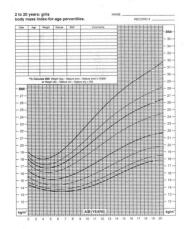

Figure 14.8 2 to 20 years: Girls body mass index-for-age percentiles.

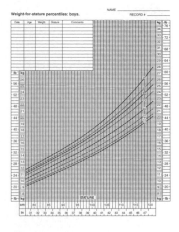

Figure 14.9 Weight-for-stature percentiles: Boys.

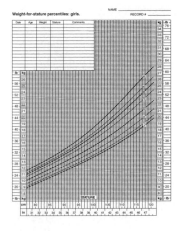

Figure 14.10 Weight-for-stature percentiles: Girls.

Chapter 15

Psychiatry

D. K. Onion

15.1 Medications

Med Let 1997;39:33; GH Clark: Practioner's Guide for Depression + Anxiety Disorders 10/02

Tranquilizers/Sleeping Medications

Med Let 2000;42:71; rv of insomnia dx and rx: Nejm 2005;353:803

> Antihistamines like diphenhydramine (Benadryl) 25-50 mg po hs; anticholinergic side effects
>
> Barbiturates; substantial OD risk
>
> Benzodiazepines (Nejm 1993;328:1398; Med Let 1991;33:43, 1988;30:26) many have long half-lives; withdrawal sx × 1-4 wk after chronic use (Nejm 1986;315:854); safest hypnotics available unless combined w alcohol abuse, but none alone work long term for sleep (Jama 1997;278:2170). All increase the likelihood of accidents (Am J Pub Hlth 1990;80:1467), especially in elderly, and especially the long-acting ones in the first week of use (Jama 1997;278:27); thus if use at all, use $\frac{1}{2}$-$\frac{1}{3}$ normal dose.
>
> **Benzodiazepines in roughly equivalent po doses:**
> > * short half-life, thus good hypnotic/sleep meds
> > Alprazolam* (Xanax) 0.5 mg, or XR long acting; may work for panic attacks without tolerance developing but hard

to withdraw (must do so very slowly) and recurrences
are frequent (Med Let 2005;47:5), high incidence of adverse CNS effects and high addiction potential

Chlorazepate (Tranxene) 7.5 mg

Chlordiazepoxide (Librium) 10mg

Clonazepam (Klonopin) 0.5 mg; binds similar site but since
long acting, less of a high and preferable; can also be
used to withdraw from alprazolam by switching to clonazepam for 2-3 wk while tricyclic started (J. Dreher
7/91)

Diazepam (Valium) 5 mg, also available im/iv

Estazolam (ProSom) 1-2 mg

Flurazepam (Dalmane) 30 mg

Lorazepam* (Ativan) 1-2 mg; ok for sleep if used occasionally (Med Let 1989;31:23), effective im, renal excretion

Midazolam* (Versed) iv use, syrup also available; used for se-
dation/anesthesia only

Oxazepam* (Serax) 15-30 mg; ok for sleep if use occasionally
(Med Let 1989;31:23); hepatic gluuronidation preserved
even w liver disease, so often used for DTs or lorazepam

Temazepam* (Restoril) 15-30 mg; may be best for sleep
(Med Let 1991;33:91)

Triazolam* (Halcion) 0.125-0.25 mg; higher incidence of
"blackouts"

Imidazopyridines; non-benzo's, not anxiolytic; bind benzo receptor but no tolerance, withdrawal, or REM sleep rebound
(Clin Ger Med 1998;14:67); half-lives < 2.5 hr

Eszopiclone* (Lunesta) (Med Let 2005;47:17) 1-3 mg po hs;
$3/pill any strength

Zaleplon* (Sonata) (Med Let 1999;41:93) 5 mg; very short
acting; $3/10 mg

Zolpidem* (Ambien)10 mg (5 mg in elderly); ODs aren't
bad and can be rx'd w flumazenil (Mazicon); adverse effects: nausea and vomiting, rare psychotic reactions;
$3/10 mg

Others:

Buspirone (BuSpar) 5-10 mg t-qid, for chronic anxiety, not a
benzodiazepine, no abuse potential or interactions with driving or alcohol; not for panic disorder or sleep; takes several
weeks to work like tricyclics (J. Dreher 7/91); levels increased a lot by erythromycin and itraconazole; $10/wk
(Med Let 1986;28:117)

Chloralhydrate (Noctec) 500 mg po hs; OD risk, rapid entry into
CNS increases dependence and abuse, tachyphylaxis

Ethchlorvynol (Placidyl); substantial OD risk, and rapid entry
into CNS increases dependence and abuse

Antidepressants like trazodone or amitriptyline; but OD risk,
anticholinergic side effects w latter

Non-rx/herbal hypnotics:

Kava root extract, herbal equivalent of benzodiazepines; adverse
effects: hepatotoxicity

Melatonin (Nejm 1997;336:186; Med Let 1995;37:962) 2 mg sustained release, or 1-5 mg po hs; helpful to allow chronic hs
benzo taper, 5 mg po qd × 2+ d helps jet lag (ACP J Club
2001;135:97) and useful to entrain blind people in a 24-hr
cycle (Nejm 2000;343:1070,1114); adverse effects:
hypothermia, gonadal inhibition

Valerian root 200-900 mg po hs; sold as Alluna w hops

Cognitive behavioral rx for sleep (Jama 2001;285;1850):

- Educate re normal age-specific sleep patterns
- Sleep in bed; no reading, TV, etc
- Establish standard wake-up time
- Get up during extended awakenings
- Stop daytime naps
- Set time in bed = avg sleep time + 30 min; increase or de-
crease by 15 min q 1 wk if sleep efficiency > 85% or < 80%

Antipsychotics

Med Let 1991;33:47; Nejm 1996;334:34

Older types:

Table 15.1   Older Types of Antipsychotics

Name	Equivalent Potency
Phenothiazines	
Chlorpromazine (Thorazine)	100 mg
Thioridazine (Mellaril)	100 mg
Perphenazine (Trilafon)	8 mg
Trifluoperazine (Stelazine)	5 mg
Other	
Clozapine (Clozaril)	50 mg
Haloperidol (Haldol)	5 mg
Molindone (Moban)	50 mg
Thiothixene (Navane)	5 mg

Common adverse effects:

- Acute dystonic reactions; rx with antihistamines, or antiparkinsonism meds;
- Akathisia (restlessness, inability to sit still)
- Neuroleptic malignant syndrome (p 17)
- Parkinsonism; rx with anticholinergics like benztropine (Cogentin), trihexyphenidyl (Artane), etc
- Tardive dyskinesia (p 778)

Atypical antipsychotics (Med Let 2005;47:81): All have fewer extrapyramidal side effects than older antipsychotics and often cause weight gain; neuroleptic malignant syndrome occurs w all, hyperprolactinemia only w risperidone

Aripirazole (Abilify) (Med Let 2003;45:15) 10-30 mg po qd; lacks weight gain, diabetes, hyperlipidemia, long QT syndrome, hyperprolactinemia of other atypicals; $300/mo for 15 mg qd

Clozapine (Clozaril) (Jama 1995;274:981; Med Let 1993;35:16) 12.5 mg po qd gradually increasing to 300-400 mg qd; a tetracyclic, works without increasing prolactin or causing Parkinsonism so can use in those pts (Nejm 1999;340:757); adverse effects: sedation, anticholinergic, seizures, and fatal agranulocytosis (Nejm 1993;329:162), which recurs if rechallenged, so q 1 wk CBC monitoring for 1st 6 mo, rare tardive dyskinesia; drug alone costs $250 (generic) to $350/mo for 100 tid + costs of CBCs ($300/mo for q 1 wk); interacts w phenytoin by decreasing blood levels, w benzodi-azepines by causing respiratory arrest, and w carbamazepine (Tegretol) by worsening agranulocytosis risk

Olanzapine (Zyprexa) (Med Let 1997;38:5) 5 (in elderly) to 20 mg po/im qd; for schizophrenia; adverse effects: postural hy-potension, somnolence, constipation, weight gain and dia-betes, increased LFTs; no agranulocytosis, rare tardive dyskinesia, less anticholinergic than risperidone; $400/mo for 15 mg qd

Quetiapine (Seroquel); adverse effects: sedation, dizziness; $300/mo for 200 mg bid

Risperidone (Risperdal) (Med Let 1994;36:33), start at 0.5-1 mg po bid, increase to 2 mg po bid max, im depot form also available; low doses help Alzheimer's hallucinations and psy-choses; helps negative sx of schizophrenia (eg, apathy) much better than phenothiazines or haloperidol but not as good as clozapine, also helps the positive sx as well, with only rare tardive dyskinesia and no agranulocytosis; adverse effects: asthenia, extrapyramidal sx esp at doses > 6 mg, sedation, occasional orthostatic hypotension, weight gain, prolactin elevations, sexual dysfunction; cost: $260/mo for 4 mg qd

Ziprasidone (Geodon) (Med Let 2001;43:51) 20-80 mg po bid, im form available; less weight gain than w others; adverse effects: long QT syndrome, more than others in class; cost $250/mo for 40 mg bid

Antidepressants

Nejm 2000;343:1942; Ann IM 2000;132:738,743; Med Let 1999;41:33)

All types of roughly equal efficacy and have similar dropout rates (Am J Med 2000;108:54); taper shorter-acting ones over 2-4 wk to avoid withdrawal side efects

Mixed serotonin and norepinephrine reuptake inhibitors tricyclics:
Start low and increase by 25 mg q 4-5 d; give 2-3 hr before hs; 80% improve sleep within 1st wk; check levels 10-12 hr after last dose; if asx after 6 mo, taper by halving dose × 4 mo, then tapering by 25 mg/wk to avoid cholinergic hyperactivity w abrupt withdrawal. Safe in pregnancy (Nejm 1997;336:258). Levels increased by aging, weight loss, inflammatory diseases, cimetidine, morphine, steroids, alkaline urine; levels depressed by smoking, hyperlipidemia, barbiturates, anticonvulsants, acid urine, and antipsychotics; hence *beware* use w phenothiazines, which increase TCA levels, especially Mellaril, which lengthens QT intervals as well and thus can cause ventricular arrhythmias (Med Let 1978;20:49). Appetite stimulated by amoxapine, amitriptyline, and doxepin; suppressed by protriptyline, imipramine, and desipramine. Adverse effects: see Table 15.2; all can worsen heart-block and increase arrhythmias like class I antiarrhythmics slightly (Am J Med 2000;108:2); overdose (p 33); anticholinergic effects of dry mouth, urinary retention, blurry vision, and sexual dysfunction; psych sx (Med Let 2002;44:59) like mania, delirium, hallucinations, paranoia

Amitriptyline (Elavil); start at 50 mg hs, increase by 25 mg q 2-3 d to 150 mg qd; much lower doses in elderly, eg, 10 mg po qd

Amoxapine (Asendin); quite stimulating, especially of appetite, cf Ritalin; adverse effects: metabolite can cause tardive dyskinesia

Table 15.2 Common Side Effects of Antidepressants

Drug	Central Nervous System			Cardiovascular		Gi Distress	Other
	Anticholinergic[1]	Drowsiness	Insomnia/Agitation	Orthostatic Hypotension	Cardiac Arrhythmia		Weight Gain (Over 6 kg)
Amitriptyline (Elavil, Endep)	4+	4+	0	4+	3+	0	4+
Desipramine (Norpramin, Pertofrane)	1+	1+	1+	2+	2+	0	1+
Doxepin (Adapin, Sinequan)	3+	4+	0	2+	2+	0	3+
Imipramine (Janimine, Tofranil)	3+	3+	1+	4+	3+	1+	3+
Nortriptyline (Aventyl, Pamelor)	1+	1+	0	2+	2+	0	1+
Protriptyline (Vivactil)	2+	1+	1+	2+	2+	0	0
Trimipramine (Surmontil)	1+	4+	0	2+	2+	0	3+

(continues)

Table 15.2 (continued)

| | Side Effect | | | | | | | |
| | Central Nervous System | | | Cardiovascular | | | | Other |
Drug	Anticholinergic[1]	Drowsiness	Insomnia/ Agitation	Orthostatic Hypotension	Cardiac Arrhythmia	Gi Distress		Weight Gain (Over 6 kg)
Amoxapine (Asendin)	2+	2+	2+	2+	3+	0		1+
Maprotiline (Ludiomil)	2+	4+	0	0	1+	0		2+
Trazodone (Desyrel)	0	4+	0	1+	1+	1+		1+
Bupropion (Wellbutrin)	0	0	2+	0	1+	1+		0
Fluoxetine (Prozac)	0	0	2+	0	0	3+		0
Paroxetine (Paxil)	0	0	2+	0	0	3+		0
Sertraline (Zoloft)	0	0	2+	0	0	3+		0
Monoamine oxidase inhibitors	1	1+	2+	2+	0	1+		2+

0 = absent or rare; 2+ = in between; 4+ = relatively common.
1. Dry mouth, blurred vision, urinary hesitancy, constipation.
Reproduced with permission from Rush AJ. Depression in primary care: detection, diagnosis and treatment. Am Fam Phys 1993;47:1784

Clomipramine (Anafranil) 50-150 mg po qd; also helps obsessive-compulsive behaviors, especially trichotillomania (Nejm 1989;321:497); adverse effects: seizures, much anticholinergic effect, weight gain, sexual dysfunction

Cyclobenzaprine (Flexeril) 10 mg po qd-tid; esp for muscle and neuropathic pain, rarely used for depression and no studies to show it is an effective antidepressant

Desipramine (Norpramin); same dosing as amitriptyline; least sedating, fewer anticholinergic side effects

Doxepin (Sinequan); sedating; use this or trazodone (Desyrel) in elderly (UCLA 1/92)

Imipramine (Tofranil), start low to 200 mg po qd

Nortriptyline (Pamelor, Aventyl), start low to 100 mg po qd, titrate to blood levels of 50-150 ng/cc

Protriptyline (Vivactil) 5 mg tid-10 mg qid po

Selective serotonin and norepinephrine reuptake inhibitors:
Duloxetine (Cymbalta) (Med Let 2004;46:81) 60 mg po qd; renal excretion; not clearly better than venlafaxine or SSRIs; $102/mo

Venlafaxine (Effexor) 25-100 mg po bid or as Effexor XR (Med Let 2004;46:15; Jama 2000;283:3082) 37.5 mg gradually increased to 75-225 mg po qd; especially effective for anxiety-type depression, better than buspirone; adverse effects: activation and hypertension, also occur for 3 d w cessation of drug or even one missed pill so must taper; $115/mo for 75 mg bid

Tetracyclics: Maprotiline (Ludiomil)

Serotonin antagonists: Mirtazapine (Remeron) (Med Let 1996; 38:113) 15-60 mg po hs; adverse effects: sedation, weight gain, rare agranulocystosis; $60/mo for 30 mg qd

Mao inhibitors (rarely prescribed because of food restrictions and many drug interactions, especially bad ones w tricyclics):

Phenelzine (Nardil) 15 mg qd × 1, 30 mg qd × 3 d, then 30 mg
b-tid; best for generalized social phobias, refractory panic
d/o, and intrusive sx of PTSD; avoid specific foods (Med Let
1980;22:38); *beware* concomitant use of meperidine
(Demerol) and all opiates, which causes severe sedation; sexual dysfunction

Tranylcypromine (Parnate) 20-50 mg po qd but start at 10; no
drowsiness or sedation

Selective serotonin reuptake inhibitors (SSRIs) (Med Let 2003;
45:93): Except for fluvoxamine, all equally useful for panic d/o,
depression (Jama 2001;286:2947), bulimia, and OCD; all ok in
children? (Med Let 2003;45:53); all free of anticholinergic side
effects, safer if taken in OD than but equal in efficacy to TCAs
(BMJ 1993;306:683); safe in pregnancy (Jama 1998;279:609;
Nejm 1997;336:258) in 1st and 2nd trimesters but at least w fluoxetine, increase perinatal cmplc in 3rd trimester as well as incidence of low birth weight (Nejm 1996;335:1011); and safer to
use post-MI than TCAs (Jama1998;279:287); all have half-lives
< 24 hr except fluoxetine, for which is 90 hr (Mayo Clin Proc
1994;69:1069) and an active metabolite lasting 1 wk; no increased suicide w initiation (Jama 2004;292:338)

Adverse effects: nausea, diarrhea, sleepiness, bruxism, sexual
dysfunction in 70% of both men and women but rx'able w sildenafil (Jama 2003;289:56), weight gain w most but least w fluoxetine; drug interactions: increase TCAs, haloperidol, clozapine, warfarin, metoprolol, **serotonin syndromes** (p 18); all
$66-86/mo, generics $1/2-2/3$ of that cost

Fluoxetine (Prozac, Sarafem) (Nejm 1994;331:1354; Med Let
1990;32:83) 20-40 mg po qd in am, 60 mg q 1 wk may work,
long-acting forms not worth it (Med Let 2001;43:27); 7 d
half-life, takes 3 wk to plateau, hence after started can go to
40-60 mg q 1 wk; least sedating, an "upper," even 20 mg qd
may be too much for some pts; not too useful in the elderly

(long half-life); can use in children. Sold in combination w olanzapine as Symbyax but is not useful (Med Let 2004; 46:23).

Citalopram (Celexa) (Med Let 1998;40:113) 20-80 mg po qd; adverse effects: interacts w MAO inhibitors, increases levels of β-blockers, TCAs; levels increased by cimetidine; long QT syndrome at high doses

Escitalpram (Lexapro) (Med Let 2002;44:83) 10 mg po qd; active L-isomer of citalopram; probably fewer drug interactions than fluoxetine or paroxetine but still some sexual dysfunction

Paroxetine (Paxil) (Med Let 1993;35:24) 20-40 mg po qd; most sedating and weight gain ("packing the pounds w Paxil")

Sertraline (Zoloft) (Med Let 1992;34:47) 50-150 mg po qd, or even 200 mg (Jama 1998;280:1665); used often in elderly and in children (Jama 2003;290:1033), can decrease aggressive behavior (Mike Tyson); adverse effects: diarrhea

Fluvoxamine (Luvox) (Med Let 1995;37:13) 50-200 mg po hs; for obsessive-compulsive disorder; adverse effects: serotonergic ones as above, dangerous ODs w hypotension and seizures, toxic epidermal necrolysis (Lancet 1993;342:304), slows metabolism of benzodiazepines, warfarin, phenytoin, propranolol, theophylline, TCAs, etc.

Serotonin antagonists and reuptake inhibitors:

Nefazodone (Serzone) (Med Let 1995;37:33) 100-300 mg po bid; similar to trazodone; adverse effects: sedating, atropine effects, bad LFT effects, lots of drug interactions and w grapefruit

Trazodone (Desyrel) 100-300 mg qd, 25-100 mg in elderly for sleep; mixed serotonergic effects; no anticholinergic problems; can use w SSRIs especially if sleep disturbance, 3.5-hr half-life; adverse effects: priapism (Med Let 1984;26:35); more sedating than TCAs; may increase phenytoin, digoxin levels; appetite suppression; postural hypotension sometimes; w ginko, can cause coma

Dopamine and norepinephrine reuptake inhibitors: Bupropion (Wellbutrin, Zyban) (Med Let 1993;35:25) 100 mg po tid; no anticholinergic side effects or sexual dysfunction; adverse effects: agitation, insomnia; sometimes anticholinergic sx; seizures, esp at dose > 450 mg qd and esp if h/o bulimia

Other antidepressants:

St. John's wort? (Med Let 1997;39:107) 300 mg po tid; potency and efficacy still unclear, maybe for mild depression, no effect in moderate depression by RDBCT (Jama 2002;287: 1807, 2001;285:1978); adverse effects: photosensitivity and secondary neurotoxicity can cause neuropathic pain in sun-exposed areas; increases cataracts; drug interactions (Med Let 2000;42:56) w nearly half of all meds (Jama 2003;290: 1500) via induction of CP450 enzymes, including digoxin, warfarin, SSRIs, indinavir; possibly w oral contraceptives (decreases effect), theophylline, TCAs

Lamotrigine (Lamictal) 50-100 mg po qd; adverse effects: rashes, rare Stevens-Johnson syndrome risk

Mood stabilizers: For hyperarousal, anxiety, and irritability

Lithium (Eskalith) (Nejm 1994;331:591) 0.3-0.6 gm po tid to serum level = 0.8-1.0 mEq/L 12 hr after last dose (Nejm 1989;321:1489); usually used for bipolar pts with prominent manic component to illness, good response for acute mania in 70%; adverse effects: tremor; nausea, vomiting, diarrhea; teratogenic; many drug interactions; goiter in 15%, lowered T_3T_4 with elevated TSH in 5%, similar to I_2 load; worsens COPD (Nejm 1983;308:319); nephrogenic DI in 20-70%, rx with amiloride 5-10 mg bid (Nejm 1985;312:408) or other thiazide; hypokalemia and PVCs (Nejm 1972;287:867); elevated calcium and PTH (Ann IM 1977;86:63); drug toxicities worsened by ACEIs and loop diuretics (J Am Ger Soc

2004;52:794); $8/mo generic, $20/mo for Eskalith at 1200 mg qd

Valproate (Depakote)/divalproex (Depakene) (Med Let 1994; 36:74) 250-750 mg po b-tid to level of 50-125 µgm/cc; prevention of manic sx and used for hypomania especially in rapid cycling; adverse effects: nausea and vomiting, weight gain, rash, alopecia, ataxia; $94/mo for 1500 mg qd

Carbamazepine (Tegretol) ~1000 mg po qd; used for hypomania especially in rapid-cycling bipolar pts; $37/mo generic, $52/mo trade

15.2 Psychiatric Diseases

Alcoholism and Withdrawal

Nejm 1998;338:592, 1989;321:442

Cause: Multifactorial including genetic (cross fostering studies: Nejm 1988;318:180) and/or behavioral characteristics leading to addiction

Epidem: Males/females = 3:1. Acute and chronic complications of alcohol may occur more often in women than men due not to size differences but to gastric mucosa alcohol dehydrogenase activity (Nejm 1990;322:95).

Pathophys: gi and pancreatic acute and chronic toxicity (Ann IM 1981;95:198). Withdrawal sx due to increased noradrenergic activity (Ann IM 1987;107:875) and long-term changes in GABA and glutamate receptors.

Sx: H/o significant trauma (70%: Ann IM 1984;101:847), eg, motor vehicle accident (Nejm 1987;317:1262)

Standardized questionnaires (Ann IM 1998;129:353; Jama 1998;280:166, 1994;272:1782) like MAST, AUDIT, TWEAK (Tolerance measured by ability to "hold" ≥ 6 drinks or "high" on ≥ 3 drinks; Worried friends; Eye openers; Amnesia hx; Kut down plans), and the short test CAGE questions (Have you tried to Cut down; are you Annoyed by criticism of your drinking; do you sometimes feel Guilty about your drinking; and do you sometimes have an Eye-opener drink in the morning?: Jama 1984;252:1905). TWEAK score ≥ 2 is 87% sens and specif in women, 95% sens and 56% specif in men; scores ≥ 3, less sens and more specific. CAGE score ≥ 2 has 74% sens, 91% specif (Jama 1994;272: 1782; Ann IM 1991;115:774).

Upper limit of alcohol consumption not associated w problems is < 4 drinks qd and < 14-17/wk for men, and < 3 drinks qd and < 7-12/wk for women (Jama 1995;276:1964; Am J Pub Hlth 1995;85:823)

Si:

Crs:

Cmplc: Hypokalemia, hypomagnesemia, hypocalcemia, hypoglycemia, hypophosphatemia, ketoacidosis, respiratory alkalosis (Nejm 1993;329:1927)

Increased mortality from cirrhosis, accidents, cancer, respiratory illness when > 4 drinks qd (Am J Pub Hlth 1993;83:805; Ann IM 1984;101:847); smoking-related mortality continues even if stop drinking (Jama 1996;275:1097)

Pneumonia, due to diminished macrophage function, ciliary action, and polymorphonuclear wbc responses (Nejm 1970; 282:123)

Sudden death (arrhythmias) and strokes (Curr Concepts Cerebro Dis 1986;21:24; Nejm 1986;315:1041)

Delirium tremens (DTs) including prior h/o often, agitation, tremor, disorientation, delirium, hallucinations, seizures, hyperthermia (rectal temp); 10-20% mortality

Wernicke's encephalopathy and Korsakoff's psychosis (p 316)

Seizures, as often during drinking as in withdrawal? (Nejm 1988;319:666) whenever alcohol levels are rapidly falling

Vitamin A deficiency causing impaired night vision (Ann IM 1978;88:622)

Lab: *Chem:* Blood alcohol level > 0.08 mg % = legal intoxication, but levels often > 0.02% in alcoholics w few overt si of intoxication; fatty acid ethyl esters pos up to 24 hr later (Jama 1996;
276:1152)

LFTs up, acutely GGTP, chronically AST (SGOT), GGTP, Alk Phos

Xray: CT scan of head for alcohol seizures only if evident head trauma or focal si's (Ann IM 1981;94:519)

Rx (rv: Nejm 2005;352:596): Primary prevention: Screen with GGTP, if > 50 U/L, educate once, repeat in 1 mo and 1 yr (Prev Med 1991;20:518); or ask re number of drinks/wk, if > 14 for men, > 11 for women, then educate q 1 mo × 2, this strategy decreases alcohol intake by $^1/_3$-$^1/_2$ over 1 yr (Jama 1997;277:1040)

Secondary prevention (Am J Med 2000;108:263; Jama 1998;279:1230): Structured treatment program should include anticipatory guidance by primary doctor, 12-step program (AA), and perhaps prophylaxis (Nejm 1999;340:1482) w

- Naltrexone (ReVia) (Med Let 1995;37:64 vs not effective by DBCT: Nejm 2001;345:1734) 50-100 mg po qd or 190-380 mg im q 1 mo (Jama 2005;293:1617); an opiate antagonist, hepatic metabolism; $110/mo
- Disulfiram (Antabuse) 250 mg qd (Ann IM 1989;111:943); $22/mo
- Acamprosate (Campral) (Med Let 2005;47:1; Jama 1999; 281:1318) 333-666 mg po tid; moderately effective, can use w disulfiram or naltrexone; $105/mo

Alcoholics Anonymous (AA), detoxification programs, etc; prognosis for rehabilitation better after motor vehicle accident (Nejm 1987;317:1262). With safe stable home situation, outpatient rx as good as inpatient (Nejm 1989;320:358). Nonhospital residential programs adequate and cheaper (Nejm 1990;323:844, Institute of Medicine recommendations re drug and alcohol rehab policies). Later controlled drinking controversial, < 2% can safely pull it off (Nejm 1985;312:1678).

Rx any depression (p 942) (Jama 1996;275:761) w SSRIs of withdrawal (Jama 1997;278:145)

of DTs: Hospitalize, iv lorazepam 1 mg/5 min, or diazepam 1 mg/min until BP and agitation decrease

of lesser degrees of withdrawal:

- Thiamine 100-200 mg im/iv bid × 2 d +
- Benzodiazepines

  Lorazepam (Ativan) 2 mg im q 1 hr or po q 2 hr to control si and sx, to 12 mg max

  Chlordiazepoxide (Librium) 100 mg po/im q 6 hr × 4 doses, then q 8 hr × 3 doses, then q 12 hr × 2 doses, then hs once, then stop; or 25-100 mg po q 4-6 hr prn scoring system like below results in hospital d/c > 2 d sooner (Jama 1994;272:519); beware oversedation, which takes days to recover from since has a 36+-hr half-life, or

  Oxazepam (Serax) 30 mg po q 6 hr × 7 d (Am J Psych 1989;146:617); or 30 mg po q 4 hr × 6 doses, then q 6 hr × 4 doses, then q 8 hr × 3 doses, then q 12 hr × 2 doses, then hs once, then stop; or 0-45 mg po q 4 hr (q 2 hr if no improvement after last dose) based on various scoring systems (Br J Addict 1989;84:1353) that rate tachycardia (> 100), HT (> 140/90), sweating, tremor, fever (99.6°F), insomnia, agitation, disorientation, and hallucinations (Clin Pharmacol Ther 1989;34:822), or

  Diazepam (Valium) (Clin Pharmacol Ther 1983;34:822) 0-15 mg iv/im/po q 2-4 hr based on a scoring system as above; long half-life like chlordiazepoxide

- Other meds:

  Carbamezepine

  Valproate

MgSO$_4$ 50% soln, 2 cc iv/im q 8 hr × 2 d

Thiamine 100 mg po/im tid × 3d

of seizures: Lorazepam (Ativan) 2 mg iv after 1st seizure reduces 25% recurrence rate within next 6 hr to 3% and over 48 hr from 32% to 4% (Nejm 1999;340:915)

Anxiety

Jama 2001;286:450, 2000;283:2573; Nejm 1993;329:631, 1989;321:1209

Cause: Genetic component perhaps; increased incidence in families w h/o alcoholism

Types:

- Generalized anxiety (most common)
- Panic disorder (PD)
- Phobias
- Obsessive-compulsive disorder (Nejm 2004;350:259)
- Post-traumatic stress disorder (Nejm 2002;346:108) from severe stress in adult life or childhood

Epidem: Panic disorder lifetime prevalence = 1.5-3.5%; pts ²/₃ of the time have another primary psychiatric dx, especially depression

Pathophys: In PD, dysfunctional brain neurotransmitter alarm system (Jama 2000;283:2573)

Sx: Generally onset in 20s; sx include hyperventilation, palpitations, pains, fears, flushes; h/o long medical workups, agoraphobia

Panic attack: Unfounded sudden fear, terror, sense of impending doom with associated somatic manifestations; defined as 3 such attacks within 3 wk

Post-traumatic stress disorder: Onset either immediate within 1-2 d of event or delayed months to years, manifested by numbing and avoidance sx (Oklahoma City bombing: Jama 1999;282:755); seen especially in wounded veterans and incest/abuse victims; manifested by hyperalertness and difficulty falling asleep (Nejm 1987;317:1630); often associated w confounding chemical abuse

Si: Sympathomimetic si's; obsessive-compulsive actions (Nejm 1989;321:540) in OCD types

Crs: Often chronic and disabling

Cmplc: Suicide in panic disorder debatably
r/o alcohol and/or substance abuse; **Caffeine addiction withdrawal**, especially with headache and fatigue (Jama 1994; 272:1043,1065; Nejm 1992;327:1109)

Lab:

Rx (Nejm 2004;351:675; Med Let 2005;47:5):

of generalized type:
Cognitive-behavioral therapy to train to substitute positive thoughts; perhaps relaxation therapy
SSRIs in gradually increasing doses; also helpful in panic d/o, OCD
Venlaxatine (Effexor) or nefazone (Serzone)
Kava (J Clin Psych 2000;20:84)
Buspirone 5-10 mg t-qid to 60 mg/d max; can prevent emergence of but not acute sx
TCAs like nortriptyline, imipramine
Benzodiazepines like clonazepam et al for 2-4 wk, then taper
of social phobias: Propranolol for stage fright type of anxiety, 40 mg 1.5 hr before stress, can improve performance (Med Let 1984;26:61); also helps violent outbursts in the elderly (M. Beers UCLA 1/92)
of generalized type:
SSRIs (Brit J Psych 1999;175:120; Jama 1998;280:708) like paroxetine (Paxil) 20-50 mg po qd
Phenelzine (Nardil)
Gabapentin
Cognitive-behavioral rx
of simple phobias (eg, of animals): Desensitization
of OCD (Nejm 2004;350:259): SSRIs in increasing doses, even in children and adolescents (Nejm 2001;344:1279; RCT: Jama

1998;280:1752); try several for 2-3 mo each; cognitive-behavioral rx (Jama 2004;292:1969); clomipramine (Anafranil) 50-250 mg po qd, which helps obsessive-compulsive behaviors especially trichotillomania (Nejm 1989;321:497) as do SSRIs

of panic disorder:

> Cognitive-behavioral rx helps, adds to imipramine rx (Jama 2000;283:2529)

> Antidepressants like:

- Fluoxetine (Prozac) or other SSRI in *low*, not usual, doses (Med Let 1994;36:89)
- MAO inhibitors are as effective as benzodiazepines for some anxious pts even if no depression

> Benzodiazepines, eg, alprazolam (Xanax) or clonazepam (Klonopin) for panic disorder, but addicting so taper (pts often resistant) after TCAs, SSRIs, or MAOIs on board (Med Let 2005;47:5)

Anorexia Nervosa

Ann IM 2001;134:148; Nejm 2005;353:1481

Cause:

Epidem: Females/males = 20:1; associated with bulimia and depression; prevalence of bulimia + anorexia = 5-10% of young women; prevalence increases w family h/o addictive disorders

Pathophys: Amenorrhea develops early when < 90% ideal body weight (IBW= 100 lb @ 60 in, + 5 lb for each inch over that)

Sx: Over 25% weight loss; onset before age 17; laxative use; diuretic use; excessive exercising; amenorrhea; always think self too fat no matter how thin; secretive eating

Si: Lanugo hair; thin to cachectic

Crs: 50% progress to chronic bulimarexia; 9% mortality

Cmplc: Suicide (2-5%); depression; osteoporosis/bone loss (Ann IM 2000;133:790); CHF (starvation: Nejm 1985;313:1457) r/o Addison's disease (Nejm 1996;334:46)

Lab: *Chem:* Hypokalemia; amylase elevated, sometimes due to pancreatitis, but many times due to salivary origin (lipase and pancreatic fraction normal: Ann IM 1987;106:50); hypophosphatemia

Noninv: EKG at regular intervals (Ann IM 1985;102:49) to detect myocardiopathy; long QT syndrome

Rx: Inpatient or outpatient behavioral program is only effective rx
Adjunctive:

Calcium 1200-1500 mg po qd and vitamin D to prevent osteoporosis

Periactin

Perhaps leptin injections for amenorrhea (Nejm 2004;351:987)

Bulimia

Nejm 2003;349:875

Cause: Self-induced vomiting; often use emetine and other meds

Epidem: Females/males > 20:1; usually associated with anorexia; prevalence among young women = 4-8%; 2% of college women are bulimic (Am J Pub Hlth 1988;78:1322)

Associated w childhood sexual abuse in $\frac{1}{3}$ (Am J Pub Hlth 1996;86:1082)

Pathophys: Diminished cholecystokinin production causes decreased satiety (Nejm 1988;319:683) and CNS serotonin

Sx: Onset later than anorexia; compulsive eating binges followed by intense anxiety/guilt leading to purging

Si: Callus on back of hand from emesis induction; dental caries from gastric fluids on teeth; enlarged salivary glands; thin or normal weight; postural blood pressure drops

Crs:

Cmplc: CHF from starvation and Ipecac myocardiopathy and myopathy (Nejm 1985;313:1457); aspiration pneumonias and Mallory-Weiss tears; hypokalemia and sudden death due to long QT syndrome (Ann IM 1985;102:49)

Lab: *Chem:* Amylase elevated, sometimes due to pancreatitis, but many times due to salivary origin (lipase and pancreatic fraction normal: Ann IM 1987;106:50); urinary emetine levels (Nejm 1996;334:47); lytes show: hypoK$^+$, high HCO_3, normal anion gap acidosis w laxative use

Urine qualitative Ipecac

Noninv: EKG at some regular interval (Ann IM 1985;102:49)

Rx: Replace volume and electrolytes; calcium 1200-1500 mg po qd and vitamin D to prevent osteoporosis

Fluoxetine (Prozac) 20 mg po qd and work quickly up to 60 mg po qd; or TCAs

Psychotherapy, esp cognitive-behavioral rx

Schizophrenia

Nejm 1994;330:681, 1993;329:555

Cause: Polygenic; significant genetic component by twin studies (Ann IM 1969;70:107), 10% for fraternal twins, 50% for identical twins; also multifactorial nongenetic contributors, which cause abnormalities in neural circuits and cognitive mechanisms (Njem 1999;340:645)

Epidem (Nejm 1999;340:603): < 1% of general population; incidence increased 10× if parent or sibling has schizphrenia; increased urban prevalence may be artifact of care sources distribution; and, controversially, if born in Feb or March?

Pathophys: Psychosis (hallucinations, delusions, disorder in form of thought) linked to increased brain dopaminergic activity; incidence and symptomatology similar across cultures

Limbic and temporal lobe show subtle atrophy (Nejm 1992;327:604, 1990;322:789) specifically demonstrable by MRI in the L hippocampus–amygdala and L posterior–superior temporal gyrus (Nejm 1992;327:604)

Sx: Bizarre, irrational behavior

Si: Inappropriate affect, although may be entirely appropriate to delusions and hallucinations; loose associations; primary process (nonrational, magical, childlike); diminished sociality, drive, and emotional responsiveness; ambivalence

Crs: Recurrent psychotic episodes usually beginning at age 17-24 yr, with residual sx between psychotic episodes

Cmplc: r/o chemical abuse and/or dependence, delirium (p 773), prescription drug toxicity (long list: Med Let 2002;44:59), bipolar manic disorder, brief reactive psychosis, dissociative disorders including very rare **Dissociative Identity Disorder** or multiple personality disorder (voices are those of the other personalities); metachromatic leukodystrophy (p 755)

Lab:

Rx (p 940) (Ann IM 2001;134:47; Nejm 1996;334:34; Med Let 1991;33:47):

1st:

- Olanzapine (Zyprexa) 10-20 mg/d (vs "weight gain and cost make no better than Haldol": Jama 2003;290:2693)
- Risperidone (Risperdal) (Med Let 1994;36:33), start at 0.5-1 mg po bid, increase to 2 mg po bid in 3 d; 30% relapse rate @ 1 yr compared to 60% w haloperidol (Nejm 2002;346:16)
- Quetiapine, aripiparazole, ziprazidone

2nd: Other antipsychotics (p 940) like chlorpromazine (Thorazine), fluphenazine (Prolixin), etc, and haloperidol (Haldol)

3rd: Clozapine (Clozaril) (Med Let 1993;35:16) 12.5 mg po qd gradually increasing to 300-400 mg qd, reserved for treatment-resistant cases

Bipolar Disorders (Manic-Depressive Illness)

Nejm 2004;351:476

Cause: Genetic, autosomal dominant suggested by strong family corre-lations, HLA-linked on chromosome 6 (Nejm 1981;305:1301; Jama 1972;222:1624)

Epidem: 1% lifetime incidence; 50% have positive family hx; 80% concordance in identical twins

Pathophys: Unknown; functional brain studies may be helpful someday

Sx: Grandiose plans and actions in all realms of life

Si: Depression alternating w mania

Crs: Manic spells last months to years w/o rx; rapid cyclers up to 4+ episodes/yr

Cmplc: Alcohol and drug abuse

Lab:

Rx: (Nejm 2004;351:476; Med Let 2000;42:114), in order of choice:
1st:
- Lithium 6-900 mg po qd titrated to therapeutic blood levels, if manic component, or augmentation of primary antidepressants if they alone fail (J Clin Psychopharm 1999;19:427); suicide rates $1/3$ or less than w valproate or carbamazepine (Jama 2003;290:1467)
- Carbamazepine
- Valproic acid to levels 12 hr after last dose of 50-125 μgm/cc
2nd:
- Typical antipsychotics, but don't help the depression
- Atypical antipsychotics, although not enough for severe mania; clozapine last

Depression

Ann IM 2001;134:47, 2000;343:1942

Cause: Genetic, autosomal dominant suggested by strong family correlations

Epidem: Increased incidence in postpartum females, late-middle-age and elderly pts, pts w family h/o alcoholism. Major depressive disorder onset in teens and 20s w recurrence in adulthood in $\frac{2}{3}$ (Jama 1999;281:1707). Lifetime incidence 15-25%.

Pathophys: ACTH, TSH, sleep studies, and neurotransmitter abnormalities to explain cause keep being proposed and discounted

Sx: 2+ wk of function-impairing sx including depressed mood or loss of interest, plus at least 3 changes in weight, sleep w early-morning awakening, activity level, energy, ability to think, or suicidal ideation.

Somatic complaints alone or w complaints of depression, guilt, and other psychological sx (Nejm 1999;341:1329)

Ask re suicidal thoughts (no increased risk of precipitating those thoughts if asked-Jama 2005;293:1635), previous suicide attempts, sleep disturbance lasting $\geq$ 2 wk, guilt feelings $\geq$ 2 wk, hopelessness (1 or more such sx have an 84% sens: Jama 1994;272:1757)

Si: Flat affect, sad, irritable, panic attacks; mania in bipolar d/o

Crs: Variable; may be chronic relapsing

Cmplc: Suicide (Ann IM 2002;136:302), alcoholism, mania; lower bone mineral density in women (Nejm 1996;335:1176)

r/o secondary causes like prescription drug side effects (long list: Med Let 2002;44:59), stress, bereavement, illness, alcohol/illicit drug use; **Seasonal affective disorder** (SAD) (Jama 1993;270:2717); males/females = 1:3-4, especially in northern climes in winter; sx of lethargy, increased sleep, decreased libido, weight and appetite changes; rx w $\frac{1}{2}$ hr tid 10,000 lux light box ($400), $\times$ 2 hr qd (Am Fam Phys 1988;38:173), or get outdoors at noon; many pts may have latent bipolar d/o and rx may precipitate mania

Lab:

Rx: Preventive evaluation of alcohol use, suicidality (Nejm 1997:337:910)

Brief, focused cognitive-behavioral analysis, psychotherapy as good as meds and provides additive benefit to drug rx (Jama 2004;292:807 [adolescents]; Nejm 2000;342:1462; Arch Gen Psych 1999;56:829) but probably not for severe or bipolar types

Medications (Ann IM 2001;134:47) (see p 942); rx for 6 mo after remit (Am J Psych 1998;155:1247):

1st: SSRIs, after 6-9 mo successful rx, maintenance reduces recurrence from 25% to 5% (NNT-1 = 5 by DBRCT: Jama 1998;280:1665); adjunctive benzo's for 1st 4-6 wk helpful (J Affect Disord 2001;65:173); work in children and adolescents too (Jama 2004;292:807, 2003;290:1033)

2nd: Buproprion (Wellbutrin); nefazodone (Serzone), venlataxine (Effexor), TCAs

3rd: Combinations of TCAs and MAOIs

4th: Electroshock therapy q 2-3 d × 2-3 wk is most effective antidepressant especially if suicidal or elderly (Nejm 1984;311:163); very safe; follow w lithium + nortriptyline to maintain (Jama 2001;285:1299); only relative contraindication is intracranial mass; adverse effects: transient memory loss

Others:

- Trazodone or buspirone 10-20 mg po bid possibly as adjunct to SSRIs

- T_3 (Cytomel) 25-50 μgm po qd as adjunct to SSRIs or TCAs

in menopausal women: Estrogens; NNT = 3 (Arch Gen Psych 2001;58:529)

in postpartum depression: SSRIs or TCAs ok (Nejm 2002;347:196)

Somatization Disorder (probably "Hysteria," "Neuresthenia")

Ann IM 1997;126:747; Jama 1997;278:673; Nejm 1986;314:1407

Cause:

Epidem: 0.2-2% of women and associated w positive family h/o same; < 0.2% in men

Pathophys:

Sx: Onset before age 30 yr; depressive sx; lifetime h/o 12+ (in male) or 14+ (in female) unexplained sx, often pain. Often include or merge w multiple functional gi disorders like globus hystericus, dysphagia, dyspepsia, irritable bowel syndrome, etc (Ann IM 1995;123:668).

Si: Normal exam

Crs: Lifelong

Cmplc:　　Hospitalization, procedures, and false-positive test results
　　　　　　r/o **Hysteria**, a manifestation of psychosomatic or somatiform illness including conversion reactions like hysterical paralysis or blindness, manifested by a single bizarre sx unlike the polysymptomatic pattern of somatization d/o; **Somatiform disorder**, which has fewer sx and later onset, pt will not accept reassurance, and is associated with alexithymia, an inability to discern or describe feelings (Nejm1985;312:690); **Hypochondriasis** (Nejm 1981; 304:1394), which does respond at least transiently to reassurance and cognitive-behavioral rx (Jama 2004;291:1464); other functional somatic syndromes (p 440)

Lab: Minimal

Rx: Pt reassurance, see frequently, avoid testing as much as possible

Personality Disorders

Jama 1994;272:1770

Cause: Genetics and environment

Epidem: Prevalence 6-10% of general population, ~50% of psych hospital pts

Pathophys: Pervasive lifelong character styles not viewed as pathological by pt (except in obsessive-compulsive personality d/o), unlike neurotic sx, which are. Some pts may have less extreme pathology of axis I disorders, eg, schizophrenia, manic-depressive disorders, etc.

Sx: Odd/eccentrics cluster: Paranoid, schizoid, and schizotypal types
Dramatic/emotional/erratic cluster: Antisocial, borderline, histrionic, and narcissistic types
Anxious/fearful cluster: Avoidant, dependent, obsessive-compulsive types

Si:

Crs: Onset in adolescence

Cmplc: r/o active axis I disorders, neurosis (pt can identify problem and complains about it), and chemical dependency chronic or in early recovery

Lab:

Rx: Time-limited benzodiazepines for anxiety
of self-sacrifice (dependent, passive-aggressive, and depressive types): Listen to sx and anticipate pts' ambivalence re improvement; plus antidepressants and carbamazepine for borderlines
of manipulative/antisocial types: Firm limits
of dependency and overdemandingness (dependent and borderline types): Empathetic recognition of pts need for reassurance and anxiety about being alone; plus limit-setting consistency,

clarity, and structure, and meds like olanzapine, fluoxetine, or divalproate

of obsessive-compulsiveness: Respect need for control by providing information, eg, test results asap, plus engaging pts in rx plan; meds: SSRIs, clomipramine not effective unlike in OCD

of dramatization (histrionic type): Disallow inappropriate familiarity w a respectful, professional manner without shortening time w pt

of self-importance (narcissistic type): Nondefensive acceptance of earlier consultation and referral

of detachment and paranoia (schizoid, schizotypal, avoidant types): Allow privacy, plus antipsychotics

Chapter 16

Pulmonary Diseases

D. K. Onion

16.1 Infections

Pneumonia

Nejm 2002;346:430 (children), 1995;333:1618

Cause:

< 1 month, commonly: Group B strep, *E. coli* and other gram-negative organisms, CMV.

Less commonly: *S. aureus*, RSV, *Enterobacter* sp, Listeria

1 mo-5 yr, commonly: RSV, parainfluenza virus, adenovirus, rhinovirus, influenza

Less commonly: Strep pneumoniae, chlamydia, whooping cough, staph, mycoplasma, H. flu, tbc

5-15 yr, commonly: Influenza A, adenovirus, chlamydia

Less commonly: *Mycoplasma*, *S. pneumoniae*, tbc

Adults (%'s from Nejm above): *S. pneumoniae* (50%), viral including influenza A (10%), aspiration (8%), H. flu (6%; others feel much higher, up to 30%, depending on group), *S. aureus* (4%), gram-negative organisms (6%), atypicals (15%) including mycoplasma (4%) and *Chlamydia* (5%), which have higher incidence (> 20%) in young adults, and *Legionella* (5%)

In elderly, prognosis bad if elevated BUN, hypotensive, respiratory rate > 30 (Ann IM 1991;115:428)

Epidem: Much more common in immunosuppressed pts, who constitute 60% of hospital admissions for pneumonia

Sx: Cough, fever, dyspnea, sputum production, pleurisy

Si: T° (80%); RR > 20 in adults; RR > 40 in pts age 1-5, > 50 in pts age 2-12 mo, > 60 in pts under 2 mo; in children, 70% sens and specif (Arch Dis Child 2000;82:41, 46); rales (80%), consolidation changes (30%), bronchial breath sounds, dullness, E to A changes

Cmplc: Empyema

Lab: *AGBs:* Admit if pO_2 < 60
   Bact: Blood cultures (pos in 11% overall, in 67% w *S. pneumoniae*), sputum Gram stain (50% pos in *S. pneumoniae*)
   Hem: CBC

Xray: Chest, infiltrate, although false-neg results esp in 1st 24 hr or w neutropenia or w PCP (10-30% neg); effusions (40%). Resolution in community-acquired pneumonia in elderly pts takes 12-14 wk (J Am Ger Soc 2004;52:224).

Rx   (Nejm 2002;347:2039 for hospitalization criteria; Med Let 2001;43:65):
   Outpts: Erythromycin, azithromycin, or clarithromycin; or 2nd, tetracycline at least under age 60 w/o complicating illness (Jama 1997;278:32); or a 3rd-generation fluoroquinolone alone w good antipneumococccal activity like levofloxacin, moxifloxacin, or gatifloxacin, especially if > age 60
   Inpts: 3rd-generation cephalosporin like ceftriaxone or cefotaxime w a macrolide; or 3rd-generation fluoroquinolone
   ICU pts: Imipenem + Aminoglycoside if *Pseudomonas* possible (Med Let 1996;38:25)
      Aspiration (Nejm 2001;344:665): Levofloxacin 500 mg qd or ceftriaxone 1-2 gm qd

Lung Abscess

Cause: Often mixed organisms with anaerobic bacteria (p 578) such as fusobacterium, bacteroides, peptostreptococcus, and peptococcus as well as aerobic organisms such as necrotizing gram-negative rods and staph; from aspiration of mouth organisms

Epidem: Associated w alcoholism, loss of consciousness, recent dental work

Pathophys:

Sx: Fever, sputum, weight loss

Si:

Crs:

Cmplc: Empyema, bronchopleural fistula, brain abscess

Lab:

Xray: Chest shows abscess cavities with air fluid levels; or may show a round "pneumonia" before the abscess communicates with a bronchus to create an air fluid level; r/o bronchopleural fistula or empyema from which it may be very hard to tell

Rx: Clindamycin 600-900 mg iv q 8 hr until improves then 300 mg po q 6 hr; or ampicillin/sulbactam (Unasyn)
    Bronchoscopy if doesn't resolve

16.2 Asthma and Interstitial Lung Disease

Acute Respiratory Distress Syndrome (Shock Lung)

Nejm 2000;342:1334

Cause: Direct injury: Multiple agents including pneumonia, aspiration, inhalation injury (30-40% risk), salicylate poisoning (Ann IM 1981;95:405), fat emboli, drowning (p 20), hantavirus infection in southwestern U.S. (p 697) (Nejm 1994;330:949)
Indirect injury: Bacterial sepsis (30-40% risk) most often from

intra-abdominal gi perforation, pancreatitis, neurogenic (head trauma), drug OD, transfusions, bypass

Epidem: Incidence increased by risk factors (see Table 16.1)

Table 16.1   Risk Factors for ARDS

Risk	% with Risk Who Get ARDS
Disseminated IV coagulopathy	22
Cardiopulmonary bypass	2
Burns	2
Bacteremia	4
Hypertransfusion	5
ICU pneumonia	12
Aspiration	35

If multiple risk factors, 25% get (Petty: Ann IM 1983; 98:593); most develop within 48 hr of getting risk factors; hypotension precedes in 90%. Chronic alcohol abuse doubles risk and mortality (Jama 1996;275:50).

Pathophys: Normal pressure pulmonary edema from capillary leak (Nejm 1982;306:900). Associated w decreased levels of pulmonary urokinase, which causes increased fibrin deposition and scarring (Nejm 1990;322:890), elevated cytokines and other inflammatory proteins, depressed interleukins and interleukin receptor availability

Sx: Dyspnea

Si: Hypoxia, tachypnea; PCWP < 18 mm Hg

Crs: Substantial mortality of ~45% (Jama 1995;273:306), usually not respiratory; survivors have significant impairment of exercise capacity and muscle strength even 1 yr out (Nejm 2003;348:683)

Cmplc: Barotrauma, especially if peak pressures > 70 cm water for more than a day. Pulmonary fibrosis in 30%.

r/o CHF, *Pneumocystis carinii* and other overwhelming opportunistic infections

Lab: *ABGs:* Hypoxia; $P_aO_2/F_iO_2 \leq 200$
Bact: Bronchopulmonary lavage for pathogens

Xray: Chest shows diffuse bilateral pulmonary infiltrates starting perihilar within 24 hr, often looks like CHF; may progress to "white out"

CT shows patchy involvement, the extent of which correlates w ABGs; also can show occult abscesses or barotrauma

Rx: Treat underlying disease; Swan-Ganz monitoring of PCWP and cardiac output; avoid fluid overload

Newer ventilator modes like lower volumes and permissive hypercapnia, inverse I/E, pressure control; PEEP when on ventilator, 0-30 cm water, can't use preventively (Nejm 1984;311:281,323); debate exists over maximum and minimal settings parameters (Nejm 1998;338:341,347,355,385); increases in PEEP cause decreases in cardiac output due to left shift of interventricular septum (Nejm 1981;304:387) as well as diminished venous return and elevated pulmonary vascular resistance, which increases R-to-L shunt in 15% of the population w potential ASD (Ann IM 1993;119:886)

Nitric oxide inhalation improves V/Q mismatch and arterial pO_2, but unclear if improves survival (Nejm 1993;328:399,431)

Steroids perhaps 2 mg MePrednisolone/kg/d (Jama 1998;280:159)

Aerosolized surfactant × 24 hr does not improve survival (Nejm 2004;351:884)

Asthma (Chronic Eosinophilic Bronchitis)

Jama 1997;278:1855; Nejm 1992;327:1928, 1992;326:1540

Cause: Innumerable allergens including house dust mites, animal dander, actinomyces in car air conditioners (Nejm 1984;311:1619)

and other mold spores, cockroach allergens (Nejm 1997; 336:1356), and soybean dust (Nejm 1989;320:1097)

Genetic autosomal dominant susceptibility on chromosome 5, co-inherited w atopy susceptibility (Nejm 1995;333:894), as well as various mutations of interleukin-4 and its receptor (Nejm 1997;337;1720, 1766)

Epidem: 4-5% of U.S. population, increasing overall (Nejm 1994;331:1584), and greater prevalence in low-income groups (Nejm 1994;331:1542) has led to the "hygiene hypothesis." Incidence may be decreased by increased enviromental endo-toxin exposure (Nejm 2002;347:869,911,930).

Pathophys: Airway inflammation. Multiple types including exercise-induced (Nejm 1994;330:1362), cholinergic; as well as older distinctions between "extrinsic/familial atopic" plus expo-sure by age 1 to house mite antigens (Nejm 1990;323:502); and intrinsic/idiopathic or infectious type associated with h/o bron-chiolitis (10-30% will go on to asthma: Peds 1963;31:859), bronchiectasis, chronic bronchitis, and eventually COPD and emphysema. Some argue that all are really allergic (extrinsic) (Nejm 1989;320:271) w eosinophilic and mast cell infiltration of lower airway submucosa and smooth muscle (Nejm 2002; 346:1699).

Morning wheezing due to circadian decrease in epinephrine and perhaps steroids as well (Nejm 1980;303:263). In extrinsics, IgE is sensitizing. ASA sensitivity caused by increased leukotriene production and sensitivity to it in nasal and other airway mucosa, causing asthma and nasal polyps (Nejm 2002;347:1493,1524; Ann IM 1997;127:472). Food sulfites pre-cipitate (Med Let 1986;28:74), as does first- and second-hand cigarette smoke (Nejm 1993;328:1665).

Sx: Quadrad of dyspnea, wheezing, cough, and sputum production; ex-ercise and/or cold induction caused by respiratory tract heat loss directly and through evaporation in dry air (Nejm 1979;301:763) w pattern of bronchoconstriction lasting 20+ min, 3-8 min after cessation of exercise (Nejm 1998;339:192); URI induction often; h/o occupational irritants; h/o allergen induction

Si: Wheezing, although may have only dyspnea on exertion or cough (Nejm 1979;300:633); dyspnea; cyanosis late; papilledema with acutely increased pCO_2; nasal polyps (30% of extrinsics); paradoxical pulse from "tethered heart" within the mediastinum, correlates with severity (Nejm 1973;288:66)

Crs: Annual decrement in FEV_1 % twice as great in asthmatics as in normals (Nejm 1998;339:1194). Overall mortality not increased (Nejm 1994;331:1537); acute attack prognosis worse if have diminished sensitivity to hypoxia (Nejm 1994;330:1329). 25% of child asthmatics have sx as adults (Nejm 2003;349:1414).

Cmplc: Respiratory arrest with respiratory acidosis, not arrhythmia, is most common mode of death (Nejm 1991;324:285); may be precipitated by exposure to airborne spores of *Alternaria alternata*, an IgE-producing allergen (Nejm 1991;324:359); NSAIDs, esp ASA, induce exacerbations in 5-10%, esp those with nasal polyps.

Multifocal atrial tachycardia associated with hypoxia, aminophylline, and catechol rx (Nejm 1968;279:344)

In pregnancy (rv of management: Jama 1997;278:1865); associated with premature labor and RDS of newborn (Nejm 1985;312:742)

r/o vocal cord dysfunction, a frequent mimicker; conversion reaction? (Nejm 1983;308:1566); pulmonary emboli rarely (Nejm 1968;278:999); CHF, gastroesophageal reflux disease trigger

Lab: *Chem:* Theophyllin levels to optimize dose

Hem: Eosinophil elevation correlates with severity (Nejm 1990;323:1033); sputum eosinophils also helpful to tell from COPD

Path: Mucous metaplasia of ciliated epithelial cells into goblet cells

PFTs: Before and after bronchodilators; FEV_1 % reductions. Intrinsics are rarely normal between attacks, but extrinsics are. Peak flows done at home by pt are useful in management. Methacholine challenge test for dx.

Skin testing: Basically documents if is atopic or not; may have value in deciding whether omalizumab (Xolair) recombinant human IgE antibody will work

Xray: Chest to r/o pneumothorax (Nejm 1983;309:336) and pneumonitis; atelectasis

Rx:

ACUTE (Med Let 1993;35:11):

Catechols (Med Let 1999;41:51), β_2-selective, via inhaler with spacer or via nebulizer q 1 hr × 3; all equally effective and similar cost ($30/mo) at 2 puffs q 3-6 hr (Med Let 1987;29:11); use prn sx, not prophylactically:

- Albuterol (Proventil, Ventolin, et al) 0.1-0.15 mg/kg/dose up to 5 mg/dose if > 40 lb q 2 hr (guidelines for asthma, National Asthma Education Program, NIH 1991)
- Bitolterol (Tornalate)
- Terbutaline (Brethine) 250 μgm/puff

Steroid bolus, eg, 100-300 mg iv hydrocortisone, then q 6-8 hr helps (Nejm 1986;314:150), or prednisone 2 mg/kg po; but takes 6+ hr, so no rush (Ann IM 1990;112:822); f/u up with 8+ d of tapering prednisone to prevent acute recurrence (Nejm 1991;324:788) or 10 d level (40 mg po qd) rx w no taper (Lancet 1993;341:324); not inhaled steroids (Nejm 2000;343:689)

Fluids, depending on initial hydration status, as much as 360 cc/m^2 in 1st hr, then 1500 $cc/m^2/24$ hr; too much can cause pulmonary edema (Nejm 1977;297:592); with 2 mEq KCl/kg /24 hr,

3 mEq Na/kg/24 hr, and $NaCO_3$ if pH < 7.35 and/or it takes > 1 hr to decrease pCO_2; O_2

Bipap or respirator if pH low and pCO_2 elevated and stays there despite initial efforts; beware pneumothorax

Occasionally:

- Iprotropium 500 μgm (2.5 cc) nebulizer clearly helps w severe exacerbations (Am J Med 1999;107:363; Ann EM 1999;34:8; Nejm 1998;339:1030)

- Aminophylline (Nejm 1993;119:1155,1216; Ann IM 1991;115:241,323) 5.6 mg/kg load over 20-30 min then 0.5 mg/kg/hr; but efficacy and safety in doubt (ACP J Club 2001;134:97)

- Anesthesia for status asthmaticus when all else fails

CHRONIC (Med Let 2000;42:19; 1999;41:5):

Spacers with CFC but not HFA and powder inhalers; commercial or homemade w 500 cc plastic soda bottle (Lancet 1999;354:979); may reduce compliance due to bulkiness and inconvenience

Monitor with peak-flow meters at home and have pt take short crs of steroids whenever peak flow falls > 2 standard deviations below mean for 2 out of 3 consecutive days (Ann IM 1995;123:488)

Dust-free bedroom if skin test shows sensitivity to dust or house mites; cover pillows and mattress (? not effective: Nejm 2003;349:207,225), damp-mop, cover hot air vents, all produce dramatic effects (Peds 1983;71:418); and rarely, if this fails, de-sensitization to house dust mite antigens, danders, and pollens like ragweed (Am J Respir Crit Care 1995;151:969), which has minimal (Nejm 1996;334:501,531) to no benefit (Nejm 1997;336:324)

Influenza vaccine, safe and efficacious in children and adults (Nejm 2001;345:1529)

Medications (J Allergy Clin Immunol 2002;110:5); but use of prn β-agonists may be more harmful than no use at all because of rapid tachyphylaxis (Ann IM 2004;140:803)

Step 1 for mild, intermittent sx: Short-acting β-agonist (Nejm 1996;335:841, 1995;333:499) inhaler prn, like those listed above; associated with 2× increased death rates or even higher if use > 2 canisters/mo (Nejm 1992;326:503; BMJ 1991;303:1426); in nebulizers or metered-dose inhalers (MDIs), and w inhaler devices for kids and uncooperative adults (Nejm 1986;315:870)

Step 2 for mild, persistent sx: Prn short-acting β-agonist inhaler as above + low-dose inhaled steroids (Nejm 1995;332:868) like:

Beclomethasone (Beclovent, Vanceril), triamcinolone (Azmacort), or flunisolide (Aerobid) MDI 2 puffs b-tid (Nejm 1991;325:388, 1989;321:1517; Med Let 1985;27:5); safe long term in children (Nejm 1993;329:1702) and adults? (Nejm 1994;331:700 vs 737); or

Budesonide (Pulmicort, Turbuhaler) dry-powder inhaler (DPI) (Med Let 1998;40:15) 200 μgm (low dose) to 800 μgm (high dose) qd-bid, also available in very expensive nebulizer form (Med Let 2001;43:6); adrenal suppression at 800 μgm bid (Am J Med 2000;108:269), and stunts growth at least for 1st yr in children (Nejm 2000;343:1054,1024,1113, 1997;337:1659)

Fluticasone (Flovent) (Med Let 1996;38:84) MDI or as Flovent Rotadisk DPI (Med Let 1998;40:15) in 44 (low), 110 (med), and 220 μgm/inhaler doses

Cromolyn canister (Med Let 1994;36:37) inhaler best choice in children (Nejm 1992;326:1540) and good in some adults, esp those w eosinophilia and increased IgE levels; $65/canister

Nedocromil (Tilade) (Med Let 1994;36:37, 1993;35:62), similar to cromolyn; $37/canister

Step 3 for moderate, persistent sx: Prn short-acting inhaled β-agonist as above + medium-dose (2-3 puffs t-qid) inhaled steroids as above +

- Long-acting β-agonist like:

  Salmeterol (Serevent) (Med Let 1994;36:37) 2 puffs or 1 puff of powder form (50 μgm) bid; safe and effective in children (but not as effective as beclomethasone: Nejm 1997;327:1669) can be used w other prn short-acting catechols (Am J Med 1999;107:209); dangerous if used by pts as an acute rx drug (Jama 1995;273:967) and not for monoRx (Jama 2001;285;2583,2594,2637); $60/canister unlike most others, which are $20-30/canister. Also available combined w fluticasone 100, 250, or 500 μgm as Advair Diskas powder inhaler bid (Med Let 2001;43:31); $103/mo.

  Formoterol (Foradil) (Med Let 2001;43:39; Nejm 1997;337:1405) T̄ puff powder (12 μgm) inhalation bid, or as needed (Lancet 2001;357:257)

- Theophylline (Nejm 1997;337:1405,1412, 1996;334:1380) low-dose therapy w only 250-375 mg bid despite low blood levels, used w inhaled steroids is as good as long-acting β-agonists; long-acting forms like Theo-dur, etc, 400 mg qd, can be increased to 600-800 mg qd. Long duration of action is helpful for hs use (Ann IM 1993;119:1216), as are long-acting β-agonists. Levels are increased by bcp's, erythromycin, flu shots, allopurinol, cimetidine, coffee; decreased by phenytoin, nicotine, phenobarbital. Toxic sx: seizures, tachycardia, NVD, tremor (Ann IM 1991;114:748); no impairment of school performance (Nejm 1992;327:926).

Step 4 for severe, persistent sx: High-dose inhaled steroids like budesonide or others above + whatever it takes including po steroids

Other meds:

Leukotriene receptor antagonists (LRAs) (ACP J Club 2004; 141:73) of marginal benefit:

- Montelukast (Singulair) (Jama 1998;279:1181; Med Let 1998;40:71) 5 mg (child over age 6) chewable or 10 mg po (adult) tab hs; $70/mo

- Zafirlukast (Accolate) (Ann IM 1997;127:472, 1997;126:177; Med Let 1996;38:111) 20 mg po bid, not under age 12; less effective than inhaled steroids to decrease inflammation; use esp for ASA-induced asthma and exercise exacerbations in pts already on β-agonists; adverse effects: many drug interactions, causes or unmasks (Jama 1998;279:455) Churg-Strauss eosinophilic vasculitis, rare severe hepatitis (Ann IM 2000;133:964); $60/mo

- Zileuton (Zyflo) (Med Let 1997;39:18; Jama 1996;275:931) 600 mg po qid; similarly inhibits production but not a receptor antagonist; $82/mo

Ipratropium (Atrovent) inhaler alone or w albuterol (Combivent), esp in elderly pts or for β-blocker–induced disease

Antibiotics if acute or chronic infection, like tetracycline, erythromycin (beware theophylline levels), trimethoprim-sulfa

Proton pump inhibitor like omeprazole 40 mg po qd if any reflux sx or if pt is resistant to rx, although studies don't show benefit (ACP J Club 2000;132:15)

IgE antibody, omalizumab sc q 2-4 wk, reduces exacerbations and steroid use in severe asthma, NNT = 5-7 (Cochrane: ACP J Club 2004;140:13; Peds 2001;108:E36); $10,000/yr of exercise-induced asthma (Nejm 1998;339:192):

- Chronic inhaled steroids
- Inhaled albuterol, cromolyn, or nedocromil 15 min before exercise
- Salmeterol inhalation bid (Nejm 1998;339:141), effect lasts several hours unlike similar formoterol (Foradil)

- LRAs like montelukast 10 mg po qd (Nejm 1998;339:147), better long term than salmeterol (Ann IM 2000:132:97)
- Heparin inhalation? (Nejm 1993;329:90)

of ASA-sensitive asthma and polyps (Nejm 2002;347:1493,1524), helped by oral ASA desensitization and polyps by topical nasal lysine aspirin (see Figure 16.1, p 978)

	Symptoms	Lung Function	Long-term Control Medication
Step 4 Severe Persistent	Continual Symptoms Limited Physical Activity Frequent Exacerbations Nighttime Symptoms Frequent	FEV_1 or PEF ≤60% Predicted PEF Variability >30%	Daily Medication Inhaled Corticosteroid (High Dose) and Long-Acting Inhaled β_2-Agonist and Oral Corticosteoids, but Attempt to Reduce Dose and Maintain Contol With Inhaled Corticosteroids *May Add Leukotriene Receptor Antagonist
Step 3 Moderate Persistent	Daily Symptoms Daily Use of Inhaled Short-Acting β_2-Agonists Exacerbations Affect Activity Exacerbations ≥2 Times a Week, May Last Days Nighttime Symptoms >1 Time a Week	FEV_1 or PEF >60% - <80% Predicted PEF Variability >30%	Daily Medication Inhaled Corticosteroid (Medium Dose) or Inhaled Corticosteroid (Low to Medium Dose) and Long-Acting Inhaled β_2-Agonist Especially for Nighttime Symptoms *May Add Leukotriene Receptor Antagonist
Step 2 Mild Persistent	Symptoms >2 Times a Week But <1 Time a Day Exacerbations May Affect Activity Nighttime Symptoms >2 Times a Month	FEV_1 or PEF ≥80% Predicted PEF Variability 20%-30%	Daily Medication Inhaled Corticosteroid (Low Dose) or Cromolyn or Nedocromil Alternatives: Leukotriene Receptor Antagonist, Sustained-release Theophylline
Step 1 Mild Intermittent	Symptoms ≤2 Times a Week Asymptomatic and Normal PEF Between Exacerbations Exacerbations Brief (Few Hours to Few Days); Intensity May Vary Nighttime Symptoms ≤2 Times a Month	FEV_1 or PEF ≥80% Predicted PEF Variability <20%	None

↓ Step Down
Review Treatment Every 1 to 6 Months; a Gradual Stepwise Reduction in Treatment May Be Possible.

↑ Step Up
If Control Is Not Maintained, Consider Step Up. First Review Patient Medication Technique, Adherence, and Environmental Control (Avoidance of Allergens or Other Factors That Contribute to Asthma Severity).

Figure 16.1 Stepwise approach for managing asthma in adults and children older than age 5 years. FEV_1, forced expiratory volume in 1 second; PEF, peak expiratory flow. Reproduced with permission from Busse WW. A 72 year old woman with severe asthma. J Am Med Assoc. 2000;284:2225. Copyright 2000, American Medical Association, all rights reserved.

Occupational "Asthma" (Byssinosis, Mill Fever, Etc)

Nejm 1995;333:107; Ann IM 1984;101:157

Cause: Cotton-dust bacterial endotoxin in byssinosis (Nejm 1987;317:805), hemp and flax dust, redwood sawdust, isocyanates, castor bean dust, etc. Occupational airborne exposures in factories that process raw products.

Epidem: Very common, especially in cotton-mill carding rooms, where 70% of all workers will react within 1 yr of employment, 40-50% will develop sx

Pathophys: Acute pulmonary bronchoconstriction starts on 1st work day of the week; later in the disease course, sx's persist later into the week. Occupational asthma is in contrast to allergic alveolitis, where predominant inflammation is in alveoli (p 979); mill fever may be a variant of allergic alveolitis; nylon flock worker's lung (Ann IM 1998;129:261).

Sx: Tight chest, dyspnea, cough for a day or 2 after a weekend off or other rest. Fever with mill fever.

Si: Decreased ventilation capacity during the work day

Crs: Progressive bronchospasm may lead to irreversible obstruction

Cmplc: Pulmonary HT; severe COPD, even if leave work (Ann IM 1982;97:645)

Lab: *PFTs:* Decreased FEV_1/FVC

Xray: Chest often normal, or shows hyperinflation

Rx: Prevent by improving dust removal. Pre- and post-Monday work FEV_1 checks
of sx, inhaled bronchodilators; avoid dust.

Allergic Alveolitis/Pneumonitis

Ann IM 1976;84:406; Nejm 1973;288:233

Cause: Actinomycetes, rarely other fungi (cryptococcus, aspergillus), or any organic dust

Epidem: Occupational/recreational exposures in multiple ways possible: eg, exposure to wood dust (Nejm 1972;286:977); mushroom picker's disease; cork dust (suberosis); pigeon breeder's disease (Ann IM 1969;70:457); farmer's lung disease (distinct from silo filler's disease, which is caused by NO_2 direct toxicity leading to pulmonary edema, rx with steroids); maple bark stripper's disease from cryptococcus under bark or in pulp wood (Ann IM 1970;72:907); bagassosis (moldy cane); air conditioners (Nejm 1970;283:271); aspergillosis, although more commonly causes a predominantly bronchoconstrictive disease rather than alveolitis (Ann IM 1970;72:395)

Pathophys: An individual is sensitized to 1-2 μm-sized antigens. Compared to allergic asthma, more alveolar and less bronchiolar involvement.

Sx: Cough

Si: Fever, no sputum

Crs: Often reversible with withdrawal of source; but may be chronic

Cmplc: Chronic interstitial pneumonitis, occasionally is apical and thus can look like tbc
r/o nitrofurantoin acute allergic-type pneumonitis (Nejm 1969;281:1087); nematode asthma

Lab: *PFTs:* Low normal FEV_1 % and FVC if interstitial disease, especially in chronic forms
Serol: Specific antibody testing but often not helpful because of high false-negative rates

Xray: Chest shows pulmonary alveolar infiltrates that look like pulmonary edema

Rx: Avoidance of allergen; masks for farmers if they can use during brief exposures; steroids for brief courses

COPD/Chronic Bronchitis/Emphysema

Nejm 2000;343:276

Cause: Bronchitis/hyperreactive airways from smoking, recurrent infections; cystic fibrosis (p 985); α_1-antitrypsin deficiency (α_1-ATD) (Nejm 1993;328:1392), autosomal recessive (Nejm 1977;296:1190), and usually combined with smoking in heterozygote (Ann IM 2002;136:270), occurs even w/o smoking in homozygote

Epidem: Smoker-type onset usually after age 50 yr; males > females; increased prevalence in cold, damp climates. Maternal smoking may increase incidence in offspring (Nejm 1983;309:699). α_1-ATD type: gene incidence ~ 5% in U.S. (Nejm 1969; 281:279); onset by age 45.

Pathophys: Proteases, especially elastase from polys and macrophages, are balanced by α_1-antitrypsin, the primary antielastase; hence functional deficiencies cause loss of lung elasticity; and smoke both inactivates it (Ann IM 1987;107:761; Nejm 1983;309:694) and increases polys in the lung capillaries (Nejm 1989;321:924). Thus elasticity is decreased, causing loss of connective tissue support that normally keeps bronchioles open; when expiratory pressure is increased, that loss of elastic support causes bronchiole collapse and resulting "ball valving" entrapment of air and hence emphysema, along with V/Q imbalances, end-stage hypoventilation, and increased pCO_2. Goblet cell hyperplasia may contribute to bronchiolar plugging and initiate more of above.

Classified now by global obstructive lung disease system (Am J Respir Crit Care Med 2001;163:1256)

Sx: Dyspnea on exertion of arms more than legs (Nejm 1986; 314:1485); chronic productive cough with bronchitis not emphysema

Table 16.2 Symptoms of COPD

	Sensitivity (%)	Specificity (%)
Orthopnea	19	88
Smoker	94	24
Dyspnea	82	33
Cough	51	71
Wheezing	51	84
Chronic sputum	42	89

(J Gen Intern Med 1993;8:63)

Si: Barrel chest. Two extremes: "blue bloater" (CHF, hypoxia, and hypercarbia) and "pink puffer" (weight loss, low pCO_2, moderate decrease in pO_2 at rest and left-sided CHF, which may be occult) (Nejm 1971;285:361)

Forced expiratory time over trachea > 6 sec (75% sens/specif: Jama 1993;270:731)

Table 16.3 Signs of COPD

	Sensitivity (%)	Specificity (%)
Diminished breath sounds	29	85
Wheezing	14	99
Cough	14	93
Subxyphoid PMI	4	99
Rales	1	99

(J Gen Intern Med 1993;8:63)

Crs: Pink puffer has better prognosis than blue bloater because pulmonary HT is less (Nejm 1972;286:912)

Cmplc: Polycythemia; pulmonary HT (p 988), peptic ulcer disease (Nejm 1969;281:279), acute respiratory failure; lithium worsens (Nejm 1983;308:39); hypophosphatemia, especially on ventilator, < 1 mM/L (< 1.5 mg %) impairs diaphragmatic contractility, treatable (Nejm 1985;313:420); exacerbations 3-4×/yr often caused by a new bacterial pathogen

Lab: *Bact:* Chronically infected sputum with bronchitis

Path: Emphysema, centrilobular of secondary and tertiary respiratory bronchioles most commonly; in α_1-ATD, panlobular of primary lobules and PAS-positive staining inclusions in hepatocytes (Nejm 1975;292:176)

PFTs: Diffusion capacity decreased in emphysema, not bronchitis or asthma alone, due to loss of total alveolar/capillary membrane surface area; $< 55\%$ of predicted value correlates with hypoxia on exercise (Nejm 1984;310:1218); increased total lung capacity; decreased FEV_1/FVC; 7-min nitrogen washout with O_2 is prolonged

Serol: in α_1-ATD, SPEP shows decreased α_1 peak < 0.2 gm (no false pos: Ann IM 1970;73:9)

Rx: Stop smoking (p 1007) to prevent or stabilize progression, steroid inhalers not much help if don't (Nejm 1999;340:1948); pulmonary rehab programs (Lancet 1996;348:1115; Ann IM 1995;122:823; Lancet 1994;344:1394) clearly improve quality of life and endurance (Chest 1997;111:1077; J Respir Crit Care Med 1995;152:S77). Cardioselective β-blockers safe if needed for ASHD (ACP J Club 2001;135:87).

Vaccination vs influenza, pneumococcus, and eventually maybe RSV and parainfluenza (Jama 2000;283:499)

O_2: 1-2 L/min nasal prongs or enough to maintain O_2 sats at 90% without driving up pCO_2; around-the-clock O_2 to increase survival (Ann IM 1983;99:519). CHF rx with digoxin, if L- but not if R-sided failure, helps (Ann IM 1981;95:283).

Meds (Nejm 2004;350:2689; Jama 2003;290:2301,1313):

1st: Catechol bronchodilators (p 975), especially salmeterol or formoterol bid, often used as an alternative to or w iprotropium; via nebulizers or inhalers; used prn is not safe routinely (Nejm 1992;326:560)

2nd: Steroid inhalers (p 974) (Nejm 1992;327:1413), help sx but don't slow progression (controversial: ACP J Club 2004; 140:57) and increase osteoporosis (Nejm 2000;343:1902)

3rd: Anticholinergics: • Ipratropium (Atrovent) 2-3 puffs qid (Nejm 1988;319:486; Med Let 1987;29:71); or

• Tiotropium (Spiriva) (MedLet 2004;46:41) 18 μgm powder inhaler qd, often used w Advair; $120/mo

Theophylline preparations; acutely of no benefit (BMJ 2003;327:643) but help ~50% of chronic cases (Chest 1993; 104:1101) via increased diaphragmatic muscle strength and by dampening sense of dyspnea, as can opiates (Nejm 1995; 333:1547).

Antibiotics prophylactically: Tm/S, tetracyclines, or amoxicillin at 1st si of cold, fever, or change in sputum (Jama 1995; 273:957; Med Let 1980;22:68)

Continuous O_2 if resting hypoxia $<$ PaO_2 of 60 mm Hg

Perhaps α_1-proteinase inhibitor for α_1-antitrypsin deficiency (Med Let 1988;30:29) iv weekly or monthly

Proteolytics like acetylcysteine po (not inhaled) may work (BMJ 2001;322:1271)

Surgical resection of bullae and/or severely impaired areas (Nejm 2000;343:239, 1996;334:1095,1198); can improve diaphragm and accessory muscle effectiveness; may help only pts w low inspiratory resistance (Nejm 1998;338:1181) or those w predominant upper lobe disease AND low exercise capacity (Nejm 2003;348:2055,2059,2134,2092)

of acute exacerbation (Ann IM 2001;134:595,600; Nejm 2002;346:988): Chest xray then prn O_2, bronchodilators, steroids $\times$ 1-2 wk maximum, antibiotics (ampicillin, Tcn, Tm/S); no chest PT, mucolytics, or theophyllines

Cystic Fibrosis (Mucoviscidosis)

Nejm 1997;336:487, 1996;335:179, 1993;328:1390

Cause: Genetic mutations of the CF gene on chromosome 7; autosomal with variable penetrance (Nejm 2005;352:1992)

Epidem: Caucasians have 98.4% of all cystic fibrosis; 1/30,000 whites in U.S.; heterozygotes about 5% of population. Blacks have 1.4% prevalence of heterozygote; all other racial groups have prevalence < 0.2%; only 1 reported case in Asians (Nejm 1968;279:1216).

Pathophys: Deficient Cl^- secretion and excessive Na^+ resorption across epithelial surfaces (Nejm 1991;325:533). Exocrine gland fibrosis in homozygote; pancreatic duct obstruction causes pancreatic insufficiency (Nejm 1985;312:329). Bronchi obstructed, leading to secondary infections especially with staph and pseudomonas, COPD, and pulmonary failure. Vas deferens obstruction/absence causes male sterility (98%) (Nejm 1972; 287:586); nothing analogous in female. Sweat glands obstructed causing an inability to lose heat.

Sx: COPD; heat exhaustion; malabsorption sx; sterility, esp male (90%), which may be only sx (Nejm 1995;332:1475)

Si: Meconium ileus at birth (15%); no sweat; malnourished; severe chronic bronchitis and pulmonary insufficiency

Crs: Depends on age of onset and complications; 2-yr mortality > 50% once FEV_1 % becomes < 30% of predicted, PaO_2 < 55 mm Hg or pCO_2 > 50 mm, so begin planning lung transplant then (Nejm 1992;326:1187)

Cmplc: COPD, bronchiectasis, pneumothorax (20% lifetime incidence), massive hemoptysis (7% get in lifetime); growth retardation; pancreatic insufficiency (80%); diabetes mellitus (20%) without vascular lesions (Nejm 1969;281:451); rectal prolapse, may be presenting sx; gallstones, in 50% by age 26, w common bile duct obstruction (15-20%) (Nejm 1988;318:340); modest increase in gi cancers in adulthood (Nejm 1995;332:494); osteoporosis w fx's and kyphosis in adulthood (Ann IM 1998;128:186)

Lab: *Bact:* S. *aureus* in sputum and/or nasal pharynx; pseudomonas or E. *coli* in sputum, both of which produce a mucoid material almost pathognomonic of CF (Nejm 1981;304:1445)

Chem: Sweat tests w or w/o pilocarpine stimulation; characteristically Cl > 60 mEq/L, usually > 80; r/o Addison's, atopic dermatitis, malnutrition, hypothyroidism, and a few rare others (Nejm 1997;336:487). Duodenal aspirate shows diminished pancreatic enzyme secretion and pH < 8 even after secretin stimulation.

Noninv: PFTs show diminished vital capacity, increased residual volume

Semen analysis: Azoospermia

Xray: Sinus films show opacified paranasal sinuses

Rx: Prevent by carrier detection with tissue culture (Nejm 1981; 304:1); but not practical to screen entire Caucasian population yet (Nejm 1990;322:328). In affected families, in vitro fertilization and preimplantation testing possible (Nejm 1992;327:905).

Screen newborns maybe w blood trysinogen levels since may eventually be reasonable to institute dietary and pulmonary interventions early (Nejm 1997;337:963)

Lung transplants (Jama 2001;286:2683)

Of cmplc:

- Pulmonary, rx same as COPD, consider:
  Prophylactic antibiotics like ciprofloxacin or azithromycin (Jama 2003;290:1749), which have anti-inflammatory properties, or antibiotic aerosols like tobramycin (Nejm 1999;340:23) for pseudomonas; but antibiotic management is complex esp in end stages

Amiloride (Midamor) inhaler qid slows progression, perhaps by blocking Na resorption and thinning mucus (Nejm 1990;322:1189)

Avoid smoke exposure, eg, in home (Nejm 1990;323:782)

Acetyl cysteine (Mucomyst) DNAase inhaler qd-bid, significantly thins secretions (Nejm 1994;331:637, 1992;326:812), modestly improves PFTs, and decreases infections, but inhaler without medication costs $2000 and total cost/yr used qd is $12,000 (Med Let 1994;36:34); but cheap po form may work (ACP J Club 2002;136:54)

Ibuprofen 25 mg/kg qd chronically slows progression (Nejm 1995;332:848)

- Pancreatic (p 341)
- Intestinal obstruction w Gastrografin enema, which increases gi fluid

Interstitial Pneumonias (Idiopathic Pulmonary Fibrosis, Hamman-Rich Syndrome)

Am J Surg Path 2002;26:1567; Nejm 2001;345:517; Ann IM 2001;134:136

Cause: Unknown

Epidem: Males > females; adults age 50-70 yr; rare, 7-10/100,000; associated w smoking

Pathophys: Alveolitis is due to uncontrolled response of T cells to inflammation and/or B-cell production of IgG vs collagen? Inflammatory etiology in doubt. Possibly epithelial injury and abnormal wound healing.

Exaggerated release of platelet-derived growth factor by macrophages causes abnormal scarring/fibrosis (Nejm 1987;317:202)

Sx: Dyspnea on exertion, nonproductive cough for 6+ mo

Si: "Velcro" or "cellophane" rales, clubbing, fever, cyanosis

Crs: Most fatal; mean survival = 5.5 yr (Nejm 1978;298:801); die of right heart failure (20%) or infection (80%)

Cmplc: r/o asbestosis; collagen vascular disease; **Bronchiolitis obliterans** (recurrent patchy pneumonia), may be work-related exposures (eg, butter fumes in microwave popcorn workers: Nejm 2002;347:330), has good prognosis and responds to steroids (Nejm 1985;312:152); and desquamative interstitial pneumonia

Lab: *ABGs:* At rest show mild decrease in pO_2 and pCO_2; with exercise, marked decrease in pO_2
Hem: ESR elevated, crit usually normal despite decreased pO_2
Path: Lung bx shows fibrosis w some inflammatory component plus cellular hyperplasia of epithelium; hypertrophied bronchial muscle, endarteritis, and honeycombing in end stages
PFTs: Decreased volumes and diffusing capacity
Serol: Occasionally positive ANA, rheumatoid titer, etc (all are epiphenomena)

Xray: Chest shows reticulonodular infiltrate (fibrosis) especially at bases; spiral CT

Rx: None good. Steroids may improve PFTs during acute phase but help only 11%; perhaps interferon-γ1b? (Nejm 2004;350:125 vs 1999;341:1264) for those who fail just steroids; perhaps ACE inhibitors, interferons
Lung transplant? (p 1003)

16.3 Pulmonary Hypertension

Pulmonary Hypertension: Primary and Secondary

Ann IM 2005;143:282; Nejm 2004;351:1425, 1997;336:111 (primary type)

Cause: Primary types due to autosomal dominant gene in 6% (Nejm 2001;345:319) including ones associated w HAT (Nejm

2001;345:325); maybe Kaposi's sarcoma associated w human herpes virus 8 (HHV-8)? (Nejm 2003;349:1113)

Secondary causes: COPD w hypoxia (most commonly); recurrent chronic pulmonary emboli (Nejm 2001;345:1465; Ann IM 1988;108:425); silicosis; sarcoid; CHF; mitral stenosis; L-to-R shunts, most of which worsen w vasodilator rx (Ann IM 1986;105:499); HIV infection; cocaine and/or iv drug use; cirrhosis; fenfluramine-type anorexic drugs (Nejm 1996;335:609); collagen vascular diseases like scleroderma (Ann IM 2000;132:425), where > 50% get pulmonary HT (Am J Med 1983;75:65)

Epidem: In primary, female/male = 1.7:1; peak onset at age 30-40 yr; associated w positive family hx

Pathophys (Nejm 2004;351:1655):

Vascular proliferation, vasoconstriction, and thrombosis all increase pulmonary vascular resistance. Excess platelet thromboxane A and deficient endothelial cell prostacyclin, nitric oxide, and enothelin production are associated w both primary and secondary pulmonary HT—cause or effect? Worsened by hypoxia, cocaine, and weight-loss drugs related to amphetamines.

Sx: Onset over 1-3 yr

Table 16.4　Symptoms of Pulmonary HT

	As 1st Sx (%)	Present Sometime During Crs (%)
Exertional dyspnea	60	98
Fatigue	20	73
Chest pain	7	47
Syncope or near-syncope	13	77
Edema	3	37
Palpitations	5	33
Raynaud's	?	10

Si: $P_2 \geq A_2$; RV heave; R-sided S_3; pulmonary systolic and diastolic murmur

Crs: Progressive; median survival = 2.8 yr; 68% survive 1 yr, 50% survive 3 yr, and 34% survive 5 yr, worse if mean PA pressure ≥ 85 mm Hg, mean RA pressure > 20 mm Hg, or cardiac index < 2 L/min/m^2 (Ann IM 1991;115:343). Even w prostacycline rx, still have 33% 3-yr mortality.

Cmplc: Cor pulmonale, sudden death (7%)

Lab: *ABGs:* Low pCO_2 often is the only abnormality; hypoxia later in course—first exertional, then at rest

Rx: Of secondary types: Rx the cause if possible; thrombectomy successful in chronic emboli pts even after years (Nejm 2001;345:1465; Ann IM 1987;107:560); O_2 critical if hypoxic etiology

of primary type: Avoid indomethacin and other prostaglandin inhibitors, which increase pressure (Ann IM 1982;97:480)

of both types:

Warfarin anticoagulation increases survival (Nejm 1992;327:76)

Vasodilator rx:

- Epoprostenol (Flolan) iv continuous pump infusions (Ann IM 2000;132:425,500, 1999;130:740, 1990;112:485; Nejm 1998;338:273,321, 1996;334:296; Med Let 1996;38:14); a prostacycline; $72,000/yr

- Iloprost (Ilomedia) 2.5 μgm inhalation 6-12× qd (Nejm 2002;347:322, 2000;342:1866; Ann IM 2000;132:435); a prostacycline; $60,000/yr

- Treprostinil (Remodulin) (Med Let 2002;44:80) 20 ng/kg/min sc continuous; a prostacycline; $93,000/yr

- Calcium-channel blockers help 25%; in those 25%, 5-yr survival is improved to 94% (Nejm 1992;327:76); eg, diltiazem and nifedipine 40-120 mg po qd (Ann IM 1983;99:433)

- Bosentan (Tracleer), an endothelin receptor antagonist (Med Let 2002;44:30; Nejm 2002;346:896,933) 125 mg po bid after half-dose 1st mo; adverse efffects: hepatotoxic, teratogenic; $38,000/yr

• Sildenafil (Viagra) (Med Let 2004;46:18; Ann IM 2002;136:515) 50 mg po tid; $10,000/yr

Lung transplant (p 1003)

Acute Mountain Sickness (High-Altitude Cerebral and Pulmonary Edema)

Ann IM 2004;141:789; Nejm 2001;345:107

Cause: Acute change in elevation above at least 7000-8000 ft, by going up mountains, or in unpressurized airplanes (commercial airlines pressurized at 9000 ft); and usually w associated exertion

Epidem: Increased incidence with exercise and cold weather; increased in teenagers (Nejm 1977;297:1269) and pts with congenital aplasia of right pulmonary artery (Nejm 1980;302:1070). Inhabitants of high altitudes can get just with 1-2 d at low altitudes and return. Physical conditioning before ascent has no effect on acute mountain sickness, pulmonary edema, or cerebral edema incidence. 22% incidence @ 7000-9000 ft, 42% @ 10,000 ft.

Pathophys: Cerebral edema from either cytotoxic vascular dilatation or change in blood–brain barrier permeability (Jama 1998; 280:1920). Normal pulmonary capillary wedge pressures; increased atrial natriuretic factor; increased capillary permeability (Ann IM 1988;109:796).

Sx: Onset in 6-48 hr; headache (62%); fatigue (26%) and lassitude; anorexia (11%), nausea, and vomiting; insomnia (31%); dyspnea (21%); dizziness (21%)

Si: Dyspnea; dry cough; Cheyne-Stokes respirations, especially at night. Acute pulmonary edema (4% of nonacclimatized people at 12,000-14,000 ft) without warning si's; cerebral edema w ataxia and confusion; asymptomatic retinal hemorrhages (Ophthalm 1992;99:739; Nejm 1970;282:1183).

Crs: Spontaneous resolution in 3-4 d

Cmplc:

Lab: *ABGs:* Mild respiratory alkalosis

Xray: MRI of head in cerebral edema type shows white matter edema, esp of corpus callosum

Rx:

Prevention:

- Avoid exertion for several days or acclimatize at 6000-8000 ft for 2-4 d
- O_2 at 4-10 L/min, hs and at 1st sx
- Acetazolamide 250 mg po b-tid 24-48 hr, decreases incidence by 50%
- Dexamethasone 4 mg po q 6 hr before and during exposure; perhaps decreases cerebral edema (Nejm 1984;310:683) and mountain sickness but not the physiologic consequences, ie, it may mask sx (Nejm 1989;321:1707)
- Salmeterol 125 μgm w MDI and spacer decreases pulmonary edema by > 50% (Nejm 2002;346:1631)
- Sildenafil (Viagra) 50 mg po qd (?), increases exercise capacity in hypoxic conditions (Ann IM 2004;141:169); adverse effects: headache

Rx of sx: Most importantly, descend at least 1000 ft at 1st sx; O_2

of pulmonary edema: Prophylactic nifedipine 20 mg SR po q 8 hr; decrease PA pressures (Nejm 1991;325:1284), eg, w nitric oxide 10% inhalations (Nejm 1996;334:624); morphine im to relieve anxiety and pool peripheral blood; rest and descend

of cerebral edema: Dexamethasone 8 mg po/iv, then 4 mg q 6 hr; O_2; immediate descent

Pulmonary Embolus

Nejm 2003;349:1247, 1998;339:93

Cause: Embolic clots to pulmonary arteries via systemic venous return

Epidem: Very common; probably incidence correlates best with thoroughness of postmortem exam

Associated w estrogen-containing bcp's, esp 2nd-generation (< 50 μgm estrogen + norgestrel, levonorgestrel, or norgestrienone) or, worse, 3rd-generaton (desogestrel, gestodene, or norgestionate) types; pregnancy (Nejm 1996;335:108); postmenopausal HRT; occult cancers, 15% of cancer pts will have within 2 yr (Ann IM 1982;96:556); DVT and its genetic precipitants (p 147); surgery, especially of legs; cramped air travel (Nejm 2001;345:779), end-of-trip incidence = 1.5/1 million for trips > 3100 mi, 4.8/1 million if > 6200 mi

Rare upper-extremity DVT, esp after central iv line and in athletes w repetitive arm abduction, "Paget-Schroetter syndrome" (Nejm 2002;347:1876); can even lead to fatal PE

Pathophys: Thrombophlebitis causes thrombus, which breaks free and migrates to the lungs; many pts have many small emboli chronically rather than one big one. Rarely are calves the source; most from thigh and pelvic veins (Ann IM 1981;94:439); no si or sx of DVT in 50%.

Sx: Sudden or chronic dyspnea; pleuritic chest pain w infarct; hemoptysis; fever; syncope with large emboli

Si: All uncommon; elevated JVP; high diaphragm on one side by percussion; basilar atelectasis; pleural effusion; wheezing (Nejm 1968;278:999); BP cuff test for calf pain; $P_2 > A_2$; cyanosis

Crs (Nejm 1992;326:1240):

Resolves over 10-30 d (Nejm 1969;280:1194); 80% overall survival; 60% without rx, 90% with rx; 75% of deaths occur in first 2 hr; DVT clinically resolves in $1/3$ after 3 d of heparin rx

Fatalities < 2% in yr following dx if rx'd × 3-6 mo (Jama 1998;279:458)

Cmplc: "Milk leg" from incompetent leg veins; chronic pulmonary HT in 4% (Nejm 2004;350:2257)

    r/o air embolism (Nejm 2000;342:476)

Lab (McMaster's Univ rev: Ann IM 1991;114:300, 1983;98:891):

ABGs: pO$_2$ < 80 mm Hg, 10% false negative; < 90 mm Hg, 0% false negative

Hem: Fibrin split products/D-dimer > 500 ng/cc by ELISA methods, 96% sens, 68% specif (Ann IM 2004;140:589); combined w ABG criteria above, if D-dimer negative and pO$_2$ > 80 mm Hg on RA, no false negs for PE (Thorax 1998;53: 830); or combined w alveolar dead space fraction ≤ 20%, 98% sens, 50% specif (Jama 2001;285:761)

Noninv: EKG may show S$_1$Q$_3$T$_3$, very specific but only w massive emboli (Am J EM 1997;15:310); anterior T-wave inversions (68% sens) (Chest 1998;113:850); or ≥ 3 of the following (70% sens) (Am J Cardiol 1994;73:298): RBBB or pRBBB, S in I and aVL ≥ 15 mm, poor R progression, Q in III and F not II, RAD > 90°, voltage < 5 mm in limb leads, T-wave inversions in II + F or V$_1$-V$_4$

Xray: All doable even in pregnancy (Nejm 1996;335:108)

    Chest shows infiltrates, effusions, high diaphragm, lucency

    V/Q scan to look for multiple mismatched defects (87% sens, 97% specif), but even if all defects are matched, odds of pulmonary embolus still are substantial (case: Nejm 1995;332:321; Ann IM 1983;98:891), ie, 40% (PIOPED: Jama 1990;263:2753)

    CT angiography has < 1.5% false-neg rate in high-risk pts (meta-analysis: Ann IM 2004;141:866)

    Spiral (helical) CT, neg w leg ultrasounds enough to r/o w < 2% false-neg rate; spiral study misses the 30% of PEs with only subsegmental clots (Rad 1996;199:31; Chest 1997;111:246)

MR angiography is 75% sens, 95% specif (Lancet 2002;359:1643; Nejm 1997;336:1422)

Pulmonary arteriography is diagnostic and the gold standard

To find DVT, B-mode duplex ultrasound now as good or better (Ann IM 1989;111:297) than IPGs; ultrasound positive in only ⅓ of documented pulmonary emboli cases (Ann IM 1997;126:775); venograms (Nejm 1981;304:1561; Ann IM 1978;89:162)

Rx: Prevent w warfarin or sc unfractionated q 12 hr or qd LMW heparin (p 52)

Screen for reversible causes w factor V (Leiden), homocysteine, and lupus anticoagulant (which requires more intense anticoagulation)

Heparin (p 51), LMW or unfractionated for at least 5 d if start warfarin on day 1 (Nejm 1990;322:1260). Used long term in pregnancy, keeping PTT 1.5× control at 6 hr.

Warfarin to an INR of 2-3 (p 52) for 6 (Nejm 1995;332:166) to 12 mo; 12% will recur whenever anticoagulation stopped (Ann IM 2003;139:1)

Thrombolysis rarely if severe, w thrombolytics especially if right heart failure/dysfunction or pulmonary HT w acute embolus (Nejm 2002;347:1143)

Surgical IVC plication, or Greenfield filter rarely; embolectomy (50% survival) rarely needed

Fat Emboli

Nejm 1993;329:926,961, 1967;276:1192

Cause: Fat globules, from bony fractures, via the circulation to the pulmonary arteries and other vessels? Often seem w total hip replacement (94%: Clin Orthoped Related Research 1999;355:23)

Epidem: Symptomatic emboli in 3% of all femoral shaft traumas; they are the cause of death in 5% of all trauma deaths; but 90% of emboli cause no sx or are undetected

Pathophys: Fat from marrow or from tissue enters veins to inferior vena cava, or enters the lymphatics and from there goes to the thoracic duct via the superior vena cava to the lungs and beyond to the systemic circulation; there the fat emboli are broken down by lipoprotein lipase into triglycerides and free fatty acids, which are toxic molecules

Sx: 24-48 hr latent period after femoral, pelvic, tibial, humeral, or other trauma; then nonlateralizing CNS sx's of confusion/acute brain syndrome; dyspnea and respiratory distress

Si: Fever; tachycardia; skin petechiae (85%), mantle distribution over chest, neck, and conjunctiva; cyanosis; confusion

Crs: Of those with sx, 10-20% mortality if no coma; 85% mortality if coma present

Cmplc: Adult respiratory distress syndrome (p 967)

Lab: *Chem:* Lipase elevated in 3-5 d, peaks at 5-8 d
Hem: Thrombocytopenia
Noninv: Transesophageal cardiac echo shows emboli themselves during fx repair (Clin Orthoped Related Research 1999;355:23)
Path: Bx of petechiae or kidney shows fat in capillaries with platelets about them; use frozen section, which avoids formalin dissolution of the fat. Sputum stained for fat, 80% false negative; bronchial lavage shows intracellular fat in > 33% of cells (8/8 patients: Ann IM 1990;113:583).
Urine: Fat stain positive in 60% with acid-washed glass

Xray: Chest shows bilateral fluffy infiltrates, ARDS
Lung scan shows mismatched V/Q defects

Rx: Methylprednisolone 1+ mg/kg q 6 hr × 3 d at 1st si in likely pt; prevents w/o complications (Ann IM 1983;99:439)
Supportive rx of ARDS (p 967)

16.4 Pulmonary Tumors

Mesothelioma

Nejm 2005;353:1591

Cause: Neoplasia from asbestosis

Epidem: 2.5 cases/1 million population/yr. Most (all?) from asbestos exposure (Nejm 1969;280:488).

Pathophys: Quite malignant; ~20% are abdominal (peritoneal), which are all associated with heavy asbestos exposures, unlike often transient exposures of pulmonary types

Sx: Nonpleuritic pain and/or dyspnea (95%). Pulmonary osteo-arthropathy arthritis pain (distal extremities with periosteal new bone formation), often severe; benign types of mesothelioma have pulmonary osteoarthropathy 100% of the time, and it goes away with surgical rx.

Si: Clubbing; ascites with peritoneal type

Crs: Rapid demise in < 12 mo, usually about 4 mo after dx; die from primary lesions, not metastases usually. 0-10% 5-yr survival with rx.

Cmplc: Pericardial effusions; small bowel obstructions with peritoneal types

Lab: *Chem:* Pleural fluid hyaluronic acid level > 0.8 mg/cc is diagnos-tic but > 50% false negatives

Path: Pleural fluid cytology often hard to interpret because nor-mal mesothelial cells can appear malignant; pleural bx usu-ally diagnostic

Xray: Chest shows pleural plaques (calcified); pulmonary fibrosis in 20% of pulmonary types, 50% of abdominal types; pleural effu-sions usually

Rx: Debatable (Ann IM 1977;87:618) if anything helps; perhaps chemoRx w pemetrexed (Alimta) w B_{12} and folate (Med Let 2004;46:31)

Lung Cancer

Cause: Types: alveolar cell, small (oat) cell, bronchogenic (squamous and adenocarcinoma), and large cell undifferentiated

Neoplasia; viral origin with alveolar? (cf sheep "yagshikta") although still smoking induced; carcinogens with bronchogenic types

Epidem: Epidemic now in U.S.; leading cause of cancer death in males and females although male > female w squamous type; male = female w adenocarcinoma

All are increased in smokers and those exposed to smoke as a child (Nejm 1990;323:632); asbestos-exposed workers (incidence is about 20%!) but not people living in mining areas (Nejm 1998;338:1565); radon-exposed uranium miners (Nejm 1984; 310:1481,1485), and homeowners (Nejm 1994;330:159). Smoking multiplies the radon effect.

Pathophys: Alveolar type is multicentric in origin; rarely metastasizes, but rather presents as pneumonitis from its local invasion. Oat or small cell type is extremely malignant. Bronchogenic types are of endobronchial origin, then locally invade and eventually metastasize via the lymphatics.

Sx: Hemoptysis, often intermittent but late in course may be massive; pain, pleuritic or simply a deep sense of abnormality often when cancer is in the mediastinum; weight loss; cough; dyspnea; arthritis (pulmonary osteoarthropathy)

Si: Wheeze unilaterally; clubbing; hoarseness from recurrent laryngeal nerve paralysis; pulmonary osteoarthropathy (10%); Pancoast's syndrome (Nejm 1997;337:1359,1370): Horner's syndrome, shoulder and arm pain from $C_8 T_1 T_2$ root compression in brachial plexus that radiates down ulnar nerve with vasomotor changes in the hand, plus first rib erosion on chest xray

Crs (Nejm 2004;350:379): Coin lesions found incidentally have a 30% 5-yr survival

Table 16.5   Presenting Distribution and Survival of Treated Non-small Cell Lung Cancers

Stage	Distribution at Presentation (%)	5-yr Survival (%)
I: $T_1N_0M_0$	10	70
$T_2N_0M_0$		60
II: $T_2N_0M_0$ or $T_1N_1M_0$	20	50
$T_2N_1M_0$		40
IIIa: $T_3N_{0-2}M_0$ or $T_1N_2M_0$	70 (III + IV)	30
$T_2N_2M_0$		15
IIIb: $T_{1-3}N_3M_0$ or $T_4N_{1-3}M_0$		<10
IV: $T_{1-3}N_{0-3}M_1$		0

T_1 < 3 cm, T_2 > 3 cm, T_3 to chest wall.
N_0, no nodes; N_1, peribronchial and ipsilateral hilar; N_2, ipsilateral mediastinal and subcarinal nodes; N_3, supraclavicular and contralateral mediastinal nodes.
M_0, no mets; M_1, distant mets.
Non-small cell: limited disease has 15-25% 5-yr survival; extensive has < 5% 5-yr survival.

Cmplc: Pneumonia and effusions; superior vena cava syndrome; CNS metastases; hormone production, especially with small cell types, eg, of ADH, PTH (also common with squamous cell), ACTH, gonadotropins causing gynecomastia (Nejm 1968;279:640); neuropathies and myopathies including autonomic dysfunction leading to pseudo-small bowel obstruction (Ann IM 1983;98:129); Eaton-Lambert syndrome (myasthenia "resistant" or unresponsive to neostigmine), caused by antibodies to calcium channels that trigger Ach release at nerve endings (Nejm 1995;332:1467); in small cell types, rare paraneoplastic limbic encephalitis (Nejm 1999;340:1788) w seizures, dementia, irritability, depression, which may precede cancer discovery in 60%, 20% of time associated w testicular Ca, due to shared antigens between tumor and limbic neuronal proteins

Lab: *Path:* Cytologies on sputa or bronchoscopy specimen; bronchoscopy bx, mediastinoscopy bx; supraclavicular node bx, often find on left with left upper lobe lesions, on right with all other locations

Xray: Chest xrays even with cytologies not worth doing as screening test (Ann IM 1989;111:232)

Coin lesion w/u (Nejm 2003;348:2535)

Bone invasion usually means it is a squamous cell type. Anterior segment upper lobe infiltrates are cancer (90+%) until proven otherwise. Paralyzed diaphragm if phrenic nerve involvement.

CT scans can help define a coin lesion as benign by finding central calcium. Stable plain films over 2 yr also can reassure that lesion is benign. Expensive PET scans also helpful for 1-4 cm nodules (Jama 2001;285:922). Integrated CT–PET scans about 90% accurate for node mets and invasion (Nejm 2003;348:2500) but may be of marginal benefit (editorial: Ann IM 2003;139:950).

Rx: Prevent by stopping smoking, although takes 3-20 yr for risk to decrease to that of a nonsmoker (Am J Pub Hlth 1990;80:954) of non-small cell:

Surgery to try to cure, unless ≥ stage IIIa, nerve involvement, massive lesion or distant metastases, bad pulmonary functions, malignant pleural effusion, contralateral mediastinal nodes. Results best at hospitals doing > 67 lung Ca resections/yr (Nejm 2001;345:181).

Radiation and chemoRx w cisplatin (marginally helpful: Nejm 2004;350:351), 5-FU (Nejm 2004;350:1713), or 2-drug regimens (Jama 2004;292:470) for advanced disease including Taxol, erlotinib (Tarceva), and gefitinib (Iressa)

of small cell types: ChemoRx and radiation cures some (45% 2-yr survival)

Palliative radiation to rx bronchial obstruction, or to give pain relief when in brachial plexus; radiation alone can never cure (Ann IM 1990;113:33)

16.5 Miscellaneous

Bronchitis, Acute

Ann IM 2001;134:518,521

Cause: Usually viral esp influenza; Bordetella sp, mycoplasma, and TWAR (C. pneumonia) are all < 10%

Sx: Productive cough

Si: No T°, tachycardia, tachypnea, or focal lung findings

Xray: Chest if cough > 3 wk

Rx: Symptomatic

Cough, Acute and Subacute

Nejm 2000;343:1715

Rx: Stop smoking is 1st rx for all
- URI: Rx w Actifed bid × 1 wk, or naproxen 500 mg po tid × 5 d, or iprotropium nasal ii t-qid × 4 d
- Allergic rhinitis: Rx w nonsedating antihistamines
- Bacterial sinusitis if tooth pain, poor transillumination, purulent nasal d/c: Rx w Actifed, oxymetazoline spray bid × 5 d, and/or antibiotics vs H. flu and strep pneumo × 3 wk if sx < 4 wk
- COPD: Rx as usual
- Whooping cough: No dx tests; if in community, rx w erythromycin 500 mg qid × 14 d

Cough, Chronic Idiopathic in Adults

Ann IM 1993;119:977

Cause: Postnasal drip from chronic sinusitis; asthma, allergic bronchitis, and/or rhinitis; gastroesophageal reflux; COPD; medications, especially ACE inhibitors

Si: Methacholine challenge test positive if asthmatic origin

Xray: Sinus films, chest xray

Rx: Stop ACEIs and smoking; rx of asthma or GE reflux if either present
    1st: Decongestant/antihistamine bid, helps 39/45; perhaps w codeine or dextromethorphan (Med Let 2001;43:23)
    2nd: Nasal steroids bid
    3rd: Albuterol inhaler; or terbutaline 2.5 mg po tid or inhale, cures $^2/_3$ (BMJ 1983; 287:940); or aminophylline, and a po β-agonist like terbutaline

Diving (SCUBA) Accidents

More common in asthmatics. Barotrauma causes pneumothorax and air emboli to brain and all organs including muscles and heart; CPK elevations that correlate w severity (Nejm 1994;330:19). Bends (gas forming in vessels as ascend) causes pain and various organ impairments. Rx w hyperbaric O_2 (call divers alert network, 919-684-8111).

Also 5× increase in strokes if patent foramen ovale (Ann IM 2001;134:21)

Expectorants

None thought clinically useful in adults now:
Acetylcysteine; via inhalation; breaks S—H bonds of mucous glycoproteins; used for trach care and in CF pts
Glyceryl guaiacolate (Robitussin) po; vagal stimulation of secretions?

Iodides (SSKI); 10-20 gtts in water po; increases glandular secretions and proteolytic enzymes, which decrease viscosity; but out of favor due to long-term toxicity concerns

Deoxyribonuclease aerosol qd-bid (Nejm 1994;331:637, 1992;326:812); used in cystic fibrosis

Hemoptysis, Differential Dx

Ann IM 1985;102:833

- Chronic bronchitis: Viral/bacterial infection, coughing
- Pulmonary vascular changes: Telangiectasias, emboli, mitral stenosis
- Nonpulmonary source: Nasopharynx, gi, mouth
- Bronchiectasis
- Tbc
- Cancer
- Coagulation abnormalities: Drug induced or acquired

Lung Transplant

Unilateral w/o heart transplant and using cyclosporine and other agents rather than steroids has 40% 5-yr survival (Nejm 1999;340:108)

Physical Therapy to Chest

Is of no value unless lots of secretions (Nejm 1979;300:1155) or neuromuscular lung disease is present

Pleural Effusion Analysis

Ann IM 1985;103:799

Transudates caused by CHF; hypoproteinemia; chronic renal failure; cirrhosis; normal vaginal delivery, $^2/_3$ have in first 24 hr (Ann IM 1982;97:852)

Table 16.6   Exudates, Sensitivities, and Specificities

Lab Test	Positive Value	Sensitivity (%)	Specificity (%)
For Exudates in General			
1. LDH	> 200 U (if normal in serum is ≤ 300)	70	100
2. Fluid/serum LDH	> 0.6	86	98
3. Protein	> 3 gm	89	91
4. Fluid/serum protein	> 0.5	90	98
1 + 2 or 4		99	98
Necessity of Surgical Drainage of Exudate			
pH	< 7.0	70	100
	< 7.2	90	87
LDH	> 1000 U	100	80
For Tuberculosis			
Culture	Positive	24	100
Culture and pleural bx	Either positive	90	100
For Carcinoma			
Cytologies and pleural bx	Either positive	68	100

Pleurodesis

Ann IM 1994;120:56

For recurrent pneumothorax or malignant effusions; use tetracycline (Jama 1990;264:2224), or doxycycline 500 mg, or minocycline 300 mg; talc even better but requires thoracoscopy; or bleomycin

Pneumothorax

Nejm 2000;342:868

Spontaneous occurs usually in male smokers age 10-40
Secondary occurs in COPD and pneumocystis-infected AIDS pts

Noninvasive Positive Pressure Ventilation

Nejm 1997;337:1747

Continuous positive airway pressure (CPAP) via endotrach tube or mask over mouth and/or nose; for acute or chronic respiratory failure, pulmonary edema, and chronic CHF

BiPAP, mask administered, 2-level pressure systems w higher inspiratory and lower positive end expiratory pressures (PEEP); for acute or chronic respiratory failure

Pulmonary Function Tests

Arterial blood gases: Spuriously low pO_2 when high numbers of platelets or wbc's (Nejm 1979;301:361)

Carbon monoxide diffusion capacity: Specific but not sensitive in predicting exertional hypoxia (Nejm 1987;316:1301)

Pulmonary Toxins

O_2: Tracheobronchitis develops with 95% O_2 within 6 hr in normals (Ann IM 1975;82:40)

Radiation toxicity: Acute reaction in 4-6 wk; rx with steroids; creates scarring in 4-12 mo (Ann IM 1977;86:81)

Diffuse Interstitial Changes on Chest Xray, Differential Dx

- Alveolar proteinosis (Nejm 2003;349:2527)

    Pathophys: Fatty substance accumulates in alveoli

    Epidem: Males > females; median age at onset = 39

    Sx: Insidious-onset DOE and cough

    Si: Rales (50%)

    Crs: Death from restrictive disease, although some spontaneous remissions

    Lab: Mild increase in LDH

    Rx: With pulmonary lavage (Nejm 1972;286:1230). Steroids contraindicated because of fungal superinfections.

- Asbestosis: Lower lobe predominant; fine streak pattern; pleural effusions (21%) (Ann IM 1971;74:178); increased incidence of mesothelioma and carcinoma
- Berryliosis: Acute or chronic for years after exposure; looks like sarcoid (Ann IM 1988;108:687); a hypersensitivity pneumonitis (Nejm 1989;320:1103)
- Chronic occupational pneumonitis (p 979) and allergic pneumonitis/alveolitis (p 979)
- Cystic fibrosis (p 985) when end stage
- Eosinophilic granuloma (p 1107)
- Idiopathic pulmonary fibrosis (p 987)
- Interstitial carcinomas: Alveolar cell, breast
- Pulmonary thesaurosis (Nejm 1974;290:660): Seen in hairdressers. Patchy infiltrates. Clears when avoid hair sprays. Nodes look like sarcoid. Lung looks like idiopathic pulmonary fibrosis.
- Sarcoid (p 1117)
- Silicosis: Eggshell calcified nodes, progressive massive fibrosis "bat wings"
- Talcosis: Increased density of pattern
- Tuberculosis (p 579)
- Tungsten carbide maker's exposure: Treatable by stopping dust exposure? from cobalt involved in process (Ann IM 1971;75:709)

Respirator Weaning

By qd trials of spontaneous breathing rather than multiple trials, intermittent mandatory ventilation, or decreasing pressure supported ventilation (Nejm 1995;332:345)

Sick Building Syndrome

Cause: 25% due to exhaust; 75% due to anaerobes, etc

Sx: Fatigue, headache, inability to concentrate

Rx: Increase outdoor air to 20+ ft³/min/person (Nejm 1993;328:821)

Smoking Cessation

Nejm 2002;346:506; Jama 1999;281:72; Med Let 1995;37:6

Nicotine, either patch or gum formulation, w concomitant education results in a 33% 2-yr discontinuation rate (Nejm 1988;318:15) vs 10-15% w placebo

- Patch (Habitrol, Nicoderm, Prostep) (Nejm 1991;325:311; Arch IM 1991;151:749) 24 hr/day in decreasing doses from 21 mg × 2-3 wk, then 14 mg × 2-3+ wk, then 7 mg × 2-3+ wk, then stop. Best 6-mo outcomes = 28% cessation, 44 mg patches may or may not be safe and effective (Jama 1995;274: 1347 vs 1353); can use gum, inhaler, or nasal spray for added jolt w patch. May be ok even in ischemic heart disease (Nejm 1996;335:1792; Arch IM 1994;54:989); coincident smoking w patch not advisable but also not dangerously risky (Nejm 1996;335:1792); cost for 8 wk = $220; or can use 16 hr 15/10/5 mg patches (Nicotrol).
- Gum (Nicorette) 2-4 mg/piece, 9-12 piece/d, max 20 piece/d; tough on teeth (Med Let 1984;26:98; Ann IM 1984;101:121); cost $100 (2 mg) to $200 (4 mg)/mo
- Inhaler (Nicotrol) 6-16 cartridges qd × 3 mo, then taper over 3 mo; predominant mouth absorption; adverse effects: asthma exacerbation; $45/42 cartridges
- Nasal spray (Nicotrol) ½ mg each nostril up to 5×/hr, < 40 sprays qd; effective when used w patch (Ann IM 2004;140:426)

Bupropion (Wellbutrin, Zyban is long-acting formulation) 150 mg LA qd, increase to bid after 1 wk × 6-8 wk; start 1 wk before quit date to build level; success at 8 wk = 45% and at 1 yr = 23%, double control rates and weight gain less (Nejm 1997;337:1195); use w nicotine formulations (Addiction 1998;93:907), eg, 21 mg

patch wk 2-7, 14 mg wk 8, 7 mg wk 9 produced a 36% 1-yr quit
rate (Nejm 1999;340:685)
Antidepressants (Nejm 1997;337:1230): Nortriptyline, doxepin,
fluoxetine (Prozac)
Clonidine po or patch may also help (ACP J Club 2005;142:12)

Chapter 17

Renal/Urology

D. K. Onion

17.1 Fluid/Electrolytes/Acid–Base

if hypovolemic, initial bolus of NS: 250-500 cc in adult, 10-20 cc/kg in child

Table 17.1   24-Hr Basal Requirements

Age	Water	Na[1]	K+	Calories
Adult	2500 cc	100 mEq	20 mEq	4-800[2]
Child < 2 yr	120 cc/kg	2-3 mEq/kg	1-2 mEq/kg	125/kg,[3] 150/kg for premie
Child > 2 yr	80 cc/kg	2-3 mEq/kg	1-2 mEq/kg	125/kg

1. Can adjust intake to needs instinctively (Nejm 1991;324:232). 2. D_5W = 200 cal/L.
3. Milk = 2/3 cal/L.

Table 17.2   Loss Requirements: Typical Adult Potential 24-Hr Losses Beyond Basal by Source

	Saliva	Sweat	Gastric	Pancreatic	Large + Small Bowel
Water (cc)	1500	Variable	2500	700	3000
Na (mEq/L)	Variable	10-50	45	110-150	100-140
K (mEq/L)	Variable	10	10	2.5-7.5	5-35
HCO_3 (mEq/L)				90-110	20-50
Cl (mEq/L)			100	50-55	
Organic anion					174 (mEq/L)

Deficit calculations: Adult body spaces of fluid and lytes for calculating deficits to be made up, usually within 24 hr

K^+: female = 35 mEq/kg, male = 45 mEq/kg presuming normal pH of 7.40

Water: 60% of body weight in kg; water deficit = 0.6 (ideal body weight) $(1 - 140/Na)$ (Nejm 1977;297:1444)

Sample calculation: A 60-kg, 20-yr-old man needs iv orders for the next 24 hr; he is euvolemic as measured by vital signs, weight, postural BP, and a central monitoring line, but he has gastric atony and is putting out over 2 L/24 hr via an NG tube, K is 3.0 mEq/L, Na is 150 mEq/L, pH is normal. Thus his 24-hr water needs are basal + anticipated loss requirements + replacement for his deficit = 2500 + 2500 + $(0.6)(60)(1 - 140/150)$ = 7.5 L. Similarly, his Na^+ needs are 100 + (45)(2.5) + 0 = 212 mEq. His K^+ needs are = 20 + 10(2.5) + 45(60)(1 - 3.0/4.0) = 720; but one can't easily give more than 40 mEq/L without damaging veins; since the pt has good kidneys, he may not need this much. His caloric requirements = 400-800 cal, and more would not hurt. Thus, 300 cc/hr of D_5 1/4 S with 40 mEq/L of KCl would be a reasonable 24-hr order, giving him 7 L water, 245 mEq Na, 280 mEq K, and 1400 cal. Given the large numbers and the imprecision of any such estimates, checking parameters and reestimating every 8-12 hr during the course of the 24-hr period would be prudent.

17.2 Oral Rehydration Solutions (ORS)

Nejm 1990;323:891; Med Let 1987;29:63; contents: Postgrad Med 1983;74:336

In mild-moderate dehydration, give at 10-25 cc/kg/hr replacement rate, then 100-150 cc/kg/d maintenance

Table 17.3 Natural Oral Rehydration Solutions

	N (mEq/L)	K (mEq/L)
Apple juice	1.7	2.6
Orange juice	0.2	38
Tomato juice	100	59
Ginger ale	3.5	0.15
Pepsi	6.4	0.8
Grape juice	0.4	31
Pineapple juice	0.2	36
Coke	0.4	13
Milk	22	36

Table 17.4 Prepared Oral Rehydration Solutions

	WHO ORS	Rehydralyte	Pedialyte/Lytren
Na (mEq/L)	90	75	50
K (mEq/L)	20	20	20
Cl (mEq/L)	80	65	40
HCO_3 (mEq/L)	30	30	30
Glucose (gm/L)	20	25	20
Form	Powder	Liquid	Liquid
Cost/qt	$0.35	$4	$3

Home-made ORS: sugar/salt = 8:1; for instance,

   2 tsp sugar + ¼ tsp salt + a squeeze of lime in 8-oz glass of boiled
      water; or 8 tsp sugar + 1 tsp salt + citrus in 1 L (three 12-oz
      Coke cans); or

   4-finger scoop sugar + 3-finger pinch salt + citrus in 1 L boiled
      water; or

   8 bottle caps sugar + 1 cap salt + citrus in 1 L boiled water

   Cereal (rice, corn, or wheat) starches 50-80 gm/L (Nejm 2000;
      342:308,345, 1991;324:517) or as rice syrup; ferment in
      colon, help Na pumps there; better than glucose/sucrose; but
      can't measure out, plus they ferment quickly in field unless
      contained in a commercial powder or syrup

17.3 Hyperalimentations/Total Parenteral Nutrition (TPN)

Use helps only the severely malnourished (Nejm 1991;325:526, 573) and doesn't prolong life (Jama 1998;280:2013)

17.4 Osmolarity

- Calculated mOsm = 2(Na) + glucose/18 + BUN/2.8 (Ann IM 1989;110:854)
- Unmeasured osmoles or osmolar gap (measured minus calculated) seen with ethylene glycol (0.05 gm % = 22 mOsm), ethanol, and abnormally elevated serum lipids or proteins, but also inexplicably in lactic acidosis and diabetic ketoacidosis (Ann IM 1990;113:580)

17.5 Anion Gap Changes

- Calculation: (Na) − (Cl + CO_3) = gap, or R fraction
- Low anion gap (< 10): Multiple myeloma, hypoalbuminemia, bromism, hypernatremia, hyperkalemia, hypermagnesemia, hypercalcemia, lithium
- High anion gap (> 15): Most metabolic acidoses, nonketotic hyperosmolar coma, hypomagnesemia, hypokalemia, hypocalcemia

17.6 Hyperkalemia

- Seen in renal failure, hemolysis, rhabdomyolisis, freshwater drownings, Addison's disease, and use of ACE inhibitors, NSAIDs, K-sparing diuretics, Tm/S especially in AIDS pts (Nejm 1993;328:703); r/o "pseudo"-hyperkalemia due to thrombocythemia, increased white cells, or fist clenching when draw blood (Nejm 1990;322:1290)

- EKG shows tall peaked Ts, evolves to wide QRS and loss of P waves, then evolves to sine wave as K increases
- Rx w CaCl ampule iv; and/or insulin + glucose drip; and/or HCO_3 iv; and K-resin binder (Kayexalate) po; and/or dialysis, hemo- or peritoneal; or albuterol via nebulizer (Ann IM 1989;110:426)

17.7 Acidosis

- pH effect on O_2 hemoglobin dissociation: Decreased pH leads to immediate R shift of hemoglobin/O_2 curve, ie, easier dissociation
- K^+ shifts = 0.6 mEq/10 nEq of H^+; pH nanoequivalents (nEq): pH 7.7 = 20 nEq, 7.6 = 25, 7.5 = 32, 7.4 = 40, 7.3 = 50, 7.2 = 63, 7.1 = 79, 7.0 = 100. Thus K^+ of 5.1 at pH 7.0 is really K^+ of 1.5 at pH 7.4.

Respiratory Acidosis

Nejm 1998;338:26

Cause: Respiratory failure, inability to breathe adequately; rapid onset of coma relative to pH, compared to metabolic acidosis, since CO_2 penetrates CSF readily and raises pH rapidly (F. Plum: Nejm 1967;277:605); CO_2 also diffuses into all tissues including myocardium, rapidly leads to electromechanical dissociation (EMD), hence HCO_3 rx of arrest unwise no matter what blood gases are; arterial gases are misleading, too (Nejm 1986;315:153)

Rx: Respiratory support

Metabolic Acidosis

Nejm 1998;338:26

Cause: Ketosis from DKA, isopropyl alcohol poisoning, lactic acidosis (alcohol, septic shock, metformin rx, hypotension, or short bowel *Lactobacillus* overgrowth [Ann IM 1995;122:839]); salicylate, methanol (formic), paraldehyde, ethylene glycol, methanol, or toluene glue poisoning; severe diarrhea,* D-lactate produced by gut flora (Nejm 1979;301:249), pancreatic fistulas*; uremia, RTA*

Lab: Salicylates, lytes, ketones, alcohol level, measured vs calculated osmoles, lactate level (Jama 1994;272:1678)

Rx: Rx of the primary disease; rx with any alkali, even HCO_3, may paradoxically worsen even if pH < 7.2 (Ann IM 1990;112:492) although helpful in "low" (normal) anion gap acidoses (= *). Dichloroacetate no help in lactic acidosis (Nejm 1992;327:1564).

*helpful in "low" (normal) anion gap acidosis

17.8 Alkalosis

Respiratory Alkalosis

Nejm 1998;338:107

Cause: Hyperventilation, voluntary or iatrogenic

Sx: Tetany

Cmplc: Rare since most never increase pH > 7.55

Rx: Increase dead space, eg, with bag breathing; or slow rate and/or depth

Metabolic Alkalosis

Nejm 1998;338:107

Cause: Vomiting, diuretics (renal H^+ loss to save K^+ and Na^+)

Pathophys: Sx and cmplc when pH > 7.6, which causes decrease in ionized calcium levels

Sx: Headache, tetany, seizures, delirium, stupor

Si: Depressed respirations

Cmplc: Supraventricular and ventricular arrhythmias; angina induction

Lab: Alkalosis, hypoK$^+$

Rx: KCl and NaCl repletion, not K-gluconate; NH$_4$Cl 10 gm = 180 mEq iv as 1-2% soln, or arginine HCl in extreme or resistant cases

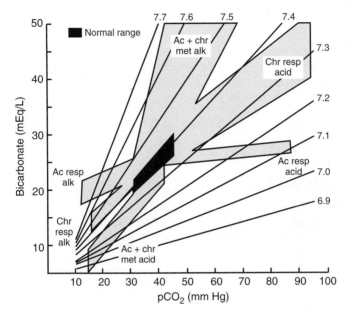

Figure 17.1 Acid–base nomogram bands: mean ±2 SD response in normals. (Reproduced with permission from Petersdorf et al, eds. Harrison's Principles of Internal Medicine, 12th ed. New York: McGraw-Hill; 1991: Table 44-1, p 290)

Hypophosphatemia

Cause: Malnutrition; aluminum-binding antacids; iv glucose, which drives intracellularly; renal tubular damage from hypokalemia, osmotic diuresis, or Fanconi's. In types without cell injury like acute DKA, hyperalimentation, or acute respiratory alkalosis, no bad consequences ensue because total body PO_4 depletion has not occurred (Nejm 1985;313:447).

Epidem:

Pathophys:

Sx: Confusion, weakness

Si:

Crs:

Cmplc: Bleeding (impaired platelet function), infections (impaired granulocyte function), rhabdomyolysis

Lab: PO_4 low

Rx: 2.5 mg elemental phosphorus/kg in NS over 12-hr iv, or po w NeutroPhos

Hyponatremia

Nejm 2000;342:1581

Cause:
- Elevated antidiuretic hormone (ADH) from:
  Syndrome of inappropriate ADH (SIADH), most commonly, or tumor (Ann IM 1985;102:165)
  Drugs: Vincristine, cytoxan, clofibrate, narcotics, nicotine, isoproterenol, vasopressin iv in ICU
  Hypovolemia
- Increased renal ADH sensitivity: Chlorpropamide and other 1st- but not 2nd-generation hypoglycemics, NSAIDs especially ibuprofen and indomethacin (Nejm 1984;310:568), thiazides, carbamazepine
- Lab error (pseudohyponatremia) (Nejm 2003;349:1465): Check osmoles, measure Na directly w ABG machine; glucose, mannitol, post-TURP glycine bladder instillation
- Free water replacement of isotonic emesis, diarrhea, blood, serum; or idiopathically post-op (Nejm 1986;314:1529)
- Hypothyroid hypo-osmolarity, Addison's disease

- Psychiatric pts with polydipsia, inappropriate ADH syndrome (SIADH), and decreased renal free water excretion (Nejm 1988;318:397)
- Post-op (1-3 d), equal sex ratio, 1% incidence; caused by high vasopressin (ADH) levels and hypotonic or sometimes even isotonic (Ann IM 1997;126:20) iv fluids, but respiratory arrest and mortality much higher in menstruating women (Ann IM 1992;117:891)

Epidem: Females > males; seen in marathon-running women from free water replacement of sweat loss (Ann IM 2000;132:711)

Pathophys: Cerebral edema causes CNS sx

Sx: Confusion, HA, N+V, muscle cramps

Si: Seizures/confusion, depressed reflexes

Crs:

Cmplc: r/o adrenal insufficiency, hypothyroidism

Labs: *Chem:* Na < 125 mEq/L; uric acid < 5 mg % with ADH-producing tumor or SIADH (Nejm 1979;301:528)

Rx: Acute: Stop drugs; give saline and furosemide (Lasix); if developed slowly, correct at < 2.5 mEq/hr, not > 10 mEq/day (Ann IM 1997;126:57) with iso- or perhaps hypertonic (3% NaCl, thus 3× normal) saline, and possibly iv furosemide, then go slowly to avoid pontine demyelination (Ann IM 1997;126:57); or go slowly over days, no benefit from rushing or using twice normal saline even when Na < 110 mEq/L (Ann IM 1987;107:656) unless symptomatic or is very acute. Dialysis (hypertonic, intraperitoneal).

Estimate effect of change in serum

$$\text{Na by 1 L fluid} = \frac{(\text{Infusate Na} + \text{infusate K}) - \text{serum Na}}{\text{Total body water (p 1010)} + 1}$$

Chronic (Na < 130 mEq/L > 2d):
if neurologic si: Avoid hypoxia, then iv saline or hypertonic saline as above to improve outcome (Jama 1999;281:2342)

if no neurologic si:
> 1st: Restrict water and, if SIADH, give liberal salt diet or
> salt tablets
> 2nd: Salt tablets + loop diuretic
> 3rd: Demeclocycline (Declomycin, a tetracycline) 0.6-1.2
> gm/d (Nejm 1978;298:173)
> 4th: Lithium 300 mg po t-qid

Hypernatremia/Hyperosmolar States

Nejm 2000;342:1493

Cause:
- Central diabetes insipidus (p 1019)
- Nephrogenic DI (p 1019), including drug induced by lithium, demeclocycline (Declomycin), foscarnet
- Dehydration from:
  Inability to drink
  Betadine rx of burns
  Diminished urine concentration and diminished thirst in elderly (Nejm 1984;311:753) especially when have adult-onset diabetes and leads to nonketotic hyperosmolar coma (Nejm 1977;297:1452)

Epidem: Most common in infants and debilitated elderly pts

Pathophys:

Sx: Confusion

Si: Confusion, stupor, coma; hypotension, dehydration

Crs:

Cmplc: Mortality > 40% in elderly pts (Ann IM 1987;107:309); seizures

Lab: *Chem:* Na > 150 mEq/L or > 300 mOsm/L, measured or calculated (p 1012)

Rx: Acutely replace water, but not > 12 mEq/24 hr (brain swelling), w D_5W, ¼ normal saline (0.225%), or ½ normal saline

(0.45%); water deficit calculation (p 1010), or estimate effect of change in serum

$$\text{Na by 1 L fluid} = \frac{(\text{Infusate Na} + \text{infusate K}) - \text{serum Na}}{\text{Total body water (p 1010)} + 1}$$

Chronically rx w thiazides and/or carbamazepine, which increase renal sensitivity; or vasopressin nasal or im (p 1020)

Diabetes Insipidus (Central and Nephrogenic)

Cause: Central: Idiopathic (30%); pituitary tumor (Nejm 2000; 343:998), sarcoid or eosinophilic granuloma; any CNS insult, eg, tumor, trauma, surgery; alcohol ingestion, transient, aggravates all other causes
Nephrogenic:
- Genetic: The "*Hopewell* hypothesis," the ship on which two Scots came to U.S. and spread via sex-linked recessive gene (Nejm 1988;318:881); but now know at least 2 different genes involved and may not be true (Nejm 1993;328:1534)
- Drug induced: Lithium (occurs in 20-70% who take Li); demethyltetracycline
- Transient in pregnancy due to increased vasopressinase (Nejm 1987;316:1070)
- Renal tubular damage from hypercalcemia, hypokalemia, chronic pyelonephritis, chronic partial obstruction, sickle cell anemia, aging, lead poisoning, renal tubular acidosis

Epidem: Pregnancy may unmask (Nejm 1991;324:522)

Pathophys: Vasopressin (ADH) deficiency or resistance; normally it dilates splanchnic arterioles, increases renin, and stimulates factor VIII clotting factors; in kidney, causes water resorption (Nejm 1988;318:881). Idiopathic central DI associated w lymphocytic infiltration of neurohypophyseal area and probably immune in etiology (Nejm 1993;329:683).

Sx: Excessive thirst and urination

Si: Hypovolemia

Crs:

Cmplc: Mental retardation due to infantile dehydration
              r/o **Psychogenic water drinker** who can partially concen-
       trate urine with fluid restriction (Nejm 1981;305:1539)

Lab: *Chem:* Na > 145 mEq/L, at least when limit water po. Serum va-
              sopressin decreased a little in psychogenic water drinker,
              markedly in central DI; elevated significantly in nephro-
              genic DI. 24-hr urinary ADH in U/hr is decreased in central
              DI, and elevated in nephrogenic DI. Uric acid elevated.
       Urine: Specific gravity < 1.019. If complaining of increased thirst
              but serum Na normal, then water-restrict and thereby dehy-
              drate until q 1 hr urine specific gravities plateau; then com-
              pare this specific gravity with that after ADH (vasopressin)
              injection; or water-restrict to hypernatremia, getting coinci-
              dent urine and serum osmoles. True DI pt will not get urine
              osmoles much > 300, unlike psychogenic water drinker who
              can get urine osmoles ≥ 600.

Xray: IVP shows dilated collecting system in genetic nephrogenic DI
              MRI of pituitary in central type

Rx: Acutely replace water deficit (p 1010) at less than 12 mEq
       Na increase/24 hr
              Of central type: Desmopressin (vasopressin analog) 5-20
       μgm nasal, sq, or iv q 4-20 hr for complete type (Ann IM
       1985;103:229). Desmopressin is resistant to vasopressinase (Nejm
       1987;316:1070). For incomplete type, treat the same or treat like
       nephrogenic.
              Of nephrogenic type: Thiazides, carbamazepine (Nejm
       1974;291:1234), or chlorpropamide (Nejm 1970;282:1266);
       amiloride 5-10 mg bid helps at least lithium type (Nejm
       1985;312:408)

17.9 Acquired Renal Diseases

Renal Stones

Nejm 2004;350:684 (acute), 1992;327:1141

Cause: Calcium oxalate (75%), from hyperparathyroidism (10+%) but probably mostly (> 50%) idiopathic (rarely sarcoid) hypercalciuria, which is genetic in most cases with autosomal dominant inheritance; struvite (10-15%), from UTIs w urease-producing organisms; urate (5%); hydroxyapatite or brushite (5%), cystine (1%)

Epidem: Incidence = 100/100,000 men, 36/100,000 women; 3-5% of U.S. population will get sometime in life; incidence higher in southeastern U.S.

Pathophys: 80% of stones are calcium type, associated with a red blood cell and probable renal tubular oxalate excretion defect (Nejm 1986;314:599) or a deficit of the Ca/Mg pump (Nejm 1988;319:897); another 10% are associated with hyperparathyroidism

Increased calcium absorption may also play a role, either primary or by bringing out deficits like those above, eg, in sarcoid (Nejm 1984;311:116). Uric acid stones may also precipitate calcium on themselves.

Calcium oxalate stones are increased in colectomy, blind loop syndrome, and intestinal bypass pts due to bacterial breakdown of bile salts leading to absorption of glycolytic acid (Ann IM 1978;89:594)

Struvite stones are caused by ammonia from urea-splitting proteus in pts with chronic UTIs due to indwelling Foley catheters and/or quadraplegia

Sx: Pain radiating into groin; hematuria gross and/or microscopic

Si:

Crs: Acutely, $^2/_3$ pass within 4 wk; if not passed by 8 wk, unlikely to do so later. Recurrence after first stone is 15% at 1 yr, 35% at 5 yr, 50% at 10 yr (Ann IM 1989;111:1006).

Cmplc: Pyelonephritis behind the obstruction. Cmplc rate increases to 20% after 4 wk of impaction.

r/o renal artery embolism pain (Ann IM 1978;89:477) and rare primary hyperoxaluria w oxalosis as renal failure develops (Nejm 1994;331:1553)

Lab: *Chem:* Serum calcium and uric acid w 1st stone

For recurrent stone, 24-hr urine for creatinine clearance, Na, calcium, urate, citrate, oxalate; or spot urine ratios

24-hr urine calcium $\geq$ 300 mg in men, $\geq$ 250 mg in women

Calcium/creatinine ratio $\geq$ 0.2 mg Ca/1 mg creatinine

Uric acid > 1 gm/24 hr; or

$$\frac{\text{urine urate} \times \text{serum creat}}{\text{urine creat}} > 0.7$$

24-hr urine oxalate > 40 mg (Nejm 1993;328:880)

Path: Stone analysis in all

Urine: Rbc's (90%), crystals (pictures: Nejm 1992;327:1142)

Xray: Spiral CT w/o contrast (96% sens, 100% specif); or IVP (87% sens, 94% specif); or ultrasound (15% sens, 90% specif), especially in pregnancy

Plain film/KUB to see if stone is radio-opaque (80%) so can follow its course

Rx: Dietary (Nejm 2002;346:77): Drink 2+ L of fluid qd, especially coffee and wine but not grapefruit juice! (Ann IM 1998; 128:534); reduce salt and protein intake; avoid calcium supplements but further decrease in dietary calcium intake is not beneficial because calcium decreases oxalate and urate absorption (Ann IM 1997;126:497; Nejm 1993;328:833,880); avoid phosphoric acid–containing soft drinks (J Clin Epidem 1992;45:911)

Thiazides help renal tubular/absorptive type, eg, hydrochlorthiazide 50 mg qd, or amiloride 5 mg po qd (Nejm 1986;314:599, 1984;311:116)

Allopurinol 300 mg po qd decreases calcium oxalate stone recurrence if there is an increased 24-hr urine rate (Nejm 1986; 315:1386)

Polycitra K 20 mEq po b-tid, Na bicarb, or citrate in lemon juice as lemonade to alkalinize urine to pH > 6.5 and thereby dissolve urate

Na cellulose PO_4 5 gm po qd-tid to get 24-hr urine calcium < 300 mg (Med Let 1983;25:67); blocks gi calcium uptake

Pyridoxine 2 gm po qd for oxalate stones? (Nejm 1985; 312:953)

Cholestyramine po for secondary oxalic aciduria (Nejm 1972;286:1371)

Surgical percutaneous dissolution of renal pelvis stones over 1-3 wk (Nejm 1979;300:341); basketing via cystoscope; or surgical excision. Extracorporeal shock wave lithotripsy, $2 million machine, requires anesthesia (Ann IM 1985;103:626) but very effective especially for calcium oxalate stones.

of acute stone: NSAIDs (ketorolac iv or diclofenac po) better than narcotics (BMJ 2004;328:1401); narcotics; possibly desmopressin; and moderate iv fluids, but decreased urine flow relieves pain

Chronic Kidney Disease

Cause: Multiple, especially diabetes and hypertension (Nejm 1996;334:13); nephrosclerosis; silent lead intoxication (Nejm 2003;348:277); chronic Tylenol and/or ASA use (Nejm 2001;345:1801)

Pathophys:
- Acidosis from decreased renal ability to secrete hydrogen ion
- Ca/P imbalances (Nejm 1987;316:1573, 1601) from uremic suppression of vitamin D effect and decreased renal conversion

to active forms, decreased degradation of PTH; decreased phosphate clearance leads to CaP precipitation in vessels, skin, kidneys, heart, and further hypoCa; all these lead to osteomalacia or secondary hyperparathyroidism.

- Potassium high or low depending on intake alone, since distal tubular excretion by remaining nephrons is already maximal
- Anemia, mostly from decreased erythropoietin, bleeding from impaired clotting and dialysis losses
- BP changes: Hypertension from Na overload, increased sympathetic tone and/or increased renin (Nem 1992;327:1912); hypotension due to end-organ resistance to ADH and aldosterone
- Neuropathies, peripheral and autonomic, from demyelination
- Delayed hypersensitivity immune suppression
- Pruritus probably caused by histamines (Nejm 1992;326:969)

Sx: Lassitude, pruritus, nausea/vomiting, anorexia, muscle cramps, sleep disturbance

Si: Distinctive breath (Nejm 1977;297:132), increased pigmentation, anemia, absent tendon reflexes and other peripheral neuropathies

Cmplc: Fractures and osteomalacia, acidosis, metastatic calcifications, infections especially viral pericarditis (Nejm 1969;281:542), renally excreted drug toxicities; sleep apnea, helped by nocturnal hemodialysis (Nejm 2001;344:102)

Lab: Disease level staged by GFR (Ann IM 2003;139:137):
Stage 1 = GFR > 90 cc/min/1.73 M^2
Stage 2 = GFR 60-89 cc/min/1.73 M^2
Stage 3 = GFR 30-59 cc/min/1.73 M^2
Stage 4 = GFR 15-29 cc/min/1.73 M^2
Stage 5 = GFR <15 cc/min/1.73 M^2

Rx: of anemia: Recombinant erythropoietin iv tiw (Ann IM 1991; 114:402) or sc (Nejm 1998;339:578) to maintain hct at

30-35%, higher not necessary even if heart disease (Nejm 1998;339:584); adequate iron replacement and dialysis facilitate erythropoietin response

of bleeding (Nejm 1998;339:245): Desmopressin sc or nasally (p 473), erythropoietin

of edema: Furosemide up to 500 mg any route; 0.5-2 gm can be used but risk of transient or permanent nerve damage, especially auditory; or bumetanide 2-6 mg bolus q 12 hr; or either, in similar doses as continuous infusions, eg, bumetanide 1 mg/hr safer and as effective (Nejm 1991;115:360)

of hyperkalemia (p 1012)

of malnutrition/fatigue: Androgens like nandrolone 100 mg im q 1 wk (Jama 1999;281:1275)

of pruritus: Antihistamines; erythropoietin rx helps (80%) (Nejm 1992;326:969); ultraviolet tan (Ann IM 1979;91:17); iv lidocaine (Nejm 1977;296:261); activated charcoal (Ann IM 1980;93:446); parathyroidectomy

of HT: ACEIs preferable; keep systolic BP < 110-130 mm Hg to slow worsening renal function and proteinuria (Ann IM 2003;139:244,296)

of calcium/phosphate abnormalities (Nejm 1995;333:166): Parathyroidectomy now rarely needed; $CaCO_3$ (Tums) binds PO_4 and improves Ca × P product better than AlOH binders (Nejm 1991;324:527), which increase aluminum levels leading to anemia, dementia, and bone changes (Nejm 1997;336:1557); rx Al toxicity with deferoxamine (Nejm 1984;311:140; Ann IM 1984;101:775); low-phosphate diets plus $CaCO_3$ or Ca acetate po given with meals to minimize absorption of dietary PO_4 (Nejm 1989;320:1110); vitamin D as calcitriol 0.25 μgm po qd, or injectable, or paricalcitol (Nejm 2003;349:446), if Ca < 10.5 and PTH high to prevent secondary hyperparathyroidism; calcimimetics like cinacalcet 30-180 mg po qd to decrease PTH (Nejm 2004;350:1516)

of azotemia:

- Diet: Protein restriction to < 0.4-0.6 gm/kg/day (BMJ 1992; 304:214; Nejm 1989;321:1773), but is controversial because malnutrition predicts poor prognosis, and phosphate restriction to 1 gm qd (Nejm 1991;324:78); along w tight lipid and BP control to slow renal failure progression (Nejm 1994;330:877)

- ACE inhibitors slow progression (Ann IM 2002;136:604; Nejm 1996;334:939), esp if used early when creatinine clearance = 40-60 cc/min and if proteinuria present; even in polycystic disease; unrelated to decrease in BP; use of receptor antagonists enhance effect

- Dialysis (Nejm 1998;338:1428):
  Peritoneal
  Hemo: Survival not as good as cadaveric transplant (Nejm 1999;341:1725) and dialysis significantly worsens renal transplant survival (Nejm 2001;344:726); adverse effects: folate deficiency, EKG artifacts with fistula/cannula arm (Nejm 1978;298:1439); mortality = 10-20%/yr; Zn deficiency causes primary gonadal impairment, reversible with 25 mg po qd (Ann IM 1982;97:357); amyloidosis; Fe deficiency; increased ASHD prevalence; gynecomastia; hepatitis B rarely now w immunization available but still chronic hepatitis C common

- Transplantation graft survival 90+% at 1 yr and 80+% at 5 yr and rapidly improving (Nejm 2002;346:580, 2000;342:605): HLA-type matched or mismatched from living or cadaver donors, 50% 10-yr survival (Nejm 2000;343:1078). Immunosuppression with cyclosporine then prednisone + azathioprine (Nejm 1988;318:1499) or mycophenolate (CellCept) in 1st yr; adverse effects: increased tumors (decreased surveillance), esp squamous cell and basal cell carcinomas of skin (Nejm 2003;348:1681, 1995;332:1052), increased ASHD (Ann IM 1979;91:554), CMV infections prevented w valacyclovir (Nejm 1999;340:1463) or ganciclovir

Acute Tubular Necrosis

Ann IM 2002;137:744; Nejm 1996;334:1448

Cause: Often multiple
- Shock, simple or that associated w muscle breakdown/myoglo-binuria, eg, traumatic crush injury (Nejm 1991;324:1417), exercise, or hypothermia; open heart surgery ($^1/_5$ get some, 3% get full ATN, correlates with pump time: Ann IM 1976;84:677), abdominal aneurysm repair with aortic cross-clamping, etc (Ann IM 1976;85:23)
- Nephrotoxins including heavy metals, CCl_4 and other organic solvents, drugs (eg, gentamicin, amphotericin), snake venom
- Intravascular hemolysis
- IVP or CT contrast material, especially in elderly pts whose creatinine > 2 mg % (Nejm 1989;320:143) or pts w multiple myeloma

Epidem:

Pathophys: GFR decreases before tubular function decreases; fortunate, otherwise would dehydrate quickly. Tubular necrosis → interstitial edema → more oliguria due to increased extra tubular pressure.

Sx:

Si: Oliguria usually, although nonoliguric form very common now with rapid fluid rx

Crs: Recovery in 10-30 d if maintain with dialysis; 30-40% will be left with diminished GFR or concentrating ability

Cmplc: (p 1023); CHF
r/o other causes of acute oliguria (Nejm 1998;338:671) like obstructive disease; other intrinsic renal diseases like acute GN and interstitial nephritis, especially drug (NSAID)-induced type; and prenatal causes including hypovolemia and low cardiac output syndromes

Lab: *Path:* Gross shows swollen kidney; congested medullary pyramids with pale cortex; microscopic shows tubular necrosis, especially proximally with poisons; interstitial edema; regenerating tubules by day 3

Urine: Smell absent, unlike prerenal azotemia (Nejm 1980;303:1125)

Urine osmoles < 350-400, in contrast to prerenal azotemia where > 500; osmole/plasma osmole ratio < 1.7; Na > 40 mEq/L, unlike < 20 in prerenal azotemia; urea nitrogen < 3× plasma, unlike > 8 in prerenal azotemia; creatinine < 20× plasma, unlike > 40 in prerenal azotemia; volume < 400 cc/24 hr, 50% false neg but that's more benign type anyway

UA sediment shows tubular casts

Rx: Avoid diuretics, which can worsen prognosis and don't help (Jama 2002;288:2547)

Supportive with protein limitation to < 30 gm/day; water to 400 cc plus urine output + insensibles; watch K^+ by avoiding old blood if transfuse, and treat elevations with Na polystyrene (Kayexalate); peritoneal or hemodialysis, especially if muscle breakdown, peritoneal less good than hemo at least if ATN caused by infection (Nejm 2002;347:895,933)

In myoglobinuria from rhabdomyolysis after crush injury (Nejm 1991;324:1417), rx w iv fluids + mannitol to keep output > 100 cc/hr + alkalinize urine w iv $NaHCO_3$; or w iv fluids + furosemide

When radiocontrast used in pt w creatinine > 1.2 or creatinine clearance < 50 cc/min:
- d/c NSAIDs × 3-4 d, hold metformin × 2 d, stop diuretics
- 1 L normal (154 mEq/L) $NaHCO_3$ at 200 cc/hr × 1 before procedure and 70 cc/hr to follow (Jama 2004;291:2328, 2376) decreases incidence to < 2%, best choice; or

- NS combined w acetylcysteine 600 mg (3 cc of 20% soln) taken w soft drink po bid day before and day of, decreases incidence to < 2-4% (J Am Coll Cardiol 2003;41:2114; Jama 2003;289:553; Nejm 2000;343:180,210); or 150 mg/kg in 500 NS over 30 min just before procedure; or
- NS at 1 cc/kg/hr × 12 hr just before and after angiography (Arch IM 2002;162:329); or
- Peri-procedure hemofiltraton (Nejm 2003;349:1333)
    Prophylactic dopamine infusion no help (Jama 2003;290:2284); mannitol and furosemide of equally doubtful help (Nejm 1994;331:1416). Anaritide (atrial natiuretic peptide) iv acutely may help oliguric form but worsens dialysis-free survival in anuric cases (Nejm 1997;336:828).

Nephrotic Syndrome

Nejm 1998;339:894, 1998;338:1202, 1994;330:61

Cause:

Primary types:
- Membranous GN (p 1033); the cause in 7% of children with nephrotic syndrome, and in 40% of adults
- Minimal change GN (p 1034); the cause in 76% of children and 20% of adults
- Chronic proliferative GN (40%); the cause in 4% of children and 7% of adults
- Focal, segmental GN; the cause in 8% of children and 15% of adults
- Other cause in 5% of children and in 18% of adults
    Secondary types:
- SLE and other collagen vascular diseases
- Amyloid (especially in rheumatoid arthritis; multiple myeloma; familial Mediterranean fever; chronic infections like SBE, hepatitis B, and HIV)
- Bee bites and snake venom

- Diabetic Kimmelstiel-Wilson disease
- Heavy-metal drug rx, eg, gold
- Chronic iv heroin use (Nejm 1974;290:19; Ann IM 1974;80:488)
- Cancer, eg, lung, probably by paraneoplastic antibody–antigen complexes (Nejm 1993;328:1621), colon, prostate, breast

Epidem:

Pathophys: Protein losses in urine lead to all si and sx and lab abnormalities. Caused by 2 types of pathologic processes: generalized uniform basement membrane thickening or damage as seen in membranous GN, and minimal lesion types caused by an elutable small protein deposited on the glomeruli (Nejm 1994;330:7); and spotty deposition of immune complexes as seen in poststreptococcal nephritis, SBE, SLE, and serum sickness

Elevated lipids; LDL is increased by slowed metabolism and an increase in apoprotein B production (Nejm 1990;323:579)

Sx: Edema, periorbital in the morning and pedal in the afternoon

Si: Edema, anasarca

Crs:

Cmplc: Infections, if IgG loss; acquired factor IX deficiency (Ann IM 1970;73:373); renal vein thrombosis (Ann IM 1976;85:310); hypercoagulable states in 50% lead to pulmonary emboli, etc; malabsorption of food and meds due to bowel wall edema; accelerated ASHD

r/o myeloma and primary renal (AL) amyloidosis w urinary immunoelectrophoresis

Lab: *Chem:* LDL cholesterol is increased (Ann IM 1993;119:263); hypoalbuminemia

Path: Renal bx usually shows etiology; foot process fusion by electron microscopy in minimal lesion GN; "wire loops" by light microscopy in membranous GN; increased mesangial cells without polys in proliferative GN

Serol: Serum protein electrophoresis (SPEP) shows decreased IgG in membranous GN type ("big holes" let IgG leak out); decreased complement; increased α_2- and β-lipoprotein

Urine: 24-hr protein > 3-3.5 gm; "oval fat bodies" (fat-laden tubular cells in sediment). Protein/creatinine ratio on random urine as good or better than 24-hr urine; < 0.2 is normal, $\geq$ 3.5 is nephrotic.

Rx: Diuretics and severe Na restriction
Captopril and other ACE inhibitors improve lipids (Ann IM 1993;118:246) and lower protein excretion
Antihyperlipidemia rx
Anticoagulation w warfarin or at least ASA
Specific rx to etiologic diagnosis

Acute Proliferative Glomerulonephritis

Nejm 1998;339:891

Cause:

- Idiopathic
- Circulating immune complexes
- Poststreptococcal (Ann IM 1979;91:76), types 4, 12, 57, and Redlake (Nejm 1970;283:832) from skin lesions or throat; these types never cause acute rheumatic fever (Nejm 1970;283:561)
- Postviral, including coxsackie B, echo, influenza A and B, and adenovirus pharyngitis infections cause 4% (Ann IM 1979;91:697)

Epidem: In adults, < 50% are poststreptococcal; more commonly due to skin infections when does occur. In children, > 95% are post-strep, often in epidemics. Males > females among children.

Pathophys: Circulating ag/ab complexes deposited in "lumpy" way in basement membrane

Sx: History of strep infection 10-14 d before; abrupt onset; malaise; headache; facial edema; flank pain; cloudy urine

Si: Hypertension, periorbital facial edema, hematuria, oliguria

Crs: Correlates with anuria and bx; best when strep cause; better with younger age; once healed, no later deterioration (Nejm 1982; 307:725); microhematuria can persist for up to 1 yr afterward

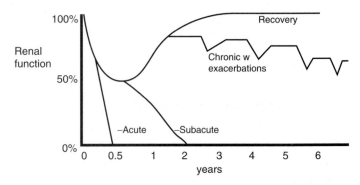

Figure 17.2 Course of AGN. Acute = 2% children; subacute = 4% children; chronic with exacerbations = 4% children, 40% adults; recovery = 90% children, 50% adults. (Nejm 1978;298:767; Ann IM 1974;80:342)

Cmplc: Hypertensive crisis; can recur in renal transplants (Nejm 2002;347:103)

r/o SBE, hypersensitivity angitis, polyarteritis nodosa, Goodpasture's, SLE, anaphylactoid purpura

Lab:

Chem: Elevated creatinine and BUN; proteins normal

Hem: ESR elevated

Path: Renal bx shows grossly swollen, "flea-bitten" kidneys; microscopically, focal or diffuse (SLE) glomerular involvement, diagnostic infiltration by polys, and lumpy deposition of immune complexes; rapidly progressive GN in anti-BM antibody (Goodpasture's) or small-vessel vasculitis (p 1142) etiology has diagnostic crescent formation, and linear immunofluorescent antibody deposition in antibasement membrane type

Serol: ASO titer > 400 Todd U is diagnostic of strep, > 125 U is suggestive; $C_3 < 100$ mg % via alternate pathway and in contrast to normal CH_{50} and C_4 (Nejm 1992;327:1366)

Urine: Hematuria with rbc casts; r/o collagen vascular disease, SBE, vasculitis, severe HT, ATN, vascular occlusion, trauma, hereditary nephritis; **Goodpasture's syndrome** w antibasement membrane type IV collagen antibodies (Nejm 2003;348:2543) and hemoptysis, rx'd w plasma exchange, Cytoxan and steroids (Ann IM 2001;134:1033)

Proteinuria > 30 mg but < 6 gm/24 hr; resolution doesn't guarantee no permanent damage

Creatinine clearance low

Rx: Penicillin $\times$ 2 wk acutely, no value as prophylaxis; supportive of renal failure

Membranous Glomerulonephritis

Cause: Idiopathic, hepatitis B (Nejm 1991;324:1457; Ann IM 1989;111:479), captopril use, NSAID use (Jama 1996;276:466), malignancy (Am J Kidn Dis 1993;22:5)

Epidem: Primarily in adults

Pathophys: Increased BM thickness in glomerular tuft by electron and light microscopy

Sx: Few, feel well, insidious onset

Si: Of nephrotic syndrome (p 1029)

Crs: 80% 5-yr survival

Cmplc: Nephrotic syndrome; renal failure

Lab: *Path:* Renal bx shows increased BM thickness on light microscopy, especially with PAS stain, and on electron microscopy

Urine: Hematuria (40%)

Rx: No rx beyond diuretics, lipid lowering, and antihypertensives justified; no renal failure in 88% after 5 yr, 73% after 8 yr, and 65% recover in 5 yr (Nejm 1993;329:85)

Steroids and cytotoxic drug roles controversial, usually reserved for pts w 24-hr urine protein > 10 gm, and/or elevated but not progressive creatinine elevations; methylprednisolone, or alternate with chlorambucil q 1 mo × 6 mo (Nejm 1992;327:599); or cyclophosphamide + prednisone × 1 yr (Ann IM 1991;114:725); or prednisone alone as good (Ann IM 1992;116:438)

In hepatitis B glomerulonephritis, α-interferon (very expensive) for 4 mo (Ann IM 1989;111:479) although recurrence when off rx and side effects substantial

Minimal Change ("Lipoid") Nephritis

Cause: Unknown

Epidem: Children, rare in adults

Pathophys: Increased podocyte processes and fusion (Ann IM 1968;69:1171)

Sx:

Si: Of nephrotic syndrome

Crs: Most resolve completely in both adults (Ann IM 1974;81:314) and children

Cmplc:

Lab: *Path:* Renal bx shows no abnormalities on light microscope; on electron microscopy, increased number and fusion of foot processes

Urine: Proteinuria enough to diagnose nephrosis (ie, > 3.5 gm)

Rx: Prednisone 60 mg/m^2/d, taper over 2+ mo

Cyclosporine if steroids alone inadequate or relapses occur

Chronic Glomerulonephritis

Nejm 1998;339:895

Cause: Sequel of membranous and proliferative glomerulonephritis (GN) and idiopathic

Epidem: 50% probably membranous GN, 20% probably proliferative GN, 30% unknown etiology including IgA nephropathy, 10% of all end-stage renal disease, higher in older men

Pathophys: Gradual progression of initiating disease leads to glomerular hyalinization with secondary tubular atrophy, and interstitial fibrosis leads to renal failure

IgA deposits are presumed immune complexes

Sx: Nephrotic syndrome (p 1029)

Si: Of nephrosis, HT

Crs: Slowly decreasing renal function over many years, usually > 20 yr

Cmplc: Of renal failure (p 1023)

Lab: *Chem:* BUN and creatinine elevated
Path: Renal bx shows scarring, focally or diffuse
Urine: Proteinuria

Rx: Supportive (p 1023), including aggressive ACE inhibitor rx of HT

of IgA nephropathy: Fish oil 12 gm qd may slow progression by preventing damage by mediators like protaglandins, etc

IgA Nephropathy

Nejm 2002;347:738, 1998;339:890, 1994;331:1194

Cause: Altered regulation of production or structure of IgA

Epidem: High prevalence in western Pacific Rim, low in U.S. and Europe; males > females, esp under age 25; most common form of GN worldwide, most common cause of asx hematuria

Pathophys: IgA immune complexes deposited in glomeruli, diffuse mesangial deposits; Henoch-Schönlein purpura similar morphologically, maybe etiologically

Sx: Goss hematuria, esp associated w URI or gastroenteritis

Si: Hematuria (60%), asx (30%); AGN, or nephrotic syndrome (10%)

Crs: 20-40% progress to chronic renal failure

Cmplc:

Lab: *Serol:* Elevated IgA levels
Urinanalysis: Hematuria, proteinuria

Rx: Fish oil; ACE inhibitors; steroids

17.10 Inherited Renal Diseases

Polycystic Kidney Disease

Nejm 2004;350:151, 1993;329:332

Cause: Genetic, autosomal dominant; at least 2 different gene sites (Nejm 1988;319:913), most commonly (90%) on chromosome 6; rare (1/20,000) autosomal recessive type

Epidem: Most diagnosed in early adulthood, although infantile type does occur and presents as large kidneys at birth, die within months. Peak onset at age 45; 100% get by age 90; female/male ratio equal; prevalence = 1/400-1000.

Pathophys: Tubular cysts increase in size by secretion of solutes and compromise renal function (Nejm 1969;281:985), thereby increasing renin-aldosterone systems, which cause hypertension (Nejm 1990;323:1091); also occur in liver

Sx: Flank/back pain (61%); positive family hx (60%); dysuria (8%); gross hematuria (12%); nocturia (8%); headache (20%); nausea (5%)

Si: Hypertension (62%); palpable kidney (52%); palpable liver (27%); abdominal tenderness (20%); peripheral edema (10%); systolic murmur (10%)

Crs: 5-10 yr after BUN starts to increase

Cmplc: Hepatic cysts (40%), increasing incidence with age; also in pancreas and spleen; berry aneurysm (4%), screen pts w family h/o aneurysm w CT or MRI and operate if > 10 mm (Nejm 1992;327:916,953); aortic and mitral valve dilatations (Nejm 1988;319:907); Na wasting, occasionally renal tubular acidosis r/o other renal cystic disease (Ann IM 1978;88:176):

- Multicystic renal disease, which consists of benign, common retention cysts
- Multicystic dysplasia: Compatible with life if unilateral, most not hereditary, associated with urethral atresia, rarely autosomal dominant and associated w deafness and hypoparathyroidism (Nejm 1992;327:1069)
- Medullary cystic disease (Nejm 2004;350:151) with anemia, severe Na wasting, renal failure, and death in teens; autosomal dominant
- Medullary sponge kidney with tubular ectasia, benign except for stones and pyelo, worst in women (Nejm 1982;306:1088), small stones in cysts (r/o nephrocalcinosis and tbc), associated with Ehlers-Danlos syndrome, also with autosomal recessive renal–retinal dysplasia with retinitis pigmentosa (Ann IM 1976;84:157)
- Hypokalemia-induced medullary cysts, reversible (Nejm 1990;322:345)

Lab: *Chem:* BUN and creatinine increase late in course
Path: Dilated nephrons and tubules lead to cysts
Urine: Am specific gravity < 1.015; proteinuria, pyuria

Xray: IVP shows large cystic kidneys
Ultrasound is most sensitive test, and can look for hepatic cysts, too (40%); most abnormal by age 20 in carriers

Rx: of renal failure
Tight BP control may retard progression, ACE inhibitors can be used cautiously but precipitate acute renal failure (Ann IM

1991;115:769); avoid catheterization at all costs since can lead to rapidly fatal infection; avoid hypokalemia, which can increase cyst growth rate

Occasionally need surgical relief of pressure from bloody cystic compression of adjacent structures

Renal Tubular Acidosis

Cause: Types I (classic) and II; both types may be genetic, autosomal dominant, or induced in a renal transplant (Ann IM 1973;79: 352; 1969;71:39); type IV is the most common

of type I: Amphotericin B, dose related (Nejm 1968;278:124); hyper-IgG states, especially with collagen vascular diseases; hepatic cirrhosis (Nejm 1969;280:1); toluene glue sniffing (Ann IM 1981;94:758); nephrocalcinosis

of type II: Sulfonamides; old tetracycline; carbonic anhydrase inhibitors; Fanconi syndromes (p 1039)

of type IV: Diabetes via hyporeninemia/hypoaldosteronism

Epidem:

Pathophys: Type I is caused by distal tubular damage, which leads to an inability to acidify urine, which then leads to general cation loss, hyperchloremic acidosis, calcium loss, and renal stone formation. "Complete" syndrome is continuous acidosis no matter what the po intake is; "incomplete" syndrome requires an acid load to bring out.

Type II is caused by a proximal tubular defect in bicarbonate resorption so that there is a lowered serum threshold for bicarbonate loss in the urine (T_{max}) but no problem otherwise, even with an acid load

Hyperchloremia maintains ionic balance of blood. In most other acidotic states, another anion such as lactate, acetate, or formate takes the place of depleted HCO_3.

Sx: Hypokalemic weakness, hypocalcemic tetany

Si: Hyperventilation and other signs of metabolic acidosis

Crs: Genetic types have onset at school age

Cmplc: Rickets and osteomalacia; nephrolithiasis and calcinosis

Lab: *Chem:* Acidosis, hypokalemia, and hyperchloremia, but r/o other causes (Nejm 1977;297:816) of hyperchloremic metabolic acidosis with normal anion gap (p 1012), like diarrhea, NH_4Cl intake, acetazolamide (Diamox), or other carbonic anhydrase inhibitors, and obstructive uropathy (Nejm 1981;304:373); or with a low anion gap as seen in multiple myeloma (Nejm 1977;296:858), and aldosterone deficiency
Urine: Elevated phosphates, potassium, calcium; and in type II, glucose. Urinary pH in type I always > 5 over 8 hr, even after 0.1 gm NH_4Cl/kg po; r/o Na depletion, which will prevent kidney from excreting enough H^+, ie, Na^+ distal absorption takes priority over H^+ and K^+ absorption (Nejm 1987;316:140). Urinary pH in type II < 5 in severe acidosis but > 5 when serum bicarbonate still < 20 mEq/L, eg, after the above NH_4Cl load.

Urinary anion gap (gap = Na + K − Cl) is positive, unlike negative gap seen in diarrhea (Nejm 1988;318:594)

Rx: K-gluconate or other potassium-containing replacement without chloride; or $NaHCO_3$; or Shohl's solution of citric acid and sodium citrate

Fanconi Syndrome

Causes: Primary adult Fanconi's syndrome is genetic, autosomal recessive

Secondary causes include inherited diseases such as cystinosis (p 1040), tyrinosis (onset at age 4-6 mo, associated with hepatic cirrhosis, and rapidly fatal), glycogen storage diseases, galactosemia, Lowe's syndrome (oculo-cerbro-renal syndrome), and Wilson's disease (p 362); and acquired conditions like multiple myeloma (p 503), renal damage from old tetracycline, heavy metals like lead and mercury

Epidem: Rare

Pathophys: Proximal tubular damage results in resorptive defects and subsequent loss of small molecules like bicarbonate, amino acids and low molecular weight proteins, glucose, phosphate, Mg, K, carnitine, water, calcium, and uric acid. Type II renal tubular acidosis (p 1038), vitamin D-resistant rickets and osteomalacia, and insulin-resistant hypophosphatemic diabetes (Nejm 1980;303:1259), nephrolithiasis, and calcinosis result

Sx: Polyuria

Si: Dehydration

Crs:

Cmplc: RTA, rickets and osteomalacia, diabetes, renal stones; acute and severe peripheral neuropathies (Nejm 1990;322:432)

Lab: *Chem:* Low phosphate, potassium, uric acid (r/o aspirin rx, Wilson's disease, Hartnup's and Israeli syndromes: Ann IM 1974;80:482); hyperchloremic acidosis; hypophosphatemia
   Urine: Elevated phosphate, calcium, ammonia, uric acid, potassium, glucose, amino acids, pH

Rx: Rarely in cases of toxic renal damage, with renal transplant, occasionally recurs (Nejm 1980;286:25)
   of rickets: High-dose vitamin D_3 (50,000-400,000 IU qd) and po PO_4 (Nejm 1980;303:1023)
   of RTA: Alkali or K-gluconate

Cystinosis

Nejm 2002;347:111; Ann IM 1988;109:557

Cause: Genetic, autosomal recessive on chromosome 17

Epidem: 100,000-200,000 births

Pathophys: Fanconi syndrome (see above) due to damage to proximal renal tubules
   Ocular (adult-onset) variant pts have partial gene preservation and have only eye findings, no renal involvement

Sx: Onset as early as 4-6 mo in childhood type, or in adulthood

Si: Rickets, hepatosplenomegaly, corneal opacities (cystine deposition), peripheral retinal patchy depigmentation in children only

Crs: Children die uremic death in < 10 yr; adults have a benign course

Cmplc: Increased mental retardation (Nejm 1970;283:783); myopathy (Nejm 1988;319:1461) including swallowing dysfunction (Nejm 1990;323:565); Fanconi syndrome; renal tubular acidosis

Lab: *Path:* Rectal bx shows cystine crystals (Nejm 1969;281:143)

Rx: Prevent by detection of carriers (Nejm 1982;306:1468)
Cysteamine (Cystagon) (Med Let 1994;36:116) or phosphocysteamine rx started before age 2 yr for 7+ yr prevents renal disease, then pt has a good renal prognosis (Nejm 1993;328:1157)
Renal transplant

Table 17.5 Other Renal Tubular Defects

Disease	Amino Acid/Sugar	Presenting Sx
Homocystinuria	Homocystine	(p 317)
Cystinosis (Ann IM 1988;109:557)	Cystine	Rickets, hepatosplenomegaly, corneal opacities, retinopathy, uremia, mental retardation, myopathy including swallowing dysfunction (Nejm 1990;323:565), Fanconi syndrome, RTA; rectal bx diagnostic; rx by detecting carriers and treating pts w cystamine
Cystinuria (Nejm 1992;327:1141)	Cystine (the sulfide, of cysteine), arginine, ornithine	Calcified hexagonal renal stones and renal calcinosis; false-pos urine acetone tests; rx with alkalinization of urine, and decreasing dietary methionine; salt restrict (Nejm 1986;315:1120); then D-penicillamine or tiopronin (Med Let 1989;31:7)

(continues)

Table 17.5   Continued

Disease	Amino Acid/Sugar	Presenting Sx
Hartnup's	Val, Leu, Tryp, Tyr, Ala, Ser, isoL, Glut, His, Threon, Asp	Diarrhea, dementia, dermatitis; pellagra disease and neurologic ataxia in attacks that are improved by nicotinamide po
Iminoglycinuria	Gly, Pro, Hpro	Deafness (Nejm 1968;278:1407)
Methionine	Met	Mental retardation, white hair, foul stools (malabsorption); rx w low-met diet
Joseph's syndrome	Pro, Hpro, Glyc	Convulsive infant, die young
Histadinemia	Hist	Benign (Nejm 1974;291:1214)
Pentosuria	Pentoses	Not a renal defect; systemic defect in pentose–phosphate shunt; 1/50,000 Jews (Nejm 1970;282:892)
Maple syrup urine disease	Branched-chain amino acid metabolism defect	Growth failure and psychomotor retardation; rx with dialysis and branched-chain amino acid–free diet (Nejm 1991;324:175)

17.11 Infections

Female Cystitis/Urethritis

Nejm 2003;349:259; J Am Ger Soc 1996;44:1235 (elderly)

Cause (K. Holmes: Nejm 1980;303:409): 70% due to coliforms at $>$ 10^5/cc in urine; 11%, coliforms at $<10^5$/cc in urine; 5%, *Chlamydia trachomatis*; 1%, *S. saprophyticus* (often misread as *S. epidermidis* or *albus* by labs); 4% (Jama 1999;281:736), gc; *H. simplex*

Epidem: Incidence, up to perhaps 20% of all women get each year; increased with catheters, mostly from perimeatal invasions of urethra along outside of catheter (Nejm 1980;303:316); increased with sexual activity, h/o previous episodes, and spermicides + diaphragm use (Nejm 2000;343:992, 1996;335:468); not prevented by various hygiene habits except voiding after sex (Ann IM 1987;107:816)

Pathophys: Recurrent disease, due to a possible inherent defect in epithelial cell membrane leading to easier adherence by bacteria (Nejm 1986;314:1208, 1981;304:1062)

Sx: Dysuria, frequency; stuttering onset over days with chlamydia type OTC home kits specific but quite insensitive, many false negs

Si:

Crs: Many resolve without rx and many are subclinical (asx) (Nejm 2000;343:992); catheter-induced UTIs have 2-4 times the mortality of non–catheter-induced UTIs (Nejm 1982;307:637) and only $\frac{1}{3}$ resolve after removal without rx, 90% will with single dose or 10 d rx (Ann IM 1991;114:713)

Cmplc: r/o vaginitis, herpes, and subclinical pyelo, which can be diagnosed when it relapses eventually; reflux nephropathy in children w renal US + VCUG debatably w 1st documented UTI; chronic interstitial (idiopathic) cystitis (Med Let 1997;39:56)

Lab: *Bact:* Culture of midstream urine (clean catch unnecessary: Nejm 1993;328:289), $> 10^5$ organisms in only 50% of truly infected women with sx; 10^2 is a better criterion when have sx (Ann IM 1993;119:454; Holmes: Nejm 1982;307:463)
Urine: UA shows pyuria, > 5-6 wbc/hpf (10% false neg, 50% false pos when have sx: Nejm 1982;307:463); hematuria (often not with chlamydia); dipstick nitrite tests have high false-pos rates so cultures much better (Ped Infect Dis J 1991;10:651). Sens/specif of all such tests vary greatly by pretest likelihood, eg, w < 5 wbc/hpf, sens/specif = 60%, if > 5 wbc, sens = 100%, specif =22% (Ann IM 1992; 117:135).

Xray: IVP and cystoscopy of no value to w/u recurrent UTIs in adult women (Nejm 1981;304:462)

Rx: Prevent in postmenopausal women w recurrent UTIs w estriol 0.5 mg cream (Ovestin) qd × 2 wk then biw, helps w/o significant estrogen absorption (Nejm 1993;329:753)

Prophylaxis w Tm/S ½ a single-strength (40/200) pill qd hs (Nejm 1974;291:597), or postintercourse; is cost-effective if ≥ 3 UTIs/yr (Ann IM 1981;94:250)

Antibiotics (Med Let 1999;41:98):

Regular rx of UTI: Tm/S single-strength bid, ciprofloxacin 250 mg po bid or other fluoroquinolone, or amoxicillin 250-500 mg po tid × 7-10 d, if no gonorrhea, chlamydia, or vaginitis (Nejm 1981;304:956). 20% resistance to cephalothin, sulfa, amoxicillin (Jama 1999;281:736).

3-d regimens in uncomplicated pts also reasonable (Ann IM 1989;111:906), eg, Tm/S DS bid × 3 d gives 82% cure vs 67% cure for amoxicillin 500 mg po bid × 3 d (Jama 1995;273:41); or a fluoroquinolone

Single-dose regimens: Tm/S 160/800 (DS), 1-2 pills (1st choice: Ann IM 1988;108:350), as good when take prn at home as prophylactic use (Ann IM 1985;102:302); amoxicillin 2-3 gm po; or sulfasoxazole 1-2 gm po

Bladder anesthetics: Phenazopyridine (Pyridium) 200 mg po tid × 2 d; stains urine dark orange

of asx bacteriuria: No rx indicated, although it correlates w worse prognosis, rx does not improve (Ann IM 1994;120:827)

of catheter-associated UTI: D/c catheter if can, rx if sx; can't clear UTI if catheter still in place

Acute Pyelonephritis

Ann IM 1989;111:906

Cause: Gram-negative rods (95%), most commonly *E. coli* (especially a few uropathic strains: Nejm 1985;313:414), and next most frequently, *Proteus* sp; more rarely, gram-positive cocci (5%), staph, and enterococcus. Possibly ascend from a cystitis, or come from hematogenous seeding.

Epidem: Increased incidence in pts w urinary retention; females age < 18 mo and of childbearing age; pts w gu instrumentation (Nejm 1974; 291:215); and w papillary necrosis in sickle cell disease and diabetes

Pathophys: Possible predisposition to infection of renal medulla due to increased osmotic pressures, which cause white cell inhibition, decreased blood flow, and NH_3 inhibition of complement

Sx: Fever, flank pain; frequency, urgency, dysuria, and hematuria

Si: CVA punch tenderness

Crs: Of significant bacteriuria: $^1/_3$ have sx; 80% recurrence over 2 yr with new organism, then stable; later, with marriage and pregnancy may recrudesce (Nejm 1970;282:1443)

Cmplc: Renal failure, chronic pyelo
r/o cystitis, intercourse-induced increased bacteriuria (Nejm 1978;298:321), cystitis with congenital vesicoureteric reflux by doing a voiding cystourethrogram if recurrent and/or abnormal ultrasound (Nejm 2003;348:195), acute interstitial nephritis (Ann IM 1980;93:735)

Lab: *Bact:* Urine culture $\geq 10^2$ col/cc; antibody-coated bacteria may distinguish from cystitis, but unreliable and not available (Ann IM 1989;110:138)

Gram stain of unspun urine shows ≥ 1 bacterium/oil immersion field

Xray: IVP shows dilated calyces and ureter acutely; r/o peritonitis (Nejm 1972;287:535)

Rx: Repair of vesicoureteral reflux, but may not alter course (BMJ 1983;287:171)

Antibiotics: Ciprofloxacin (Jama 2000;283:1583) × 1 wk, or gentamicin + ampicillin or Tm/S (J Infect Dis 1991;163:325) × 2 wk or until have sensitivities since 30% of *E. coli* now are resistant to amoxicillin alone

Chronic Interstitial Nephritis and Chronic Pyelonephritis

Cause (Ann IM 1975;82:453):

- Drug-induced (20%) analgesic nephropathy (Nejm 2001; 345:1801, 1998;338:446), direct toxicity with papillary necrosis, from acetaminophen (Nejm 1989;320:1238) and other NSAIDs (Nejm 1994;331:1675), especially men > 65 yr old (Ann IM 1991;115:165); often ongoing clandestine use even after dx (J Clin Epidem 1991;44:53)
- Vascular disease causing nephrosclerosis (10%)
- Hypercalcemia and hyperuricemia (11%) w or w/o stones
- Idiopathic (10%: Ann IM 1975;82:453)
- Infectious: Rarely in women with asx bacteriuria renal failure even with many recurrences (Nejm 1979;301:396); same is true in elderly although bacteriuria is a marker for other potentially fatal illness (Nejm 1986;314:1152); bacteria are usually *E. coli* and *Proteus* spp
- Diabetic or sickle cell–induced papillary necrosis
- K^+ depletion, especially due to increased aldosterone (Nejm 1990;322:345)
- Sjögren's syndrome (Ann IM 1968;69:1163)
- Hereditary nephritis
- Reflux nephropathy

Epidem:

Pathophys:

Sx: Often none until end-stage renal failure; hypertension

Si:

Crs:

Cmplc: Renal failure; bladder cancer in phenacetin type (Ann IM 1980;93:249)

r/o allergic reactions, w fever and/or rash, to penicillin (Nejm 1968;279:1245), furosemide (Nejm 1973;288:124), NSAIDs esp naproxen (Nejm 1979;301:1271), cimetidine (fever and acute sx: Ann IM 1982;96:180), methoxyflurane anesthesia (Jama 1970;223:1239); only in NSAID-induced type, proteinuria and eosinophils in urine by Hansel's stain (90%) (Wright's stain doesn't work on urine); rx w steroids if drug cessation not enough

Lab: *Urine:* UA shows low specific gravity (present in all diseases that affect tubules, including hydronephrosis and infection) pyuria and casts; never significant proteinuria

Xray: IVP shows calyceal clubbing; CT shows characteristic changes in analgesic nephropathy (Nejm 1998;338:446)

Rx: Discontinue any potential drug cause; rx associated disease; rx bacterial infection with appropriate antibiotic but no benefit in rx of asx bacteriuria in elderly males (Nejm 1983;309:1420); if sx, then Tm/S ½ tab qd (Nejm 1977;296:780), nitrofurantoin 50 mg qid or methenamine 1 gm qid with vitamin C 500 mg

Male Prostatitis/Cystitis

J Am Ger Soc 1996;44:1235 (elderly); Ann IM 1989;110:138

Cause: *E. coli* (25%); other gram-negative organisms (25^+%), including proteus and providencia; enterococci and *S. epidermidis* (20%)

Epidem: Rare unless obstruction by BPH, foreign body like catheter or stone, bladder tumors, or urethral strictures
Increased incidence in elderly men, mainly due to BPH, so that by age 65 UTI incidence is same as in women

Pathophys:

Sx: Urethritis syndrome: Dysuria, frequency, and urgency
Obstructive syndrome (with prostatic involvement): Hesitancy, nocturia, dribbling, slow stream, and inability to void; terminal dysuria to penile tip

Si: Fever, with prostatitis but not cystitis
Rectal exam shows tender swollen prostate in prostatitis

Crs:

Cmplc: Pyelonephritis, chronic prostatitis, epididymitis (see below), prostatic abscess

r/o gonorrhea, chlamydia, orchitis

Lab: No w/u of occult urinary tract lesions indicated with 1st UTI in adult men; 1st episode should be worked up in boys and male infants w renal US and VCUG to r/o urethral valves and reflux

Bact: Culture of urine, $> 10^3$ col/cc with single or predominant organism (97% sens/specif); $> 10^5$ col/cc if taken from condom catheter, reliable if clean glans, new catheter, and take urine within 2 hr of placing catheter. "4-glass" (first, mid, terminal void, and postprostatic massage specimens) cultures showing $> 10\times$ higher colony counts in last 2 compared to first 2 is diagnostic of prostatitis.

Rx: of asx bacteriuria: No rx indicated; although it worsens prognosis in elderly, rx doesn't improve prognosis (Ann IM 1994; 120:827)

of cystitis and acute prostatitis: Tm/S 160/800 bid; or if resistance suspected, ciprofloxacillin; all for 7-10 d first time, but for 6-12 wk for recurrence

of chronic prostatitis: Tm/S, ciprofloxacin especially if *Pseudomonas aeruginosa* (Nejm 1991;324:392), doxycycline, or aminoglycoside; all for 6-12 wk; still have 30-40% failure rates probably because much chronic prostatitis is abacterial and unresponsive to rx (Ann IM 2004;141:581, 2000;133:367)

Epididymitis

Cause: Under age 35-40, most are due to chlamydia, occasionally gc or ureaplasmas spread venereally; over age 35-40, most due to gram-negative bacterial infections (Nejm 1978;298:301) caused by reflux of infected urine

Epidem: Rare under age 18 yr; peak incidence at age 32

Pathophys: Inflammation localized to epididymis only, testes spared

Sx: Gradual onset, although may first notice when hit lightly and report traumatic etiology

Si: Swollen, tender epididymis with normal, nontender testicle below

Crs: May last 7-10 d with rx, longer without bed rest

Cmplc: Abscess, chronic pain, infertility
r/o orchitis, usually viral; **Testicular torsion** (usually under age 18, average age of onset is 14, often have had episodes in past, and more acute onset often w N+V; must operate within 4- 5 hr to save 70%, only 15% saved at 10 hr: Nejm 1977; 296:338)

Lab: *Bact:* Urine culture
Urine: UA to r/o infection

Rx (Med Let 1999;41:86):
Ofloxacin 300 mg po bid × 10 d; or ceftriaxone 250 mg im × 1 then doxycycline 100 mg po bid × 10 d
Bed rest, scrotal support, NSAIDs

17.12 Tumors/Cancers

Benign Prostatic Hypertrophy

Cause:

Epidem: Common, 30% prevalence by physical exam at age 40-50, 35% of all men eventually will have sx requiring meds or surgery (Prostate 1996;6[suppl]:67); 50% over age 70, although only 25% have sx

Pathophys: Usually lateral and median lobes around the urethra lead to obstructive sx by a ball-valve effect

Sx: Irritative: Frequency, urgency, nocturia, ± urge incontinence
Obstructive: Diminished stream/flow, hesitancy, postvoid dribbling, straining, incomplete emptying

Si: Enlarged prostate, median furrow filled in on rectal exam

Crs:

Cmplc: Obstructive uropathy, chronic cystitis, bladder calculi; no increased risk of prostate cancer except that incurred by age (Ann IM 1997;126:480)

Lab: *Noninv:* Bladder scan PVR if sx of incomplete emptying; peak urine flows: > 20 cc/sec = WNL, 15-20 cc/sec = mild, 10-15 cc/sec = moderate, < 10 cc/sec = severe (Nejm 1995;332:99)

Rx (Nejm 1995;332:99):

Medical: Avoid caffeine, alcohol, antihistamines, and OTC meds w ephedrine; relaxed voiding; possibly saw palmetto (*Serenoa repens* and *Sabal serrulata*) herbal rx (ACP J Club 1999;130:61; Med Let 1999;41:18; Jama 1998;280:1604), but preparation compositions vary; may inhibit testosterone production (Nejm 1998; 339:785)

1st: α-Blockers hs:

- Terazosin (Hytrin) (Nejm 1996;335:533,586), start w 1 mg, go to 5-10 mg po qd, improves flow within 2 wk; adverse effects: runny nose, impaired ejaculation, dizziness and postural hypotension (Med Let 1994;36:15); $62/mo
- Prazosin
- Doxazosin (Cardura) 2 mg qd to start, increase up to 8 mg po qd; $35/mo
- Tamsulosin (Flomax) (Med Let 1997;39:96) 0.4-0.8 mg $\frac{1}{2}$ hr pc po qd; less hypotensive effect than others; $60-120/mo
- Alfuzosin (Uroxatral) (Med Let 2003;46:1) 10 mg po qd; less hypotension than doxazosin and terazosin and less ejaculatory dysfunction than tamulosin; $56/mo

2nd:

- Finasteride (Proscar) 5 mg po qd (Nejm 2003;349: 2387,2449); prevents conversion of testosterone to dihydrotestosterone; may or may not (Nejm 1996;335:533,586) be worth a 6-mo trial if moderate or worse sx and large gland; if works, continue it since improvement continues > 4 yr; for prevention of acute retention or surgery, NNT-4 = 16 (Nejm 1998;338:612); cmplc: impotence and decreased libido in 6-8% vs half that rate in controls, better after 1 yr (men w these sx dropped out); lowers prostate Ca incidence but increases Gleason score? (Nejm 2003;349:213,215,297); $63/mo

* Dutasteride (Avodart) (Med Let 2002;44:110) 0.5 mg po qd; similar to finasteride

3rd:

* Nafarelin 400 μgm sc qd suppresses testosterone by blocking LH release; works but requires continuous use and it medically castrates

Surgical:

TURP, required in 10%, if retention and/or severe sx; cmplc = 4% incontinence, 5% impotence at 1 yr (J. Wennberg: Jama 1988;259:3010,3018,3027) but later VA study found incontinence and sexual dysfunction same in watchfully waiting pts as in operated pts and thus operation for pts w moderate sx may make sense although no harm in waiting (Nejm 1995; 332:75); and unexplained 2.5× increased death rate after TURP compared to open surgery, mostly MIs (J. Wennberg: Nejm 1989;320:1120; controversial: Nejm 1989;320:1142)

Suprapubic prostatectomy for large glands > 100 gm

TUNA (transurethral needle ablation), output procedure, less effective than TURP

Transurethral microwave thermotherapy possible (Lancet 1993;341:14; BMJ 1993;306:1293), although much less effective than TURP (Med Let 1996;38:53)

Laser prostatectomy

Simple incision

Stenting occasionally in high-risk pt

Testicular Carcinomas (Seminoma, Embryonal [Germ] Cell Carcinoma, Teratoma, Choriocarcinoma)

Nejm 1997;337:242

Cause: Neoplasia

Epidem:

Seminoma: Peak incidence age 35-45. Increased in undescended testicle even after operative repair; lifetime incidence of some malignancy is 1/80 for inguinal undescended testicles, 1/20 for abdominal testicles.

Non-seminoma types: Peak incidence age 20-40. Increased in Klinefelter's syndrome and in undescended testicles even postrepair; malignancy occurs in 1/80 inguinal, 1/20 abdominal undescended testicles over lifetime.

Pathophys:

Seminoma: Rarely highly invasive; metastasizes via lymphatics to retroperitoneal nodes and lung

Non-seminoma: Includes teratomas, embryonal cell carcinomas, and choriocarcinomas; highly malignant; hematogenous and lymphatic spread. Probably the source of a significant number of "undifferentiated" tumors found metastatic in body without primary tumor located.

Sx: Testicular mass, but not always palpable in non-seminoma types

Si: Testicular mass; gynecomastia if increased HCG or estrogen production (Nejm 1991;324:317) in non-seminoma types; reactive hydrocoel sometimes

Crs: Seminoma: Excellent prognosis even with distant metastases

Cmplc: Paraneoplastic limbic encephalopathy (p 1000)
r/o orchitis and epididimytis, which improve w 7-10 d of antibiotic rx

Lab: *Chem:* In non-seminoma types, HCG levels increased in 40%, esp chorio, embryonal cell, and seminoma; can use as way to follow success of chemoRx (Ann IM 1984;100:183); α-fetoprotein increased in embryonal, teratocarcinoma, and yolk sac types

Path: In non-seminoma types: Gross looks irregular and cystic; microscopic shows many tissue types and totally undifferentiated cells; teratomas have all 3 germ layer types; choriocarcinomas have syncytiotrophoblasts with pleomorphic nuclei

In seminoma: Gross shows lobulated, smooth tumor; microscopic shows irregular, round nuclei, clear cytoplasm, lymphocytic infiltration with granuloma formation

Xray: CT for retroperitoneal nodes; chest xray or CT for lung mets

Rx: Seminoma: Radical orchiectomy, rarely need node exploration; + radiation (very radiosensitive); 90% 5-yr survival

Non-seminoma: Radical orchiectomy, often w retroperitoneal node exploration for staging, esp if present by CT

ChemoRx w adjuvant course × 2 if positive nodes; prevents recurrence in ½ (Nejm 1987;317:1433); or curative (Ann IM 1981;94:181). Cisplatin, bleomycin, and vinblastine or etoposide (Nejm 1987;316:1435); or ifosfamide with others, after failure with 1st crs (Ann IM 1988;109:540)

Prostatic Carcinoma

Nejm 1995;333:1401, 1994;331:996, 1991;324:236; Ann IM 1996;125:118,205

Cause: Neoplasia

Epidem: 10% of all male cancer deaths; 40,000 deaths/yr in U.S., 2nd after lung; peak incidence at age 60-70. Histologic prevalence at postmortem = 10% at age 50, increasing to 70% at age 85; since lifetime chance of clinical prostatic cancer is only 6-8%, most must remain asx; histologic cancer is equally present in all races and environments, but clinical incidence very variable (Ann IM 1993;118:793), so blacks > whites > Asians; racial survival by tumor grade is equal (Jama 1995;333:1599).

If present in a 1st- and a 2nd-degree relative, risk is increased 8×; risk may also be elevated in pts w BRCA-1 gene mutation (Nejm 1997;336:1401). No increased risk in BPH (Ann IM 1997;126:480).

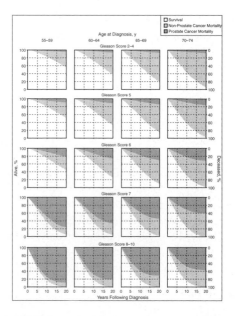

Figure 17.3 Survival (white lower band) and cumulative mortality from prostate cancer (dark-gray upper band) and other causes (light-gray middle band) up to 15 years after diagnosis, stratified by age at diagnosis and Gleason score. Percentage of men alive can be read from the lefthand scale, and percentage of men who have died from prostate cancer or from other causes during this interval can be read from the righthand scale.

Stage A_1: Well differentiated and single site, found at BPH surgery

Stage A_2: Poorly differentiated and/or multiple sites, found at BPH surgery

Stage B: Nodule without bone or epididymal invasion, or increased acid phosphatase; 80% 5-yr survival

Stage C: Extracapsular extension; acid phosphatase ok and no bone mets; 60% 5-yr survival; C_1 to seminal vesicles, C_2 fixed to pelvic wall

Stage D_0: Elevated acid phosphatase

Stage D_1: $\leq$ 3 pelvic nodes

Stage D_2: Distant bony and soft tissue mets; 15% 5-yr survival

Incidence decreased by finasteride (Proscar, ? Propecia) use (relative risk reduction = 25%, absolute risk reduction = 6%) but for some reason increases the Gleason grade of those tumors that do occur (Nejm 2003;349:215, 213,297)

Pathophys: Peripheral origin in gland (androgenic zone); slow growth, local invasion first, later metastasizes. High testosterone levels may make latent cancer clinical.

Sx: Often asx; obstructive sx (p 1049)

Si: Mass on rectal exam in prostate, very firm to rock hard, nontender (30% found this way)

Crs: Correlates with age at dx, tumor volume (Jama 1996;275:288), and Gleason grade 10 yr mortality clearly worse w watchful waiting compared to surgery, under age 65 at onset (Nejm 2005; 352:1977). After 15 yr, there is an apparent benefit to radical rx since benign tumors often eventually transform into malignant (Jama 2004;291:2713,2757 vs. not so Jama 2005;293:2095,2149).

Cmplc: Local invasion; painful mets to bone (blastic >>> clastic) often, lung, etc.

Lab: *Chem:* Acid phosphatase, prostatic fraction increased in 67% with metastatic disease; false positive with hepatic impairment (Nejm 1980;303:497,499)

Prostate-specific antigen (PSA) as screen (p 925); or to monitor disease, like CEA for bowel cancer; rectal exam may transiently elevate. Pre-op rate of rise $\geq$ 2 ng/cc/yr predicts worse prognosis after prostatectomy (Nejm 2004; 351:125,180). % free helpful in mildly increased levels (4-10).

Path: Needle biopsy. Histologic/cytologic grades (Jama 1995; 274:626); Gleason score (sum of 2 most common types scored up to 5 each: 2-4, best; 5-7 progressively worse; 8-10, worst) correlates w survival when overlaid on staging system (Nejm 1994;330:242).

Stanford alternative scoring system (Jama 1999; 281:1395): Total % tumor Gleason grade 4 or 5; if < 10%, excellent prognosis

Xray:

- Plain films for bony mets, blastic and clastic; look like Paget's
- Ultrasound transrectally as a bx directing or perhaps as a screening tool
- MRI before and after paramagnetic iron nanoparticles may be able to ID node mets very accurately (Nejm 2003;348:2491)
- Bone scan if PSA > 20, for mets

Rx: Preventive interventions (p 925)

of advanced disease and metastases, esp if Gleason grade score ≥ 5: May be worthwhile, need studies (Jama 1999;281: 1642, 1997;277:467)

of Stage A-B, localized disease (Jama 1998;280:969, 975,1008; Nejm 1994;330:242 vs opinion in Ann IM 1996; 125:118): Prognosis depends on age, Gleason score, and whether tumor was found by PSA or nodule detection on rectal. Correct strategies unclear, await RCT; watchful waiting may be enough (Jama 2000;283:3258).

Radical prostatectomy, brachytherapy (radiation implant), external beam radiation, and/or antiandrogen rx all promoted, decrease cancer recurrence but survival over 10-15 yr is not improved by aggressive rx (Nejm 2002;347:781,790,839) and cmplc of rx related to sexual, bladder, and bowel functions are significant (Jama 1995;273:129), eg, 65% impotence rate although that helped by sildenafil if nerve-sparing procedure done, 8% incontinence rate 18 mo after radical prostatectomy (Jama 2000; 283:354). Perhaps salvage radiation rx if increased PSA post-op (Jama 2004;291:1325).

of Stage C: Radiation to control sx, helps in 90%; hormonal rx as below of Stage D: Antiandrogen rx, certainly if disease progression, perhaps immediately (Med Let 2004;46:22; Nejm 1999;341:1781,1837):

Luteinizing (gonadotropin)-releasing hormone (LHRH) analogs; initially (1-2 wk) to stimulate LH, FSH, and testosterone via pituitary receptors, which are then blocked; all induce osteoporosis. All as effective as castration (Ann IM 2000;132:566); improve 5-yr survival, when given before or w radiation, from 50% to 85% in locally advanced disease (Nejm 1997;337:729); 6 mo rx enough (Jama 2004;292:821):

- Leuprolide (depot Lupron) 7.5 mg im q 1 mo, $650/mo; or as Viadur 65 mg im q 12 mo, $685/mo
- Goserelin (Zoladex) 3.6 mg sc q 1 mo (Med Let 1990;32:102); $500/mo
- Triptorelin (Telstar depot) 3.75 mg im q 1 mo; $420/mo
- Abarelix (Plenaxis) (Med Let 2004;46:22)

Antiandrogens; cmplc include anemia, erectile dysfunction (80%), and osteoporotic fracture risk, NNT-5 yr = 14, ie, 7% more pts fx a bone within 5 yr of rx than if don't use (Nejm 2005;352:154):

- Flutamide (Eulexin) (Med Let 1996;38:56); $445/mo
- Bicalutamide (Casodex); or nilutamide (Nejm 1989;321:413), also used with antiGnRH rx (leuprolide) (Nejm 1989;321:413,419) to eliminate adrenal androgens and to mitigate initial testosterone flare; but no added benefit after medical (Lancet 2000;355:1491) or surgical orchiectomy (Nejm 1998;339:1036); adverse effects: hepatotoxicity (Ann IM 1993;119:860), gynecomastia, gi sx; $420/mo
- Nilutamide (Nilandrone) (Med Let 2004;46:22) 150 mg po qd; $345/mo
- Castration and/or, in the past, diethylstilbestrol 1 mg, which suppresses testosterone to castration level in 75%; 3 mg suppresses in 100% but increases cardiovascular risk beyond cancer risk (Ann IM 1980;92:68)

of bone pain from osteoblastic mets: Strontium-89 (Metastron) or samarium-153 (Quadramet) (Med Let 1997;39:83)

Bladder Carcinoma

Nejm 1990;322:1129

Cause: Transitional cell carcinoma (90%) in bladder or rarely from ureter or kidney pelvis; squamous cell carcinoma (5%); adenocarcinoma (5%)

Epidem: Carcinogens: smoking (increases incidence 2×: Nejm 1971;284:129); cyclophosphamide (Cytoxan) rx (5% risk at 10 yr, 10% at 12 yr, 16% at 15 yr), esp if had hemorrhagic cystitis (Ann IM 1996;124:477); occupational aniline dye exposure; phenacetin users (Nejm 1985;313:292); pelvic radiation rx; chronic indwelling catheter; schistosomiasis, which causes squamous cell type only

   Possible carcinogens include cyclamates and saccharin (Nejm 1980;302:537), and chronic infections and stones
   Male/female = 3:1; most over age 50
   Lifetime incidence: 20/100,000
   High fluid intake decreases incidence (Nejm 1999; 340:1390)

Pathophys: In some pts, IgG-induced killer T-lymphocyte control of the cancer occurs locally (Nejm 1974;291:637)

Sx: Intermittent gross hematuria, painless, often only last drops of urine may cause irritative sx like frequency and urgency; obstructive sx if low in bladder; fever and pain of pyleonephritis

Si:

Crs: 80% 5-yr survival with superficial type, 20% with invasive type

Table 17.6   Bladder Cancer, Invasive Type: 5-Yr Survival Breakdown by Stage and Type of Rx

Stage	Radiation Rx (%)	Cystectomy (%)
T_1/A	72	70
T_2/B_1	40	65
T_3/B_2, C	30	30
T_4/D	15	15

Cmplc: Ureteral obstruction; pyelonephritis; metastases locally, often without si or sx. Often misdiagnosed as UTI since $1/3$ are infected when present.

Lab: *Path:* Urine cytologies useful to pick up carcinoma in situ or high-grade tumors when are hard to see on cystoscopy (Nejm 1972;287:86); may be helpful to screen high-risk groups; $\geq$ 20% false negatives, $\geq$ 5% false positives

  Cystoscopy and bx indicated for gross hematuria and/or in older smokers

Chem: Alkaline phosphatase to r/o liver mets

Urine: Hematuria, gross (cancer more likely than if only microscopic) or microscopic (2% will have bladder cancer, 0.5% will have renal cell cancer)

  Survivin (an inhibitor of apoptosis) levels present; 100% sens, 95% specif (Jama 2001;285:324)

Xray: CT w and w/o contrast to r/o upper tract disease; chest xray to r/o mets

Rx: of superficial: Transuretheral resection. Adjuvant intrabladder chemoRx, eg, BCG (Nejm 1991;325:1189; Med Let 1991;33:29) (beware of tbc skin testing, which will show severe reactions), or mitomycin or doxorubicin, or intrabladder valrubicin (Valstar) (Med Let 1999;41:32) in pts w high-grade tumors, CIS, or recurrent superficial disease.

of invasive: Radical cystectomy w radiation and w cisplatin
chemoRx (Nejm 1993;329:1377, 1420)
of metastatic disease: ChemoRx

Renal Cell Carcinoma

Jama 2004;292:97; Nejm 1996;335:865

Cause: Neoplasia; some are genetic and familial (Ann IM 1993;
118:106) from change in chromosome 3p: von Hippel-Lindau
disease, hereditary papillary renal carcinoma, familial oncocy-
toma, and hereditary renal carcinoma

Epidem: 4 (women) to 10 (men)/100,000/yr incidence (Jama
1999;281:1628); peak incidence at age 60-80; increased incidence in von Hippel-Lindau disease (40%), smokers, obesity, and
HT (Nejm 2000;343:1305). 31,000 new cases/yr in U.S.
Male/female = 3:1

Pathophys: Frequent vascular metastases

Sx: Hematuria (70%); renal colic due to clots (50%); costovertebral
angle pain. Asx in 25-40%.

Si: Flank mass (30-60% on presentation); anemia (41%); fever
(17%); polycythemia (4%); hypertension; accessory nipples
(20%) (Ann IM 1981;95:182); IVC obstruction if on right;
left varicocele due to left spermatic vein obstruction (2%) if on
left

Crs: Without metastases, 88% 5-yr survival if > 7 cm, 95% if < 7 cm.
With single resected met, 35% 5-yr survival; with multiple mets,
4% 5-yr survival.

Cmplc: Hypercalcemia due to increased parathormone, amyloidosis

Lab: *Chem:* Alkaline phosphatase increased (produced in tumor)
Path: Clear cell (75%), papillary (15%), chromophobic (5%),
collecting duct (2%) types

Xray: IVP or CT, mass; only 6% will be cancer (Rad 1974; 113:153); noninvasive (CT) w/u is 90% accurate (Am J Roentgenol 1987; 48:59)

Occasionally ultrasound with diagnostic tap if complex cystic lesion; if solid, do angiography or CT

Rx: Surgical partial or total resection; resection of multiple mets doesn't improve survival; no chemoRx or radiation rx helpful

of metastatic disease: After resection of primary, interleukin-α2b rx (Nejm 2001;345:1655); or interleukin-α2a (Nejm 1998; 338:1272); not interferon-γ1b (Nejm 1998;338:1265)

17.13 Miscellaneous

Foley Catheter Use

Foley for less than 24 hr with orthopedic surgery better than intermittent catheterization (Nejm 1988;319:321)

Hematuria

Associated with hypercalcemia (possibly through microstones) especially in children (Nejm 1984;310:1345); when asx, unassociated with another abnormality (proteinuria or HT), and under age 40, not worth pursuing (Nejm 2003;348:2330). Differential dx: GN, infection, clotting disorder, stones, exercise induced, drugs, trauma, cancer, benign familial, sickle cell disease, HUS, HSP. W/u: UA, urine cytology, IVP/CT, cystoscopy (see algorithm: Nejm 2003;348:2336).

Hormone Replacement in Men

Testosterone rx controversial (J Am Ger Soc 2003;51:101), perhaps in men w testosterone levels < 2 μgm %; UCLA Solomon 9/02 said replace under 2 μgm % for sure, probably under 3 and maybe even < 4.75?

Impotence (Erectile Dysfunction and Other Sexual Dysfunction)

Jama 2004;291:2994; Nejm 2000;342:1802; male and female: Jama 1999;281:537

Cause: Drugs including thiazides, β-blockers, clonidine, alpha-methyldopa (Aldomet), cimetidine, psychiatric medications, chemoRx of cancer, and a long list of others that occasionally do it (Med Let 1987;29:65; Ann IM 1976;85:342); diabetes (Nejm 1989;320:1025); other endocrine etiologies (Ann IM 1983;98:103), prolactin tumors, male menopause, hypogonadism (high FSH and LH, low testosterone); endothelial dysfunctiion, prostatectomy, prostate irradiation

Epidem: Prevalence = 39% at age 40, 67% at age 70 (J Urol 1994; 151:54); vs 7% at age 25, 11% at age 45, 18% at 55 (Jama 1999; 281:537). In healthy thin men, < 5% at age 50, 10% at 60, 20% at 70, 60% at 80 (Ann IM 2003;139:161).

Si: Rectal exam for prostate nodules, neurologic and vascular exams

Cmplc: r/o ejaculatory dysfunction, decreased libido

Lab: *Chem:* Testosterone, total and free; prolactin; LH; FSH; FBS; PSA

Rx (Jama 1997;277:7):
   Testosterone 200 mg:
   - Im q 2 wk
   - Patch (Nejm 1996;334:710; Med Let 1996;38:49) as scrotal (Testoderm) 4-6 mg or nonscrotal (Androderm) 2.5-5 mg patch q 24 hr
   - Topical gels like Testim (Med Let 2003;45:70) 50 mg qd or Androgel (Med Let 2000;42:49)
   - Buccal Striant (Med Let 2003;45:70) 30 mg bid
     Above for men if testosterone deficient, but also help women w post-BSOO sexual dysfunction at 300 μgm/d? at least

short term (Nejm 2000;343:682,730). Adverse effects poorly studied (Nejm 2004;350:482).

Bupropion 150 mg po qd-bid helps 30% including women; often used w antidepressants, which decrease sexual function

Vasoactive drugs:

- Alprostadil (MUSE) (prostaglandin E) 250-1000 μgm intrau-rethral pill, works ≤ ⅔ of the time (Nejm 1997;336:1); or 5-40 μgm intracavernously, or w papaverine and phentolamine (Trimix); cmplc: local pain (33%), hypotension (3%); $20/dose

- Papaverine up to 60 μgm intracavernous, along with phento-lamine, or alprostadil (prostaglandin E_1) (Nejm 1996;334:873; Med Let 1995;37:83) at 1.25 μgm if neurogenic, 5-10 μgm usually enough except higher doses to 60 μgm needed often in vascular impotence, erections should last < 60 min, ≤ 1/d, < 3/wk; $20/shot (10 or 20 μgm/cc); help 86%; self-adminis-tered with insulin syringe; cmplc: priaprism (Med Let 1987; 29:95), and penile fibrotic nodules, which are less common with alprostadil but transient testicular pain is common; costly (Med Let 1990;32:116)

- Selective phosphodiesterase inhibitors: Block enzyme that metabolizes vasodilating nitric oxide via cyclic quanosine monophosphate (cCMP). Adverse effects: Transient visual changes; severe hypotension if given w nitrates, alpha blockers, or HIV protease inhibitors; mild headache; facial flushing; in-digestion; ok w other (non-nitrate) antianginal and HT meds (Nejm 2000;342:1622) and in pts w ASHD if not on nitrates (Jama 2002;287:719):

  Sildenafil (Viagra) (Med Let 1998;40:51; Nejm 1998;338:
  1397) 50-100 mg po (25 mg if on erythromycin, ketoconazole, or itraconazole, or in renal or hepatic failure) 1 hr before anticipate intercourse, onset in 25 min, duration of 4
  hr; helps 70+% (50-60% of diabetics: Jama 1999;281:

421); avoid within 4 hr of α-blocker meds; adverse effects: angina, MI, shock, esp in pts on nitrates; also ischemic optic neuropathy (Med Let 2005;47:49) $10/tab but all 3 strengths cost same so can buy 100 mg pills and break in half

Vardenafil (Levitra) 2.5-20 mg po prn; onset in 25 min, duration of 4 hr; don't use w α-blocker meds at all; $9/pill no matter size

Tadalafil (Cialis) (Med Let 2003;45:101) 5-20 mg po prn; onset in 45 min, duration of 36 hr; $9/pill no matter size

Vacuum/constriction devices: Vacuum devices (Erectaid), or adjustable bands (Actis or Rejoyn) work but are clumsier

Prostheses, permanent or inflatable, surgically inplanted

Prerenal Azotemia and Compensatory Mechanisms

Nejm 1988;319:623

Proteinuria

Ann IM 1983;98:186

< 2 gm/24 hr: Transient in 10% with severe medical disease or stress (Nejm 1982;306:1031)

Orthostatic proteinuria: None with 1st morning urine; benign even over 50 yr (Ann IM 1982;97:516; Nejm 1981;305:618)

Obesity associated: Due to focal GN, decreases w weight loss or ACEI rx (Nephron 1995;70:35); or due to sleep apnea w no GN and reversible w rx of sleep disorder (Arch IM 1988;148:87)

Sexually Transmitted Diseases (STDs) Causes:

Viruses
HIV
Hepatitis A, B, and C
Human papillomavirus
Herpes simplex viruses
Cytomegalovirus
Molluscum contagiosum virus

Protozoans
Trichomonas vaginalis
Giardia lamblia

Entamoeba histolytica
Ectoparasites
  Phthirus pubis
  Sarcoptes scabiei
Bacteria
Neisseria gonorrhoeae
Treponema pallidum

Haemophilus ducreyi
Calymmatobacterium granulomatis
Gardnerella vaginalis (?)
Mobiluncus sp

Ureaplasma urealyticum
Shigella sp
Campylobacter sp
Group B *Streptococcus* (?)
Chlamydia trachomatis
Mycoplasma hominis

24-Hr Urine Collection Adequacy

Total creatinine should be 20-26 mg/kg/d (J. B. Henry, *Clinical Diagnosis and Management by Laboratory*. Philadelphia: WB Saunders 1984:1439)

Vasectomy

Reversal even when successful leads to fertility only about half the time because of permanent testicular damage (Nejm 1985; 313:1252,1283) and perhaps sperm antibodies. In vitro fertilization possible at least in cases of congenital absence of vas (Nejm 1990; 323:1788).

Chapter 18

Rheumatology/Orthopedics

D. K. Onion

18.1 Nonsteroidal Anti-inflammatory Drugs (NSAIDs)

All inhibit prostaglandin synthetase COX (cyclooxygenase) COX types 1 and 2. All except for salicylates are associated w Na retention, 2-8× increase in end-stage renal disease (Nejm 1994;331: 1675), and membranous GN nephrotic syndrome (Jama 1996;276: 466). All but nonacetylated salicylates cause platelet dysfunction, which is irreversible w ASA but reversible w all others. All cause gastric irritation to varying degrees (Nejm 1999;340:1886):

Low risk: Nonacetylated salicylates, nabumetone, sulindac, etodolac

Moderate risk: Ibuprofen, naproxen, ASA, ketoprofen, diclofenac

High risk: Piroxicam, indomethacin, flurbiprofen

Acetylsalicylic acid (ASA) 1-3 gm po qid, therapeutic level = 20-30 mg %, 3-8-hr half-life; analgesic effect potentiated by caffeine (Arch IM 1991;151:733); for all arthritis except septic and gout as well as for anticoagulant effect at 75-300 mg po qd doses but which is blocked by ibuprofen (Med Let 2004;46:61); adverse effects: tinnitus, delirium/confusion, asthma/anaphylaxis esp in pts w eosinophilia and nasal polyps, increased bleeding time for 2 d, platelet dysfunction for 7-10 d; cheap

Nonacetylated salicylates (Trilisate, Dolobid, Disalcid) 0.4-1.2 gm po qid; for all arthritis except septic; adverse effects: similar to ASA but no effect on platelets or gastric mucosa; $8-$50/mo generic, $100/mo trade names

Celecoxib (Celebrex) 100-200 mg po qd-bid; only over age 18; for DJD and RA; compared to other NSAIDs, less gi irritation (Jama 2000;284;1247) and no antiplatelet effects, similar renal and allergic effects; adverse effects: dose-dependent increases in MI/CAD/thromboembolic disease (Nejm 2005;352:1071,1081,1092,1131,1133); sulfa based so sulfa allergies; drug interactions w warfarin, zafirlukast, fluconazole, fluvastatin, and w some β blockers, antidepressants, and antipsychotics; 100 mg bid costs $75 for 200 mg/mo

Diclofenac (Voltaren) 50-75 mg po bi-qid; or w 200 μgm misoprostol as Arthrotec; or as topical gel (J Rheum 1999;26:2659); $46/mo generic, $88/mo Voltaren

Etodolac (Lodine) (Med Let 1991;33:79; J Intern Med 1991;229:5) 300 mg po b-qid; less gastric irritation than naproxen but 3× as expensive as ibuprofen; $50/mo generic, $90/mo trade for tid

Flurbiprofen (Ansaid) (Med Let 1989;31:31); no better than others; more expensive, $38/mo generic, $102/mo trade names

Ibuprofen (Motrin, Advil) 0.4-1.2 gm po qid, 3-hr half-life; in children (Med Let 1989;31:109) as antipyretic, 5 mg/kg for T° < 102°F, 10 mg/kg for T° > 102°F (no Reye's syndrome reported); for all arthritis except septic, as strong an analgesic as Tylenol 3; adverse effects: diarrhea, gi intolerance but lowest of all NSAIDs (BMJ 1996;312:1563), renal failure (Ann IM 1990;112:568), Na^+ retention with hypertension, mental status changes, rash, platelet dysfunction for 1 d; $2/d generic, $22/mo trade names

Indomethacin (Indocin) 25-50 mg po t-qid, 3-hr half-life; 75 mg bid for slow-release type, which is better tolerated; for all arthritis except septic, may be especially good for hip DJD,

shoulder tendonitis, and gout; adverse effects: usual +
headache, dizziness, mental status changes/confusion, rash,
pancytopenia, visual changes, acute oliguric renal failure especially when used with triamterene (Nejm 1984;310:565),
platelet dysfunction for 1 d; $17/mo generic, $60/mo Indocin

Ketoprofen (Orudis) (Med Let 1993;35:15) 50-75 mg po t-qid;
adverse effects: usual NSAID ones; $38/mo generic,
$140/mo trade names

Ketorolac (Toradol) (Med Let 1990;32:79) 10-30 mg im q 6 hr;
used as a short-term pain med, not as an anti-inflammatory;
as effective as 12 mg morphine without respiratory depression, gi constipation, or addiction; adverse effects: usual
NSAID ones especially gi bleed esp if > 90 mg/d × 5 d
(Jama 1996;275:376), anaphylaxis in ASA-sensitive pt,
and especially renal failure more frequent if used > 5 d
(Ann IM 1997;126:193); $5 per dose vs $0.50 for
morphine

Meloxicam (Mobic) (Med Let 2000;42:47) 7.5-15 mg po qd; for
DJD; adverse effects: diarrhea, N+V, no platelet effect, increased lithium levels, may increase warfarin levels; $2/pill

Nabumetone (Relafen) (Med Let 1992;34:38) 1000-2000 mg po
qd; adverse effects: usual NSAID type but gi toxicity only
0.02-0.9% compared to 2-4% ulcers/yr for other NSAIDs in
aggregate; $71/mo

Naproxen (Naprosyn) 250 mg po qd to 500 mg tid, 13-hr
half-life; potentiated effects when used with ASA; for all
arthritis except septic; adverse effects: usual + tinnitus,
mental status changes, hepatitis, platelet dysfunction for 1 d;
$20/mo generic, $52/mo trade names

Oxaprosin (Daypro) (Med Let 1993;35:15) 600-1800 mg po qd;
adverse effects: usual NSAID ones; $44/mo

Piroxicam (Feldene) 10-20 mg qd, takes 11 d until reach steady
state w 44-hr half-life; for all arthritis except septic; adverse
effects: usual + photosensitivity rash, tinnitus, platelet

dysfunction for 2-4 d, confusion in elderly complicated by
long half-life; $32/mo generic, $83/mo Feldene

Sulindac (Clinoril) 100-200 mg po tid, 13-hr half-life; for all
arthritis except septic; adverse effects: usual + headache,
mental status changes/confusion, hepatotoxic, rash, pancytopenia; $50/mo

18.2 Narcotics

All have addiction potential and cause respiratory depression and
constipation (hence should prophylact for constipation); iv
patient-controlled devices work well, cost $40-1500 (Med Let
1989;31:104); selective blocking of gi motility inhibition w experimental drug may be possible (Nejm 2001;345:935). Rv of chronic
pain use/strategies (Med Let 2005;47:21; Nejm 2003:349:1943).

Buprenorphine (Med Let 1986;28:56) 0.3 mg iv/im q 6 hr; partial
antagonist like butorphanol and pentazocine

Butorphanol (Stadol) (Med Let 1993;35:105; Nejm
1980;302:381) 1.5-2.5 mg im, similar nasal doses as good and
last longer; as strong as 10 mg im morphine, less respiratory
depression; adverse effects: a narcotic antagonist so can precipitate withdrawal in addicted pts, addiction in migraine pts

Codeine 30-60 mg po q 3-6 hr w ASA (Empirin Cmpd) or acetaminophen (Tylenol 3); analgesia inhibited by cimetidine,
fluoxetine (Prozac), and quinidine

Dezocine (Dalgan) 11-30 mg iv/im; like pentazocine (Med Let
1990;32:95)

Dihydromorphone (Dilaudid) 1-2 mg po q 3-4 hr; $125/mo for 25
mg/3 d patch; or as sustained-release Palladone 12-32 mg
caps, which, if broken or abused iv, are very dangerous;
$210/mo for 12 mg qd

Fentanyl (Duragesic) transdermal patch 25, 50, or 100 μgm/hr,
lasts 72 hr (Med Let 1992;34:97), or as experimental DPCA
transdermal pump (Jama 2004;291:1333), or as lozenge lol-

lipop (Actig) (Med Let 1994;36:24) 200-1600 μgm, esp if
can't take po; or as fast-acting lozenge (Actig) 100+ mg up
to tid; dangerously long-acting in elderly and fatal to children if mistake for lollipop

Levorphanol po for cancer pain, long (16 hr) half-life

Meperidine (Demerol) 50-150 mg iv/im, 3-hr duration; irritating
im/sc; beware fatal encephalopathy and serotoninergic syndromes (p 18) when used w MAO inhibitors or SSRIs; toxic
metabolite w 20-hr half-life esp in renal failure can cause
dysphoria and even seizures

Methadone (Dolophine) 10-20 mg po and LAAM (methadol)
both used for rx of heroin addicts and available only through
federal clinics (Med Let 1994;36:52)

Morphine SO$_4$ (MS) 5-15 mg iv/im, or 1 mg intraarticular, eg,
postarthroscopy (Nejm 1991;325:1123), or po 20 mg/cc w
4-hr duration or 15+ mg bid if given po as long-acting form
(MS Contin, Oramorph bid, Kadian bid, Avinza qd) supple-
mented w immediate-release prn breakthrough pain at $^1/_3$ the
single long-acting dose q 2 hr prn, readjust long-acting dose
q 24 hr by total MS past 24 hr and give $^1/_2$ that dose bid as
LA and $^1/_3$ that dose q 2 hr as immediate release; twice as
effective if given with 5-10 mg amphetamine (Nejm
1977;296:712) but rarely done

Oxycodone 5-10 mg po q 3-6 hr w ASA (Percodan) or acetaminophen (Tylox, Percocet); or Oxycontin, long-acting,
often abused form

Pentazocine (Talwin) 40-60 mg iv, im, po q 3-4 hr; adverse
effects: depresses respirations, morphine antagonist like
nalorphine

Propoxyphene (Darvon) (Nejm 1972;286:813) 30-65 mg po q
4-6 hr; adverse effects: abuse and death (Jama 1973;223:
1125), rx OD with nalorphine (Med Let 1973;15:61)

Tramadol (Ultram) (Med Let 1995;37:59) 50-100 mg po q 6 hr prn
pain; as good as codeine + ASA, hepatic/renal excretion,

unscheduled; adverse effects: seizures and serotonin syndromes, esp w concomitant MAO inhibitors, antipsychotics, or antidepressants; $60/100 tab

18.3 Analgesic Enhancers

Caffeine 65-200 mg po, used w NSAIDs
Hydroxyzine (Vistaril) 50-100 mg im, used w parenteral narcotics

18.4 Disease Modifying Antirheumatic Drugs (DMARD)

Med Let 2000;42:57

Azathioprine (Imuran) (p 442)
D-Penicillamine (Depen) (Nejm 1979;300:274) 125-1000 mg po
    qd divided; "go low, go slow"; used in scleroderma; adverse
    effects: rash, itch, nephrosis, depresses polys and platelets;
    $62/mo generic, $123/mo Depen
Gold compounds (p 1086)
Hydroxychloroquine (Plaquenil) (J Clin Rheum 1997;3:1;
    Rheum Dis Clin N Am 1994;20:243), < 3.5 mg/lb; used for
    discoid lupus, SLE, RA; stabilizes lysozymal membranes and
    decreases interleukin-2 and macrophage production of TNF;
    adverse effects: depigmentation of skin and hair; retinopathy
    with bull's-eye red patch, irreversible, dose-related (Nejm
    1967;276:1168), prevent w q 6 mo ophthalmology visits;
    reversible cataracts; $25/mo generic, $40/mo Plaquenil
Methotrexate (Rheumatrex) 2.5-25 mg po q 1 wk; adverse ef-
    fects: nausea and vomiting, hepatitis; rarely marrow suppres-
    sion, pulmonary fibrosis, and hepatic fibrosis; $50/mo
Steroids, like prednisone 5 mg qd, is physiologic unstressed re-
    placement, up to 120 mg qd to rx arthritis and other diseases
    (steroid equivalents in order of diminishing mineralocorti-
    coid component: hydrocortisone 20 mg, prednisone 5 mg,
    methylprednisolone 4 mg, dexamethasone 0.75 mg); adverse
    effects (even w 10 mg prednisone qd): subcapsular cataracts,

osteoporosis so pts on long-term rx even low dose (5 mg/d) should get at least $CaCO_3$ + vitamin D (Ann IM 1996;125:964) and probably biphosphonates, infections because inhibits polymorpho-leukocyte diapodesis, aseptic necrosis of hip, peptic ulcers if used with NSAIDs (Ann IM 1991;114:735)

New RA drugs:

- Anakinra (Kineret) (Med Let 2002;44:18) sc qd, interleukin-1 receptor antagonist for RA; probably less effective than TNF agents
- Leflunomide (Arava) (Nejm 2004;350:2167) 100 mg po qd × 3 d then 20 mg po qd; pyrimidine synthesis inhibitor
- Rituximab (Rituxan) (Nejm 2004;350:2572), anti-B-cell rx for RA

Tumor necrosis factor agents (Nejm 2001;344:907, 1999;340:310, 1997;337:141); all about equal clinically (Nejm 2000;343:1640) so choose among by frequency, route of administration, and insurance coverage (iv forms covered by Medicare); check PPD for latent tbc first (Nejm 2001;345:1098); may cause or worsen CHF (Ann IM 2003;138:807); all about $1300/mo

- Adalimumad (Humira) (Med Let 2003;45:25) 40 mg sc every other week
- Etanercept (Enbrel) (Ann IM 1999;130:478; Nejm 2000; 342:763, 1999;340:253; Med Let 1998;40:110) 0.4 mg/kg up to 25 mg sc biw for up to 3 mo; recombinant TNF blocker/binder; for disease resistant to mtx, and may be marginally more effective and therefore better choice than mtx (Nejm 2000;343: 1586); adverse effects: local irritation, serious infection, theoretical increase in autoimmune disease; $1100/mo
- Infliximab (Remicade) (Med Let 1999;41:19, 1998;40:110) 3-10 mg/kg iv q 4-12 wk; anti-TNF monoclonal antibody; used for Crohn's disease and RA; adverse effects (Nejm 2004; 350:934): hypersensitivity reactions including fever and

urticaria, increase in autoimmune antibodies, increase in tumors/lymphomas; $1100-3300/dose

ACTH, rarely indicated; maybe in children, acute gout, myasthenia, or in diagnostic testing

18.5 Collagen Vascular Diseases

Ankylosing Spondylitis (Marie-Strümpell Disease)

Cause: Genetic, HLA association suggests close link to primary gene or immune interaction between antigen and agent, eg, klebsiella antigens (Bull Rheum Dis 1989;39(2):1)

Epidem: Male/female = 3:1; 0.1-0.2% prevalence in whites; associated with HLA B27

Pathophys: Tendonitis, periostitis, and ligamentous inflammation and calcification lead to bony hyperplasia and ankylosis

Sx: Hip and foot arthritic sx, although can involve any joint; onset at age 15-35, or in late childhood

Back pain that improves with exercise, worsens with inactivity, unlike chronic low-back syndrome; sacroiliitis early and constant

Anorexia and weight loss, fever, sciatica (10% have it when first present)

Si: 10-cm mark on LS spine stretches on flexion only to < 15 cm; chest expansion ≤ 2.5 cm (Ann IM 1976;84:1)

Painful SI joints on palpation

Crs: Relatively benign, rarely die of disease, but overall mortality is 4× normal (Nejm 1977;297:572)

Cmplc: Iridocyclitis (25%); aortic insufficiency (5%); mitral insufficiency (Nejm 1978;299:1448) and abnormal cardiac conduction including heart block (8%); kyphosis, fracture of cervical spine; pneumonitis (1%) that can look like old tbc r/o other seronegative spondyloarthropathies all with similar HLA B27 association and clinical syndromes, eg, Reiter's syndrome, regional enteritis, ulcerative colitis, psoriatic arthritis, post-*Yersinia* colitis (Nejm 1989;321:16)

Lab: *Hem:* ESR increased (80%)

Serol: HLA B27-positive; 10% false negative, 8% false positive. 20% (Bull Rheum Dis 1981;31:35) of positive people with positive family hx get ankylosing spondylitis; of those who are HLA B27-positive but with negative family hx, only 2% get the disease.

Xray: Bilaterally symmetric sacroiliitis with subchondral sclerosis (100%), osteitis of symphysis pubis, anterior spinal ligament calcification, late "bamboo spine" with bony fusion of spine and osteophytes are parallel not perpendicular to spine. Calcification of tendons and heels (cf Reiter's syndrome).

Rx: Exercise program most important to prevent fusion in kyphosis

NSAIDs

Sulfasalazine (Br J Rheum 1990;29:2)

Steroids only for eye cmplc

Perhaps TNF-α antagonists like etanercept (Enbrel) sc biw (debatable: ACP J Club 2004;140:71; Nejm 2002;346:1349 vs 1399)

Dermatomyositis (DM), Polymyositis (PM), and Inclusion Body Myositis (IBM)

DM/PM: Nejm 1991;325:1487; Ann IM 1995;122:715; IBM: Nejm 1991;325:1026

Cause: Multiple autoimmune, usually involving CD_8 killer T cells (Nejm 1991;324:877); plastic surgical bovine collagen injections (Ann IM 1993;118:920)

Epidem: Incidence of all 3 is about 1/100,000/yr

DM: Females > males in both children and adults

PM: Adults only

IBM: Male/female = 3:1; Caucasians > blacks; most pts > 50 yr old

Pathophys: Perhaps autoimmunity to own muscle protein. In DM, immune complex activation and vessel damage via complement (Nejm 1986;314:329); in PM and IBM, autoimmunity is T cell mediated.

Sx: Fever for weeks; proximal muscle weakness manifested by falling, trouble standing up, or with stair climbing, gradually progressive over weeks to months, occasionally pseudohypertrophic; painless (if painful, r/o polymyalgia rheumatica); dysphagia and regurgitation in 50%; never eye muscle involvement; Raynaud's syndrome. IBM may affect fine distal motor early as well; finger flexor or toe extensors impaired in 50%.

Si: Proximal > distal muscle weakness, palatal paralysis; periungual hyperemia and telangiectasias, r/o hot water; minimal joint involvement; reflexes preserved unless muscle totally gone, as often is the case with quadriceps in IBM

In DM, above plus facial edema and dusky erythema especially in sun-exposed areas; heliotrope (purplish) eyelid, periorbital, and facial coloring; rash w macular scaling plaques, especially in exposed areas and knuckles; scalp involvement (Jama 1994;272:1939)

Crs: Weeks to months usually. IBM may be very slow over years and mimic limb-girdle muscular dystrophy.

Cmplc: Respiratory failure from muscle weakness; amyloidosis; 10% get interstitial pneumonitis and fibrosis (Am Rev Respir Dis 1990;141:727); myocardiopathy; heart block (Ann IM 1981;94:41). Cancer associated in 10% of PM pts and 15% of DM pts (Nejm 1992;326:363) vs 20% and 40% (Ann IM 2001;134:1087). DM appears in overlap syndromes with other connective tissue diseases.

r/o other causes of muscle weakness, including inflammatory myopathies, colchicine myo/neuropathy (Nejm 1987;316:1562); drug-induced myopathies (Semin Arth Rheum 1990;19:259) from penicillamine, AZT, ipecac, cimetidine, chloroquine, steroids, statins; and infectious myopathies from parasitic diseases, Lyme disease, and legionella

Lab: *Chem:* AST (SGOT), LDH, aldolase, and CPK increased (r/o muscular dystrophy)

Noninv: EMG, diagnostic small-amplitude action potentials and fibrillations

Path: Muscle bx shows segmental necrosis, enlarged central nuclei, regeneration (myoblasts, myocytes, basophilic myofibrils), focal inflammation especially around vessels

Serol: ANAs positive (83%); anti-Jo-1 in 40% polymyalgia (Bull Rheum Dis 1985;35:6) and if positive, > 50% have interstitial lung disease; anti-KJ; anti-Mi-2, etc (Ann IM 1995;122:715)

Rx (Ann IM 1995;122:715): Steroids, eg, 60 mg prednisone qd × 3 mo, then taper to 5-10 mg q 1 mo as muscle strength increases and enzymes decrease; helps 80% (D. Dawson, HMS 3/85)

Azathioprine if steroids fail; also chlorambucil and cyclophosphamide

Methotrexate if lungs will tolerate it

Colchicine po may help inflammation with calcinosis in childhood type

Immunologic w immune globulin 2 gm/kg iv q 1 mo; expensive but clearly helps DM and may help PM and IBM (Nejm 1993;329:1993); plasma exchange and leukophoresis no help (Nejm 1992;326:1380)

Mixed Connective Tissue Disease

Cause: Autoimmunity, perhaps an SLE variant

Epidem:

Pathophys: Antibodies to ribonucleoprotein (J Clin Immunol 1991;11:297)

Sx: Arthralgias/arthritis (95%), Raynaud's (85%), myositis (63%), scleroderma skin changes (33%), dyspnea

Si: Impaired esophageal motility (67%), impaired pulmonary diffusion capacity (67%), lymphadenopathy (39%), rash (38%), fever (33%), splenomegaly (19%), hepatomegaly (15%)

Crs:

Cmplc: Renal failure (5%), sicca syndrome (7%), Hashimoto's (6%)

Lab: *Serol:* Anti-RNP, extractable nuclear antigen ANAs positive; elevated in 100% MCT but not specific since also increased in $\frac{1}{2}$ of SLE pts and occasionally in scleroderma pts

Rx: NSAIDs, steroids if must
of Raynaud's: Calcium-channel blockers

Polyarteritis Nodosa (PAN) (Systemic Necrotizing Vasculitis)

Rheum Dis Clin N Am 1990;16:251

Cause: Idiopathic autoimmune

Epidem: Associated with hypertension, hepatitis B (Nejm 1997;337:1739), and other medical diseases; males >> females

Pathophys: Immune complex deposition leads to fibrinoid necrosis of vessel wall and thrombosis. An acute necrotizing vasculitis of small and medium-sized vessels; focal lesions may lead to thrombosis or aneurysmal dilatation at site (Arthritis Rheum 1990;33:1065).

Less acute renal disease and more chronic renal disease and/or amyloidosis as go in the spectrum of disease from PAN to SLE to RA to SS to dermato/polymyositis (Petersdorf 11/68)

Sx: Fever, weight loss, arthralgias/arthritis, abdominal pain, headache, smokey urine, blindness

Si: Myalgias and myositis (39%), splenomegaly (34%), petechiae and purpura (20%), skin necrosis, urticaria, hypertension, mononeuritis multiplex, fever, fundal vessel damage, cutaneous and visceral nodular aneurysms, ulcers of corneal limbus

Crs: ⅓ die in < 1 yr; in hepatitis B surface antigen–associated type, disease burns out in 1 yr if survive

Cmplc: Renal involvement or failure (85%), infections, infarcts, and hypertension in 50%; hepatic infarcts and cirrhosis (66%); cardiac (76%) infarcts and conduction abnormalities; pancreatic (35%) cysts and hemorrhage, blindness from retinal artery occlusion; gi tract (51%) ulcers, hemorrhage, and perforations; aneurysms of mesenteric vessels (25%); asthma (29%); Cogan's syndrome (bilateral 8th cranial nerve palsies and eye keratitis)

Lab: *Hem:* ESR elevated, eosinophilia (20%)
Path: Biopsies (pos if show involvement of nutrient vessels) of kidney (also shows GN); sural nerve, especially if slowed nerve conduction velocities; liver; gastrocnemius or other muscle; testicular; skin
Serol: Complement levels depressed; rheumatoid titers elevated; antineutrophil cytoplasmic autoantibodies, r/o Wegener's (Ann IM 1990;113:656)

Xray: Diagnostic microfusiform aneurysms on renal and hepatic angiography (Nejm 1970;282:1024)

Rx (Ann IM 1992;116:488):
Steroids perhaps qod + cyclophosphamide or azathioprine

Relapsing Polychondritis

Ann IM 1998;129:114

Cause:

Epidem: Male/female = 1:3. Associated with systemic vasculitis (10%), RA (7%), SLE (5%), Hashimoto's (4%), other fibrosing syndromes (9%).

Pathophys: Autoimmune

Sx: Onset at age 13-84, median age is 51; arthritis (52%); ocular (51%); laryngotracheal sx (48%); saddle nose (29%); hearing loss (26%); vertigo (13%)

Si: Auricular chondritis (85%); nasal chondritis (54%); laryngotracheal sx (48%); fever (40%); skin changes (28%); episcleritis

Crs: 5-yr survival = 74%, 10-yr survival = 55%; fluctuating progressive course

Cmplc: Systemic vasculitis death (5%), pneumonia (5%), airway collapse (2%)

Lab: *Hem:* ESR elevated (82%), anemia (55%)
Urine: Hematuria (26%), proteinuria (14%)

Rx: Steroids, 60% respond (Nejm 1978;299:1203); possibly methotrexate, dapsone, cyclophosphamide, azathioprine

Raynaud's Disease/Syndrome

Nejm 2002;347:1001

Cause:

Primary: 15% have positive family hx, in which case is almost never associated with collagen vascular disease

Secondary: Prodrome or concomitant w other collagen vascular disease; systemic sclerosis (especially CREST syndrome types), more often than SLE, which is more common than RA; the 10% who will develop usually manifest it within 2 yr

Occupational (most common): 125 cps vibrations, noise, and cold

Epidem: Males >> females for vibration-induced type; increased incidence w estrogen replacement rx, but not w estrogen/progesterone combo HRT (Ann IM 1998;129:208). 3-5% prevalence.

Pathophys: Autonomic dysfunction causes small-vessel spasm with later development of permanent vessel impairment?; hand small vessels shown to have diminished constrictive and dilating response to normal cold and warm stimuli; may be because vessels respond abnormally to normal levels of sympathetic discharge; may be due to platelet receptor abnormalities (Rheum Dis Clin N Am 1993;19:53)

Sx: Idiopathic or cold-induced fingertip blanching, painful

Si: White fingers

Crs: May precede si and sx of associated collagen vascular disease by up to 10 yr

Cmplc: Fingertip ulcers, no gangrene, migraine headaches (61%: Ann IM 1992;117:985)
r/o systemic sclerosis (scleroderma) and SLE, which are distinguished by their dilated nail capillaries and associated sx of other organ systems

Lab: ESR and ANA/RA titers to r/o collagen vascular disease

Xray: Ba swallow shows motility changes in many pts, rarely do they have sx. Arteriography of hand vessels normal after si and sx return to normal, in contrast to what happens in collagen vascular diseases.

Rx (Curr Opinion Rheum 1997;9:544):
Decrease noise, vibration, and cold exposure by mitten use
Biofeedback; centrifugal arm swing
Plasmaphoresis q 1 wk × 4 wk may yield long remissions
Meds:
1st: Calcium-channel blockers like amlodipine or nifedipine 20-60+ mg po qd (Nejm 1983;308:880); 50-60% decrease in attacks
2nd: Prazosin 1 mg po bid (Ann IM 1982;97:67), then increase perhaps nitrate skin patches or paste; reserpine 0.25-1.5 mg po qd

Acute Rheumatic Fever

Alto: Am Fam Phys 1992;45:613; Nejm 1968;278:183

Cause: Group A hemolytic streptococcus (rarely group A non-hemolytic: Nejm 1971;284:750), type irrelevant but presence of m-protein probably key, eg, nephrogenic strains especially skin ones, lack m-protein and never lead to ARF (Nejm 1970;283:561). Poststrep infection × 2-3 wk, although bacteria must still be present. Genetic susceptibility in some populations? (Bull Rheum Dis 1993;42:5)

Epidem (Nejm 1991;325:783): Children, peak incidence at age 5-15 yr; female/male = 3:1; incidence = 61/100,000/yr in NYC (Jama 1973;224:1593), marked decrease since use of penicillin (Nejm 1988;318:280), increased 3× among the poor. Recent outbreak in Rocky Mt states (Nejm 1987;316:421).

Pathophys: Autoimmune theories, like strep A and humans share antigens, or at least haptens, so strep infections develop cross-reacting antibodies. But not the complete explanation, as L. Weinstein points out, because only strep pharyngitis causes ARF, not strep infections elsewhere in body, unlike AGN.

Sx: Jones criteria to make the dx requires 2 major criteria, or 1 major + 2 minor, + positive ASO titer or culture or h/o scarlet fever; major criteria = carditis, polyarthritis, erythema marginatum, subcutaneous nodules, chorea; minor criteria = fever, arthralgias, distant h/o ARF, elevated wbc ESR or CRP, long PR interval or other EKG abnormalities. Members of same family tend to have same major sx (Nejm 1968;278:183).

Arthralgias, transitory; Sydenham's chorea, may follow other si and sx by weeks or months

Si: • Erythema marginatum, associated with carditis
  • Murmurs, valvular or middiastolic nonvalvular, associated with pericarditis;

- Subcutaneous nodules at bony prominences, associated with carditis (94%);
- Pneumonitis;
- Serositis;
- Polyarthritis of large joints, may be only si (Ann IM 1978;89:917)

Crs: < 10-12 wk in 80-90%. Murmurs all (95%) appear by 2 wk of sx onset.

Cmplc: Chronic cardiac valve disease; mitral regurgitation with Jaccoud's arthritis (ulnar deviation that pt can voluntarily correct: Ann IM 1972;77:949); transient glomerulonephritis (Ann IM 1981;94:322)

Lab: *Hem:* Elevated ESR
Noninv: EKG: PR interval increased
Serol: Streptozyme test (Med Let 1974;16:41); ASO (antistreptolysin O) > 400 Todd U, means had β-strep, < 125 U means didn't, 80% sensitivity; anti-DNAase titer; anti-streptodornase titer

Xray: Chest shows interstitial, nonbacterial pneumonitis

Rx: Preventive: Penicillin as pen V 250 mg po bid in adults or qd in children; or sulfasoxazole, or benzathine penicillin im q 1 mo most effective (Nejm 1971;285:646)

Table 18.1 Rx of Acute Rheumatic Fever

	If No Murmur	If Severe Carditis	If Sick/No Murmur
Penicillin	Yes	Yes + years of prophylaxis	Yes
ASA	Yes	Yes	Yes
Steroids	No	Yes	Optional unless has pneumonia then should rx (Weinstein)

Rheumatoid Arthritis

Nejm 1990;322:1277

Cause: Genetic, associated w HLA DRB_1, DR_1, and DR_4 (Ann IM 1992;117:801, 869)

Epidem (Epidem Rev 1990;12:247):
Adult female/male = 3:1, onset at age 25-50

Pathophys: Collagenase produced by granulation tissue (Nejm 1977;296:1017)

Suppressor T-cell defect; doesn't suppress EBV antibody production normally, leads to chronic EBV antibody production? (Nejm 1981;305:1238); rv of all theories including EBV ones (Ann IM 1984;101:810)

Diagnostic criteria (Bull Rheum Dis 1988;38(5):1) have 90% sensitivity and specificity if have ≥ 4 of following criteria: (1) early-morning stiffness > 6 wk; (2) arthritis involving 3 or more joints > 6 wk; (3) wrist mcp or pip joint involvement; (4) symmetric arthritis; (5) rheumatoid nodules; (6) positive rheumatoid titer; (7) bony xray changes

Sx: Fever > 102°F, erratic (1%); joint pain (100%), monoarticular arthritis (8%); insidious onset

Si: Subcutaneous (rheumatoid) nodules over pressure points; evanescent rash (6%); arthritis and thick synovium

Crs: Chronic over decades; often improves during pregnancy (Nejm 1993;329:466)

Cmplc:
- Peptic ulcers
- Septic arthritis, subtle (Ann IM 1969;70:147)
- Scleral malacia perforans and uveitis
- Pulmonary interstitial pneumonitis and fibrosis, empyema, pleuritis
- Pericarditis and aortic valvulitis (Nejm 1973;289:597)
- Sjögren's syndrome (p 1090)

- Felty's syndrome (J Rheum 1989;16:864) [depressed white counts (p 491), frequent infections, sometimes splenomegaly, skin ulcers]
- Odontoid ligament rupture (Rheum Dis Clin N Am 1991;17: 757; J Rheum 1990;17:134) (10%) (if on xray have > 4 mm separation, should have surgery) and other tendon/ligamentous rupture

Lab: *Joint fluid:* Wbc ~ 40,000, poor mucin clot, protein = 4-5 gm %, C′ decreased

Pleural fluid: Low glucose (< 30 mg %); elevated LDH, protein > 4 gm %, C′ decreased (distinguishes from cancer)

Serol: Rheumatoid factor titers

Rx (Nejm 2004;350:2591):

Start w methotrexate (Ann IM 1996;124:699) or NSAID + gold, chloraquine, or follow with buttoning or shoe-tying time, and BP cuff grip strength test with cuff starting at 30 mm (Ann IM 1994;120:26)

Medications (Ann IM 2001;134:695; Med Let 2000;42:57):

1st: Methotrexate (mtx) 5-20+ mg po q 1 wk (Med Let 1994;36: 101; Ann IM 1991;114:999; Nejm 1985;312:818), sc or im possible if po not helping; w 1 mg folate po qd helps toxicity w/o decreasing efficacy (Ann IM 1995;122:833); no cancer risk (Ann IM 1987;107:358); adverse effects: nausea and vomiting, pulmonary fibrosis, 10% get liver disease (Am J Med 1991;90:711)

2nd: Mtx w hydroxychloroquine 200 mg bid (retinopathy unlikely at < 3.5 mg/lb) + sulfasalazine 500 mg bid (72% improved vs 50% at 1 yr: Nejm 1996;334:1287)

3rd: Mtx w other drugs:

- Steroids, into joints, and po low-dose prednisone 5-10 mg only; 7.5 mg po qd × 2 yr causes fewer osteoporotic changes (Nejm 1995;333:142) and 10 mg qd × 1st 6 mo of rx helpful by DBCT (Ann IM 2002;136:1)

- Gold, 10 mg im, then 50 mg im q 1 wk × 20 wk, then decrease gradually to q 1 mo; rare used now because of doubts about efficacy (Ann IM 1991;114:437); adverse effects: rash, depressed wbc and/or platelets, proteinuria (10%), pulmonary infiltrates. Or oral-form auranofin (Ridaura) 3 mg bid or 6 mg qd to 3 mg tid after 6 mo; less effective than injectable (Arth Rheum 1990;33:1449); adverse effects: bowel sx especially diarrhea (50%); $100/mo for 3 mg bid.
- Cyclosporine ~3 mg/kg/d po divided into bid doses (Nejm 1995;333:137)
- Azathioprine
- Tetracyclines like minocycline or doxycycline 100 mg po bid (Ann IM 1995;122:81)
- D-Penicillamine (Ann IM 1986;105:528) < 1 gm qd, start at 250 mg qd, increase q 3 mo; rarely used because of adverse effects: rashes, depressed wbc and platelets, proteinuria, Goodpasture's

4th: Mtx w tumor necrosis factor antagonists (p 1073); safe and effective (Ann IM 2002;137:726); or other new RA drugs like anakinra, leflunomide, or rituximab (p 1072)

Experimental: Plasmapheresis over a protein A column (Prosorba) (Med Let 1999;41:69) to absorb antibodies

Juvenile Rheumatoid Arthritis (Juvenile Chronic Arthritis)

Jama 2005;294:1671

Cause:

Epidem: Incidence = 1.4/10,000 children/yr; prevalence = 1/1000 children in U.S.

Pathophys (J Rheum 1990; 21[suppl]:1):
Rubella virus present in ⅓ of cases (Nejm 1985;313:1217)

Sx & Si: Polyarticular type (45%): Onset at later age, occasionally rheumatoid factor positive; arthritis in ≥ 5 joints; no systemic sx or si

Pauciarticular type (30%): Arthritis in < 4 joints; often ANA positive; iridocyclitis leads to blindness often even when arthritis is inactive; eye disease often asx (Clin Exp Rheum 1990;8:499)

Systemic type (25%): Intermittent fever < 39.4°C (103°F), no arthritis; Still's disease variant: diurnal fevers, salmon-colored reticular rash, high ESR, pleuropericarditis, but rare or late arthritis

Crs: 20% still crippled at 10 yr

Cmplc: Growth impairment (Clin Orthop 1990;259:46)
r/o (Rheum Rev 1991;1:13) juvenile ankylosing spondylitis with positive HLA B27 (Bull Rheum Dis 1987;37(1):1); child abuse; neoplasms; infections (viral, endocarditis, Lyme disease); granulomatous disorders (Crohn's, sarcoid); connective tissue diseases like PAN, SS, giant cell arteritis, rheumatic fever, and SLE

Lab: No good diagnostic test
Hem: Anemia and leukocytosis
Serol: ANA often positive in pauciarticular type. HLA studies 90% positive for B27, cf Reiter's and ankylosing spondylitis

Rx (Clin Orthop 1990;259:60):
Physical rx (Rheum Dis Clin N Am 1991;17:1001) and NSAIDs like ASA or tolmetin; these alone enough in 50-60%, mostly the pauciarticular type
Methotrexate up to 1 mg/kg/wk
Tumor necrosis factor antagonists (p 1073)
Gold (p 1086)

Reiter's Syndrome

Bull Rheum Dis 1987;37(1):1

Cause: Autoimmune

Epidem: Triggered by chlamydial urethritis and enteric pathogens like *Shigella, Salmonella* Yersinia, campylobacter, and HIV infection

(Bull Rheum Dis 1990;39(5):1). Associated w HLA B27-like ankylosing spondylitis (Ann IM 1976;84:8). Male/female = 9:1.

Pathophys:

Sx: 2-4 wk incubation period after trigger (see above). First urethritis (85%), cervicitis, and/or prostatitis; then red eye (conjunctivitis); then weeks later, arthritis and arthralgias (99%), especially peripheral and in lower extremities, especially heels, knees, ankles, low back.

Si: Peripheral arthritis and purulent urethral discharge (95%); red eye from conjunctivitis (40%) or uveitis (8%); fever (37%); painless skin or mucous membrane lesions (32%) especially circinate balanitis and keratodermia blennorrhagia (looks like pustular psoriasis)

Crs: Some resolve after 4-12 mo, but many go on to be chronic

Cmplc: Aortitis (1%); heart block (1%)
r/o chronic Lyme arthritis, gonorrhea, erythema multiforme variants, Behçet's syndrome, psoriasis, ankylosing spondylitis

Lab: *Joint fluid:* Wbc = 5000-50,000, mostly polys but lower % than gonorrhea with more monos
Serol: RA titer negative; HLA B27 has 60-75% sensitivity, 8% specificity

Xray: Periosteal new bone formation along shafts, eg, of phalanges

Rx: Tetracycline rx of presumed chlamydia of pt and partner (Bull Rheum Dis 1992;40(6):1)
NSAIDs as in ankylosing spondylitis (p 1074)

Behçet's Syndrome/Disease

Nejm 1999;341:1284, 1990;322:326

Cause: Vasculitis

Epidem: Some combination of environmental and genetic factors; genetic ones associated (27%) with HLA B51 and, to a lesser extent, B27; may be precipitated by *H. simplex* or parvovirus B19.

Highest prevalence along ancient silk route w highest rates in Turkey and Turkish descendants. Male/female = 1.7:1 in eastern Mediterranean type, $\frac{1}{2}$ in U.S. at Mayo Clinic.

Pathophys: An immune-complex small-vessel vasculitis

Sx: Onset in 20s-30s. Blurred vision, photophobia, eye pain and tearing; painful oral and/or genital lesions.

Si: Recurrent:

- Oral aphthous ulcerations, deep, painful, numerous, may scar
- Genital ulcers: Scrotal, prepuce, or glans; labial or cervical; usually painful but not always
- Uveitis, red eye; hypopyon, anterior as well as retinal scarring
- Erythema nodosum, acneiform lesions, superficial thrombophlebitis, and "delayed hypersensitivity reaction" to saline or any shot

Crs: Each attack lasts 1-4 wk. CNS disease has bad prognosis.

Cmplc:

- Blindness (Bull Rheum Dis 1985;35(5):1), rx often titrated, therefore, to the uveitis
- Cardiovascular: Cardiac (Ann IM 1983;98:639), DVT, aneurysms
- Inflammatory mono- or polyarthritis with polys > 200,000
- Neurologic: Aseptic meningitis and MS-like syndromes
- Colitis

Lab: *Hem:* ESR elevated

Serol: Increased acute-phase reactants

Skin tests: Positive delayed hypersensitivity reaction to a saline shot is diagnostic

Rx: Anti-inflammatory meds like ASA, indomethacin, pentoxifylline (Trental) 300 mg po bid (Ann IM 1996;124:891), colchicine, or thalidomide 100 mg po qd (Ann IM 1998; 128:443); cmplc: teratogenicity in pregnant women, polyneuropathy

Steroids, high dose, often w azathioprine (Nejm 1990;
322:281), cyclophosphamide, chlorambucil, or interferon-α2a

Sjögren's (Sicca) Syndrome

Rheum Dis Clin N Am 1992;18(3); Bull Rheum Dis 1988;30:1046

Cause: Autoimmune?; a retrovirus?; impaired response to cholinergic
stimluli (Ann Rheum Dis 2000;59:48); primary, or secondary to
scleroderma, rheumatoid arthritis, SLE, primary biliary cirrhosis,
vasculitis, thyroiditis, hepatitis C (J Hepatol 1999;31:210), etc

Epidem: Females >> males; 2nd most common collagen vascular disease after RA. Associated w HLA B8 (54%) and HLA DR$_W$3
(75%).

Pathophys: Lymphocyte-mediated destruction of exocrine glands leads
to mucosal dryness; an immune-complex small-vessel vasculitis

Sx: Primary type: Raynaud's (20%); sicca syndrome with dry eyes and
mouth and secondary caries, thirst; dry cough with frequent upper and lower respiratory infections; dysphagia; dyspareunia
Secondary type: Other collagen vascular disease present

Si: Primary type: Parotid enlargement (80%); pseudolymphoma;
caries; positive Schirmer test (< 5 mm/5 min filter paper ascent
from eyelid) but many false positives and negatives, and hence
not worth doing (Br J Rheum 1993;32:231)

Crs:

Cmplc: Primary type: Obstructive and restrictive lung disease; gastric
atrophy; pancreatitis; interstitial renal disease and Fanconi's syndrome; B-cell lymphomas (Nejm 1987;316:1118) and perhaps
other cancers; staph conjunctivitis; blindness (Bull Rheum Dis
1985;35:5), and other MS-like syndromes in 20% (Ann IM
1986;104:322)

r/o other causes of sicca syndrome (Cornea 1999;18:625):
Type IV and V hyperlipidemia, sarcoid, hemachromatosis, amyloid, local irradiation, HIV infection that can be associated with

as well as cause secondary Sjögren's (Bull Rheum Dis 1992; 40(6):6)

Lab: *Hem:* ESR elevated (Semin Arth Rheum 1992;22:114)

Path: Lip salivary gland bx shows lymphocytic infiltration (94%) (Nejm 1987;316:1118)

Serol: Positive RA titer (90%), ANA (50-80%), SSA, SSB (p 1135)

Rx: Methylcellulose eye gtts and mouthwash, or "Lacrisert" methylcellulose lid insert q 12 hr; perhaps cyclosporine 0.05% ophth gtts bid (Med Let 2003;45:42) for Sjögren's and idiopathic, marginal help for $6/d

Steroids if marked parotid swelling or other life-threatening complications

of aphthous ulcers: Tetracycline oral rinse

of dry mouth (Med Let 2000;42:70):

- Methylcellulose mouthwash, frequent sips of water, sugar-free gum, hard candy
- Pilocarpine (Salagen) 5 mg po qid; helps xerostomia, at least radiation-induced type (Nejm 1993;329:390); $160/mo
- Cevimeline (Evoxac) 30 mg po tid; similar to pilocarpine, a cholinergic agonist; adverse effects: sweating, NV+D, rhinitis, worsens asthma, decreases night vision; $120/mo

Scleroderma (Progressive Systemic Sclerosis) and CREST* Syndrome

Cause: Genetic? Autoimmune?

Epidem:

Predominant in middle age, peak age 65 yr; 2.7 new pts/1 million population/yr; female/male = 8:1; recently rising incidence (Arthritis Rheum 1989;32:998)

Pathophys: Fetal Y chromosomes found in some skin lesions, suggesting it may be a fetal graft-vs-host disease at least in some women (Nejm 1998;338:1186)

Collagen deposition in skin and muscles, especially smooth muscle, associated w increased mast cells (Ann IM 1985;102: 182); debate if fibrosis or vascular disease is primary (J Rheumatol 1999;26:938)

Progressive sclerosis of skin, esophagus, and rest of gut, lung, heart. Cardiac sx due to microvascular changes causing fibrosis (Nejm 1986;314:1397), which can be cold induced (Ann IM 1986;105:661). gi cmplc all due to bacterial overgrowth from diminished large and small bowel motility.

Sx: Dx criteria (Bull Rheum Dis 1981;31:1): major = proximal scleroderma (proximal to mcp joints), 91% sens, 99% specif; minor = sclerodactyly,* digital pitting, basilar pulmonary fibrosis (30% false neg, 2% false pos)

Raynaud's* (86%); esophageal reflux,* dysphagia (75% gi involvement) w eventual nonmotile esophagus, pulmonary sx especially cough (50%), cardiovascular sx (20%), polymyositis, arthritis

Si: Pitting edema early, brawny nonpitting later, then thin mummy-like skin with increased pigmentation; periungual telangiectasias* (r/o constant hot-water exposure); subcutaneous calcinosis*

Crs: 5-yr survival is 68%, worse if renal > heart > lung involvement (Ann IM 1993;118:602)

Cmplc: Renal disease, progressive but reversible (60%: Ann IM 2000;133:600), 76% 1-yr survival with ACE inhibitor rx (Ann IM 1990;113:352); amyloid; malabsorption/digestion; Sjögren's (17%: Ann IM 1977;87:535); progressive acute and chronic pulmonary failure and HT (Arthritis + Rheum 1999;42:2638); primary hypothyroidism (Ann IM 1981;95:431); heart block and arrhythmias (Ann IM 1981;94:38); MIs and microcirculatory changes (J Rheumatol 2000;27:155); impotence

r/o sclerodactyly from air hammer use or ergot; porphyria cutanea tarda; **eosinophilic fasciitis** (Ann IM 1980;92:507) w "peau d'orange" skin and flexion contractures esp of upper extremities and complicated by carpal tunnel syndrome (Arthritis Rheum 1995;38:1707); and **eosinophilic/myalgia syndrome** caused by contaminated tryptophan, spares hands and feet, no Raynaud's (Nejm 1990;323:357; Ann IM 1990;113:124); similar syndrome related to increased 5-HT with pyridoxine, tryptophan, and carbidopa rx: Nejm 1980;303:782)

Lab: *Path:* Skin bx shows increased collagen, epidermal degeneration

Serol: C' normal, SPEP shows increased IgG, rheumatoid titer elevated (25%), cryoglobulins, false-positive serologic tests for syphilis. ANA positive (see p 1135), especially speckled (centromere-staining antibodies) type, which is present in 70% of CREST; antinucleolar antibodies positive in 54% but 26% of SLE pos and 10% of RA. Scl-70 specific but nonsensitive, positive in only 20%.

Xray: Hand films show distal phalanx tuft resorption (cf psoriasis) with periarticular calcification. UGIS shows esophageal dysmotility and reflux. BE shows "wide mouth" diverticula.

Rx (Semin Arth Rheum 1993;23:22, 1989;18:181):

Physical therapy

Steroids

Relaxin, human recombinant type (Ann IM 2000;132:871) 25 μgm/kg sc qd; slows skin thickening and perhaps lung fibrosis

D-Penicillamine 500-1500 mg po qd; helps skin, organs, and survival (Ann IM 1982;97:652) but ⅓ can't tolerate (Ann IM 1986;104:699) and fell out of favor in the 1990s

ACE inhibitors, prevent renal failure if BP elevated

Nifedipine for cardiac changes (Nejm 1986;314:1397) and Raynaud's

Octreotide, a somatostatin analog, po helps gi motility (Nejm 1991;325:1461)

Minocycline (Lancet 1998;352:1755)

Colchicine perhaps

of GERD: Proton pump inhibitors (p 334)
of pulmonary fibrosis: Cyclophosphamide (Ann IM
2000;132:946)

Systemic Lupus Erythematosus

Ann IM 1995;123:42; Nejm 1994;330:1871

Cause: Idiopathic type is multifactorial in etiology but clearly there
is a genetic predisposition that has several HLA type linkages
(Ann IM 1991;115:548)

Drug-induced type (Bull Rheum Dis 1991;40:4):
Procainamide (40% of pts become ANA positive but a much
smaller % develop SLE), especially slow-release preparation
(Ann IM 1984;100:197); hydralazine (10% become ANA positive: Ann IM 1972;76:365); INH (20% become ANA positive);
rarely quinidine (Ann IM 1984;100:840), methyldopa, chlorpromazine, penicillamine (Ann IM 1982;97:659); etc. Occurs sooner
in slow acetylators (autosomal recessive) than in rapid acetylators
(Nejm 1978;298:1157).

Epidem: Female/male = 9:1 in idiopathic types; equal in drug-induced
type. Black/white = 3-4:1. Prevalence = 40/100,000; seen especially in women during childbearing years.

Pathophys: Tissue damage is from immune-complex vasculitis, thrombocytopenia, and antiphospholipid antibody-induced thrombosis.
The autoantibodies are from abnormally intolerant B and T cells
(Nejm 1991;115:548). Renal disease occurs in idiopathic types
only, not drug-induced types (Nejm 1972;286:908).

Sx: H/o stress, eg, UV exposure, pregnancy; facial rash; fever; visual
sx; oligoarthritis (95%), episodic, pain > objective findings

Si: Rash, facial butterfly rash (33%), sun sensitive, and unlike discoid
lupus scarred delineated rash especially on ears, and differs from
seborrheic rash in same area by sparing nasolabial folds; periungual atrophy; corneal staining (88% by fluorescein: Nejm 1967;

276:1168); rheumatoid nodules (Ann IM 1970;72:49); lymphadenopathy (30%), especially with suppressed T-cell type (Nejm
1985;312:1671)

Crs: 90% 10-yr survival, worse w hypertension and/or nephritis;
peripheral neuropathy usually regresses

Cmplc:

- Infections, most common cause of death
- Nephritis, w nephrotic syndrome (prognosis no worse if have:
  Nejm 1983;308:187), and renal failure
- Serositis with pleuritis, pericarditis, and effusions
- Hemolytic anemia (Am J Med 2000;108:198), agranulocytosis
  (Ann IM 1984;100:197) and thrombocytopenia
- Neurologic vasculitis, peripheral neuropathy, visual cortex
  (Ann IM 1975;83:163) and diffuse CNS involvement often
  cause seizures (Ann IM 1974;81:763), transverse myelopathy
  (Ann IM 1976;84:46), chorea
- Nasal septum ulceration and perforation (Nejm 1969;281:722)
- Liebman-Sachs endocarditis (Nejm 1988;319:817) with AI
  and MR; present in > 50%? and associated w 22% incidence
  of cmplc (Nejm 1996;335:1424)
- Newborn heart block (Nejm 1983;309:209), fetal distress and
  loss from lupus anticoagulant
- Thromboses, venous and arterial, from lupus anticoagulant, an
  antiphospholipid antibody (p 147)
- Sjögren's
- Bleeding from factor IX and XI inhibition (Ann IM
  1972;77:543)
- Pneumonitis and fibrosis from immune complexes (Ann IM
  1979;91:30)
- Cystitis (Ann IM 1983;98:323)
- Tendon rupture
- Ischemic heart disease incidence increased 2.5× (Nejm
  2003;349:2399,2407)

Lab: *Hem:* Thrombocytopenia, leukopenia, hemolytic and ncnc anemia (Ann IM 1977;86:220); ESR elevated

Path: Skin bx shows specific IgG immunofluorescence at epidermal–dermal junction in all skin, in contrast to only affected skin in discoid lupus (Ann IM 1969;71:753)

Renal bx (Nejm 1974;291:693; Ann IM 1970;73:929) may show:

- Benign focal proliferative glomerulonephritis (may progress to b)
- Diffuse proliferative GN with elevated BUN and nephrotic syndrome
- Membranous GN with nephrotic syndrome

Serol: ANAs (p 1135):

- Total ANA > 1/64 in 95% over time, especially peripheral pattern; in drug-induced types, diffuse/homogeneous patterns most common
- Anti-Sm, very specific but not sensitive (present in 20-35%)
- Anti-Ro
- Anti-RNP (soluble nuclear antigen antibodies; elevated in 50%), but also elevated in mixed connective tissue disease, levels correlate with SLE psychosis (Nejm 1987;317:265)
- Antihistones positive in many cases of drug-induced SLE, 50% of other SLE, 20% in RA
- Anti-DNA antibodies against double-stranded (natural) DNA are specific but not sensitive (miss half of cases), associated w renal disease
- Anti-DNA against single-stranded DNA is nonspecific
    STSs: VDRL falsely positive; FTA falsely positive
    Complement levels decreased, $C_3' < 100$ mg % and $CH_{50} < 50$ U, especially with renal disease

Rx: Flu shots, don't cause flareup (Ann IM 1978;88:729)
ASA (or indomethacin) to tinnitus-producing levels

OH-chloroquine 250 mg qd, < 3.5 mg/lb relatively safe
(p 1072)

of renal disease (Nejm 2004;350:971,1044): Systemic
steroids and 7 mo of iv cyclophosphamide, then maintenance
with mycophenolate mofetil (Nejm 2000;343:1156), or azathioprine; renal transplant, rarely recurs in transplant (Ann IM 1991;
114:183)

of rare bullous eruption: Dapsone (Ann IM 1982;97:165)

Temporal Arteritis (Giant Cell Arteritis; Granulomatous Arteritis) and Polymyalgia Rheumatica

Nejm 2003;349:160, 2002;347:261; Ann IM 2003;139:505

Cause: Autoimmune

Epidem: TA = 15-25/100,000; female/male = 5-17:1; usually in pts
> 60 yr old, peaks in age 70-80 decade. Cyclic incidence w 10-yr
peaks (Ann IM 1995;123:192). Occasionally associated w
HLA DR_4 (J Rheum 1983;10:659). Incidence over age 50 of
PMR = 1/133.

Pathophys: Large-vessel vasculitis (r/o Takayasu's arteritis: Ann IM
1985;103:121); exists in a spectrum ranging from a little patchy
involvement of medium vessels with arteritis in PMR to much
more w TA. Muscle pain is probably claudication.

Sx: Fever; polymyalgia syndrome w muscle aches and weakness esp in
quads (33%) (Ann IM 1995;123:192); headache (77%) and scalp
pain; sore throat and cough (Ann IM 1984;101:594); leg, tongue,
and jaw claudication; weakness, malaise, and weight loss; synovitis, shoulder and hip pain

Si: Fever (27%) up to 103°F; mild muscle tenderness, asx knee effusions (8/18), tender indurated temporal arteries (67% sens, 99%
specif in TA: Ann IM 2002;137:232), cherry-red macular spot of
retinal artery occlusion

Am Coll Rheum criteria (Arthritis Rheum 1990;33:1122) require 3 of 5 findings:

- Age > 50
- New localized headache
- Temporal artery tender or diminished pulse
- ESR > 50 mm/hr
- Biopsy pathology positive

Crs: PMR and TA resolve in ±2 yr; 30-50% recurrence. No increased mortality with PMR (Ann IM 1978;88:162).

Cmplc: Sudden cranial nerve defects (17%), especially blindness, preventable with steroids and occurs in first 12 wk if going to; psychosis; MI and CVA are the most common causes of death; aortic dissections and thoracic aneurysms (Ann IM 1995;122:502); hypothyroidism (5%) (Brit J Rheum 1991;30:349)

Lab: *Chem:* Normal muscle enzymes, negative rheumatoid titer; liver function tests often slightly elevated

Hem: ESR elevated [increased α_2-globulin > 40 mg % (97%)], usually > 100, often only abnormal test; elevated CRP; crit = 30-40% in 14/18, hgb < 11 gm % (23%)

Path: Muscle bx normal; temporal artery bx (take 3-4 cm) shows patchy (easily missed) giant cell arteritis, which remains positive even after 14 d of prednisone rx (Ann IM 1994;120: 987); do it if palpably abnormal arteries or claudication sx in their distribution

Urine: UA usually normal

Xray: Color duplex US of temporal arteries shows hypoechogenic edema around arteries, "halo sign" (73% sens, ? 100% specif) (Nejm 1997;337:1336,1385) vs much worse (meta-analysis: Ann IM 2005;142:359)

Annual chest xray to watch for thoracic aneurysm
MRI of joints shows synovitis

Rx: Prednisone 40-60 mg (10-15 mg for PMR) po qd × 12 wk, then decrease to control sx's; keep up at least for 2 yr (Ann IM 1972;77:845); qod doesn't work (Ann IM 1975;82:613); use calcium and vitamin D to prevent osteoporosis biphosphonates if bone densities diminished

Methotrexate 10 mg po q 1 wk allows lower steroid doses (Ann IM 2001;134:106; Arthritis + Rheum 1991;345:A43) in TA; not clearly helpful in PMR (Ann IM 2004;141:493,568)

Wegener's Granulomatosis

Nejm 1997;337:1512; Ann IM 1992;116:488

Cause: *Staphylococcus aureus* nasal carriage associated w relapses possibly through induction of autoimmunity (Ann IM 1994;120:12)

Epidem: Rare, but all forms of ANCA-associated small-vessel vasculitis are the most common type of vasculitis in adults

Pathophys: ANCA-associated necrotizing granulomatous vasculitis of small blood vessels of the upper and lower respiratory tract (90%) and kidney (80%, although < 20% on presentation)

Sx: Purulent rhinitis; sinusitis; insidious onset; fever; arthralgias, pneumonitis

Si: Pneumonitis, sinusitis, otitis media, rhinitis, peripheral neuropathies, purpura, arthritis

Crs: Fatal in 80% at 1 yr, and 93% at 2 yr without rx; 95% survival with rx (Ann IM 1983;98:76)

Cmplc: Pulmonary insufficiency (20% of fatalities), massive pulmonary hemorrhage, tracheal sclerosis w stridor (15% adults, 50% children); renal failure (80% of fatalities)

r/o **midline granuloma** with local facial erosion, rx with xray (Ann IM 1976;84:140); malignant or benign **lymphomatoid angiitis and granulomatosis**; other ANCA-associated vasculitis (see below)

Lab: *Chem:* Creatinine elevated, IgA increased in blood and secretions, normal IgG and IgM

Hem: ESR elevated, eosinophilia

Path: Bx of nose, throat, and lung show focal angiitis with granulomas; bx of kidney shows GN

Serol: IgG antineutrophil cytoplasmic antibodies (p-ANCA or c-ANCA) elevated, 66% sens, 98% specif (Ann IM 1995; 123:925), can use to follow rx; but as many as $^1/_3$ of positive pts may have polyarteritis or idiopathic renal vasculitis? (Ann IM 1990;113:656); r/o other ANCA-associated small-vessel vasculitis: microscopic angiitis, Churg-Strauss syndrome, and drug-induced type

Urine: Red cell casts

Xray: Cavitating pulmonary nodule

Rx: Rapid rx, crucial to survival, w methotrexate or cyclophosphamide ~2 mg/kg/d to keep polys count $\geq$ 3000 + prednisone iv at 7 mg/kg/d at first then tapering to 1 mg/kg/d then change to qod over 3-4 mo; 93% complete remission, 30% cure? with good long-term survival. Azothiaprine maintenance safer and as good as cyclophosphamide (Nejm 2003;349:36) for all ANCA-associated vascultis? Etanercept no help (Nejm 2005;352:351).

Tm/S DS given bid as prophylaxis decreases recurrences by preventing immune-stimulating infections (Nejm 1996;335:16) esp by staph, helps 90%? (Ann IM 1987;106:840); decreases pneumocystis infections in pts on cyclophosphamide

18.6 Crystal Diseases

Gout

Cause: Hyperuricemia, with pain due to wbc ingestion of crystals? Primary type is due to a transferase deficiency (normally salvages urate); may be genetic, sporadic. Secondary type is due to tissue breakdown or decreased renal tubular excretion or urate.

Epidem: Primary type more common in higher social classes; male/female = 20:1; peak onset in males age ~30 yr and post-menopausally in women

Secondary type seen w leukemia especially when being rx'd, polycythemia, hemolytic anemia, starvation even in obese, diuretic rx, moonshine drinkers due to lead in alcohol (Nejm 1969; 280:1199), alcoholics because of increased urate production and perhaps decreased excretion

Pathophys: In kidneys, uric acid is normally 100% filtered, 100% resorbed, 100% excreted in distal tubule but may be competitively inhibited by lactate, ETOH, ketone bodies. Podagra from traumatically increased synovial fluid from which water is resorbed at night faster than urate, leading to a gouty attack (Ann IM 1977; 86:230,234).

Sx: Family hx (50%); podagra (inflammation/swelling of 1st mp joint of big toe) (84%) or other severely painful arthritis; low-dose ASA (< 4 gm) precipitates and/or worsens

Si: Arthritis including podagra, tophi (ear > elbow > finger > foot)

Crs: Acute attacks last 1-14 d, sx free between attacks but increasing frequency over years; without rx, permanent damage ensues

Cmplc: DJD; no increase in pseudogout; renal stones, but nephropathy is associated only with lead-related gout (Nejm 1981;304:520)

r/o sarcoid arthritis, which also improves with colchicine (Nejm 1971;285:1503); Reiter's; septic joint; RA; pseudogout; DJD; rare hyperuricemic X-linked recessive **Lesch-Nyhan syndrome**, characterized by choreoathetosis, dystonic spasticity, and self-mutilation (Nejm 1996;334:1568)

Lab: *Chem:* Uric acid > 10 mg %, r/o other causes:
- Idiopathic without gout (10% of Framingham population have)
- Hemolysis
- Leukemia

- Diuretics
- Psoriasis
- Fanconi's syndrome
- Chronic beryllium disease
- Down's syndrome (never get gout)
- Starvation
- Lead poisoning
- Alcoholism

> False depressions of uric acid from uricosurics, eg, ASA,
> allopurinol, radiocontrast agents (Ann IM 1971;74:845);
> false increases from methyldopa, Ld-opa

Joint fluid: With polarizing scope, long thin urate crystals, some
inside wbc's, negatively birefringent (yellow when parallel to
red filter axis, blue when perpendicular)

Urine: 24-hr urine acid $\geq$ 1 gm; urate/creatinine ratio > 0.75;
$urate_u/creat_u \times creat_s/creat_u > 0.7$ = high excretor on am
spot urine (Ann IM 1979;91:44)

Xray: Soft tissue swelling; in chronic type, DJD and punched-out areas
of bone

Rx (Nejm 1996;334:445):

Prevention: No need to rx asx mild increases in uric acid

> Diet: Minimize dairy products, minimize meat and seafood
(Nejm 2004;350:1095)

> Meds:

- Colchicine 1-2 mg po qd
- Probenecid 1-3 gm po qd divided, start with 0.5 gm; or
- Sulfinpyrazone 800 mg po qd divided; both prevent 100%
  resorption, use especially if 24-hr urine urate < 600 mg
- Allopurinol 200-400 mg po qd if 24-hr urate > 600 mg, or renal
  disease (decrease dose to 100 mg qd in anuria to prevent rash/
  fever/hepatitis syndrome, or tophi; can precipitate an attack)

> Acute: if attack < 10 d old:

- Colchicine 0.6 mg po q 1 hr up to 7 mg; renal excretion, inhibits microtubular (actin) formation and hence decreases

lysozymes, which cause inflammation; adverse effects: NV+D, B_{12} malabsorption from ileum (Nejm 1968;279:845), alopecia, decreased wbc's; myo- and neuropathies (Nejm 1987;316: 1562); or

- Indomethacin 50 mg po t-qid until relief then rapid taper over a week; or
- Steroids intra-articularly or systemically; or ACTH 80 IU im/iv, then 40 mg 12 hr later (Arthritis Rheum 1988;31:803) especially if sx > 10 d

Pseudogout

Cause: Calcium pyrophosphate crystals

Epidem: Increased incidence in hemochromatosis, hypothyroidism, hypoMg^{2+}, hyperparathyroidism, gout, RA, DJD

Pathophys: Poly ingestion of crystals results in enzyme release in the joint and subsequent inflammation

Sx: Acute arthritis

Si: Knee > mcp > wrist > shoulder

Crs:

Cmplc: r/o calcium oxalate deposition in renal failure (Ann IM 1982;97:36)

Lab: *Joint fluid:* With a polarizing scope, calcium pyrophosphate crystals (rhomboid, positively birefringent in red filter) (p 1102), may be small and require oil immersion lens to see

Xray: Semilunar calcifications of joint cartilages

Rx: Indomethacin; local steroid joint injections or systemic steroids

18.7 Inherited and Other Rheumatologic Diseases

Amyloidosis

Nejm 2002;346:1786,1818, 1997;337:902

Cause: Deposition of short-chain proteins in many parts of the body; several proteins are responsible for such deposition:

AL: Immunoglobulin light-chain amyloidosis (primary type): patients with B- or plasma cell disorders like multiple myeloma or Waldenström's; idiopathic

AF: Abnormal familial protein subunit found in affected families, usually present in middle or late life as myocardiopathy or neuropathy (Nejm 1997;336:466)

AA: Amyloidosis (secondary type) associated w SAA protein, an acute-phase reactant: collagen vascular diseases, Crohn's disease, cystic fibrosis, iv drug use, chronic infections (tbc, familial Mediterranean fever, osteomyelitis, etc)

AH: β_2-microglobulin accumulated in serum of dialysis pts

AP: Normal serum protein

Epidem:

Pathophys: Infiltration of organs by protein; in all types: kidney, liver, spleen, gi tract, skin; in AL type, predominantly vessels, heart, marrow, lung infiltration with hemoptysis, joints (synovium), peripheral nerves, factor X deficiency, pancreatic islets (in myeloma, light chains taken up by macrophages, then excreted into interstitium where polymerized: Nejm 1982;307:1689)

Sx: Exertional muscle pain (due to arteriole infiltration and ischemia); fatigue; carpal tunnel syndrome

Si: Hepatosplenomegaly; raised skin plaques, if rubbed results in purpura, "greasy nose syndrome" (amyloid infiltration); "shoulder pad" deposition associated with arthropathy (Nejm 1973;288:354); RA-like acute arthritis; "scalloped pupils" in familial type

(Nejm 1975;293:914); macroglossia (AL type only; sensory and autonomic neuropathy)

Crs: AA-type amyloidosis may revert, especially the nephrotic syndrome, with rx of the primary disease (Nejm 1970;282:128)

Cmplc: Functional asplenia; nephrotic syndrome; CHF; water-losing nephropathy (r/o DI and postobstructive syndrome); factor X deficiency, which rx with splenectomy (Nejm 1981;304:827); peripheral or polyneuropathy (Nejm 1991;325:1482); atrial thrombi and embolization (Nejm 1992;327:1570)

Lab: *Path:* Rectal or other tissue bx shows protein infiltration with green birefringence on polarizing scope exam with Congo red staining; in AA type, Congo red affinity can be leached out by K-permanganate unlike AL type. Normal-appearing skin will be positive in ~ half of all pts with either type.
Urine: 24-hr protein > 3 gm and thus nephrotic

Xray: Chest shows cardiomegaly if cardiac infiltration. Serum amyloid P scan (Nejm 1990;323:508).

Rx: AA type: Rx primary disease
AL type: Rx with melphalan + stem cell transplant, 40% 1-yr cure (Nejm 2004;140:85). Plasma exchange helps neuropathies (Nejm 1991;325:1482).
AF type: Liver transplant (Ann IM 1997;127:618)
In cardiomyopathy, avoid calcium-channel blockers and digoxin (Am J Cardiol 1985;55:1645)

Familial Mediterranean Fever

Nejm 2001;345:1748

Cause: Autosomal recessive MEFV gene on chromosome 16

Epidem: Eastern Mediterraneans, especially Sephardic Jews and Armenians; gene prevalence in some of these populations is as high as 1/14-1/21 (Nejm 1992;326:1509)

Pathophys: Diffuse serositis in abdomen, chest, and joints; associated with deficiency of a serosal protease that is a C_{5a} inhibitor (Nejm 1984;311:287, 325) and deficiency of interleukin-8

Sx: Onset in childhood or adolescence; positive family hx (30%)

Intermittent fever, abdominal pain lasting usually < 1 day, pleurisy (40%), monoarticular joint pains without residua especially in knees, acute scrotal attack (5%), myalgias for 6 wk

Si: Acute abdomen (peritonitis), splenomegaly, big kidneys

Crs: Death from amyloidosis before age 40 yr without rx

Cmplc: Amyloidosis (40%) with nephrosis, less in U.S. than in Europe, colchicine rx helps (Nejm 1986;314:1001; Ann IM 1977;87:568); drug addiction, depression; infertility

r/o similar hyper-IgD syndrome, and TNF receptor-associated periodic syndrome

Lab: *PCR:* Amplification refractory mutation system (ARMS) identifies 80% (Ann IM 1998;129:539)

Hem: ESR elevated, fibrinogen and other acute-phase reactants increased

Joint fluid: Poor viscosity, polys > 5000 and up to 10,000

Xray: Periosteal new bone about femoral condyles (pathognomonic)

Rx: Colchicine 0.6 mg q 1 hr up to 4-6 pills for acute attack; works in $> \frac{1}{2}$ (Ann IM 1977;86:162), then 0.6-1 mg po qd-qid to prevent (Ann IM 1974;81:792; Nejm 1974;291:832,934); 1-2 mg po qd × 15+ yr works and is safe even in pregnancy (Semin Arth Rheum 1991;20:241). Colchicine decreases polys migration rate so can't clump so fast to exceed C_{5a} inhibitor activity (Nejm 1984;311:287); prevents amyloid long term (Nejm 1986;314:1001).

Langerhans Cell Histiocytosis (Histiocytosis X), Letterer-Siwe Disease, Hand-Schuller-Christian Syndrome, and Eosinophilic Granuloma

Nejm 1994;331:154

Cause: None are genetic

Epidem: Several dozen/yr at Boston Children's Hospital

Pathophys: Spectrum ranges from lethal Hans-Schuller-Christian (HSC) leukemia-like disorder primarily affecting infants to curable solitary lytic lesions of bone (eosinophilic granuloma, [EG]). A monoclonal, probably neoplastic proliferation of histiocytes that look like Langerhans giant cells; these invade lung, marrow, pituitary, liver, bone, and subcutaneous areas.

Sx: Letterer-Siwe (LS): In infants only; rash
HSC: Youngest onset
EG: Oldest onset; often asx; or cough, weight loss, hemoptysis, chest pain

Si: LS: Papular/vesicular rash with white center and red rim, also on mucous membranes; lymphadenopathy; hepatomegaly; xantholasmata, xanthomas, even infiltration into cornea; saddle nose
HSC: Triad of (1) exophthalmus, (2) diabetes insipidus, and (3) punched-out bone lesions
EG: Localized often, eg, in lung, or in bone especially head and pelvis; fever

Crs: Histocytosis X: In adults (Nejm 2002;346:484), median survival = 12.5 yr from dx; die of respiratory failure; 60% mortality when occurs in infants
LS: Rapidly fatal
HSC: More slowly fatal
EG: 50% recover, 50% progress

Cmplc: In all, diabetes insipidus in 40% by 5 yr (Nejm 1989;321:1157)

EG: Spontaneous pneumothorax (10%) in pulmonary variety; skin invasion

Lab: *Noninv:* PFTs in EG show obstructive and restrictive mixed pattern, impaired diffusion capacity; pO_2 may be normal at rest but decreases with exercise

Path: Skin bx of rash shows histiocytes in LS; fibrosis, sclerosis, cholesterol phagocytosis in HSC; eosinophils in EG. Scalene node or lung bx even in asx pt will usually show diagnostic changes in EG.

Xray: In EG, chest shows diffuse reticular pattern, bone survey shows lytic lesions

Rx: Steroids may help at least pulmonary forms
Radiation if in skin or single organ, eg, bone lesion
Marrow transplant (Nejm 1987;316:733)

Marfan's Syndrome

Cause: Genetic, autosomal dominant on chromosome 15 (Nejm 1994;331:148, 1992;326:905); however, 15% of cases are sporadic

Epidem:

Pathophys: Defect in elastic collagen caused by a defect in microfibrillar fibers on which elastin is laid (Nejm 1990;323:152); cystic medical necrosis of thoracic aorta (95%)

Sx: Positive family hx; tall; frequent joint dislocations with minor trauma

Si: Arachnodactyly, arm span > height; hernias; lenticular dislocations (80%) upward, unlike downward in homocystinuria; aortic insufficiency (60%) with click, also mitral insufficiency due to posterior leaflet prolapse; arched palate

Crs: Average age at death is 32 yr, most from aortic root dilatation causes such as dissection, rupture, and aortic and mitral insufficiencies (Nejm 1972;286:804)

Cmplc: Aortic dissection (12%), accounts for 90% of deaths (Nejm 1986;314:1070); SBE; vascular rupture during pregnancy (Ann IM 1995;123:117)

r/o homocystinuria (p 317); **Ehlers-Danlos syndrome** (Nejm 2001;345:1167, 2000;342:675, 730) due to genetic collagen defects; all types have skin fragility, bruising, DJD; type IVs die from aortic, arterial, bowel, or uterine rupture; not usually associated w hyperextensibility types

Lab:

Xray: Chest; echocardiogram

Rx: Of scoliosis (p 881)

of ascending aortic aneurysm: Propranolol qid po or other β-blocker to keep exercise P < 100, slows progression of aortic disease (Nejm 1994;330:1335); or surgical when 6+ cm

Osteoarthritis

Cause:

Endogenous factors:

- Changes in articular cartilage like increased brittleness, decreased water binding, decreased chrondroitin sulfate, perhaps increased protein/polysaccharide ratio
- Lubrication and viscosity failure
- Genetic defects in procollagen (Nejm 1990;322:526), which are autosomal dominant

Exogenous factors:

- Trauma, including injuries decades before (Ann IM 2000;133:321)
- Congenital anomalies
- Metabolic diseases like gout and ochronosis
- Endocrine diseases like acromegaly
- Inflammatory joint diseases
- Obesity, increases knee DJD especially (Am J Med 1999;107:542)

Epidem: Older pts

Pathophys: Rv of pathophys (Nejm 1989;320:1322)

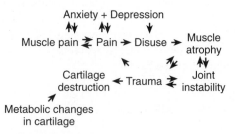

Figure 18.1 Pathophysiology of DJD.

Quadriceps weakness may precede and somehow cause knee arthritis (Ann IM 1997;127:97)

Pain due to adjacent marrow space edema (Ann IM 2001;134:541, 591)

Sx: Post-rest stiffness, pain on motion. Joints most frequently involved are great toe and thumb mcp's, knee, hip, sacral and cervical spine.

Si: Motion preserved but local tenderness. Bony enlargement at dip joints called Heberden's nodes, or at pip joints called Bouchard's nodes. Local inflammation occasionally, especially in erosive osteoarthritis variant with hot joints seen in middle-aged women.

Crs:

Cmplc: CNS sx's from cord or vertebral artery compression **(cervical spondylosis)** occasionally causing paraplegia; but neck, head, and shoulder pain all common

r/o avascular necrosis: of femoral head, especially in pts on steroids, alcoholics, or with sickle cell disease; of knee, medial femoral condyle, or tibia in elderly pts (Bull Rheum Dis 1985;35:42)

Lab: *Path:* Synovial bx shows fibrous cartilaginous degeneration especially at points of stress

Xray: Hypertrophic changes, eg, osteophytes, sclerosis, and bone cysts without cortical bone changes unlike RA; MRI shows marrow edema (Ann IM 2003;139:330)

Rx (Rheum Dis Clin N Am 2003;29:4; Ann IM 2000;133:726): Braces, exercise (Ann IM 2000;132:173 vs 2003;138:613), weight reduction, psychiatric rx, patellar taping (DBRCT: BMJ 2004;327:135)

Calcium + vitamin D po to prevent osteoporosis and slow progression (Ann IM 1996;125:353)

Acupuncture by DBCT (Ann IM 2004;141:901)

NSAIDs of debatable efficacy (NSAIDs for OA of hip, 2003; Cochrane Library issue 4); acetaminophen helps pain (Nejm 1991;325:87)

Glucosamine sulfate 500 mg po tid OTC dietary supplement may help (Med Let 2001;43:111) but may worsen diabetic control and variable purity of OTC products

Chondroitin sulfate may also help (Jama 2000;283:1469) but studies not rigorous, as w glucosamine

Intra-articular:
- Steroid injection may help as long as joint is stable
- Hyaluronic acid (Hyalgan, Synvisc) (ACP J Club 2003;138:20; Rheumatol 1999;38:602; Med Let 1998;40:69) weekly × 3-5; of dubious benefit by meta-analysis (Jama 2003;290:3115); $700

Surgical arthroplasties, joint replacements (hip: Nejm 1990;323:725; knee: Nejm 1990;323:801), arthroscopic lavage and/or debridement at least in knee no help by DBCT (Nejm 2002;347:81)

Experimental: Leeches 4 at a time q 3 mo better than topical NSAIDs! (? Ann IM 2003;139:724)

Osteomyelitis

Nejm 1997;336:999

Cause: *S. aureus* (60%), tuberculosis, group A strep, haemophilus, pneumococcus, salmonella, gonorrhea, enterobacter, fungal; in neonates, group B strep, *E. coli*; pseudomonas in drug addicts, in sneaker wearers who step on nails

- Hematogenous via bacteremia, especially in children with open epiphyses, starts in metaphysis
- Compound fractures and other open injury with bone contamination, eg, surgery
- Direct extension from adjacent infected tissue, eg, joint

Epidem: 85% of cases are children; salmonella osteomyelitis very frequent in sickle disease; also common in diabetics w foot ulcers (Nejm 1994;331:854) and pts w decubitus ulcers (Arch IM 1983;143:683)

Pathophys: Bacteremia results in bacteria being picked up by slow blood flow area of metaphysis; infection can't penetrate epiphysis so moves down bone via haversian and Volkmann's canals; may rupture through thin metaphyseal cortical bone; sequestration of dead bone prolongs recovery. Persistence may be a result of intracellular survival especially w tuberculosis.

Sx: Localized pain; antalgic use of limb; fever

Si: Often nothing besides fever; may have local redness, swelling, drainage

Crs: 20% mortality without antibiotics; chronicity in 15% even with rx

Cmplc: Altered (increased or decreased) epiphyseal growth of one limb due to changes in blood supply, Brodie's abscess, sequestration and reactivation years later, acute glomerulonephritis (Ann IM 1969;71:335), amyloidosis, local epidermoid carcinoma in 0.5%

Lab: *Bact:* Blood cultures; if negative, bone aspiration is positive in 60%, bone bx is positive in 90%. Culture of draining sinus unreliable.

Hem: ESR elevated (but not always: Nejm 1987;316:763)

Xray: MRI or CT very sensitive, esp early before changes on plain films

Plain films may show gross deformities with lytic and blastic activity after 2-4 wk

Bone scan positive within weeks, 50-75% false pos, 70-90% sens (J Gen Intern Med 1992;7:158)

Rx: Appropriate long-term parenteral antibiotics (see Table 18.2) and surgical removal of sequestrum

Table 18.2 Antibiotic Treatment of Osteomyelitis in Adults[1]

Microorganisms Isolated	Treatment of Choice	Alternatives
S. aureus Penicillin-sensitive	Penicillin G (4 million units every 6 hr)	First-generation cephalosporin (e.g., cefazolin, 2 g every 6 hr), clindamycin (600 mg every 6 hr), or vancomycin (1 g every 12 hr)
Penicillin-resistant	Nafcillin (2 g every 6 hr)	First-generation cephalosporin, clindamycin (as above), or vancomycin (as above)
Methicillin-resistant	Vancomycin (1 g every 12 hr)	Teicoplanin (400 mg every 24 hr; first day, every 12 hr intravenously or intramuscularly)‡
Various streptococci (group A or B β-hemolytic or *Streptococcus pneumoniae*)	Penicillin G (4 million units every 6 hr)	Clindamycin (as above), erythromycin (500 mg every 6 hr), vancomycin (as above), or ceftriaxone (2 g once a day)
Enteric gram-negative rods	Quinolone (ciprofloxacin, 750 mg every 12 hr orally)	Third-generation cephalosporin (e.g., ceftriaxone, 2 g every 24 hr)

Serratia or *Pseudomonas aeruginosa*	Ceftazidime (2 g every 8 hr) (with aminoglycosides for at least the first 2 wk)§	Imipenem (500 mg every 6 hr), piperacillin–tazobactam (4 g and 0.5 g, respectively, every 8 hr), or cefepime (2 g every 12 hr) (with aminoglycosides for at least the first 2 wk)§
Anaerobes	Clindamycin (600 mg every 6 hr intravenously or orally)	Amoxicillin–clavulanic acid (2.0 and 0.2 g, respectively, every 8 hr) or metronidazole for gram-negative anaerobes (500 mg every 8 hr)
Mixed aerobic and anaerobic microorganisms	Amoxicillin–clavulanic acid (2.0 and 0.2 g, respectively, every 8 hr)	Imipenem (500 mg every 6 hr)¶

*All antibiotic treatments are given intravenously unless otherwise stated.

†In Europe, fludoxacillin is the treatment of choice.

‡Teicoplanin is currently available only in Europe.

§Aminoglycosides may be given once a day or in multiple doses.

¶Imipenem should be given when infection is due to aerobic gram-negative microorganisms resistant to amoxicillin–clavulanic acid.

RHEUMATOLOGY/ORTHOPEDICS

Paget's Disease

Nejm 1997;336:558

Cause: Benign neoplasia of bone remodeling unit?

Epidem: 3% of population will develop it sometime in lifetime, although severe disease much less common

Pathophys: Excessive formation and destruction of bone constantly; normally sequence is increased osteoclast activity followed by increased osteoblast activity; in Paget's, the rate of this progression is markedly increased (Nejm 1973;289:15). High blood flow due to idiopathic shunting at a capillary level, no true arteriovenous shunts (Nejm 1972;287:686). Increased vertebral size leads to neural compression syndromes.

Sx: Fractures; knee, hip, and other joint arthritis; bone pain

Si: Angioid streaking of retina (r/o sickle cell disease and pseudoxanthoma elasticum) (p 183); deformed long bones; head enlargement

Crs:

Cmplc: CNS compression syndromes including deafness from calvarial deformities (eg, Beethoven), pathologic fractures, high-output CHF, osteogenic sarcoma (2%), renal stones especially with immobilization, heart block due to bundle calcifications

Lab: *Chem:* Alkaline phosphatase increased markedly, highest values of any disease, r/o osteomalacia (Am J Med 2000;108;296)
Urine: Calcium and phosphate levels elevated

Xray: Sclerotic bone, expanded bone size (only Paget's will do this); bone scan hot spots correlate with pain sx better than plain film changes (Ann IM 1973;79:348)

Rx:

1st: Bisphosphonates (p 413)
- Alendronate (Fosamax) 40 mg po qd; $120/mo
- Etidronate (Didronel) 5-20 mg/kg/d po × 6 mo (see Nejm 1990;323:73 for use in osteoporosis), can cause fractures at high doses (Ann IM 1982;96:619)

- Pamidronate (Aredia) 60 mg iv over 24 hr q 1-3 yr (Med Let 1992;34:1)
- Risedronate (Actonel) (Med Let 1998;40:89) 30 mg po qd × 2 mo; $763
- Tiladronate (Skelid) (Med Let 1997;39:65) 400 mg po qd; $450/mo

2nd: Calcitonin, human 0.5 mg sc, $177/mo (Med Let 1987; 29:47); or salmon calcitonin (Calcimar) (Jama 1972;221: 1127) 50 U sc qd until asx, then tiw, $81/mo. Both inhibit osteocyte progenitor duplication and speed conversion of clasts to blasts (Ann IM 1981;95:192).

Others: Gallium nitrate? iv/sc for weeks (Ann IM 1991;114:846)

Sarcoidosis

Jama 2003;289:3300; Nejm 1997;336:1224

Cause:

Epidem: 10-50/100,000/yr in U.S.; black/white = 1:6; associated with regional enteritis

Pathophys: Activated T cells (also seen in Crohn's disease, perhaps same pathophysiology) and macrophages, unclear why activated. Granuloma formation without necrosis or inflammation, often involves lung, skin, and RES; occasionally bone, kidney, eye, gi tract. Hypercalcemia due to increased vitamin D sensitivity.

Sx: Fatigue, weight loss, fever/malaise

Si: Dyspnea, cough, rales; neurologic (Ann IM 1977;87:336); uveitis, anterior chamber tissue masses, corneal precipitant and band keratopathy; splenomegaly, lymphadenopathy; skin lesions blanch with pressure, residual brown pigment, erythema nodosum on shins without scarring

Crs: 75-90% spontaneous resolution without rx in 2 yr

Cmplc: Restrictive lung disease (r/o chronic berylliosis: Ann IM 1988; 108:687); pulmonary cavities with aspergillus; pleuritis occasionally with exudative lymphocytic effusions (Ann IM 1974;81:190); hypercalcemia and hypercalciuria with renal stones; meningitis with low sugar; pituitary tumors with thirst and diabetes insipidus; Bell's palsy; arthritis especially of knees and ankles

r/o primary biliary cirrhosis overlap syndrome; berrylliosis; Wegener's granulomatosis; tuberculosis; histoplasmosis; and **Löfgren's syndrome**, a sarcoid variant in young person w erythema nodosum, bilateral hilar adenopathy, and bilateral ankle arthritis that is self-limited in 6 mo w no residua (Am J Med 1999;107:240)

Lab: *Chem:* Elevated angiotensin converting enzyme, but very nonspecific; elevated Ca^{++}

Noninv: PFTs show decreased volumes, decreased diffusion capacity, pO_2 often ok at rest but decreases with exercise

Path: Bx of minor salivary gland, supraclavicular node, or transbronchial (95% positive) shows noncaseating granuloma

Xray: Hilar adenopathy and interstitial pattern (one or both present in 90%)

Gallium scan positive over lung (macrophages) and nodes; very nonspecific

Rx: Steroids, eg, prednisone 30-40 mg po qd × 8-12 wk, then taper to 10-20 mg qod over 6-12 mo; possibly anti-tumor necrosis factor (TNF) meds like infliximab (Ann IM 2001;135:27)

of skin: Chloroquine 250 mg po bid

of elevated calcium and/or renal calcium stones: Steroids, decrease vitamin D intake, chloroquine as above (Nejm 1986; 315:727)

18.8 Entrapment Syndromes

Anterior Compartment Syndrome, Chronic

Cause: Genetic predisposition?; or trauma

Epidem: Males in their 20s; trauma to anterior legs

Pathophys: Anterior tibial compartment claudication from congenitally or traumatically edematous small compartment, which prevents normal vascular engorgement of exercising muscles

Sx: Anterior shin pain especially if walking on heels, usually bilateral. Relief by walking on toes or resting; can run ok.

Si: BP can be auscultated after exercise over dorsalis pedis pulse without BP cuff. Muscle hernias through anterior fascial compartment.

Crs:

Cmplc: Ischemic necrosis of anterior tibial muscles possible even without pain

r/o **Shin splints** caused by periostitis and microfractures of bone; bone scan is positive; more frequent in osteoporotic athletes (Ann IM 1990;113:754); rx by discontinuation of running trauma

Acute anterior compartment syndrome after trauma, w acute swelling that, if not relieved surgically, can lead to ischemic death of anterior compartment muscles

Lab: *NIL:* Measurement of compartment pressures during exercise

Rx: Cross-friction massage; fasciotomies of anterior tibial compartments rarely indicated but fails only if don't expose all compartments

Low-Back Syndromes

Nejm 2001;344:363; Ann IM 1990;112:598

Cause: Ruptured herniated intervertebral disc; musculoligamentous strains/trauma; osteoarthritis of facet joints; perhaps leg length discrepancies; in elderly, vertebral compression fractures

Epidem: 65% of the population have low-back sx sometime in their lives; males = females; onset at age 30-50

Pathophys: Myofascial, skeletal, disc, and/or ligamentous entrapment/compression of nerve conduction/vascular flow, causing secondary edema, spasm and contracture, and/or neurosensory hyperstimulation or deficits

Sx: Focal (segmental) pain; distal radiation of burning/shooting pain and/or parestheisas, often worsened by cough; decreased range of motion due to pain and/or muscular restriction

Si: Rv of exam (Bull Rheum Dis 1983;33:4)

Straight leg raising $< 60°$ on affected side induces sx; if SLR on opposite side induces, this positive "crossed-leg sign" is highly specific for central disc rupture

Levels: Depression or loss of knee jerk = L_{3-4} (L_4 root); ankle jerk = L_5-S_1 (S_1 root); toe extensors especially extensor hallucis longus (big toe extensor) and sensation loss in medial foot especially between first and second toes = L_{4-5} (L_5 root)

Crs: Most ($> 90\%$) improve with conservative rx over several days to weeks and no w/u is required unless motor loss is present and does not improve or worsens over this time period. $^2/_3$ recur within 1 yr; pain lasts 2 mo on average (Spine 1993;18:1388).

Cmplc: Worker's compensation (Ann IM 1978;89:992); cauda equina syndrome w rectal or bladder dysfunction

r/o **Spinal stenosis**: pain, pseudoclaudication, numbness, worse with hips extended, eg, walking downhill; bilateral in $^2/_3$ (Ann IM 1985;103:271)

Lab:

Xray: MRI/CT good if observed abnormality correlates with sx and si, but $^1/_3$ of pts' CT interpreted as abnormal (Spine 1984;9:549); and, in normal asx people, bulges (50%) and protrusions (25%) are present on MRI (Nejm 1994;301:69). Initial plain films adequate (Jama 2003;289:2810).

Scanograms for leg length are the only way to measure but rarely needed; tapes are inaccurate (Spine 1983;8:643)

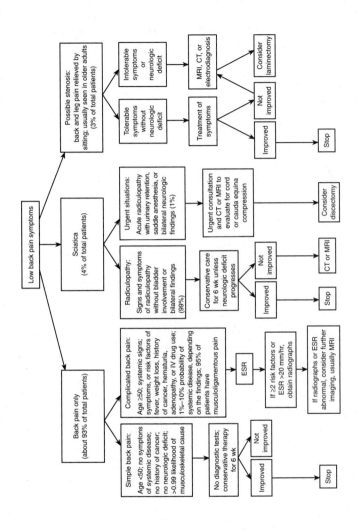

Figure 18.2 Suggested algorithm for the diagnostic evaluation of patients with low-back pain. Reproduced with permission from Jarvik JG, et al. Diagnosis evaluation of low back pain with emphasis on imaging. Ann Int Med 2002;137:593.

RHEUMATOLOGY/
ORTHOPEDICS

Rx: Prevention: Exercise programs w aerobic conditioning and leg/back strenghthening helps; back belts no help (Jama 2000; 284:2727)

Primary care strategy (Ann IM 1994;121:187), 70% better by 1 mo:

- Educate re chronic/recurrent nature but that severe flareups are time-limited
- Pain rx only as time-limited, scheduled regimens, not prn; limited (< 2 d) bed rest
- Referral for surgical evaluation only for abnormal neurologic findings
- Graded increasing activity even if pain not better/resolved
  Education and/or lumbar supports of questionable value (Jama 1998;279:1789)

Bed rest: Even 2 d bed rest slows recovery, as do exercises; best strategy is continued normal activity as tolerated (Nejm 1995;332:351), true even if have sciatic sx (Nejm 1999;340:418); hard bed/bed board not helpful? (Lancet 2003;362:1599)

NSAIDs; tricyclics, tetracyclics; heat; massage; muscle strengthening and flexibility exercises as well as a progressive fitness program (BMJ 1995;310:151); manipulation probably speeds recovery of acute and subacute types by 10-20% (RAND meta-analysis: Ann IM 1992;117:590). Exercise rx of acute pain is no help (Spine 1993;18:1388) but is helpful when chronic (> 4 wk) (BMJ 1999;319:279). Steroid injections no help (Nejm 1997;336:1634, 1991;325:1002). TENS no help in chronic back pain (ACP J Club 2001;135:99).

Manipulative techiques if not better in 3 wk, including high-velocity, low-amplitude; strain/counter strain; and craniosacral. Chiropractic or PT care of acute low-back pain is more expensive although more satisfying for pt w same result as primary care physician care (meta-analysis: Ann IM 2003;138:871; Nejm 1998;339:1021, 1995;333:913)

Surgery if worsening motor weakness after 2 wk; better than chymopapain injection (Spine 1992;17:381) or microsurgery, but long term the latter comes out the same if combined with medical rx (J Gen Intern Med 1993;8:487)

Of chronic low-back pain: Percutaneous electrical nerve stimulator (PENS) 30 min tiw × 3 wk helps (Jama 1999;281:818); magnets no help (Jama 2000;283:1322); multidisciplinary pain center referral; opioids not that helpful

Carpal Tunnel Syndrome

Jama 2000;283;3110, 2002;346:1807

Cause: Local swelling and entrapment of median nerve at wrist

Epidem: Associated with occupational repetitive hand movements (but not computer keyboard use?: Jama 2003;289:2963) in ⅔, also pregnancy, myxedema, amyloidosis, tumor, rheumatoid arthritis, tenosynovitis, acromegaly, diabetes, wrist fracture, gout, myeloma, ganglia, renal failure with chronic dialysis

Female/male = 2:1 usually, but in an occupational setting ratio is equal (Am J Pub Hlth 1991;81:741). Prevalence = 125-500/100,000 adults; but up to 15/100 in high-risk occupations; perhaps as high as 2+% (Jama 1999;282:153,186).

Pathophys: Swelling within the carpal tunnel formed by the transverse carpal ligament impairs blood flow to median nerve

Similar entrapment syndromes can occur elsewhere but are very rare, eg, very similar **tarsal tunnel syndrome** in lateral foot; in the pronator teres (Nejm 1970;282:858); or of the ulnar nerve at the wrist, usually sx there only after sx's in median nerve distribution first

Sx: Numbness in median nerve distribution of the hand; worse at night (77%), shaking and/or hanging improves; pain and paresthesias often radiate proximally to elbow and shoulder; later, weakness of pincer grip, eg, holding a cup

Si: No pain, position or touch loss objectively, but often hypesthesia in median nerve distribution. Thenar wasting (15%) from loss of all but short thumb flexor.

Tinel's sign (60% sens, 67% specif) = paresthesias when tap over median nerve at wrist; or Phalen's sign (75% sens, 47% specif) = paresthesias with forced wrist flexion for 60 sec; or median nerve paresthesias with 1 min of BP cuff pumped up above systolic pressure

Crs: Slowly progressive, or may wax and wane

Cmplc: Permanent loss of thenar median nerve function, weakness and/or numbness

r/o other causes of similar sx including Raynaud's, cervical arthritis w radiculopathy, bursitis of shoulder, thoracic outlet syndrome, and ulnar neuropathy from elbow entrapment, which is less easily helped by local measures (Nejm 1993;329:2016)

Lab: *Noninv:* EMG nerve conduction velocities markedly decreased (90% sens, ?% specif)

Rx: NSAIDs; steroids (BMJ 1999;319:884) 4 mg of methylprednisolone or 25 mg hydrocortisone locally injected proximally improves 80% at 1 mo, 50% at 1 yr; diuretics; splinting; change jobs; yoga program × 8 wk helps more than splint (Jama 1998;280:1601)

Surgical, especially if thenar wasting present, or if pt plans to continue heavy work, or when conservative rx has failed

De Quervain's Tenosynovitis

By James Glazer

J Am Acad Orthop Surg 2001;9(4):246-252; Clin Sports Med 1992;11:77

Cause: Overuse

Epidem: Common in occupational setting, throwers, racket sports

Pathophys: Tenosynovitis of tendons in 1st dorsal wrist compartment: one or both of extensor pollicus longus/brevis

Sx: Pain with gripping, lifting, movement of thumb. May have audible "squeak."

Si: TTP radial side of wrist, positive Finklestein's test (pain with flexion of thumb under clenched fingers with ulnar deviation at wrist)

Crs: Gradual or acute onset, usually associated with increase in activities involving wrist motion

Cmplc: May become chronic if untreated

Rx: Initially, anti-inflammatory modalities. Immobilize in thumb spica wrist splint. PT necessary to increase strength, ROM after acute inflammation resolved. Surgical synovectomy only in extreme resistant cases.

Gamekeeper's Thumb (Ulnar Collateral Ligament Sprain)

By James Glazer

J Am Acad Orthop Surg 2001;9:389-400

Cause: Forced valgus loading of the metacarpo-phalangeal joint of the thumb

Epidem: Fall on pole while skiing, classically gamekeepers twisting heads off birds

Pathophys: Sprain/rupture of ulnar collateral ligament or bony avulsion at insertion onto proximal phalanx

Sx: Immediate pain following fall. Weakened grasp.

Si: Swelling and redness at mcp. May be able to palpate avulsed tendon early in course before swelling. Pain and opening with valgus loading of mcp joint in 80° flexion.

Crs: Grade I-II (partial tears): Immobilize in thumb spica splint for 6 wk, longer if pain and laxity persists

Grade III (complete tear, no endpoint to valgus stressing):
   Surgical repair (see below)

Cmplc: Stener's lesion, related to complete UCL tear in which ligament end becomes trapped beneath palmar aponeurosis and does not heal

Xray: PA, lateral and oblique views of the finger. Valgus stress views only to r/o fracture. Stress angulation difference greater than 15° is positive for UCL sprain.

Rx: 6 wk immobilization; modified thumb spica cast vs splint. Surgery for grade III.

Jersey Finger (Flexor Digitorum Profundus Avulsion)

By James Glazer

Am Fam Phys 2001;63:1961; Hand Clin 2000;16:359

Cause: Forced extension of the distal interphalangeal joint

Epidem: Jersey tackle in football, lifting car door latch, ball sports. Digit 4 most commonly affected.

Pathophys: Rupture of flexor digitorum profundus or bony avulsion at FDP insertion onto distal phalanx

Sx: May be painless. H/o forced extension. Often presents late.

Si: Swelling and redness at DIPJ, inability to actively flex DIPJ while middle phalanx immobilized. Do not test strength in flexion—can cause retraction of tendon into wrist and complicate surgery. Pain and/or palpable bony deformity on volar aspect of distal phalanx.

Crs: Needs surgery for full recovery

Cmplc: Permanent DIPJ dysfunction if untreated. Refer to hand surgeon immediately. Delay leads to tendon retraction into wrist.

Xray: PA, lateral and oblique views of the finger. Splint and refer to hand.

Rx: Surgical tendon reattachment in all cases

Mallet Finger (Baseball Finger, Drop Finger)

By James Glazer

Fam Physic 2001;63:1961; Hand Clin 1995;11:373

Cause: Forced flexion of the distal interphalangeal joint

Epidem: Ball sports, falling. Digits 2 and 3 most commonly affected.

Pathophys: Rupture of extensor digitorum longus or bony avulsion at EDL insertion onto distal phalanx

Sx: May be painless. H/o forced flexion; pt may hear popping sound as injury occurs.

Si: Fexion deformity at DIPJ, inability to actively extend DIPJ. Pain and/or palpable bony deformity on dorsal aspect of distal phalanx.

Crs: Full recovery if treated

Cmplc: Permanent DIPJ dysfunction if untreated. Refer to hand surgeon if extensor lag present after 6-8 wk of splinting.

Xray: PA, lateral and oblique views of the finger. Refer to hand for avulsion fx involving > 30% of the articular surface. Post-reduction radiographs if applicable.

Rx: Splinting of the DIPJ in slight hyperextension for 6 wk, 8 wk for older adults, athletes. Reduce avulsion fx with dorsal pressure prior to splinting, needs only 4 wk splint. Finger must never fall into flexion; resplint for 6 wk if it does. Evaluate for extensor lag only after 6-8 wk (see above).

Plantar Fasciitis

By James Glazer

Nejm 2004;350:2159; Glazer/Brukner: Phys Sportsmed, 2004;32

Cause: Overuse, rapid increase in training load or intensity

Epidem: May be athletic or sedentary

Pathophys: Repetitive stress leads to microfracture; progresses to fasciosis with dysfunctional inflammatory response

Sx: Pain with weight bearing, worse with first steps in morning. May be relieved after some ambulation, then worse with continued weight bearing. Often bilateral, although only one side may be affected on presentation.

Si: Tenderness along plantar fascia, worst plantar medial on calcaneus. Worse with "Windlass test": dorsiflexion at ankle and extension of toes.

Crs: Generally self-limiting; most cases resolve spontaneously with rest. Can become chronic.

Cmplc: Chronicity. Plantar fascia rupture in small number of cases, causes resolution of symptoms without negative effect on foot biomechanics.

Xray: Plain films often show calcaneal spur, which results from the condition. Excising the spur does not help.

Rx: Activity modification
Footwear change (14% response rate) and prefabricated orthoses (95%)
Dorsiflexion night splints (80%)
Plantar-specific stretching
Corticosteroid injection (70%)
Surgical plantar release only if all other modalities fail (65-96%)
Shock wave ultrasound is new, expensive, and controversial

Stress Fractures

By James Glazer

Am J Sports Med 2001;29:100; Med Sci Sports Exerc 1999;37:S48; Phys Sportsmed 1999;27:57

Cause: Overuse, rapid increase in training load or intensity

Epidem: May be athletic or sedentary

Pathophys: Repetitive stress leads to bony microfracture; may progress to overt fracture with overload event

Sx: Pain with weight bearing, relieved with unloading. Night pain typical.

Si: Tenderness, swelling, ecchymosis. May be able to palpate area of focal tenderness and periosteal swelling. Tuning fork vibration transmits along bone and felt as pain at fracture site.

Crs: Generally recovers if load modified so that pain free

Cmplc: Nonunion. Progression to complete fracture, open fracture (rare). Anterior tibial "dreaded black line" heals only after surgery because of distraction bowing with loading of tibia.

Xray: Plain films may be normal or show localized periosteal reaction. Bone scintography nonspecific, virtually 100% sensitive. MRI may show bony edema and fracture line, sensitivity same as bone scan but more specific (Phys Sportsmed 1998;26:31). CT best for visualizing actual fracture line in foot bones.

Rx: Activity modification and splinting for 2-6 wk, or until comfortable weight bearing. Gradual return to activity with pain as guide.

Foot: 1st, 2nd metatarsal most common, cast (hard sole) shoe for 6 wk. 5th metatarsal at distal $\frac{1}{3}$ needs NWB short leg cast boot vs pin to heal.

Tarsal: Common in runners. Non-weight-bearing cast for 6-8 wk. Danger of nonunion—discuss with surgeon. Refer for prolonged pain after cast removed or for displaced fx.

Tibia: Use high leg aircast or walking boot for pain-free ambulation for 6 wk. Anterior, middle $\frac{1}{3}$ fx through cortex needs referral for possible pin.

Femoral neck: Common in runners. Superior (compression) surface heals with rest, toe touch crutch ambulation for 6-12 wk, inferior (distraction) surface fx needs referral because may need operation (Clin Sports Med 1997;16:307).

Thoracic Outlet Syndrome

Nejm 1993;329:2017

Cause: See Pathophys

Epidem: Associated with cervical ribs and malformations of 1st rib

Pathophys: Compression of vessels or nerves between 1st rib and clavicle, cervical rib, bony anomalies, muscles, etc. Vascular compression: of subclavian vein causes edema and venous distention leading to thrombosis; of subclavian artery results in loss of pulse, claudication, and arterial thrombosis; of sympathetic nerves causes Raynaud's; of peripheral nerves causes pain, paresthesias, and weakness.

Sx: Arm edema, claudication, Raynaud's, pain, paresthesias, weakness

Si: Loss of pulse at "attention" or with other maneuvers no longer felt helpful (Jama 1966;196:109) because also found in 15% of normal persons; motor nerve impairments, especially of intrinsic hand muscles plus ulnar sensory losses

Crs:

Cmplc: r/o carpal tunnel (p 1123)

Lab: *Noninv:* EMG shows impaired nerve conduction velocities subclavian fossa to hand (normal = 68-75 m/sec)

Rx: Passive range of motion, physiotherapy, posture changes, occupational health evaluation, and/or manipulation techniques (J Am Osteop Assoc 1990;90:686,810, 1989;89:1046), alone if NCV > 60 m/sec; if less, then consider surgical decompression, eg, resect 1st rib. RCT of surgery clearly better than splinting (Jama 2002;288:1245).

18.9 Bony Tumors

Chondrosarcoma

Cause: Neoplasia, genetic in 10%

Epidem: Older pts

Pathophys: Neoplastic transformation of adult cartilage cells, often from enchondromas or osteochondromas, especially in genetic type; most commonly arises from metaphysis side of epiphyseal plate area; ribs often involved; may calcify

Sx: Pain after trauma

Si:

Crs: Very benign even with metastases since such a slow grower; easily live years even without rx

Cmplc: Local and pulmonary mets; surgical excision may start metastatic implants

Lab: *Path:* Large chondrocytes, multinucleate, little cytoplasm; less intercellular matrix than normal or than a benign tumor

Xray: Flecks of calcification next to joints

Rx: Surgical excision. Little reponse to radiation.

Ewing's Sarcoma

Nejm 1999;341:342

Cause: Neoplasia from chromosome 11 and 22 translocation

Epidem: Children 5-15 yr; 2/million children/yr; no correlation w radiation exposure

Pathophys: Marrow reticular cells become neoplastic. Usually begins in bony shaft; 40% in axial skeleton.

Sx: Local pain or swelling in bone or joint for months

Si: Fever, tumor mass

Crs: Highly malignant; lung mets occur quickly; 60% 5-yr survival w rx, 20% if mets at diagnosis

Cmplc: r/o osteomyelitis

Lab: *Hem:* Elevated wbc

Path: Neoplastic reticular cells with little cytoplasm extending beyond marrow space through haversian system out subperiosteally, where elicits periosteal callus reaction

Xray:

Rx: Radiation to primary w multiagent chemoRx w vincristine, dactinomycin, doxorubicin + cyclophosphamide, or others like osfamide and etoposide (Nejm 2003;348:694) to cover micromets

Giant Cell Tumor

Cause: Neoplasia

Epidem: Associated with irradiation; older pts, most age >20 yr

Pathophys: Connective tissue cell hypertrophy with fusion resulting in abnormal osteoclasts. Many are benign but are hard to distinguish from malignant ones.

Sx: Painful joint swelling

Si:

Crs:

Cmplc: r/o similar less malignant **fibrosarcoma**

Lab:

Xray: "Expanding bubble" within bone

Rx: Surgical resection

Rhabdomyosarcoma

Nejm 1999;341:342

Cause: Genetic translocations

Epidem: 4-7/1 million/yr in children < 15 yr old

Pathophys:

Sx: Painless soft tissue mass

Si:

Crs: 70-80% cure unless mets, then 20% 5-yr survival

Cmplc:

Lab: *Path:* Embryonal (good prognosis) or alveolar cell types

Rx: Surgical removal, then chemoRx

Osteosarcoma

Nejm 1999;341:342, 1991;324:467

Cause: Neoplasia from suppressor gene inactivation

Epidem: Incidence in males twice that in females; 900/yr in U.S.; more common under age 20 yr. Associated with Paget's, radiation exposure (takes 12+ yr) especially in children rx'd for Ewing's sarcoma and retinoblastoma with chemoRx and radiation (Nejm 1987;317:588). Not associated with trauma, although trauma often leads to discovery of the tumor.

Pathophys: Osteoid, lytic, and sclerotic forms may all coexist, or one may predominate. Bloodborne metastases usually, lymphatic spread rare; may involve joints in persons with mature epiphyses; originate in metaphysis; and spread via haversian system; double q 34 d.

Sx: Cachexia, local pain and swelling. 90% in distal femur, proximal tibia, and proximal humerus.

Si:

Crs: 20-40% relapse, mostly within 1 yr, all who will relapse do so within 2 yr; 80-90% relapse in the 20% with gross metastases on presentation; relapse correlates w p-glycoprotein presence, which is associated w drug resistance (Nejm 1995;333:1380)

Cmplc: Metastases

Lab: *Path:* Osteoid, lytic, and/or sclerotic osteoblasts seen in wild formations, no longer lined up along bony trabeculations (contrast myositis ossificans)

Xray: "Ray" formation subperiosteally in sclerotic form; calcified area expands constantly in time

Rx: Surgical radical excision, although limb-sparing techniques may work; plus adjuvant multidrug chemoRx (Nejm 1986; 314:1600)

18.10 Miscellaneous

Ankle and Foot Injuries

Si: Distinguish sprain vs fx and need for xray ("Ottawa ankle rules"; see diagrams: Jama 2000;284:80, 1994;271:827) only if
1.   Can't bear weight,
2.   Bone tenderness over edge or tip of medial or lateral malleolus (ankle), or
3.   Bone tenderness over base of 5th metatarsal laterally or over navicular medially (foot).

   When applied, this protocol decreases xrays by 25% and misses no significant fx's (Jama 1997;278:1935)

Table 18.3 Autoantibodies and Clinical Disease Correlates

Autoantibody	Clinical Disease Correlate
Antinuclear antibody (ANA)	Nonspecific
Anti-dsDNA (double-stranded DNA)	High specific for SLE
Anti-ds and ss (single-stranded) DNA	Active SLE, especially renal
Antihistones	Drug-induced SLE and RA
Anti-Sm (Smith)	High specificity, 10% sensitivity for SLE, no correlation w disease activity
Anti-SM (smooth muscles)	Autoimmune hepatitis
Anti-Ro/SSA	Neonatal lupus (w anti-La/SSB); photosensitivity; subacute cutaneous lupus
Anti-La/SSB	Neonatal lupus (w anti-Ro/SSA); Sjögren's
Antiphospholipids	Inhibition of in vitro coagulation tests; thrombosis; recurrent fetal abortion/wastage; focal neurologic deficits; thrombocytopenia
Anticentromere	Limited cutaneous scleroderma (CREST)
Scl_{70} (antitopoisomerase)	Diffuse scleroderma
Anti-Jo_1 (antitransfer RNA)	Polymyositis

Calcium Levels, Corrected in Serum

Normal = total: 8.6-10.4 mg %; or 2.15-2.60 mEq/L; unbound: 4.5-6.0 mg %

Corrections for protein levels: at normal protein levels (4 gm % albumin), 47% is free and is the level by which parathormone adjusts feedback to parathyroids and bone. To correct, increase or decrease by 0.8 mg % (total)/gm albumin; or corrected $Ca^{++} = Ca^{++} - (albumin) + 4$.

Hallux Valgus

Cause: Shoes

Epidem: 33% adult prevalence, although most mild

Si: Lateral deviation of 1st MP joint of foot

Rx: Chevron ostotomy, 90% successful and better than orthotics (Jama 2001;285:2475)

Joint Fluid

Use heparin for cell counts (rv: Nejm 1993;329:1013)

Table 18.4   Joint Fluid Analysis

Dx	Viscosity	Mucin Clot	Wbc/mm^3	% Polys	Other
Traumatic	High	Good	< 200	< 25%	Fat in joint
Osteoarthritis	High	Good	< 2000	< 25%	Red cells often
Lupus	High	Good	~5000	10%	LE cells in joint fluid
Rheumatic fever	Low	Good	10,000-12,000	50%	
Pseudogout	Low	Good to poor	1000-5000	25-50%	Positively birefringent crystals
Gout	Low	Poor	10,000-12,000	60-70%	Negatively birefringent crystals
RA and HLA B27 disease incidence of Reiter's	Low	Poor	15,000-20,000	50-60%	Occasional cholesterol crystal
Tuberculosis	Low	Poor	25,000	75+%	AFB positive
Septic (Nejm 1985;312:764)	Low	Poor	80,000-200,000 (95% >20,000)	75+%	Gram stain positive and culture; glucose low in 50%

Reproduced with permission from J. Hollander, ed. Arthritis and allied conditions; a textbook of rheumatology. 8th ed. Baltimore: Lippincott, Williams and Wilkins, 1972, p72 (www.lww.com).

Knee Injuries and Rx

Ann IM 2003;139:575; Nejm 1988;318:950

In acute injury, xray only if age > 55, tender head of fibula, isolated patellar tenderness, can't flex ≥ 90°, or can't bear weight; 100% sensitivity (Ottawa knee rules: Jama 1997;278:2075, 1996;275:611)

- Anterior cruciate tear: Caused by anterior subluxation injuries usually involving forward motion on planted foot with a twisting motion; sx = "trick knee." Test by (1) anterior drawer si at 30° flexion + (2) pivot/shift si = 20° flexion, relaxed quad, then axial or valgus force on knee and knee is flexed + extended, if cruciate deficient will go in and out of subluxation. ⅓ resolve, ⅓ are functional although sx, ⅓ go on to progressive damage. Repair early if young or avulsed insertion on lateral tibial condyle apparent on xray.
- Meniscal injury may occur acutely or later when they are trapped because anterior cruciate doesn't keep femur and tibia aligned; 60% incidence w ACL tear. Sx = "locked knee," pain, "popping." Test for by Apley compression test prone, McMurray test, and lateral medial/lateral grind test, although sens and specif poor for all, esp in older pts (J Fam Pract 2001;50:938). Repair or partial resection better than total resection.
- Medial collateral tear. Test: Knee opens medially when extended. Rx: Conservative with immobilization and ROM and strengthening exercises × 3-6 wk; or if severe, hinged brace locked at 30° × 3 wk then full ROM × 3-5 wk additional.
- Posterior cruciate tear: Caused by posterior subluxation injuries, eg, dashboard or fall on flexed knee. Leads to early DJD, especially of medial femoral condyle, and damage to medial meniscus. No good rx yet available; conservative rx if isolated, surgical if associated w multiple ligamentous injuries

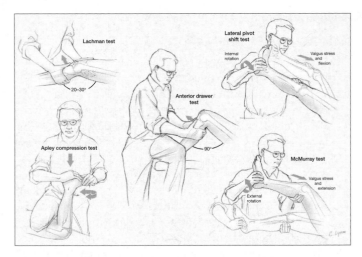

Figure 18.3 Knee injury examination maneuvers. Reproduced with permission from Solomon DH, et al. Does this patient have a torn meniscus or ligament of the knee. J Am Med Assoc 2001:286:1610. Copyright 2001, American Medical Association, all rights reserved.

Anterior knee pain syndromes:

- Lateral facet compression syndrome; rx w patellofemoral rehab or arthroscopic lateral release
- Chronic patellar subluxation in pts with valgus knees or lateral tracking of patella; rx w rehab or quadriceps realignment
- Inflamed synovial plica; rx w NSAIDs, steroid injections, rehab, or arthroscopic plicectomy
- Patellar tendonitis, "jumper's knee" (Nejm 1988;318:950); rx'd w NSAIDs and rehab; r/o **Osgood-Schlatter disease**, inflammation of anterior tibial tubercle apophysis in adolescent
- Anterior fat pad impingement; rx w rehab, steroids

Lymphedema

Cause: Mastectomy, filariasis, inflammation, lymphatic agenesis, idiopathic

Rx: Conservative measures like PT and compressive stockings
Benzopyrone 400 mg po qd (Nejm 1993;329:1158)

Polyarthritis with Fever, Differential Dx

Nejm 1994;330:769

- Infectious
  Bacterial: Septic arthritis (gc/staph),
  SBE, Lyme, tbc, fungal
  Viral: hep B, parvovirus, rubella, HIV
- Reactive: Enteric infection, Reiter's, rheumatic fever, IBD,
  Whipple's
- RA/Still's
- Vasculitis
- SLE
- Crystal diseases
- FMF
- Acute leukemias/lymphomas
- Dermatomyositis
- Behçet's
- Henoch-Schönlein purpura
- Kawasaki's
- Erythema nodosum
- Erythema multiforme
- Pyoderma gangrenosum
- Pustular psoriasis
- Sarcoid

Scaphoid Fractures

Phys Sportsmed 1996;24:60

Sx: Fall on outstretched hand

Si: Tender snuff box w thumb extended; pain w axial compression and
w resisted wrist pronation

Cmplc: Avascular necrosis

Xray: Fracture, distal, waist or proximal types

Rx: if no fx but has pain, thumb spica × 2 wk, then re-xray; if still neg but still sx and suspicious, then CT or bone scan

Surgery for waist or proximal types

Thumb spica × 6-8 wk for distal types

Shoulder Syndromes

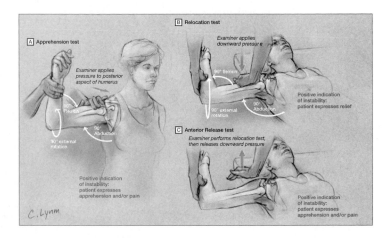

Figure 18.4 Clinical tests to evaluate anterior instability of the shoulder.
Reproduced with permission from Luime, JJ, et al. Does this patient have an instability of the shoulder or a labrum lesion. J Am Med Assoc. 2004;292:1989. Copyright 2004, American Medical Association, all rights reserved.

A: Apprehension test, although of limited clinical value because of its low specificity, is included as part of a sequence of tests for shoulder instability. It is conducted with the patient sitting or standing, with the arm placed in 90° abduction and 90° external rotation and the elbow flexed 90°. Pressure is applied to the posterior aspect of the humerus.

B: Relocation test, performed to relieve symptoms (pain and apprehension) of instability, is conducted with the patient supine and the arm abducted to 90° and externally rotated to 90°. Downward (posterior) pressure is applied to the humeral head.

C: The anterior release test is conducted in a similar manner as the relocation test, then the examiner's hand is removed suddenly, releasing pressure on the humeral head.

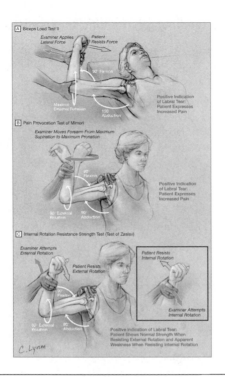

A: Biceps load test II is performed with the patient supine, the arm is placed in 120° abduction (90° abduction in biceps load test I), and the elbow is placed in 90° flexion. The patient is asked to resist the lateral force applied by the examiner.

B: In the pain provocation test of Mimori, the arm is placed in 90° abduction, the elbow in 90° flexion, and the forearm in maximum supination. To provoke symptoms, the examiner moves the forearm into maximum pronation.

C: Internal rotation resistance strength test (test of Zaslav) is conducted with the patient standing or sitting, the humerus in 90° abduction and 80° external rotation. The patient is asked to resist an external rotation force applied by the examiner, then to resist an applied internal rotation force.

Tendonitis (vs Tendinosis?) (Calcific Tendonitis)

Big debate re absence of inflammation and doubt about efficacy of NSAIDs and steroids in these syndromes (Clinics Sports Med 2003;22:(4)

- Injecting the functional structure and causing pain with steroids and lidocaine is much better than pain trigger points (75% vs 20% success: BMJ 1983;287:1339)
- Shoulder tendonitis (Nejm 1999;340:1582); rx w NSAIDs, steroid injections, or, if that fails, ultrasound (Nejm 1999;340: 1533) by high-energy extracorporeal shock wave (beneficial for calcific tendonitis by DBCT: Jama 2003;290:2573)
- Tennis elbow; rx w cessation of repetitive motion and NSAIDs, later steroid injection; all w equal outcome at 1 yr (BMJ 1999;319:964)

Bursitis

- Greater trochanteric bursitis
- Prepatellar and olecranon bursitis occasionally infected with staph and may need tap, I + D, and antibiotics (Ann IM 1978; 89:21), but rarely

Vasculitis Etiologies

Jama 1997;278:1962; Nejm 1997;337:1512

Large vessel: Giant cell and Takayasu's arteritis
Medium-sized vessels: Polyarteritis and Kawasaki's disease
Small vessel:
- ANCA (antineutrophil cytoplasmic autoantibodies)-associated types: Microscopic polyangiitis, Wegener's Churg-Strauss, drug induced
- Immune complex types: Henoch-Schönlein purpura, cryoglobulinemic vasculitis, SLE, RA, Sjögren's, Behçet's, Goodpasture's, serum sickness, drug induced, infection induced
- Paraneoplastic
- Inflammatory bowel disease

Whiplash Injury of Neck

Cmplc: Chronic cervical pain from zygapophyseal joints

Rx: Hourly range-of-motion exercises, started within 4 d of injury helps diminish long-term sx (Spine 2000;25:1782). Rarely, w needle radiofrequency neurotomy (Nejm 1996;335:1721).

Functional Somatic Syndromes (Medically Unexplained Physical Sx [MUPS])

Ann IM 1999;130:910

Multiple manifiestations, some of which may have some physiologic basis, eg, chemical sensitivities, sick building syndrome, chronic whiplash, silicone breast implant syndrome, chronic irritable bowel syndrome, chronic food allergies, mitral valve prolapse, chronic mononucleosis, etc (see somatization d/o p 962). Overall strategy (Am Fam Phys 2000;61:1073,1423) is to r/o organic disease, look for depression and panic disorder especially to rx, set functional not curative goals, and apply cognitive-behavioral rx and/or antidepressants (J Fam Pract 1999;48:980), see regularly and avoid repetitive w/u's.

Chronic Fatigue Syndrome

Jama 1998;280:1094, 1997;278:1179; Ann IM 1994;121:953, 1988;108:387

Cause: Biologic vs psych causes debated; lots of circumstantial evidence for biologic connections (T. Kamaroff: Am J Med 2000; 108:169,172). Associated w neurally mediated hypotension always (70% have abnormal tilt table test w/o pharmacologic precipitation); thus rx for that may help (p 753, 158) (Jama 1995; 274:961).

May be equivalent to old dx of "neurasthenia," but unlikely that caused by EBV, and more likely that the EBV antibodies are the result not the cause of the syndrome. Acyclovir rx no help

(Nejm 1988;319:1692). Other purported causes: candida (Nejm 1990;323:1165,1717), hypoglycemia, fibrositis, depression, Lyme disease (Ann IM 1993;119:503,518), human herpes virus type 6 (Ann IM 1992;116:103); no evidence of a retrovirus (Ann IM 1993;118:241).

Sx: Fatigue $\geq$ 6 mo, normal labs (chem 20, CBC, ESR, TSH, UA) and $\geq$ 4 of the following sx: impaired memory/concentration, sore throat, tender cervical/axillary nodes, myalgias, arthralgias, headache, poor sleep, post-exertion malaise

Cmplc: r/o depression; fibromyalgia overlaps; alcoholism

Lab: Chem panel, CBC, ESR, UA; optionally ANA, cortisol, RA titer, SPEP, IPPD, Lyme titer, HIV serology

Rx (Jama 1995;274:961):

Cognitive-behavioral rx (Lancet 2001;357:841) and graded exercise programs (BMJ 2001;322:387) help

Avoid salt restriction, diuretics, vasodilators, TCAs; increase salt in diet; fludrocortisone (Florinef), but RCT doesn't confirm efficacy (Jama 2001;285:52); β blockers; anticholinergics like disopyramide (Norpace), all in that order. Avoid low-dose steroids, which are of minimal help but cause adrenal suppression (Jama 1998;280:1061).

Gulf War Syndrome

No increase in hospitalization or medical illness but increase in accidental death, ? related to depression or greater risk taking (Nejm 1996;335:1498,1505); may be caused by organophosphate poisoning and/or DEET exposure, causing chronic measurable neuropsych dysfunction (Jama 1997;277:215,223,231,238,259); but other studies find no such correlations (Am J Med 2000;108:695; Jama 1998;280:981). Rx w cognitive-behavioral rx and exercise (Jama 2003;348:1396).

Fibromyalgia Syndrome

Ann IM 1999;131:850; Post Grad Med 1996;100:153

Cause: Unknown, possibly related to chronic fatigue syndrome

Epidem: Females >>> males

Pathophys: Increased sensitivity to pain; otherwise not understood

Sx: Musculoskeletal pains and stiffness, sleep disturbances, headache, fatigue

Si: Multiple tender areas/points

Cmplc: r/o spondyloarthropathy (Am J Med 1997;103:44)

Lab: r/o other diseases w CBC, chem panel, TSH, ESR, CPK

Rx   (Jama 2004;292:2388): Exercise, education, cognitive-behavioral rx; maybe biofeedback, hypnotherapy, acupuncture

Amitriptyline 25-50 mg po hs qd; or cyclobenzaprine (Flexeril) 10-30 mg po bid (Arthritis Rheum 1994;37:32); and/or SSRIs like sertraline (Zoloft), which probably just help latent depression unlike TCAs

Pain meds like tramadol (Ultram), lidocaine injections of trigger points; clonazepam (Klonopin) for sleep

Index

Copolymer I in MS, 748
Coral stings, 29
Cordarone, 58
Coreg, 57
Corgard, 56
Corkscrew hairs, 319
Corlopam, 66
Corneal abrasion, 860
Corneal burns, 857
Coronary artery bypass grafting, 78
Coronavirus, 682
Cortical basal ganglionic
  degeneration, 739
Cortisol levels, 248
Corvert, 59
Corynebacterium diphtheria, 529
Cosopt, 854
Cosyntropin test of adrenal reserve,
  251
Cough
  acute, 1001
  chronic, 1002
Coumadin, 52
Councilman bodies in dengue, 706
Coxa plana, 880
Coxiella burnetii, 601
Coxsackie virus A and B, 684
Cozaar, 64
CPAP, 1005
CPK-MB, 82
Crabs, 659
Cradle cap, 207
Craniopharyngioma, 771
C reactive protein elevations, 512
Creatine phosphokinase in MI, 82
Creeping eruption, 652
CREST syndrome, 1091
Crestor, 280
Cretinism, 302
Creutzfeldt-Jakob disease, 430
Crigler-Najjar syndrome, 867

Crixivan, 663
Crocodile tears, 751
Crohn's disease, 379
Crotamiton (Eurax), 627
Croup, 886
  emergent rx, 9
  membranous, 529
Crowe sign, 182
Cruciate ligament injury, knee,
  1137
Cruex, 170
Cryoglobulinemia, 516
Cryptococcosis, 619
Cryptococcus neoformans, 619
Cryptorchid testicle, 876
Cryptosporidiosis diarrhea, 404
Cryptosporidium spp, 632
CSF, increased protein, 773
CSF eosinophilia, 773
Currant jelly sputum, 553
Cushing's disease, 247
Cushing's syndrome, 247
Cutaneous nerves distributions, 774
Cyanide poisoning, 39
  from combustible plastics, 39
Cyclobenzaprine (Flexeril), 945
Cyclooxygenase inhibitors, 1067
Cyclophosphamide (Cytoxan), 442
Cyclospora cayetanensis, 409, 633
Cyclosporine, 444
Cylert, 885
Cymbalta, 945
Cystadane, 319
Cystic acne, 174
Cysticercosis, 647, 648
Cystic fibrosis, 985
Cystinosis, 1040
Cystitis
  female, 1042
  male, 1047
Cytarabine, 442